APPLIED IMMUNOHISTOCHEMISTRY FOR THE SURGICAL PATHOLOGIST

APPLIED IMMUNOHISTOCHEMISTRY FOR THE SURGICAL PATHOLOGIST

Edited by

ANTHONY S-Y. LEONG

MB, BS, MD, FRCPath, FRCPA, FCAP

Director, Division of Tissue Pathology
Institute of Medical and Veterinary Science and
Clinical Professor of Pathology
University of Adelaide

Edward Arnold
A member of the Hodder Headline Group
LONDON BOSTON MELBOURNE AUCKLAND

First published in Great Britain 1993

Distributed in the Americas by Little, Brown and Company, 34 Beacon Street, Boston, MA 02108

British Library Cataloguing in Publication Data

Leong, Anthony S-Y.
Applied Immunohistochemistry for the
Surgical Pathologist
I. Title
616.99

ISBN 0–340–55148–8

Typeset by "Anneset", Weston-super-Mare, Avon.
Printed and bound in Great Britain for Edward Arnold, a division of Hodder Headline PLC, Mill Road, Dunton Green, Sevenoaks, Kent TN13 2YA by Butler and Tanner Ltd, Frome and London.

Dedication

This book is dedicated to Wendy, Joel and Trishe

PREFACE

The past decade has witnessed tremendous progress in the field of immunohistochemistry. Innovative technological advances have resulted in new diagnostic techniques and the availability of a continually expanding range of antibodies of increased sensitivity and specificity has, in a short space of time, entrenched immunohistochemistry as the mainstay of ancillary investigations for the surgical pathologist. The technique is now frequently employed in many laboratories, both in large and small medical centres, often contributing important and essential information in many aspects of surgical pathology. Its pace of growth has been so rapid that one could justifiably be considered courageous (or foolish, depending on one's point of view) to be associated with the production of a volume devoted to diagnostic immunohistochemistry. Nevertheless, I have undertaken the task of editing this book with the support of my friends and colleagues who are fellow *aficionados* of the subject and experts in different fields, as I am of the firm belief that immunohistochemistry as a discipline has come of age and its numerous contributions are sufficiently extensive and significant to warrant documentation. While some of the techniques and procedures described in this book will undoubtedly be modified, improved, and added to in the near future, and new and better reagents will continue to be produced, the basic approach adopted by the contributing authors will not see fundamental changes.

Several monographs on immunohistochemistry have been published, but these have not always approached diagnostic problems in a manner familiar to or practical for the surgical pathologist. Furthermore, they may not always have contained the pertinent information required to answer the questions which may have been raised during the morphological examination of the specimen. This book is intended to make up for such deficiencies. It is written by practising surgical pathologists who are experts in their various disciplines and it is written for both the experienced pathologist as well as those in training. Diagnostic problems are handled in a manner similar to that adopted by the surgical pathologist when confronted with a difficult biopsy. The clinical and morphological features are discussed in the context of the differential diagnoses which are arrived at following examination of the morphology and correlation with the clinical features, so that throughout the text, immunohistochemistry is employed as an extension of the process of morphological examination. The text concentrates on the use of immunoenzyme techniques applied to paraffin sections which are still the basic substrate of surgical pathology, and with few exceptions, only commercially available antibodies and reagents form the basis of discussion. Fluorescence immunostaining is only discussed briefly as there are other excellent texts on the use of this technique in traditional areas such as glomerular disease and the dermatoses.

The major areas in which immunohistochemistry has an established diagnostic role are covered. These include the 'solid' tumours, lymphoproliferative diseases, renal diseases, cutaneous tumours and central nervous system tumours as well as some of the newer prognostic markers used in the evaluation of carcinomas. In addition, the applications of immunohistochemistry in cytology, flow cytometry and image analysis are discussed and chapters on the theoretical and practical aspects of immunohistochemistry are included, as well as a chapter devoted to the setting up of a diagnostic immunohistochemistry service with practical hints on tested reagents, their sources and their application. All chapters are extensively illustrated with photomicrographs of light microscopic and immunohistochemical features.

Anthony S-Y. Leong, MD
Adelaide, 1992

Acknowledgment

I am most grateful to my secretary, Mrs Margaret Elemer, who employed initiative and her extensive word processing skills in the preparation of this monograph.

Contents

THE EDITOR

Anthony S-Y. Leong, graduated from the University of Malaya in 1969 with MB,BS and obtained a Doctorate in Medicine from the University of Adelaide. He is a Fellow of the Royal College of Pathologists of Australasia and the United Kingdom and of the College of American Pathologists, as well as an Honorary Fellow of the College of Pathologists of Hong Kong.

Professor Leong is currently Clinical Professor of Pathology at the University of Adelaide and Director of the Division of Tissue Pathology at the Institute of Medical and Veterinary Science in Adelaide. He is also head of the Immunohistochemistry Laboratory and he has wide-ranging interests in diagnostic and research pathology, particularly in the areas of tumour pathology, immunohistochemistry and laboratory technology, including the laboratory applications of microwave irradiation. He has contributed over 200 scientific papers on cancer research and laboratory procedures to books and international medical journals and has been an invited lecturer to many international symposia and medical centres at home and abroad. He has co-authored and edited three books on lymphoid malignancies, cancer and diagnostic immunohistochemistry and has served as guest editor on special topics in medical journals. Professor Leong sits on the editorial boards of several prestigious international journals of pathology, namely, *Pathology, Journal of Pathology, Diagnostic Cytopathology, Pathology, Research and Practice* and *Applied Immunohistochemistry*. He has also acted as scientific adviser to World Health Organisation on diagnostic electron microscopy and immunohistochemistry.

List of Contributors

Carlos W.M. Bedrossian MD,FIAC Professor of Pathology, Wayne State University; Chief of Cytopathology, Detroit Medical Centre, Detroit, Michigan USA.

John P. Dowling MB,BS,FRCPA,FRCPath Deputy Director of Pathology, Department of Anatomical Pathology, Royal Melbourne Hospital, Parkville, Victoria, Australia.

David W. Ellis MB,BS,FRCPA Director, Department of Anatomical Pathology, St Vincent's Hospital, Fitzroy, Victoria, Australia.

Michael F. Gonzales MB,BS,FRCPA Consultant Neuropathologist, Director, Neuropathology Research Laboratory, Department of Anatomical Pathology, Royal Melbourne Hospital, Parkville, Victoria, Australia.

Allen M. Gown MD Professor of Pathology, Director of Immunocytochemistry Laboratory, University of Washington, Seattle, Washington, USA.

Anthony S-Y. Leong MB,BS,MD,FRCPath,FRCPA,FCAP Director, Division of Tissue Pathology, Institute of Medical and Veterinary Science, Clinical Professor of Pathology, University of Adelaide, Adelaide, South Australia.

Shahla Masood MD Associate Professor of Pathology, College of Medicine, University of Florida, Jacksonville, Florida, USA.

James Milios HT Senior and Supervising Technical Officer, Immunohistochemistry Laboratory, Institute of Medical and Veterinary Sciences, Adelaide, Australia.

Paul E. Swanson MD Assistant Professor of Pathology, Lauren V. Ackerman Laboratory of Surgical Pathology, Department of Pathology, Washington University School of Medicine, St Louis, Missouri, USA.

Mark R. Wick MD Professor of Pathology and Director of Surgical Pathology, Washington University School of Medicine, St Louis, Missouri, USA.

1 ◆ *Immunohistochemistry – theoretical and practical aspects*

Anthony S-Y. Leong

Introduction

The development of the immunoperoxidase and the introduction of hybridoma techniques represent two of the most important technological advancements in surgical pathology in recent times. After Coons et al. (1941) applied the fluorescent antibody method to tissue sections, pathologists began to recognize the potential value of a method that would permit specific identification of cells according to their antigenic constituents or cellular products. Although immunofluorescence methods were very successful in some areas of pathology, such as the study of renal diseases, they did not achieve widespread appeal among surgical pathologists. This lack of general utility stemmed largely from two principal disadvantages, viz. its unsuitability for use in conventional formalin-fixed, paraffin-embedded tissues, and the poor morphological detail obtained when immunofluorescence methods were applied to cryostat sections. Furthermore, there was the necessity for fresh frozen tissue, and the technique did not provide permanent preparations. While immunofluorescence techniques are still used extensively in the study of renal and skin diseases, the inability to study the fine morphological features of 'tissues that glow in the dark' is a major handicap to the surgical pathologist who traditionally bases diagnosis and identification of cell type on cytomorphological details which sometimes can be subtle.

By substituting horseradish peroxidase for fluorescein-isothiocynate as the label of the specific antibody, it became possible to stain for the horseradish peroxidase by adding a suitable chromogenic substrate which produced a coloured reaction product, visible by ordinary light microscopy. This technique was pioneered by Nakane and Pierce (1966), and Sternberger et al. (1970) subsequently developed the peroxidase-antiperoxidase technique. Several years later, when Kohler and Milstein (1975) gave us the hybridoma monoclonal antibody technique, they provided the super fuel required to propel immunohistochemistry into a new era of exponential growth which has been called the 'brown revolution'. This new modality of examination has already produced an enormous impact on the diagnosis and classification of tumours. It has also greatly expanded our understanding of many diseases and neoplastic processes, including those of the lymphoid, neuroendocrine, cutaneous, renal, neural and soft tissues.

These developments in immunolabelling have come at a time when increasing sophistication of cancer treatment modalities has made it necessary to have a more precise morphological diagnosis prior to the selection of the optimal therapeutic regimen. Refinements in cancer therapy make the diagnosis of 'undifferentiated tumour' and similar uncommitted diagnostic labels untenable, so that the surgical pathologist may need to employ ancillary investigations to aid his or her morphological observations.

While immunoperoxidase histochemistry may justifiably be viewed as 'magic markers', it is important to realize that the technique is beset by many technological and interpretative pitfalls. Whether pathologists elect to perform immunostaining themselves or to send their cases to a reference laboratory, it is important that they have some knowledge of the kinds of problems encountered with the technique, particularly those concerned with initial specimen handling. This chapter deals with the common immunolabelling techniques and their associated problems.

Immunofluorescence techniques

Fluorescence and phosphorescence are emissions of light following its absorption from a non-thermal source of energy such as ultraviolet or visible light. Unlike fluorescence which persists only as long as the stimulating light is present, phosphorescence persists after the source of energy or stimulating light ceases. The most commonly employed light source in fluorescence microscopy is a high pressure mercury vapour lamp that supplies an intense ultraviolet radiation. Other light sources such as tungsten halogen, tungsten and xenon can also be utilized. Fluorescence microscopes use either transmitted light in which the exciting light is transmitted through the specimen, or incident light in which the exciting light is reflected off the specimen, the latter being a superior technique.

In the transmitted light fluorescence microscope, the light first passes through an exciter filter which selectively blocks out wave lengths other than those most effective for stimulating fluorescence in the fluorochrome-stained specimen. The exciting light contacts the undersurface of the specimen and the emitted light or fluorescence is then transmitted through to the objective. Exciting light that is not absorbed by the specimen will enter the objective but is excluded from the eyepieces by a barrier filter. This exciting light needs to be suppressed otherwise it would obscure the comparatively low intensity fluorescence emitted by the specimen.

In the incident light fluorescence microscope, the exciting light, which is located above the specimen, passes through an exciter filter before contacting a dichroic beam-splitting mirror which reflects the light down through the objective onto the upper surface of the specimen. The fluorescence emitted from the specimen, in turn, passes upwards, back through the objective and through the dichroic beam-splitting mirror to the eyepieces. The splitting mirror forms an efficient barrier to block the exciting light from passing to the eyepieces. Prolonged exposure to the exciting light may cause the fluorochromes to exhaust their capacity to fluorescence. This process, known as quenching, is more rapid with transmitted light than with incident light excitation as a larger portion of the specimen is exposed.

Fluorochrome labelling can be used to detect antigens in a wide variety of tissue and cell preparations. Cells obtained by mechanical disruption of tissue specimens, or exfoliated cells, exudates, aspiration biopsies, blood and tissue culture cells can be stained by immunofluorescence. They may also be prepared as fresh-frozen or fixed tissue sections, imprints, viable cells in suspension, cyto-centrifuge preparations, tissue culture monolayer preparations, cells air-dried onto slides, and smears of micro-organisms.

Compared to the bridge-amplified immunoenzyme techniques discussed below, direct immunofluorescence microscopy is relatively less sensitive, so that it is mostly performed on fresh-frozen tissues or cell preparations that have not been fixed with cross-linking fixatives such as formalin. Sometimes, brief fixation with acetone, ethanol, or methanol is used to improve tissue morphology or to inactivate pathogens. The methods for freezing fresh tissues for immunofluorescence microscopy are similar to those described below for immunoenzyme techniques.

The direct immunofluorescence staining technique is most commonly used because of speed and simplicity. Immunofluorescence staining results from the specific reaction of the fluorochrome-labelled antibody to the antigen in the substrate. This is achieved by exposing the substrate, in the form of tissue sections or cells, to fluorochrome-labelled antibodies. The specific antibody-antigen recognition allows the binding of the fluorochrome-labelled antibody to the section or cell preparations at the sites where the antigen is present. Unbound antibodies are washed from the preparation with neutral buffer and the sites of antibody binding are identified by fluorescence microscopy.

The most commonly used fluorochromes for immunofluorescence microscopy are fluorescein and rhodamine. These fluorochromes can be covalently linked to antibodies without destroying their biologic activities. Fluorescein absorbs blue light and emits green light, whereas, rhodamine absorbs green light and emits red light.

More than one antigen can thus be simultaneously identified in the same section or smear by using antibodies conjugated to different fluorochromes. For example, in the detection of κ and λ-secreting plasma cells, the anti-κ antibody can be labelled with fluorescein and the anti-λ antibody with rhodamine. The distribution of the fluorescein labelled κ-secreting cells is evaluated after blue excitation, whereas, the distribution of rhodamine labelled λ-secreting cells is identified by red emission after green excitation.

The immunofluorescence technique has the main advantage of relative ease of use of the reagents and simplicity of the procedure. Only washing steps are required after antibody labelling, and no further reagents are required as they are in the case of enzyme immunohistochemical procedures. The major disadvantages of immunofluorescence techniques include the need for an expensive specialized microscope, the lack of permanency of the preparations and the poor visualization of cytomorphological features. Furthermore, the autofluorescence of some biologic tissues, particularly connective tissue, contributes to the background fluorescence, posing additional difficulties in interpretation, and the need for fresh frozen tissue limits the application of immunofluorescence methods in surgical pathology where most specimens are fixed and paraffin-embedded. Fluorescent labelling is also impermanent and will fade with quenching and the direct immunofluorescence technique requires greater concentrations of primary antibody, each primary antibody having to be conjugated to a fluorochrome, adding to costs.

Immunoenzyme techniques

Immunoenzyme techniques are based on the attachment of an enzyme to a specific antibody. The enzymatic activity induces a visible colour change in the substrate and chromogen at the sites of localization of the antibody-enzyme complex within the tissue, i.e. the sites of specific antibody-antigen reaction. Horseradish peroxidase is the prototype of the immunoenzyme method but other enzyme systems such as glucose oxidase and alkaline phosphatase have also been successfully used. Many commercial sources offer enzyme-conjugated antibodies, chromogens, as well as kits which contain matched reagents for the common types of multilayered immunoenzyme staining procedures.

Direct immunoenzyme staining

This technique utilizes an enzyme-conjugated antibody to bind an enzyme to antigens in the section (Fig. 1.1). The section is then incubated with an appropriate substrate such as hydrogen peroxide, and chromogen, such as, diaminobenzidine, to produce a brown reaction product which is identifiable by light microscopy. While the direct immunoenzyme technique is simple, it is less sensitive than the multilayered bridge techniques and is not the method of choice for routine diagnostic use.

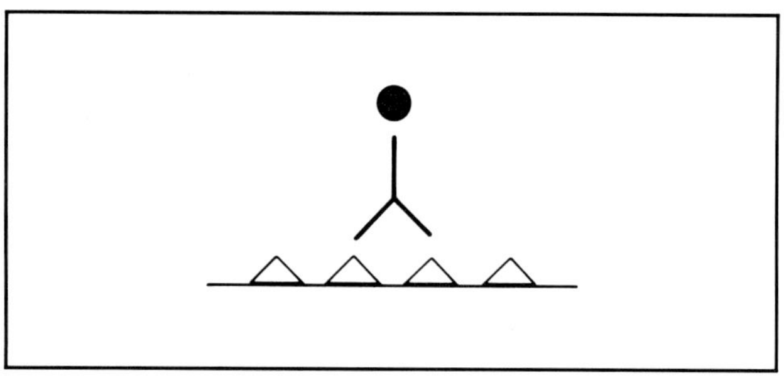

Fig. 1.1. Direct immunoenzyme technique. The enzyme label, represented by the solid circle, is directly attached to the antibody which binds to the tissue antigen for which it has specificity against. If the enzyme peroxidase is employed, incubation with hydrogen peroxide and a chromogen such as diaminobenzidine, produces a brown reaction product localized to the site of the antigen.

Bridge techniques

Bridge techniques have the main advantage of increasing the sensitivity of the immunoenzyme stain by increasing the amount of reaction product deposited at the antigen sites. They also increase the versatility of the technique in that a single conjugated antibody can be used with different primary antibodies to different antigens, obviating the need for enzyme-conjugating each primary antibody.

Indirect immunoenzyme staining

This technique requires the initial incubation of the section with a primary antibody specific for the antigen being sought. The section is then rinsed and incubated with an enzyme-conjugated secondary antibody which is specific for immunoglobulin from the species which was the source of the primary antibody (Fig. 1.2). The advantage of this indirect procedure is the ability to use one enzyme-conjugated antibody preparation to bind to an unlimited variety of primary antibodies derived from a given species.

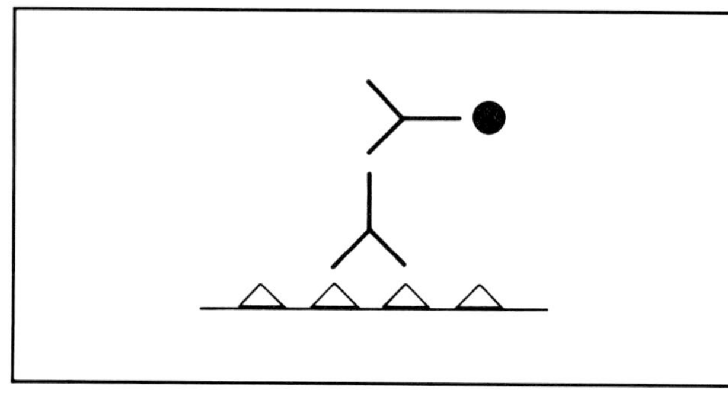

Fig. 1.2. Indirect immunoenzyme technique. In this case, the primary antibody is unlabelled. It binds to the antigen for which it has specificity and is detected by a labelled secondary antibody with specificity against the primary antibody, i.e., the secondary antibody has specificity against immunoglobulin from the species which was the source of the primary antibody.

Enzyme-antienzyme techniques

In these techniques the primary antibodies are not labelled. Instead, antienzyme antibodies are used to form a bridge between the primary antibody and the enzyme, avoiding the necessity of conjugating enzyme to antibodies, a procedure which can reduce antigen-binding avidity and is often technically difficult.

Sternberger et al. (1970) was the first to employ the peroxidase antiperoxidase system (PAP), reported to have a sensitivity of 100 to 1000-fold greater than comparable conjugate techniques. In the PAP technique, the PAP complex which is the tertiary reagent, consists of a soluble and stable preformed complex of antibody against horseradish peroxidase and horseradish peroxidase antigen. There is evidence that this immune complex typically consists of two antibody molecules and three horseradish peroxidase molecules in a cyclic complex. The primary antibody, raised against the human antigen, binds to the tissue antigen through its Fab portion. The secondary or bridge reagent, in turn, forms a molecular bridge between the primary antibody and the immunoglobulin incorporated into the PAP complex (Fig. 1.3). Both the primary antibody and the PAP reagent have to be of the same species, so that the bridge reagent, derived from a second species, can have specificity for the constant components of both primary and tertiary reagents.

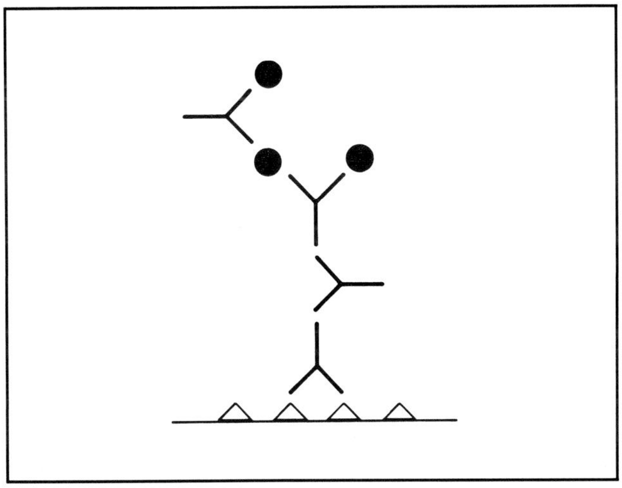

Fig. 1.3. Peroxidase antiperoxidase (PAP) technique. In this three-stage procedure, the primary antibody binds to the tissue antigen through its Fab portion. The secondary, or bridge antibody, is raised against the primary antibody. Thus, by binding the secondary to the primary antibody and after washing away excess unbound secondary antibody, one free valency of the secondary antibody is available to react with the PAP complex which is subsequently added. The PAP complex comprises a soluble and stable preformed mixture of antibody against horseradish peroxidase and horseradish peroxidase antigen. A pre-requisite for the technique is that the primary antibody and PAP complex have to be from the same species so that the secondary antibody can bind specifically for the constant components of the primary and tertiary reagents.

In the PAP immunostaining procedure, endogenous peroxidase in the sections has first to be blocked with hydrogen peroxide or a mixture of hydrogen peroxide and methanol. Non-specific binding is next blocked with diluted non-immune serum from the same species from which the bridging antibody was obtained. The bridging antibody is then added in excess so that free antigen-binding sites will remain for linkage to PAP complexes. The bridging antibody must react with determinants in the constant region of both the primary antibody as well as the antibodies in the PAP complex. Unbound bridging antibody is rinsed away before soluble PAP complexes are incubated with the specimen. The final step is the reaction of the PAP complex with substrate and chromogen to form a product visible by light microscopy which will identify the site of antigen in the tissue section.

The alkaline-phosphatase-antialkaline phosphatase (APAAP) (Cordell et al., 1984; DeJong et al., 1985; Ormanns and Schaffer, 1985) and glucose oxidase-antiglucose oxidase (GAG) (Suffin et al., 1979) are claimed to produce less background staining because of the restricted tissue distribution of these respective endogenous enzymes. These systems are similar to that of PAP except that the tertiary reagents (antibody-chromogenic enzyme complexes) comprise two IgG molecules bound to alkaline phosphatase or glucose oxidase in place of horseradish peroxidase.

Avidin-biotin technique

The avidin-biotin procedure exploits the high affinity binding between biotin and avidin. Biotin, a low molecular weight vitamin, can be covalently linked to the primary antibody to produce a biotinylated conjugate which, when added to the tissue section, localizes to the sites of antigen in the section. The egg-white glycoprotein avidin, has four avid binding sites for biotin. Avidin, therefore, can be used as bridges between the components of multilayered immunoenzyme stains. The addition of avidin, chemically conjugated to horseradish peroxidase will allow tight binding of avidin to the biotinylated antibody, thus locating the peroxidase moiety at the site of antibody antigen reaction in the tissue section (Fig. 1.4). This

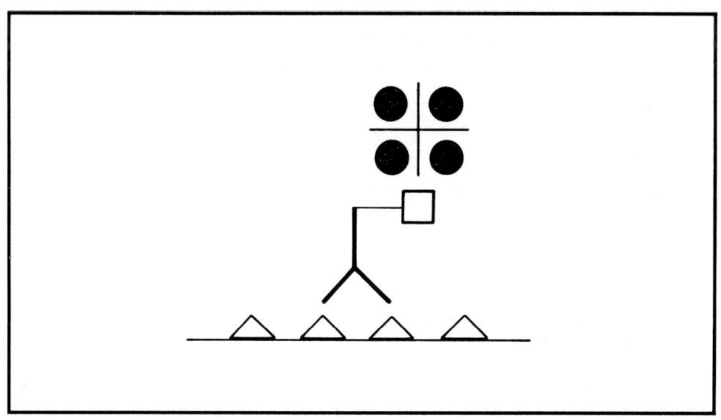

Fig. 1.4. Biotin-avidin technique.Biotin, represented by the open square, is covalently linked to the primary antibody which binds to the tissue antigen. Avidin, represented by the +, has four avid binding sites for biotin and can be chemically conjugated to horseradish peroxidase, represented by the solid circles. The addition of peroxidase-conjugated avidin as a secondary reagent will allow tight binding of the complex to the biotinylated primary antibody, localizing to the site of antibody-antigen reaction.

method is rapid and may be used as an indirect procedure but is apparently not as sensitive as the PAP method.

A further development to the avidin-biotin system is the avidin-biotin-peroxidase complex (ABC) system of Hsu et al. (1981). The ABC system employs a preformed complex of avidin bound to biotinylated peroxidase molecules. The method is largely used as an indirect technique, whereby the primary antibody is linked to the avidin-biotin-peroxidase conjugate by a biotinylated secondary antibody (Fig. 1.5). The complex is a lattice-like, three-dimensional formation and serves to localize several molecules of horseradish peroxidase at the site of antigen in the section, endowing the technique with a higher sensitivity than the PAP procedure (Hsu et al., 1981).

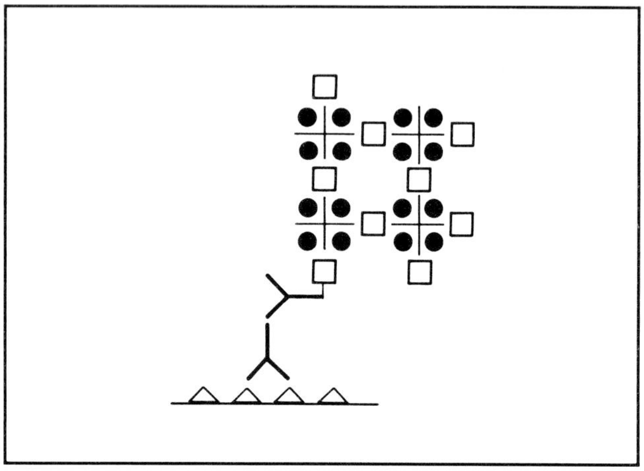

Fig. 1.5. Avidin-biotin-peroxidase complex (ABC) technique. This sensitive technique employs a primary antibody with specificity against the antigen under study, a secondary biotinylated antibody, and a tertiary, ABC complex. The latter comprises a complex, lattice-like three-dimensional formation of avidin-biotin-peroxidase molecules which serves to localize several molecules of horseradish peroxidase at the site of antibody-antigen reaction in the tissue section.

The ABC procedure has been further refined by the introduction of streptavidin. As a substitute for avidin, streptavidin which has a neutral charge (pI = 5) at physiological pH, does not produce the non-specific binding associated with egg-white avidin, which has a positive charge (pI = 10) at physiological pH. Many commercial sources of ABC reagents are available and we have tested some of these streptavidin-biotin peroxidase kits and found that they can be applied at strengths many times less than the manufacturers' recommendations, allowing considerable cost savings (Milios and Leong, 1988). Recently released kits such as the Elite ABC kit (Vector PK6100) and the Super Sensitive kit (Biogenix ZP000-UM) are claimed to be more sensitive and modifications to the unlabelled antibody procedure such as sequential overlaying of the ABC-stained section with an avidin-rich and biotin-rich complex (Cattoretti et al., 1988), employment of a streptavidin or avidin-horseradish peroxidase conjugate (Giorno, 1984; Cartun and Pedersen, 1989; Elias et al., 1989) and sequential application of the PAP and ABC techniques (ABPAP) (Swanson et al., 1987) have been described to be more sensitive than the ABC method.

A potential problem with biotin-avidin procedures is the presence of endogenous biotin that may bind the avidin peroxidase complex directly to produce non-specific or false positive staining. This can be blocked by first incubating the specimen with free avidin followed by free biotin (Wood and Warnke, 1981).

Protein-A-peroxidase conjugate method

Staphylococcal protein A has the remarkable ability to bind with the constant portion (Fc) of immunoglobulin molecules from several different species. This binding capability has been used to develop a simple and rapid immunoperoxidase procedure in which protein A is substituted for the secondary antibody in the PAP staining procedure (Fig. 1.6). Because protein A has the ability to bind to most IgG molecules, it is able to bridge between primary antibodies and antiperoxidase antibodies derived from different species. In cryostat sections, however, the protein A-peroxidase conjugate will bind not only to the Fc

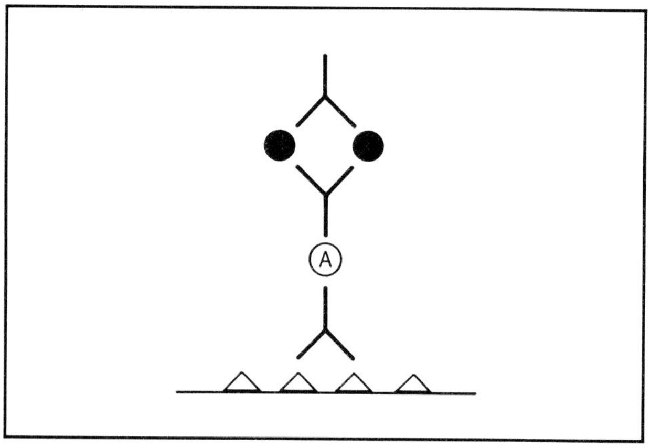

Fig. 1.6. Protein-A-peroxidase conjugate technique. Protein-A has the ability to bind with the constant portion of immunoglobulin from several species. In this technique, unlabelled protein-A is used as the bridging reagent between the primary antibody and the peroxidase-anti-peroxidase complex.

component of the primary antibody but also to the Fc fragments of intrinsic immunoglobulins within the section. This does not appear to be a problem in the staining of paraffin sections.

Immunogold-silver staining

Several metal irons and metal-protein complexes such as ferritin, gold and mercury have been used as markers of immunohistochemical reactions because they are visible by light microscopy when deposited in tissue. Other metals can be superimposed on such complexes to enhance their visibility after they have been bound to tissue. The most popular of these is the immunogold-silver technique. The method described by Holgate et al. (1983) is a highly sensitive indirect method in which the secondary antibody is adsorbed to colloidal gold particles. The gold particles employed are usually of the range of 5–10 nm, and generally not visible by ordinary light microscopy. Silver, in solution, is used to enhance the gold particles which turn black with the silver precipitation. The black granules of the immunogold-silver precipitate are clearly visible in the light microscope. The immunogold-silver technique can also be used in double labelling procedures in combination with chromogens with which the black granules are clearly contrasted against. The immunogold-silver precipitate stands out clearly against the brown reaction product of 3,3′-diaminobenzidine (DAB) or the red of the alkaline phosphatase technique (Schaumburg-Lever and Tronnier, 1989).

Biotinylated oligonucleotide probes for *in situ* hybridization

Polyclonal and monoclonal antibodies coupled with any of the detection systems described above form accurate methods of identifying specific cell types. Cellular antigens and other protein components are dependent upon nucleic acids, both DNA and RNA, of specific base-pair sequences for their synthesis and their expression may be relatively late and represent only incidental changes in the histogenesis of the disease or neoplasm. In place of identifying the cellular protein, the ability to detect specific nucleic acid sequences is a much more specific technique with the added advantage that the nucleic acid target, when DNA, is much more stable than the protein antigen, surviving both fixation and paraffin embedding. Using cloned genes, obtained through the latest recombinant DNA technology, as probes, and relying on the property of DNA to bind only to their own complementary sequences through hydrogen bonds, it is possible to detect many genes in pathological specimens. Until recently, such hybridization reactions were performed using highly radioactive DNA probes and subsequent autoradiography on target DNA immobilized on filter membranes. It is now possible to label DNA probes by non-radioactive methods and to perform *in situ* hybridization directly on the tissue sections and cytologic smears (Grody et al., 1987; Rijntjes et al., 1988).

While it may be argued that *in situ* hybridization is not an immunohistochemical procedure, the use of non-radioactive DNA probes is analogous to that of immunohistochemistry in that the DNA probe is rendered immunologically detectable by the attachment of a hapten molecule which can be recognized by specific antibodies. For example, N-acetoxy-2-acetyl-aminofluorene (AAF) which reacts with guanine residues in nucleic acid can be incorporated directly into a pre-existing DNA or RNA probe, or immunogenic proteins can be bound covalently to DNA and detected by antibodies following hybridization. By linking nucleoside analogues to fluorescent dyes such as fluorescein and rhodamine, it is possible to produce one-step detection systems in which the visual signal-generating moiety is itself directly incorporated into the DNA probe. Horseradish peroxidase and alkaline phosphatase can also be conjugated covalently to single-stranded DNA resulting in probes capable of generating their own chromogenic reaction at the site of hybridization. Such techniques have not been popular because AAF is a carcinogen and fluoresceinated probes are less sensitive than other methods and fluorescent procedures have inherent deficiencies and inconveniences discussed previously. The peroxidase and phosphatase enzymes tend to lose their activity under the high temperatures required for the hybridization reaction.

Biotin can be conjugated directly to nucleic acids so that the avid biotin-avidin binding properties can be employed, as in immunohistochemical reactions, for the detection, labelling and identification of nucleic acids (Burns et al., 1985; Pringle et al., 1988; Guerin-Reverchon et al., 1989; LLoyd et al., 1990). The direct incorporation of biotin into the nucleic acid probe itself in the form of biotinylated derivatives of uridine triphosphate and deoxyuridine triphosphate allow these analogues to be substituted in place of uridine triphosphate and thymidine triphosphate in

RNA and DNA respectively. Detection of the hybridized biotinylated DNA probe can be accomplished, therefore, by using either antibiotin antibodies or avidin complexed with fluorescent molecules, chromogenic enzymes, or electron-opaque plastic spheres. Other reporter molecules which have been shown to be promising are bromodeoxyuridine (Jirikowski et al., 1989) and digoxigenin (Murray et al., 1992). Commercial sources of biotin labelled probes are available to various organisms including adenovirus 2, cytomegalovirus, Epstein–Barr virus, hepatitis B virus, herpes simplex viruses types I and II, chlamydia, *trachomatis*, human papilloma virus and some oncogenes (Bethesda Research Laboratories, Maryland; Enzo Biochem, New York; Vector, California; Tako Inc., California).

Briefly, *in situ* hybridization with biotinylated probes is performed on deparaffinized tissue sections following proteolytic digestion of the formalin-fixed tissue to exposed intracellular nucleic acid targets. Brief post-fixation in paraformaldehyde assures that the targets remain anchored in the tissue and this is followed by denaturation of probe and target DNA at high temperatures, hybridization at physiologic temperature, and detection of hybridized probe using either a two-step avidin-peroxidase complex, or four-step goat antibiotin antibody followed by biotinylated anti-goat antibody and avidin-peroxidase complex procedure. Other optimized non-radioactive reporter molecules such as digoxigenin and bromodeoxyuridine can be used with diaminobenzidine or alkaline phosphatase to produce results of equivalent or enhanced sensitivity compared to radioactive methods (Warford and Lauder, 1991). They have been employed with probes to a wide variety of viruses, chromosomes (Arnoldus et al., 1991) and mRNA (Pringle et al., 1990; Murray et al., 1992) and combined immunohistochemistry and *in situ* hybridization procedures have been performed for the simultaneous detection of cellular antigens and nucleic acids (Sollberg et al., 1991; Mullink et al., 1991).

Chromogens

Different chromogens are available for the different enzyme systems. DAB is currently the most widely used chromogen (Marcollet et al., 1980; Tubbs and Sheibani, 1981; Trojanowski et al., 1983; Sheibani and Tubbs, 1984; DeJong et al., 1985; Scopsi and Larsson, 1986). Its brown reaction product is clearly visible and is alcohol-fast, making it suitable for use with a wide range of counterstains and mounting media. Its suspected carcinogenicity, however, has prompted the introduction of other reagents. One of the most popular of these alternatives is 3-amino-9-ethylcarbazole (AEC) (Graham et al., 1965; Tubbs et al., 1979; Trojanowski et al., 1983). This chromogen produces a cherry-red colour which is soluble in organic solvents and therefore requires special aqueous media for mounting. The reaction product is labile and gradually looses its intensity with storage. More recently, as with diaminobenizidine, aminoethylcarbazole has also become a suspected carcinogen, so that there is no longer a valid reason for its use as an alternative. Other chromogens include tetramethylbenzidine (Sheibani et al., 1981; Tubbs and Sheibani, 1981), *p*-phenylenediamine-pyrocatechol (Hanker-Yates reagent) (Hanker et al., 1977; Tubbs et al., 1979; Sheibani et al., 1981), 4-chloro-1-naphthol (Sheibani and Tubbs, 1984), α-naphthol pyronine (DeJong et al., 1985; Scopsi and Larsson, 1986) and homovanillic acid (DeJong et al., 1985). All these chromogens allow the final visualization of antibody binding in the immunohistochemical procedure. They are dependent on the ability of peroxidase to mediate an oxidation-reduction reaction in the presence of hydrogen peroxide with the insoluble, oxidized chromogen precipitating at the sites of tissue-bound antibody-enzyme complexes.

Enhancement methods

Metallic ions or organic compounds may be used to enhance the visibility of the insoluble, oxidized chromogen products. Immersion of immunostained sections in solutions of 0.5 per cent copper sulphate, 0.125 per cent osmium tetroxide, 1 per cent cobalt chloride, or 1 per cent nickel ammonium sulphate will enhance the chromogen staining (Hsu and Soban, 1982; Johansson and Backman, 1983; DeJong et al., 1985), altering the colour of the reaction product according to the solution used. We do not employ enhancement methods routinely in our laboratory as we prefer the distinct golden brown colour of DAB which one learns to recognize even when staining is only faint.

Imidazole enhancement

The peroxidation of DAB by horseradish peroxidase can be boosted by a variety of nitrogenous compounds of which imidazole is one of the most effective (Straus, 1982; Fu-Kuo and Fridoruch, 1988). Imidazole elevates the rate of oxidation of DAB by peroxidase several-fold at neutral pH, and has the added advantage of inhibiting the pseudoperoxidase activity of haemoglobin (Straus, 1980). The addition of 0.01 M imidazole to the DAB-peroxidase medium enhances the staining for oestrogen receptors as well as surface membrane staining of lymphocytes and in one study provided the most sensitive of eight different chromogen protocols (Trojanowski et al., 1983).

Enhancement by repeated application of reagents

Another method of enhancing immunostaining in situations where the amount of tissue antigen is low is to employ repeated applications of the primary antibody. The initial incubation can be short, followed by washing in PBS, a re-application of the antibody at the same concentration and overnight incubation at 4°C. The sequence can be reversed with an initial overnight incubation at 4°C or at room temperature, PBS washing, reapplication and incubation at 37°C for 1 to 2 hours. Such manipulations can be employed to the PAP, the APAAP, GAG as well as ABC complex methods (Vacca et al., 1980; Cordell et al., 1984; Lansdorp et al., 1986; Swanson et al., 1987; Wick, Hagen and Frizzera, 1987; Pfreundschick et al., 1988; Elias et al., 1989).

Fixation

Fixation is a key issue as the quality of immunostaining is only as good as the fixation. There is good evidence that current methods of tissue processing as well as paraffin-embedding reduce the amounts of immunohistochemically detectable antigen (Hancock et al., 1982; Leong et al., 1988; Leong and Gilham, 1989). Some tissue antigens, particularly cell surface antigens, detectable in small amounts in fresh frozen tissue, may be completely lost during routine processing and embedding and frozen section remains the gold standard for antigen preservation. Lymphocyte surface antigens are particularly labile and cryostat sections are required for their demonstration. Thus, the availability of the most suitable tissue for antigen demonstration is ensured only if a portion of each biopsy specimen is frozen in its fresh state, especially in anticipated problem cases.

Freezing techniques

Snap freezing may be performed by placing a selected piece of fresh tissue of appropriate size on a frozen section chuck and covering the tissue with OCT compound. This may then be directly immersed into liquid nitrogen or into a mixture of liquid nitrogen and isopentane. A mixture of solid carbon dioxide and alcohol may also be used. The tissue block thus frozen is prised free from the chuck, wrapped in aluminium foil and stored at −20°C or −70°C until required.

Material that is not frozen must be promptly fixed to avoid drying-out, a process which will cause denaturation of antigens. Tissue samples should be thinly sliced otherwise the cells in the centre of the block will not be preserved. Since antigens may be destroyed after excessive time in fixative, tissues destined for immunohistology should be embedded promptly after fixation is complete.

Formaldehyde fixation

Formaldehyde has remained the most widely used fixative in diagnostic laboratories, however, antigen preservation is inversely related to the duration of exposure to formaldehyde. We have applied a wide range of antibodies, commonly used for diagnostic purposes, to multitissue blocks containing a variety of non-neoplastic tissues which were fixed in 10 per cent buffered formalin for periods of 30 min, 1, 2, 4 and 8 h as well as 1, 3, 7, 14, 17 and 30 days (Leong and Gilham, 1989). Antisera to bovine keratin, callus keratin, cytokeratin, CAM 5.2, vimentin, desmin, α-1-antichymotrypsin, muramidase, serotonin, chromogranin, carcinoembryonic antigen, Factor VIII-related protein, S100 protein, neuron specific enolase, leucocyte common antigen and α-1-antitrypsin were used with an avidin-biotin-peroxidase complex technique. There was a distinct fall-off in the staining for some antigens after three days fixation and of most antigens after 7 days fixation. The intermediate filaments vimentin and desmin were poorly preserved even after one day of formalin fixation. Cytokeratins could be 'rescued' to some extent with enzyme digestion prior to staining. It was possible to detect changes of antigen staining in tissues fixed in formalin for a duration as short as 30 min. Such tissues showed a distinct rim of reduced antigen preservation in the periphery of the block where formalin had penetrated (Fig. 1.7). These findings indicated that cellular antigens are lost even with short periods of exposure to formalin and biopsy tissues retrieved from the fixative after several days, or autopsy material which have been similarly fixed for longer periods, may not be useful for immunoperoxidase staining.

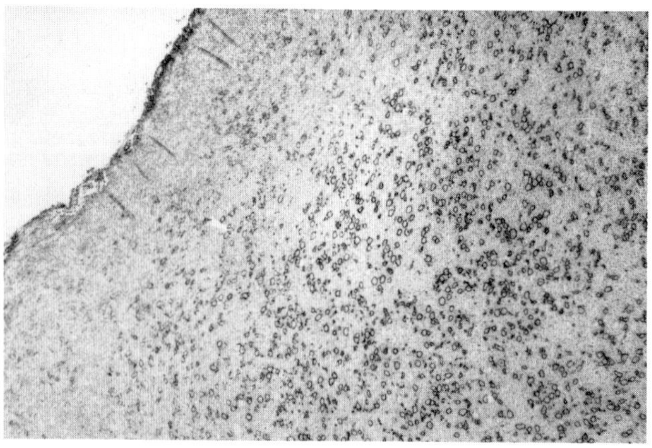

Fig. 1.7. Lymph node with a T-cell rich, B-cell lymphoma. The 15 × 10 × 8 mm node was inadvertently immersed in 10 per cent buffered formalin for about 30 min before arrival in the laboratory whereupon it was immediately retrieved, sliced into 1.5 mm thick slices, microwave-fixed at 62°C and processed through a 3½ h automated cycle of graded alcohol and chloroform before embedding. CD 20 (L26) labels large atypical cells and reveals a distinct rim of antigen loss in the periphery of the block where formalin had penetrated. A similar pattern of loss was observed for other lymphocyte antigens (anti-CD 20, X 16).

Heavy metal salts

Transitional metal salts such as zinc can be potent protein precipitants, forming insoluble complexes with polypeptides so that the use of zinc formalin as a fixative was suggested to enhance immunostaining (Jones et al., 1981). In studying the effects of a 1 per cent solution of zinc sulphate in 3.7 per cent unbuffered formalin, Herman et al. (1988) concluded that the solution produced no deleterious effects or damage on automated tissue processors and zinc formalin-fixed tissue had superior antigen preservation over that of neutral buffered formalin-fixed tissue after automated processing. There is some suggestion that post-fixation in zinc sulphate may also improve immunostaining (Abbondanzo et al., 1990) and the introduction of zinc formalin (1 per cent zinc sulphate in 3.7 per cent unbuffered formalin) into automated tissue processors was reported to result in superior antigen preservation (Herman et al., 1988).

Microwave fixation

In the past seven years, microwave irradiation has been the primary method of tissue fixation in our laboratory (Leong et al., 1985; Leong and Duncis, 1986). We find that this substitute for formalin is not only a rapid and clean method of fixation, but is also superior to formalin for the preservation of cellular antigens (Leong et al., 1988).

Specimens continue to be transferred in buffered formalin as a precaution against autolysis which may occur with delays and other mishaps during transportation of fresh specimens. On arrival in the laboratory, the specimens may have been emersed in formalin for periods ranging from a few minutes to longer. Irrespective of their state of fixation, these tissues are examined and sampled as 2 mm thick blocks and irradiated in batches of 40 to a temperature of 62° C in normal saline. They are then processed through several cycles of absolute alcohol (75 min), chloroform or xylene (50 min), and wax (50 min) in a vacuum-assisted autoprocessor (Shandon Hypercentre II). It is possible, in this manner to run several 'short cycles' of 3½ hours each during the working day so that stained sections are available for examination on the same day as receipt of the specimens. In the case of small specimens such as needle and endoscopic biopsies, a shorter cycle of 65 min in the auto-processor comprising four changes of absolute alcohol over 25 min, two changes of chloroform or xylene over 20 min and two changes of wax over 20 min, produces excellent results (Leong, 1991). The substitution of formalin by microwaves as a fixative and the exclusion of formalin from the autoprocessor, not only removes a noxious and potentially toxic reagent, but also allows the rapid preparation of good quality diagnostic sections from all tissues with the possible exception of large pieces of skin and other dense tissue such as the myometrium. We have found that the immediate irradiation of such tissues may sometimes produce unsatisfactory sections and it has been necessary for all blocks taken from such tissues to have a minimum of 30 min immersion in formalin prior to microwave irradiation.

We have compared the preservation of a wide range of tissue antigens in material fixed by microwave irradiation and those conventionally fixed by formalin (Leong et al., 1988). Tissues were microwave irradiated to 62° C and processed through changes of absolute alcohol, xylene and wax in a 10½ hour cycle. Adjacent pieces of the same tissues were fixed in 10 per cent neutral buffered formalin for periods of 5 and 17 h before processing in an identical manner. With the exception of S100 protein, staining for a wide range of commonly examined tissue antigens demonstrated superiority of immunostaining in microwave-fixed tissues. Besides displaying intense immunostaining, morphologic preservation in irradiated sections was excellent. There was a significant drop-off in staining intensity after 17 h of fixation in formalin and after 5 h in formalin, a lesser degree of immunostaining was obtained when compared with irradiated tissues. In addition, microwave fixation allowed the demonstration of many labile lymphocyte antigens which do not normally survive formalin fixation and paraffin embedding.

With the exception of the cytokeratins and desmin, microwave-fixed tissues did not require enzyme pre-treatment. Microwave fixed tissues were sensitive to proteolytic digestion so that only low concentrations of enzymes were used and only for short periods. We employed only 0.25 mg/ml Trypsin II for 6 min at 22°C .

Other methods of fixation

Non-cross linking fixatives

While no one fixative is ideal for all antigens, satisfactory results for many different antigens can be obtained following fixation in buffered formalin, provided that the exposure to this fixative is for no more than a few hours (Leong and Gilham, 1989). It appears that different mordants afford dissimilar preservation of a variety of antigens. For example, ethanol, Carnoy's solution (60 per cent ethanol, 30 per cent chloroform, 10 per cent glaceal acetic acid) and methacarn (60 per cent methanol, 30 per cent chloroform, 10 per cent acetic acid) appear to optimize the detection of intermediate filament proteins (Culling et al., 1980; Brandtzaeg, 1981; Gown and Vogel, 1984; McNutt et al., 1985), whereas, Bouin's solution provides the best preservation for neuropeptides and biogenic amines (Miller, 1972; Tubbs et al., 1980). The heavy metal fixatives such as B5 and Zenker's solutions are also preferred for the immunohistochemical detection of nuclear antigens (Epstein et al., 1984), however, in our experience, they tend to produce a consistently high level of background immunostaining.

Periodate-lysine-paraformaldehyde solution oxidizes carbohydrate moieties and cross-links them, at the same times stabilizing lipids and proteins, allowing the maintenance of morphological integrity (McLean and Nakane, 1974). This fixative is used for the preservation of leucocyte-related membrane antigens (Hancock et al., 1982) and we have found it useful for the preservation of oestrogen receptor proteins (Raymond and Leong, 1988).

The risk of antigenic denaturation is particularly high in fixatives containing acid substances, probably as a result of the destruction of the tertiary and quaternary structures of the cellular proteins. In general, the most satisfactory morphologic and antigenic preservation is obtained using fixatives near neutral or physiologic pH. The same applies to the ether reagents employed in the immunohistochemical staining procedure.

Freeze drying

Stein et al. (1985) described a method of freeze drying at −45°C, 10^{-2} torr in the presence of phosphorus pentoxide for up to 48 h before embedding in paraffin, for the preservation of labile lymphocyte antigen. While effective, we have found the method cumbersome and requiring special equipment. The resultant tissues were difficult to cut and often of suboptimal morphology. Freeze substitution with low temperature plastic embedding has been suggested as an alternative procedure which avoids the need for tissue fixation, combining the superior morphologic preservation of fixed embedded tissue with the reactivity of cryostat sections (Murray and Ewen, 1991).

The acetone-methyl benzoate-xylene (AMEX) method

The AMEX method described by Sato et al. (1986) is claimed to show better histological preservation than is possible to obtain in frozen sections, yet retaining reactivity for labile lymphocyte membrane antigens. The method required overnight fixation of tissues in acetone at −20°C, clearing in methyl benzoate and xylene before paraffin embedding. More recently, these authors (Sato et al., 1992) showed that the amount of protein extracted from tissues fixed by the AMEX method was the same as that extracted from fresh tissues.

Plastic embedding

Embedding in newer plastics following limited fixation has been shown to not only produce superior cytomorphological preservation but also good antigenic preservation (Beckstead, 1985). By employing fixatives such as paraformaldehyde, acetone or Bouin's solution and embedding in low temperature (4°C) polymerization resins such as glycol methacrylate, it has been possible to demonstrate a wide variety of haematopoietic and other cellular antigens in both normal and neoplastic tissues (Fig. 1.8) (Lazzaro et al., 1988; Casey et al., 1988; Islam et al., 1988).

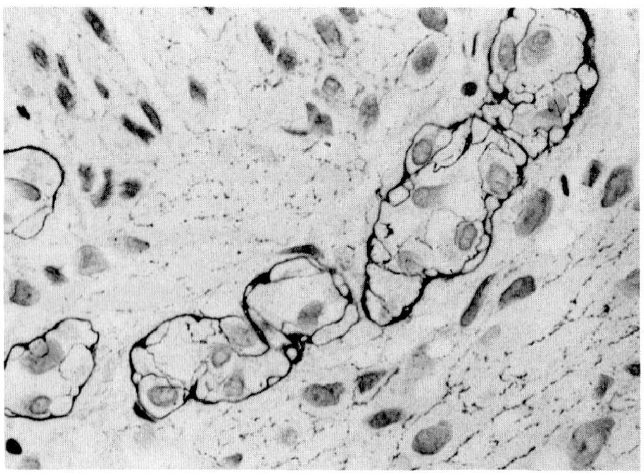

Fig. 1.8. Myometrium fixed in paraformaldehyde for 2 h and embedded in glycol methacrylate at 4°C before staining for laminin with an immunogold-silver technique. Note the exquisite labelling of the discontinuous basal lamina around individual smooth muscle cells and endothelial cells (anti-laminin, X160).

Decalcifying solutions

Reports by Matthews and Mason (1984) and by Mukai et al. (1986) suggest that neutral EDTA, 10 per cent formic acid, and 10 per cent acidic acid produces little modulation of immunoreactivity, even after periods as long as 7 weeks of decalcification. However, 5 per cent nitric acid decalcification effects a decrease in immunoreactivity, and protease treatment may help to maximize immunostaining results. These findings have been confirmed by Athanasou et al. (1987) who suggested that trichloroacetic acid was a useful one step fixation and decalcifying agent for both cryostat and routinely processed sections.

Tissue processing

Detailed studies on the effects of tissue processing on antigen preservation are lacking but temperatures of over 60°C may cause marked antigenic denaturation. In addition, there is loss of cellular morphology, particularly of nuclear detail. As such it is best that paraffin impregnation be carried out at less than 60°C, using low melting point paraffins if necessary. Recently, Wakins et al. (1990) suggested that antigens may be lost when tissue sections are heat-dried at 58°C as compared with those dried at 37°C.

Stein et al. (1985) found that the process of tissue fixation and dehydration, rather than the subsequent steps of paraffin embedding, resulted in the loss of antigenic reactivity in routinely processed paraffin sections. Their study showed that fixatives containing aldehyde groups, alcohol groups, and/or carboxyl groups (e.g. acetic acid) caused destruction of membrane antigens and fixatives like acetone and chloroform tended to preserve such antigens. Dewaxing of sections with Histoclear led to almost complete loss of antigenic activity. In contrast, xylene had no such deleterious effect. We have employed Histoclear without detectable alteration to antigen preservation.

Staining procedure

We routinely employ a streptavidin-biotin-peroxidase procedure as provided in the Appendix. Any step in the immunoperoxidase procedure may conceal a pitfall. For example, failure to block the activity of endogenous peroxidase and peroxidase-like enzymes may lead to a false positive result, particularly if fresh frozen tissue is used. Similarly, undesirable background staining, particularly of connective tissue and collagen, is a common nuisance of immunoperoxidase staining. Pre-incubation of the tissue sections with a high concentration of some protein solution like normal serum or bovine albumin may reduce background staining but it sometimes cannot be completely avoided. The use of the highest possible dilution of primary antibody may also help to reduce unwanted background reactions.

The incubation time at room temperature for most primary antibodies is 20–30 min. Increasing the temperature to 37°C may reduce the incubation time but it may also produce false negative or false positive results, and background staining is also increased, sometimes to an intolerable level. Overnight incubation of the primary antibody at 4°C requires the lowest concentration of the antibody and results in the least background staining although overnight incubation at room temperature (21°C) is the most convenient method.

At no time between incubations and washes should the sections be left to dry. Drying invariably produces false negative results. All incubations are best performed in a humidified chamber.

Microwave-stimulated staining

We have found that microwaves may be used to dry and fix cryostat sections as well as to reduce the incubation process of the primary antibody to a matter of seconds, yielding better cytomorphologic details and a clean background (Leong and Milios, 1986). We have also successfully applied microwaves to all stages of primary, secondary and peroxidase complex incubations in the staining of paraffin sections and have also been able to hasten the blocking steps by exposure to microwaves, reducing the entire staining procedure to about 16 min (Leong and Milios, 1990). As this microwave stimulated technique is labour intensive, it is used in our laboratory only for urgent or special cases.

Immunostaining of previously stained sections

Immunostaining can be performed on previously stained sections and cytological preparations. Employing a sensitive ABC technique, it was possible to immunostain a wide variety of antigens in normal and pathological tissues following removal of the cover glass and brief destaining of the haematoxylin and eosin sections in acid alcohol. There was no detectable loss of sensitivity with the procedure (Milios and Leong, 1987) and in the case of cytologic preparations, destaining was not necessary.

It is important that, for the identification of small quantities of DAB products, the counterstain employed is light. Haematoxylin or methyl green are traditionally used as nuclear counterstains. Haematoxylin counterstains yield good morphologic detail. Methyl green is inferior in this regard although it is useful for black-and-white photography as the precipitated chromogen is emphasized through the use of green camera filters. Azure B, another counterstain has similar properties to methyl green. We routinely apply a regressive haematoxylin stain employing the Lillie–Mayers technique.

Automated immunostaining

Automation of immunostaining is an inevitable phase in the development and evolution of immunohistochemistry as a diagnostic tool. The Code-On system developed by Briganti et al. (1988) was the first commercial immunostainer. The system employs the capillary action principle to apply, incubate, and sequentially removes reagents from glass microscopic slide surfaces. The system performs complete immuno assays from the dewaxing to nuclear staining stage and is capable of analysing 60 slides for 30 different antigens within 2 h and 35 min. It is claimed to save over 80 per cent of organic reagents and up to 50 per cent of immunochemicals and can be employed for *in situ* hybridization procedures. While the entire programme is driven by an IBM PC, semi-automated staining can be performed by employing the special slides and the slide holder which can be purchased separately from the fully automated system. The Code-On system is marketed by Fischer Scientific, Atlanta, USA. Another commercial product, the Cadenza, was recently marketed by Shandon Salvon Scientific Limited, Cheshire, England. It is based on a different concept in which up to 20 slides can be processed in any run, each being held in a disposable coverplate which regulates the reaction of antibody with the sections. Stark et al. (1988) developed an instrument based the controlled application of antisera from syringes and centrifugal buffer washes. A simple approach was adopted by Stross et al. (1989) who modified a standard tissue processor to automate the technique from the stage of detection of the primary antibody but performed chromogen demonstration manually. Their system had the advantage of economy by re-using reagents and reduction of man hours compared with the manual technique. MaWhinney et al. (1990) based their prototype immunostainer on a microcomputer controlled fluid transfer system, totally enclosed slide chambers and a reagent carousel, allowing flexibility in choice of primary and detection reagents for each slide. This system is currently distributed as the AS Elite system (Anglia Scientific, Cambridge, UK) and can stain up to 96 slides in each run.

It has been argued that automated immunostaining has the potential to provide savings by batch staining of a relatively large number of slides, freeing personnel to perform other manual tasks (Tubbs and Bauer, 1989). This is largely dependent on the workload of the individual laboratory as the Fischer Code-On system has a 60-slide capacity and the Shandon Cadenza can stain up to 20 slides in any run. These numbers are small compared to the ability of an experienced histotechnologist who can manually stain as many as 150 slides in a run. The cost comparison of manual and automated immunostaining provided by MaWhinney et al. (1990) indicated cost savings largely in the area of employee costs, whereas reagent costs were cheaper for manual staining.

One advantage of automated immunostaining would be in the area of standardization for laboratories which perform immunostaining infrequently. The complex immunostaining procedures that require multiple steps are prone to human errors which are minimized in the automated environment. It has been argued that automated staining would result in standardization between laboratories, however, an important aspect of any immunohistochemical procedure is the process of tissue fixation and the wide variation in methods of fixation employed by different laboratories make standardization quite impossible even with automated immunostaining.

Controls

Controls must be a part of every immunoperoxidase run. Positive controls should be included, these being selected because the antigen in question is present in the tissue. Positive controls of normal tissues with large amounts of the antigen in question can be used, but it is more appropriate to have controls of neoplastic tissues in which only small amounts of antigen are present, as these would correspond more closely to the levels present in the test section. The latter may also contain non-neoplastic tissues which express the antigen in question and can act as inbuilt controls.

A negative control is a section of tissue known to lack totally the antigen under study. Negative controls also take the form of replacing the primary antibody with either non-immune serum or any other antibody with irrelevant specificity. Abolition of positive staining by an antibody preabsorbed by the antigen under study is the most reliable control; however, this procedure is not often practical.

Reagents

The results obtained in immunoperoxidase procedures are governed by the quality of the antibodies employed. Monoclonal antibodies have given immunohistochemical techniques a new dimension. They are easy to produce and are very specific and do not show much 'batch to batch' variation. Because their reactivity is usually against an epitope rather than the whole antigen, they may be less sensitive than conventionally prepared polyclonal antibodies. In fact, some monoclonal antibodies, particularly those against cell surface antigens, may react only on cryostat sections. However, it is recommended that all new antibodies accessioned for diagnostic purposes be subjected to in-house testing for specificity and sensitivity. Primary antibodies have been known to be defective and sometimes do not conform to the manufacturers claims with respect to the characteristics of its reagents (Kuhlman and Peschke, 1985). Each laboratory must therefore thoroughly test newly accessioned antibodies on optimally processed tissues (Leong, 1992). In this regard, multitissue blocks allow a convenient and expedient way of assessing new antibodies before they are put to diagnostic use. Such multitissue blocks may be prepared according to the method of Battifora (1986) or composite blocks may be made up from 20 to 30 pieces of different types of neoplastic tissues re-embedded from previously tested paraffin blocks or tissues obtained at the time of gross specimen examination (Kraaz et al., 1988; Miller and Groothuis, 1991).

The optimal concentration of the primary antibody should also be calculated by studies on dilution. This is done by applying serial dilutions of a primary antibody to several sections of a known positive tissue. In general, three-fold to four-fold dilutions are required before differences are appreciable and it is convenient to screen doubling dilutions of the antibody. A slide with the best specific staining and the least unwanted background reaction provides the optimal dilution of the primary antibody. A list of the antibodies commonly employed in our laboratory for diagnostic purposes and their sources is given in the Appendix. The dilutions listed are optimal for the method of fixation and processing employed by our laboratory. They are provided as a guide and it is necessary for each laboratory to work out the optimal dilutions for their individual methods of fixation and tissue processing.

In order to avoid misinterpretation, one must be thoroughly familiar with characteristic staining patterns and intensity of reactions obtained with various monoclonal and conventional antibodies. Some antibodies, for example, react only on cryostat sections while others require predigestion of the sections with proteolytic enzymes (Leong, 1992).

Proteolytic enzyme digestion

The use of neutral buffered formalin as a fixative commonly results in cross linking of antigenic molecules with 'masking' of their immunoreactivity. The treatment of tissue sections with proteolytic enzymes is thought to break the methylene cross-links in the antigenic molecules, reconstituting their immunoreactivity. Bovine trypsin and pepsin are commonly used proteases for this purpose. They must be prepared fresh and in a suitable solvent such as 0.01 M NaOH-0.1 per cent calcium chloride at pH 7.8 and applied to the rehydrated deparaffinized tissue sections either at room temperature or at 37°C. The duration of digestion is dependent upon the extent of antigenic masking in the specimen. Battifora and Kopinski (1986) showed that tissues fixed for longer periods of time in formalin require longer exposure to proteolytic enzymes and were more resistant to digestion than were tissues fixed only for brief periods. The authors also indicated that formalin-fixed epithelial tissues stained weakly or failed to stain for cytokeratins unless they were treated with a proteolytic enzyme. They suggested that ethanol-fixed tissue showed excellent preservation of the antigenicity of cytokeratins and no appreciable differences in immunostaining was found with varying periods of fixation in ethanol. We have examined a comparable range of antigens in tissues fixed in 95 per cent ethanol and in formol-alcohol (90 ml of 80 per cent ethanol, 10 ml concentrated formalin and 0.22 g sodium acetate) and the results obtained were similar to those obtained with 10 per cent formalin in that most tissue antigens were lost. Although ethanol appears to be an excellent fixative for the preservation of cytoplasmic intermediate filament proteins, they do not appear to be superior mordants with respect to other antigens. Morphologic preservation in alcohol fixed tissues is suboptimal and the specimens have to be hand-processed for embedding in paraffin, making it inconvenient for most histopathology laboratories.

Enzyme digestion may reduce the background and enhance the immunoreaction for certain antibodies but false negative staining or no enhancement may be observed with other antibodies (Ordonez et al., 1988). In some instances enzyme pretreatment may result in increased background staining and false positive staining. It also has the disadvantage in that it produces a loss of adherence of tissue sections to the glass slides. Chrome-alum gel, Elmer's glue or polylysine have been used as binding agents to overcome this problem. In our laboratory we use aminoalkylsilane-treated glass slides as a 2 per cent solution of 3-aminopropyltriethoxylsilane in acetone (Rentrop et al., 1986).

Antigen retrieval

It was recently suggested that microwave heating of tissue sections in the presence of metal solutions may produce a dramatic recovery of many antigens masked by cross-linking fixatives such as formaldehyde. Shi et al. (1991) heated tissue sections in Coplin jars containing saturated lead thiocyanate or 1 per cent zinc sulphate to 100°C before immunostaining. They showed improved staining of many antigens at increased antibody dilutions or reduced incubation times and adequate immunostaining in long-term formalin-fixed tissues that failed to stain by conventional methods. Our initial experience with the technique supports their claims, although antigen retrieval was possible even in saturated sodium chloride solution and at temperatures below boiling point, such as 60°C maintained for 10 min (unpublished data).

Interpretation of staining

Patterns of staining

Interpretation of immunoperoxidase staining requires skill and experience so that the examiner should not only be familiar with the characteristics of a true positive reaction, but should also be aware of possible variability in results depending on the nature of the tissue and the type of antibody used. The causes of misinterpretation of immunoperoxidase staining are either technical or interpretative. A true positive reaction not only stains cells brown, but the most important quality of a truly positive reaction is its heterogeneity in distribution within single cells, as well as among a group of cells, and throughout the neoplasm. In individual cells, the brown granules may occupy all of the cytoplasm, the cell membrane, the perinuclear area alone, or, simply one of the poles of the cell. Diffuse, pale brown, or a monotonous yellow staining of neoplastic cells is, in all likelihood, non-specific. The majority of immunohistochemical cell markers are localized either intracytoplasmically or on the cell surface membrane with an increasing number of exceptions. Some viral antigens and oncogenes, the Ki-67 antigen, cyclin and oestrogen receptor and progesterone receptor proteins are entirely intranuclear. S100 protein, neuron specific enolase and LN2 are present both in the nuclei and cytoplasm of positive cells.

Besides the general localization of antigens to either the cytoplasmic and/or nuclear compartments of the cell, some antigens display a specific pattern of distribution which is sufficiently specific to aid in the identification of the cell type. For example, the Reed–Sternberg cell shows a characteristic cell membrane and paranuclear staining pattern with occasional cytoplasmic reactivity (Pinkus et al., 1985); the cells of Merkel cell carcinoma display juxtanuclear whorls of cytokeratin filaments and sometimes neurofilaments (Leong et al., 1986; Leong and Milios, 1987); cells of the so-called rhabdoid tumour and its simulants display a distinctive globular mass of vimentin intermediate filaments corresponding to the whorls seen by electron microscopy (Tsuneyoshi et al., 1987; Weeks et al., 1989); and the cells of malignant mesothelioma can be identified by their aberrant, circumferential and long microvilli which are labelled by monoclonal antibodies to EMA (Leong et al., 1990).

Other intrinsic and extrinsic pigments

Pigments such as formalin, melanin and haemosiderin should be differentiated from the granules of diaminobenzidine as they are different both in texture and colour. Treating the pre-stained sections with saturated alcoholic picric acid or sodium hydroxide (1 per cent) in 70 per cent ethanol resulted in removal of troublesome formalin pigment with no deleterious effect on immunoperoxidase staining. Post-treatment with the same solutions also produced similarly good results (McGovern and Crocker, 1986). The replacement of haematoxylin with azure B as counterstain results in green-blue staining of melanin, producing good contrast with the brown reaction product of DAB when staining for melanocytes in heavily pigmented melanocytic lesions (Kamino and Tam, 1991). Examination of the antibody control slide will also reveal their true character.

False-positive and false-negative staining

Mitotic cells and necrotic tissue non-specifically absorb antibodies and the latter exhibits undesirable background staining. Another problem of interpretation occurs from passive absorption or active phagocytosis of antigens by histiocytes or other cells so that they become immunoreactive even though they do not actually elaborate the antigen under study. Macrophages, for example, may pick up myoglobin from adjacent necrotic or damaged skeletal muscle cells. False positive staining is occasionally seen in the granular cells of the epidermis which show a non-specific cytoplasmic reaction regardless of the antibody used. The free edges of histological sections may at times exhibit non-specific positive reactions or may show enhanced staining in the form of an 'edge phenomena'. Similar artificial staining may be seen on the surface membrane of isolated cells floating in fluid, false-positive staining may result from contaminating antibodies in polyclonal antiserum. In cytologic specimens, additional sources of false positive staining include degenerate, crushed and necrotic cells. Lastly, it is not unusual to observe complete lack of staining for various antigens in tissues that contain them in a condensed or consolidated form. This is due to a possible failure of adequate penetration of antibodies into solidified structures like the cornified layer of the epidermis, Russell bodies and the colloid of thyroid follicles. Other causes of false-negative staining include inappropriate titre and dilution of reagents, low antigen concentration in tissue or masking or loss of antigens, and inappropriate incubation time and temperature.

Quantitation of immunostains

By identification and localization of specific antigens in tissue sections, immunohistochemistry provides information which is largely qualitative. Quantitation is currently performed most commonly by subjective grading. As the number of immunolabelled cells or structures is also of importance, immunohistochemistry can be employed to evaluate the number or proportion, i.e., volume density, of cells expressing specific antigens, but it only rarely is employed to estimate the concentration of the antigens within cells. Semi-quantitative analysis of immunolabelling in tissue sections can be represented by the product or sum of the staining intensity and percentage of positively stained cells or structures. These two values can be employed in various mathematical formulae as a method of semi-quantitative analysis (McCarty et al.,

1985), however, although this provides a numerical value, it is still largely subjectively derived. Image analysis allows the measurement of the concentration of immunostaining as a reflection of the antigen concentration in tissue sections. In the case of hormone receptor antigens, a nuclear antigen, the integrated nuclear optical density and the nuclear size can be measured; the difference in nuclear optical density between the antibody stained and unstained parallel sections being a reflection of the hormone receptor content (Franklin et al., 1987). Such methods of immunodensitometry can also be applied for the objective measurement of cellular antigens (Pappolla, 1988; Rahier et al., 1989). While such densitometric analyses can be performed with small PC-based systems, larger automated systems such as the CAS 200 image analyser (CAS Inc., Lombard, Il) and Samba 200 (Thomson TITN, Morangis, France) are also available and have been employed in various studies, particularly for the quantitation of hormone receptors (El Badawi et al., 1991; Figge et al., 1991).

A problem which is encountered in the quantitation of immunostained sections is the irregular conservation of antigen within an individual tissue sample so that uneven patterns of immunostaining are produced. This is largely the result of the unpredictable alteration of antigenic sites that is introduced by tissue fixation and processing. Battifora (1991) advocated the use of vimentin staining as an internal, or reporter molecule, to monitor the quality of tissue fixation as vimentin is a ubiquitous molecule uniformly distributed in every tissue sample. Furthermore, it is susceptible to loss or masking from poor fixation and serves not only as an indicator of the quality of antigen preservation but also allows the better selection of appropriate fields for the interpretation of other immunostains such as hormone receptors.

Photography of stained sections

The photography of immunostained sections can often pose problems, particularly with sections of low antigenicity which produce staining of low intensity. The production costs of colour plates are often prohibitive and most journals will only accept black and white prints for publication so that it is probably worthwhile to improve one's skills in the photography of immunostained sections. Metallic iron enhancement of chromogens is one way of getting around the problem of producing high contrast prints but this may not always be successful.

In black and white photography, contrast enhancement can be attained by placing various colour filters below the substage diaphragm, just above the field diaphragm in the light microscope. When the visibility of a structure exhibiting one of the primary colours, i.e., red, yellow, or blue, has to be increased, this can be achieved by placing, in the light path, a filter of complementary colour to the actual colour that has to be enhanced. However, contrast enhancement of compound colours that do not exhibit a dominant primary colour such as those with brownish hues, often gives rise to difficulties. Diaminobenzidine is probably the most widely routinely employed chromogen and it is often necessary to enhance the contrast of the brown reaction product produced with this chromogen. Moller et al. (1984) recommended the use of a combination of interference filters representing those of the primary colours green (480–500 nm) and red (575–585 nm), as well as a broader band between 385–430 nm, and showed that they resulted in contrast enhancement of 30 per cent compared to neutral grey filters. They also showed that a Kodak Wratten 80A blue absorption filter produced an increase in contrast of up to 19 per cent. We employ the Kodak Wratten 80A filter routinely in black and white photography of immunostained preparations and use Kodak Technical Pan film 2415 (ASA 100). It is possible to achieve even greater contrast by slightly over-exposing the film (in the case of automatic cameras, expose the Tech Pan 2415 (ASA100) at an ASA of 60 or 80 depending on the contrast required).

For colour photography, various colour films can be employed depending on one's preference. We employ a daylight film, Kodak Ectachrome 64. It is, however, important to remember that the intensity of brown hues can be modified by the colour temperature at which the film is exposed. Low colour temperatures produce a 'red shift' and if the colour temperature is high, a 'blue shift' results. The brown pigment of oxidized diaminobenzidine is thus somewhat enhanced in the lower colour temperature range. A handy and simple reference on photomicrography is produced by Olympus Optical Company Limited (Tokyo, Japan).

Conclusions

The contributions of immunohistochemistry are already making a major impact on the diagnosis and current classifications of neoplasms (Leong and Wright, 1987; Leong and Wannakrairot, 1992). The latter is based on traditional concepts of histogenesis and differentiation but we need to re-evaluate these concepts in the light of pertinent immunomarker studies. We actually know little about histogenesis – tumours may change patterns during their course, regardless of histogenesis; neoplasms may manifest multi-directional differentiation; cell populations with similar patterns of similar differentiation may not share related embryogenesis. Immunohistochemistry will contribute to our understanding but we cannot simplistically expect these 'magic makers' to provide all the answers and there will never be a substitute for adequate experience in clinico-pathological correlation. The interpretation of 'brown stains' still depends on cytomorphological identification and cannot replace the experience of the pathologist (Leong, 1992).

References

Abbondanzo, S.L., Allred, D.C., Lampkin, S.and Banks, P.M. (1990). Enhancement of immunoreactivity in paraffin-embedded tissue by re-fixation in zinc sulphate (abstract). *Laboratory Investigation* **63,** 2a.

Arnoldus, E.P.J., Dreef, E.J., Noordermeer, I.A., Verheggen, M.M., Tierry, R.F., Peters, A.C.B., Cornelisse, C.J., van der Ploeg, M. and Raap, A.K. (1991). Feasibility of *in situ* hybridisation with chromosome-specific DNA probes on paraffin wax embedded tissue. *Journal of Clinical Pathology* **44,** 900–4.

Athanasou, N.A., Quinn, J., Heryet, A., Woods, C.G. and McGee, J.O'D. (1987). Effect of decalcification agents on immunoreactivity of cellular antigens. *Journal of Clinical Pathology* **40,** 874–8.

Battifora, H. (1986). The multitumour (sausage) tissue block. Novel method for immunohistochemical testing. *Laboratory Investigation* **55,** 244–8.

Battifora, H. and Kopinski, M. (1986). The influence of protease digestion and duration of fixation on the immunostaining of keratins. A comparison of formalin and ethanol fixation. *Journal of Histochemistry and Cytochemistry* **8,** 1095–100.

Battifora, H. (1991). Assessment of antigen damage in immunohistochemistry. The vimentin internal control. *American Journal of Clinical Pathology* **96,** 669–71.

Beckstead, J.H. (1985). Optimal antigen localization in human tissues using aldehyde-fixed plastic-embedded sections. *Journal of Histochemistry and Cytochemistry* **33,** 954–8.

Brandtzaeg, P. (1981). Prolonged incubation time in immunohistochemistry: effects on fluorescein staining of immunoglobulins and epithelial components in ethanol- and formaldehyde-fixed, paraffin-embedded tissues. *Journal of Histochemistry and Cytochemistry* **11,** 1302–15.

Briganti, D.J., Budgeon, L.R., Unger, E.R., Koebler, D., Cuomo, C., Kennedy, T. and Perdomo, J.M. (1988). Immunocytochemistry is automated: Development of a robotic work station based upon the capillary action principle. *Journal of Histotechnology* **11,** 465–83.

Burns, V.T.W., Jonasson, J.A., Fleming, K.A., Taylor, S. and McGee, O.D. (1985). Sensitive system for visualizing biotinylated DNA probes hybridized *in situ*: Rapid sex discrimination of intact cells. *Journal of Clinical Pathology* **38,** 1085–92.

Cartun, R.W. and Pedersen, C.A. (1989). An immunocytochemical technique offering increased sensitivity and lowered cost with a streptavidin-horseradish peroxidase conjugate. *Journal of Histotechnology* **12,** 273–7.

Casey, T.T., Cousar, J.B. and Collins, R.D. (1988). A simple plastic embedding and immunohistologic technique for immunophenotypic analysis of human haemopoietic and lymphoid tissues. *American Journal of Pathology* **131,** 183–9.

Cattoretti, G., Berti, E. and Schiro, R. (1988). Improved avidin-biotin-peroxidase complex (ABC) staining. *Histochemistry Journal* **20,** 75–80.

Coons, A.H., Creech, H.J. and Jones, R.N. (1941). Immunological properties of an antibody containing a fluorescent group. *Proceedings of the Society of Experimental Biology* **47,** 200.

Cordell, J.L., Falini, B., Erber, W., Gatter, K.C. and Mason, D.Y. (1984). Immunoenzymatic labelling of monoclonal antibodies using immune complexes of alkaline phosphatase and monoclonal anti-alkaline phosphatase (APAAP) complexes. *Journal of Histochemistry and Cytochemistry* **32,** 219–29.

Culling, C.F., Reid, P.E. and Sinnott, N.M. (1980). The effects of various fixatives and trypsin digestion upon the staining of routine paraffin-embedded sections by the peroxidase-anti-peroxidase and immunofluorescence techniques. *Journal of Histochemistry* **3,** 10–19.

DeJong A.S.H., van Kessel-Van Mark, M. and Raap, A.K. (1985). Sensitivity of various visualisation methods for peroxidase and alkaline phosphatase activity in immunoenzyme histochemistry. *Histochemistry Journal* **17,** 1119–30.

El-Badawi, N., Cohen, C., Derose, P.B., Check, I.J. and Sjoutas, D. (1991). Immunohistochemical progesterone-receptor assay. Measurement by image analysis. *American Journal of Pathology* **96,** 704–10.

Elias, J.M., Margiotta, M. and Gaborc, D. (1989). Sensitivity and detection efficiency of the peroxidase antiperoxidase (PAP), avidin-peroxidase complex (ABC), and peroxidase-labelled avidin-biotin (LAB) methods. *American Journal of Clinical Pathology* **92,** 62–7.

Epstein, A.L., Marder, R.J. and Winter, J.N. (1984). Two new monoclonal antibodies (LN1, LN2) reactive in B5 formalin-fixed, paraffin-embedded tissues with follicular centre and mantle zone human B lymphocytes and derived tumours. *Journal of Immunology* **133,** 1028–34.

Figge, J., Bakst, G., Weisheit, D., Solis, O. and Ross, J.S. (1991). Image analysis quantitation of immunoreactive retinoblastoma protein in human thyroid neoplasms with a streptavidin-biotin-peroxidase staining technique. *American Journal of Pathology* **139,** 1213–19.

Franklin, W.A., Bibbo, M., Doria, M.I., Dytch, H.E., Toth, J., DeSombre, E. and Wied, G.R. (1987). Quantitation of oestrogen receptor content and Ki-67 staining in breast carcinoma by the micro TICAS image analysis system. *Analytical and Quantitative Cytology and Histology* **9,** 279–86.

Fu-Kuo, C. and Fridoruch, I. (1988). Stimulation of the activity of horseradish peroxidase by nitrogenous compounds. *Journal of Biology and Chemistry* **263,** 3811–16.

Giorno, R. (1984). A comparison of two immunoperoxidase staining methods based on the avidin-biotin interaction. *Diagnostic Immunology* **2,** 161–6.

Gown, A.M. and Vogel, A.M. (1984). Monoclonal antibodies to human intermediate filament proteins. II. Distribution of filament proteins in normal human tissues. *American Journal of Pathology* **114,** 309–21.

Graham, R.C., Ludholm, U. and Karnovsky, M.J. (1965). Cytochemical demonstration of peroxidase activity with 3-amino-9-ethylcarbazole. *Journal of Histochemistry and Cytochemistry* **13,** 150–2.

Grody, W.W., Cheng, L. and Lewin, K.J. (1987). Application of *in situ* DNA hybridization technology to diagnostic surgical pathology. *Pathology Annual* **1,** 151–75.

Guerin-Reverchon, I., Chardonnet, Y., Chignol, M.C. and Thivolet, J. (1989). A comparison of methods for the detection of human papilloma virus DNA by *in situ* hybridization with biotinylated probes on human carcinoma cell lines. Application to wart sections. *Journal of Immunological Methods* **123,** 167–76.

Hancock, W.W., Becker, J.J. and Atkins, R.C. (1982). A comparison of fixatives and immunohistochemical techniques for use with monoclonal antibodies to cell surface antigens. *American Journal of Clinical Pathology* **78,** 825–31.

Hanker, J.S., Yates, P.E. and Matz, C.B. (1977). A new, specific, sensitive and non-carcinogenic reagent for the demonstration of horseradish peroxidase. *Histochemistry Journal* **9,** 789–92.

Herman, G.E., Chlipala, E., Bochenski, G., Sabin, L. and Elfont, E. (1988). Zinc formalin fixative for automated tissue processing. *Journal of Histotechnology* **11,** 85–9.

Holgate, C.S., Jackson, P. and Pollard, K. (1983). Immunogold silver staining: new method of immunostaining with enhanced sensitivity. *Journal of Histochemistry and Cytochemistry* **31,** 983–4.

Hsu, S.M., Raine, L. and Fanger, H. (1981). Use of avidin-biotin-peroxidase complex (ABC) in immunoperoxidase techniques: A comparison between ABC and unlabelled antibody (PAP) procedures. *Journal of Histochemistry and Cytochemistry* **29,** 577–80.

Hsu, S.M. and Soban, E. (1982). Colour modification of diaminobenzidine (DAB) precipitation by metallic ions, and its application for double immunohistochemistry. *Journal of Histochemistry and Cytochemistry* **30,** 1079–82.

Islam, A., Archibaud, E., Henderson, E.S. and Han, T. (1988). Glycomethacrylate (GMA) embedding for light microscopy. II. Immunohistochemical analysis of semi-thin sections of undecalcified marrow cores. *Journal of Clinical Pathology* **41,** 892–6.

Jirikowski, G.F., Ramalho-Ortigao, J.F., Lind, T. and Seliger, H. (1989). Immunocytochemistry of 5-bromo-2'-deoxyuridine labelled oligonucleotide probes. *Histochemistry* **91,** 51–3.

Johansson, O. and Backman, J. (1983). Enhancement of immunoperoxidase staining using osmium tetroxide. *Journal of Neuroscience Methods* **7,** 185–93.

Jones, M.D., Banks, P.M. and Caron, B.L. (1981). Transition metal salts as adjuncts to formalin for tissue fixation (abstract). *Laboratory Investigation* **44,** 32a.

Kamino, H. and Tam, S.T. (1991). Immunoperoxidase technique modified by counterstain with Azure B as a diagnostic aid in evaluating heavily pigmented melanocytic neoplasms. *Journal of Cutaneous Pathology* **18,** 436–9.

Kohler, G. and Milstein, C. (1975). Continuous cultures of fused cells secreting antibody of pre-defined origin. *Nature* **256,** 495–7.

Kraaz, W., Risberg, B. and Haussein, A. (1988). Multiblock: An aid in diagnostic immunohistochemistry. *Journal Clinical Pathology* **41,** 1337.

Kuhlman, W.D. and Peschke, P. (1985). Commercial polyclonal and monoclonal histostaining PAP kits. Immunoperoxidase reagents and performance characteristics in comparison with self prepared immunoreagents. *Histochemistry* **82,** 411–19.

Lansdorp, P.M., van der Kwast, T.H. and de Boer, M. (1984). Stepwise amplification immunoperoxidase (PAP) staining: I. cellular morphology in relation to membrane markers. *Journal of Histochemistry and Cytochemistry* **32,** 172–6.

Lazzaro, B., Munger, R. and Lumb, G. (1988). Antigen localization in immunoperoxidase-stained plastic-embedded soft tissues. *Human Pathology* **19,** 902–9.

Leong, A.S-Y., Daymon, M.E. and Milios, J. (1985). Microwave irradiation as a form of fixation for light and electron microscopy. *Journal of Pathology* **146,** 313–21.

Leong, A.S-Y., Phillips, G.E., Pieterse, A.S. and Milios, J. (1986). Criteria for the diagnosis of primary endocrine carcinoma of the skin (Merkel cell carcinoma). A histologic, immunohistochemical and ultrastructural study of 13 cases. *Pathology* **18,** 393–9.

Leong, A.S-Y. and Duncis, C.G. (1986). A method of rapid fixation of large biopsy specimens using microwave irradiation. *Pathology* **18,** 222–5.

Leong, A.S-Y. and Milios, J. (1986). Rapid immunoperoxidase staining of lymphocyte antigens using microwave irradiation. *Journal of Pathology* **148,** 183–7.

Leong, A.S-Y. and Milios, J. (1987). Immunohistochemical staining in primary neuroendocrine (Merkel cell) carcinoma of the skin. *Histopathology* **11,** 668–9.

Leong, A.S-Y. and Wright, J. (1987). The contributions of immunohistochemical staining in tumour diagnosis. *Histopathology* **11,** 1295–305.

Leong, A.S-Y., Milios, J. and Duncis, C.G. (1988). Antigen preservation in microwave-irradiated tissues. A comparison with routine formalin fixation. *Journal of Pathology* **156,** 275–82.

Leong, A.S-Y. and Gilham, P.N. (1989). The effects of progressive formaldehyde fixation on the preservation of tissue antigens. *Pathology* **21,** 266–8.

Leong, A.S-Y. and Milios, J. (1990). Accelerated immunohistochemical staining by microwaves. *Journal of Pathology* **161,** 327–34.

Leong, A.S-Y., Parkinson, R. and Milios, J. (1990). 'Thick' cell membranes revealed by immunocytochemical staining: A clue to the diagnosis of malignant mesothelioma. *Diagnostic Cytopathology* **6,** 9–13.

Leong, A.S-Y. (1991). Technical note: Microwave fixation and rapid processing in a large throughput histopathology laboratory. *Pathology* **23,** 271–3.

Leong, A.S-Y. (1992). Commentary: Diagnostic immunohistochemistry – problems and solutions. *Pathology* **24,** 1–4.

Leong, A.S-Y. and Wannakrairot, P. (1992). A retrospective analysis of immunohistochemical staining in identification of anaplastic round cell and spindle cell tumours – results, reagents and costs. *Pathology* **24,** 254–60.

Lloyd, R.V., Gin, L. and Fields, K. (1990). Detection of chromogranins A and B in endocrine tissues with radioactive and biotinylated oligonucleotide probes. *American Journal of Pathology* **14,** 35–43.

Marcollet, M., Morin, J. and Lecher, P. (1980). Comparison between two chromogenic substrates for revealing an immunoperoxidase reaction of human metaphase chromosomes. *Stain Technology* **55,** 35–9.

Matthews, J.B. and Mason, G.I. (1984). Influence of decalcifying agents on immunoreactivity of formalin-fixed, paraffin-embedded tissue. *Histochemistry Journal* **16,** 771–87.

MaWhinney, W.H.B., Warfold, A., Rae, M.J.L. and Lauder, I. (1990). Automated immunochemistry. *Journal of Clinical Pathology* **43,** 591–6.

McCarty, K.S.Jr., Miller L.S., Cox, E.B., Konrath, J. and McCarty, K.S.Sr. (1985). Oestrogen receptor analyses. Correlation of biochemical and immunohistochemical methods using monoclonal antireceptor antibodies. *Archives of Pathology and Laboratory Medicine* **109,** 716–21.

McGovern, J. and Crocker, J. (1986). Effect of formalin pigment removal on peroxidase-antiperoxidase immunoperoxidase technique. *Journal of Clinical Pathology* **39,** 923–6.

McLean, I.W. and Nakane, P.K. (1974). Periodate-lysine-paraformaldehyde fixative: A new fixative for immunoelectron microscopy. *Journal of Histochemistry and Cytochemistry* **22,** 1077–83.

McNutt, M.A., Bolen, J.W., Hammar, S.P. and Vogel, A.M. (1985). Coexpression of intermediate filaments in human epithelial neoplasms. *Ultrastructural Pathology* **9,** 31–43.

Milios, J. and Leong, A.S-Y. (1987). Application of the avidin-biotin technique to previously stained histological sections. *Stain Technology* **62,** 411–16.

Milios, J. and Leong, A.S-Y. (1988). Avidin-biotin-peroxidase complex reagents for routine histological application: A comparison of 4 commercial kits. *Journal of Histotechnology* **11,** 81–3.

Miller, H.R.P. (1972). Fixation and tissue preservation for antibody studies: A review. *Histochemistry Journal* **4,** 305–20.

Miller, R.T. and Groothuis, C.L. (1991). Multitumour 'sausage' blocks in immunohistochemistry. Simplified method of preparation, practical uses and roles in quality assurance. *American Journal of Clinical Pathology* **96,** 228–32.

Moller, M., Glistrup O.V. and Olsen, W. (1984). Contrast enhancement of the brownish horseradish peroxidase-activated 3,3'-diaminobenzidine tetrahydrochloride reaction product in black and white photography by the use of interference filters. *Journal of Histochemistry and Cytochemistry* **32,** 37–42.

Mukai, K., Yoshimura, S. and Anzai, M. (1986). The effects of decalcification on immunoperoxidase staining. *American Journal of Surgical Pathology* **10,** 413–19.

Mullink, H., Jiwa, N.M., Walboomers, J.M.M, Horstman, A., Vos, W. and Meijer, C.J.L.M. (1991). Demonstration of changes in cytokeratin expression in condylomata acuminatum in relation to the presence of human papilloma virus as shown by a combination of immunohistochemistry and *in situ* hybridization. *American Journal of Dermatopathology* **13,** 530–7.

Murray, G.I. and Ewen, S.W.B. (1991). A novel method for optimum biopsy specimen preservation for histochemical and immunohistochemical analysis. *American Journal of Clinical Pathology* **95,** 131–6.

Murray, G.I., Paterson, P.J., Ewen, S.W.B. and Melvin, W.T. (1992). In situ hybridization of albumin mRNA in normal liver and hepatocellular carcinoma with a digoxigenin labelled oligonucleotide probe. *Journal of Clinical Pathology* **45,** 21–4.

Nakane, P.K. and Pierce, G.B., Jr. (1966). Enzyme-labelled antibodies: a preparation for the localisation of antigen. *Journal of Histochemistry and Cytochemistry* **14,** 929–31.

Ordonez, N.G., Manning, J.T., Jr. and Brooks, T.E. (1988). Effect of trypsinization on the immunostaining of formalin-fixed, paraffin-embedded tissues. *American Journal of Surgical Pathology* **12,** 121–9.

Ormanns, W. and Schaffer, R. (1985). An alkaline-phosphatase staining method in avidin-biotin immunohistochemistry. *Histochemistry* **82,** 421–4.

Pappolla, M.R. (1988). Computerized image-analysis microspectroscopy of tissue sections. *Archives of Pathology and Laboratory Medicine* **112,** 787–90.

Pfreundschick, M., Lehmann, M. and Steinmetz, T. (1988). Monoclonal glucose-oxidase-antiglucose oxidase (GAG) immunosandwich assay for the detection of monoclonal antibodies on routine haematological smears. *Blut* **56,** 125–30.

Pinkus, G.S., Thomas, P. and Said, J.W. (1985). LeuM1 – a marker for Reed-Sternberg cells in Hodgkin's disease. An immunoperoxidase study of paraffin-embedded tissues. *American Journal of Pathology* **119,** 244–52.

Pringle, J.H., Primrose, L., Kind, C.N., Talbot, I.C. and Lauder, I. (1988). In situ hybridization demonstration of poly-adenylated RNA sequences in formalin-fixed paraffin sections using a biotinylated oligonucleotide poly d(T) probe. *Journal of Pathology* **158,** 279–86.

Pringle, J.H., Ruprai, A.K., Primrose, L., Keyte, J., Potter, L., Close, P. and Lauder, I. (1990). In situ hybridization of immunoglobulin light chain mRNA in paraffin sections using biotinylated or hepten-labelled oligonucleotide probes. *Journal of Pathology* **162,** 197–207.

Rahier, J., Stevens, M., De Menten, Y. and Henquin, J. (1989). Determination of antigen concentration in tissue sections by immunodensitometry. *Laboratory Investigation* **61,** 357–63.

Raymond, W.A. and Leong, A.S-Y. (1988). An evaluation of potentially suitable fixatives for immunoperoxidase staining of oestrogen receptors in imprints and frozen sections of breast carcinoma. *Pathology* **20,** 320–5.

Rentrop, M., Knapp, B. and Winter, H.A. (1986). Aminoalkylsilane-treated glass slides as support for *in situ* hybridisation of keratin cDNAs to frozen tissue sections under varying fixation and pre-treatment conditions. *Histochemistry Journal* **18,** 271–6.

Rijntjes, P.J.M., Quint, W.G.V. and Herman, C.J. (1988). Nucleic acid probe techniques for the routine surgical pathology laboratory. *Progress in Surgical Pathology* **8,** 139–51.

Sato, Y., Mukai, K., Watanabe, S., Goto, M. and Shimosato, Y. (1986). The AMEX method. A simplified technique of tissue processing and paraffin-embedding with improved preservation of antigens for immunostaining. *American Journal of Pathology* **125,** 431–5.

Sato, Y., Mukai, K., Furuya, S., Kameya, T. and Hirohashi, S. (1992). The AMEX method: A multipurpose tissue-processing and paraffin-embedding method. Extraction of protein and application to immunoblotting. *American Journal of Pathology* **140,** 775–9.

Schaumburg-Lever, G. and Tronnier, M. (1989). Combination of the APAAP and IGSS techniques for double labelling with two different monoclonal antibodies. *American Journal of Dermatology* **11,** 29–32.

Scopsi, L. and Larsson, L.I. (1986). Increased sensitivity in peroxidase immunohistochemistry: A comparative study of a number of peroxidase visualisation methods employing a model system. *Histochemistry* **84,** 221–30.

Sheibani, K. and Tubbs, R.R. (1984). Enzyme immunohistochemistry: Technical aspects. *Seminars in Diagnostic Pathology* **1,** 235–50.

Sheibani, K., Tubbs, R.R. and Gebhardt, G.N. (1981). Comparison of alternative chromogens for renal immunohistochemistry. *Human Pathology* **12,** 349–56.

Shi, S., Key, M.E. and Kalra, K.L. (1991). Antigen retrieval in formalin-fixed, paraffin-embedded tissues: an enhancement method for immunohistochemical staining based on microwave oven heating of tissue sections. *Journal of Histochemistry and Cytochemistry* **39,** 741–8.

Sollberg, S., Peltonen, J. and Vitto, J. (1991). Combined use of *in situ* hybridization and unlabelled antibody peroxidase anti-peroxidase methods: simultaneous detection of type 1 procollagen mRNAs and factor VIII-related antigen epitopes in keloid tissue. *Laboratory Investigation* **64,** 125–9.

Stark, E., Faltinat, D. and van der Fecht, R. (1988). An automated device for immunocytochemistry. *Journal of Immunological Methods* **107,** 89–92.

Stein, H., Gatter, K., Asbahr, H. and Mason, D.Y. (1985). Use of freeze-dried paraffin-embedded sections for immunohistologic staining with monoclonal antibodies. *Laboratory Investigation* **52,** 676–83.

Sternberger, L.A., Hardy, P.H.,Jr. and Cuculis, J.J. (1970). The unlabelled antibody enzyme method of immunohistochemistry. Preparation and properties of soluble antigen-antibody complex (horseradish peroxidase-anti-horseradish peroxidase) and its use in the identification of spirochetes.

Journal of Histochemistry and Cytochemistry **18,** 315.

Straus, W. (1982). Imidazole increases the sensitivity of cytochemical reaction for peroxidase with diaminobenzidine, at a neutral pH. *Journal of Histochemistry and Cytochemistry* **30,** 491–3.

Straus, W. (1980). Factors affecting the sensitivity and specificity of the cytochemical reaction for the anti-horseradish peroxidase antibody in lymph tissues. *Journal of Histochemistry and Cytochemistry* **28,** 645–51.

Stross, W.P., Jones, M. and Mason, D.Y. (1989). Automation of APAAP immunocytochemical technique. *Journal of Clinical Pathology* **42,** 106–12.

Suffin, S.C., Muck, K.B. and Young, J.C. (1979). Improvement of the glucose oxidase immunoenzyme technique. Use of a tetrazolium whose formazan is stable without heavy metal chelation. *American Journal of Clinical Pathology* **71,** 492–6.

Swanson, P.E., Hagen, K.A. and Wick, M.R. (1987). Avidin-biotin-peroxidase-antiperoxidase (ABPAP) complex. An immunocytochemical method with enhanced sensitivity. *American Journal of Clinical Pathology* **88,** 162–76.

Trojanowski, J.Q., Obrocka, M.A. and Lee, V.M-Y. (1983). A comparison of eight different chromogen protocols for the demonstration of immunoreactive neurofilaments or glial filaments in rat cerebellum using the peroxidase-antiperoxidase method and monoclonal antibodies. *Journal of Histochemistry and Cytochemistry* **31,** 1217–22.

Tsuneyoshi, M., Diamaru, Y., Hashimoto, H. and Enjoji, M. (1987). The existence of rhabdoid cells in specific soft tissue sarcomas. Histopathological, ultrastructural and immunohistochemical evidence. *Virchows Archives* **411,** 509–14.

Tubbs, R.R., Velasco, M.E. and Benjamin, S.P. (1979). Immunocytochemical identification of human chorionic gonadotrophin. Comparative study of diaminobenzidine and 3-amino, 9-ethylcarbazole, a non-hazardous chromogen. *Archives of Pathology and Laboratory Medicine* **103,** 534–8.

Tubbs, R.R., Sheibani, K. and Sebeck, B.A. (1980). Immunohistochemistry versus immunofluorescence for non-Hodgkin's lymphoma. *American Journal of Clinical Pathology* **73,** 144–5.

Tubbs, R.R. and Sheibani, K. (1981). Chromogen for immunohistochemistry. *Journal of Histochemistry and Cytochemistry* **29,** 684.

Tubbs, R.R., Sheibani, K., Deodhar, S.D. and Hawk, W.A. (1981). Enzyme immunohistochemistry: Review of technical aspects and diagnostic application. *Cleveland Clinic Quarterly* **48,** 245–81.

Tubbs, R.R. and Bauer, T.W. (1989). Automation of immunohistology. *Archives of Pathology and Laboratory Medicine* **113,** 653–7.

Vacca, L., Abrahams, S.J. and Naftchi, N.E. (1980). A modified peroxidase-antiperoxidase procedure for improve localization of tissue antigens: localization of substance P in rat spinal cord. *Journal of Histochemistry and Cytochemistry* **28,** 297–305.

Wakins, J., Kellock, D., Gillet, C., Egan, M., Pontin, J.E., Millis, R.R. and Levinson, D.A. (1990). Enhancement of immunostaining (letter). *Histopathology* **17,** 185–9.

Warford, A. and Lauder, I. (1991). In situ hybridization in perspective. *Journal of Clinical Pathology* **44,** 177–81.

Weeks, D.A., Beckwith, J.B., Mierau, G.W. and Luckey, D.W. (1989). Rhabdoid tumour of the kidney. A report of 111 cases from the National Wilms' Tumour Study Pathology Centre. *American Journal of Surgical Pathology* **13,** 439–58.

Wick, M.R., Hagen, K.A. and Frizzera, G. (1987). Three immunostaining techniques for the localization of leucocyte common antigen in formalin-fixed, paraffin-embedded dermatological biopsy specimens. *American Journal of Dermatology* **9,** 250–6.

Wood, G.S. and Warnke, R. (1981). Suppression of endogenous avidin-binding activity in tissues and its relevance to biotin-avidin detection systems. *Journal of Histochemistry and Cytochemistry* **29,** 1196–201.

2 ◆ *Immunohistochemistry of 'solid' tumours: poorly differentiated round cell and spindle cell tumours I*

Anthony S-Y. Leong and Allen M. Gown

Introduction

Surgical pathologists identify and type tissues according to the appearances of their constituent cells. Cytological features such as cell size, shape, colour, cytoplasmic and nuclear characteristics, as well as the patterns produced by cell arrangements and their relationship with adjacent tissues form the basis of tissue identification. Contemporary principles of tumour classification and nomenclature are based on the resemblance of the neoplastic tissues to normal mature tissues, and tumours are named according to the normal counterpart they most closely resemble. In most instances this implies histogenetic derivation or origin from such tissues. However, it has also been eloquently argued that the resemblance, at least in some tumours, is more correctly interpreted as representing differentiation of the neoplastic cells along a particular cell line, a reflection of the genetic subsets that the cell is capable of transcribing, with no reference to its origin or derivation (Gould, 1986). In either case, for tumour diagnosis, the surgical pathologist strives to identify features of differentiation which will allow classification. A significant number of tumours, however, do not express sufficient histological features to allow their accurate identification. On the basis of H & E stained sections, such tumours remain labelled as 'undifferentiated' or 'poorly differentiated malignant neoplasms'. In the past, the surgical pathologist has had to resort to ultrastructural examination, cell culture studies, and chromosome analysis to identify additional characteristics which would enable classification. More recently, molecular biology studies have also contributed to tumour identification. While useful, these ancillary procedures are time-consuming and expensive, and perhaps, with the exception of electron microscopy, transgress beyond the scope of morphological diagnosis and represent excursions into areas which may not be familiar to the traditional surgical pathologist.

Current cancer therapeutic regimes offer a high rate of remission for many tumours, and some, including germ cell tumours, Hodgkin's disease, acute lymphoblastic leukaemia and lymphoma, osteogenic sarcoma, rhabdomyosarcoma and Wilm's tumour, have been shown to be potentially curable. With many other tumours, long-term remissions may be achieved, and yet others are amenable to significant palliative treatment. The function of the surgical pathologist in the accurate identification of tumours is thus critical, not only in their broad categorization such as distinguishing between carcinoma, lymphoma and melanoma, but also in their subclassification. This task is often based on subtle and frequently subjective features which are interpreted to indicate a particular line of differentiation in the tumour. Correct classification is also a requirement for accurate tumour statistics and epidemiology. Another important requirement of surgical pathologists is the prediction of the origin of metastatic deposits. This exercise is necessary not only for treatment but would also curtail expensive investigations which may otherwise be instituted.

Immunohistochemistry offers additional objective and reproducible findings in the examination of neoplasms and has proven to be an extremely powerful tool in tumour analysis (Osborn and Weber, 1983; Gown and Vogel, 1984; Gown and Vogel, 1985; Leong and Wright, 1987; Leong and Wannakrairot, 1992). Microscopic examination of H & E stained sections allows the ready assignment of poorly differentiated neoplasms into two broad categories based on the shape of the tumour cells, viz., a group of round cell tumours and a group of spindle cell tumours. When considered in conjunction with the clinical features, particularly the age of the patient and the site of the tumour, a list of differential diagnoses can be made. Through the application of an appropriate panel of antibodies, chosen in the light of such a diagnostic list, it is often possible to further accurately categorize the tumour. It is in accordance with this approach that we employ immunohistochemistry for the diagnosis of anaplastic neoplasms. The panel employed should include not only antibodies which would positively identify the tumour in question but also other antibodies which are known to label the remaining entities considered as differentiated diagnoses. For tumour diagnosis, therefore, antibodies should be employed in panels and not as single reagents solely for the identification of the presence of one antigenic determinant. Negative stains also make a contribution by exclusion. In this and the following chapter we present our immunohistochemical approach to an extensive list of neoplasms which may sometimes not display sufficient features of differentiation in H & E stained sections, or, which show similar morphological characteristics so that they cannot be separated or accurately identified.

Adult round cell tumours

The list of differential diagnoses for anaplastic round cell tumours in adults can be quite extensive, but the most important and common entities to be distinguished are carcinoma and lymphoma. In the case of metastatic deposits, particularly in lymph nodes, amelanotic melanoma is another consideration. The separation of these three tumours is of particular importance from both the prognostic as well as therapeutic standpoint as lymphomas are often very responsive to chemotherapy and radiotherapy (Borowitz et al., 1984) with high rates of remission and high rates of cure, especially in the case of large cell lymphomas (DeVita et al., 1988; Simon et al., 1988).

Malignant lymphoma

The immunohistochemical identification of lymphocytes and lymphoid tumours is based on the detection of leucocyte common antigen (LCA). The human LCA is a cell membrane glycoprotein of approximately 200 kiloDaltons (195–215 kD) molecular weight, and is common to all haematopoietic cells, including lymphocytes, granulocytes, thymocytes, macrophages/monocytes and immature erythroid cells. Its expression is strongest in T and B lymphocytes and appears to increase with increasing levels of differentiation. Staining of macrophages/monocytes, granulocytes and plasma cells is often weaker. Several monoclonal antibodies have been developed against human LCA, sometimes also designated the T-200 antigens (Omary et al., 1980). Among such antibodies are PD7/26 (Warnke et al., 1983; Gatter et al., 1984), 2B11 (Warnke et al., 1983) and F8-11-13 (Salter et al 1985), all of which show consistent labelling of paraffin-embedded sections as well as fresh tissue. Other monoclonal antibodies to LCA have been made but despite showing avid labelling of frozen tissue and cell suspensions, they generally display limited reactivity in fixed material. Anti-LCA antibodies are among the most specific of antibodies currently employed in diagnostic panels. When the various anti-LCA antibodies have been used as single immunostaining reagents, they consistently have failed to label non-haematopoietic neoplasms (Pizzolo et al., 1980; Warnke et al., 1983; Gatter et al., 1984; Wood et al., 1984; Salter et al., 1985). Clones PD7/26 and 2B11 are particularly useful in labelling paraffin-embedded lymphocytes. In the tonsil, PD7/26 preferentially labels B-lymphocytes and 2B11 preferentially labels T-lymphocytes (Warnke et al., 1983), so that a cocktail of the two antibodies is particularly useful for the staining of paraffin-embedded sections. Such a mixture is available as a monoclonal antibody to LCA (Dakopatts, Santa Barbara, California) which has been reported to show 100 per cent specificity (Kurtin and Pinkus, 1985). The antibody was immunoreactive with 93 per cent of paraffin-embedded T-cell and B-cell lymphomas and most cases of lymphocytic leukaemia, with the exception of CALLA-positive acute lymphoblastic leukaemia. One hundred and two non-haematopoietic neoplasms including alveolar rhabdomyosarcoma, Ewing's sarcoma, neuroblastoma, and small cell undifferentiated carcinoma were all negative for LCA. The latter tumours form a group of small cell neoplasms that are important to exclude as they can mimic lymphoma morphologically.

Bouin's fixative, B5 or Zenker's solutions and Carnoy's reagent may be used as fixatives for LCA. In our experience, neutral-buffered 10 per cent formaldehyde and microwave irradiation both produce good preservation of LCA. While it has been suggested that protease digestion prior to immunostaining may 'unmask' antigenic sites which have been obscured by the cross-linkage induced by aldehyde fixatives, we have found that enzymatic predigestion is unnecessary for the demonstration of LCA, and, indeed, may even be detrimental to the staining results (Leong and Gilham, 1989a).

It is important to appreciate that LCA is a cell membrane glycoprotein and immunostaining for this antigen should be regarded as positive only if the reaction product outlines the tumour cell membranes. While there may be a lesser degree of staining in the Golgi areas of the cytoplasm and even faint cytoplasmic staining, these are not reliable indicators of true positivity, particularly if they occur in isolation. The staining of histiocytes is probably the only exception where membranous staining for LCA is often minimal and phagocytic cells may show immunolocalization of the antigen to secondary lysosomes. The expression of LCA on granulocytes is also lower, however, stimulation of granulocytes rapidly increases the amount of LCA expressed from the intracellular stores (Thomas, 1989).

CASE 2.1: Diffuse large cell lymphoma, B-cell lineage, in the stomach, retroperitoneum and omental lymph nodes

A 68 year-old woman presented with anaemia, melaena and epigastric pain. At endoscopy, a tumour mass was found in the posterior wall of the stomach associated with ulceration in the overlying mucosa. Biopsy revealed necrotic and inflamed tissue infiltrated by a round cell tumour. The diagnosis of anaplastic carcinoma was favoured over that of lymphoma. There was insufficient material for immunohistochemical examination. At laparotomy, it was found that the posterior wall of the stomach was in continuity with a large retroperitoneal mass and several enlarged lymph nodes in both the greater and lesser omentum adjacent to the tumour were present. One of these was biopsied. The lymph node revealed infiltration of the subcapsular sinus as well as a sinusoidal pattern of infiltration by a large, round cell tumour with moderate amounts of cytoplasm and vesicular nuclei which contained two or three prominent eosinophilic nucleoli (Fig. 2.1A). There was abrupt transition of the tumour cells from the adjacent normal lymphoid tissue. The differential diagnoses were anaplastic carcinoma and diffuse large cell lymphoma. The panel of antibodies employed for these diagnoses and results of staining are shown in Table 2.1.

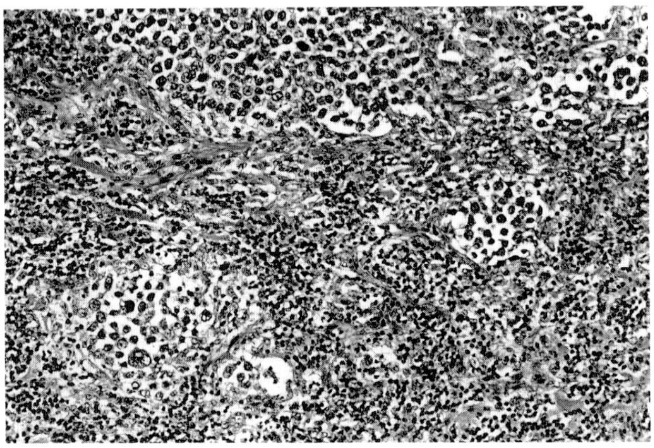

Fig. 2.1A. Greater omental lymph node showing infiltration of the subcapsular sinus and sinusoids by poorly cohesive large cells with pleomorphic, vesicular nuclei containing prominent nucleoli. There is sharp transition between the clusters of tumour cells and normal lymphoid tissue (H & E, X 40).

Table 2.1. Immunostaining results in an example of large cell lymphoma

Antibody	LCA	VIM	CK
Lymphoma	+	+	−
Carcinoma	−	−/+	+
Case 2.1	+	+	−

Membranous staining for LCA was clearly demonstrated (Fig. 2.1B) while the tumour cells were not immunoreactive for cytokeratins (CK). Scattered cells showed cytoplasmic staining for vimentin (VIM). With the confirmation of the lymphoid nature of the lesion, lineage typing was performed using UCHL1 (CD45RO), MT1 (CD43), LN1 (CDw75), L26 (CD20). The tumour cells were identified to be of follicular centre origin labelling with LN1 and L26, while both the T-cell markers were negative.

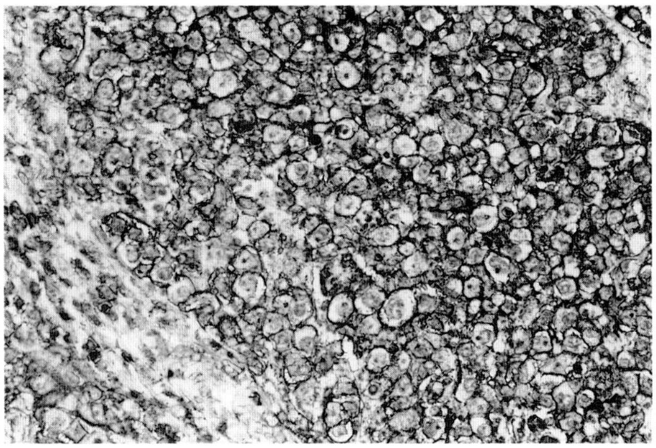

Fig. 2.1B. The tumour cells show distinct membranous labelling for LCA and lineage typing revealed positivity for LN1 (CDw75) and L26 (CD20), indicating their B-lymphocyte nature (anti-LCA, X 80).

Staining for LCA has been used for the distinction of non-Hodgkin's lymphoma from Hodgkin's disease. In contrast to the cells of non-Hodgkin's lymphoma, Reed-Sternberg cells are generally negative or only weakly reactive with anti-LCA antibodies. Furthermore, the latter are strongly positive for LeuM1 (CD15) (Hsu and Jaffe, 1984; Sheibani et al., 1986), BerH2 or Ki-1 (CD30) (Stein et al., 1982), and usually negative for epithelial membrane antigen (EMA) (de Mascavel et al., 1990).

An exception to the consistent expression of LCA in non-Hodgkin's lymphoma is the entity of Ki-1-anaplastic large cell lymphoma. Such anaplastic lymphomas may often show bizarre cytomorphology and a pattern of sinusoidal infiltration within lymph nodes which make differentiation from anaplastic carcinoma difficult. To compound the problem, only about 54 per cent of Ki-1 large cell anaplastic lymphomas stain for LCA in paraffin sections (Chott et al., 1990) and some 58 per cent of cases express epithelial membrane antigen. The phenotype of LCA−/EMA+ was found in 30 per cent of cases (Chott et al., 1990). In such cases, membranous staining for Ki-1 (CD30) is helpful in making the distinction from carcinoma, as, with very few exceptions, such as embryonal carcinoma, this antigen is expressed only by activated lymphoid cells.

CASE 2.2: Ki-1 positive anaplastic large cell lymphoma

A 17 year-old boy presented with a 3-week history of mild 'gastroenteritis-like' syndrome. Ultrasound examination revealed mildly enlarged para-aortic lymph nodes. As he responded to symptomatic treatment, a decision was made to observe him. Two weeks later, he presented with obstructive jaundice and was found to have a large epigastric mass which represented epigastric lymph nodes. These were associated with enlargement of porta-hepatic and para-aortic lymph nodes. At laparotomy, a para-aortic lymph node was biopsied.

The lymph node was infiltrated by large, poorly cohesive cells with oval pleomorphic nuclei showing prominent nucleoli and nuclear lobation. These cells showed moderate amounts of dense eosinophilic cytoplasm and displayed a striking pattern of sinusoidal infiltration (Fig. 2.2A). As carcinomas are uncommon in this age group, the provisional diagnosis was that of a pleomorphic large cell lymphoma. This was confirmed by positive staining for LCA in the tumour cells which failed to label with a broad spectrum anti-cytokeratin (anti-bovine keratin). The tumour cells, however, were labelled by anti-EMA (Fig. 2.2B) and they also showed distinct membranous staining for Ki-1 (CD30) (Fig. 2.2C), enabling the diagnosis of Ki-1 large cell anaplastic lymphoma to be made. Lineage typing revealed the lymphoma to be of T-cell lineage, staining with MT1 (CD43), Leu22 (CD43), and UCHL1 (CD45RO), while B-cell markers were negative.

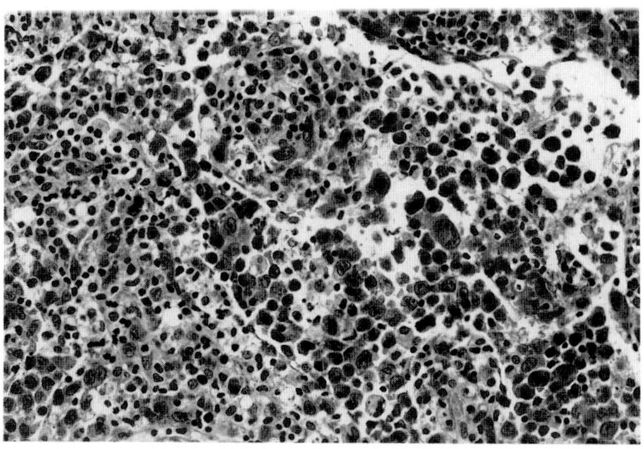

Fig. 2.2A. Poorly cohesive, pleomorphic large cells infiltrating the lymph node in a sinusoidal pattern. Note the lobated nuclei with prominent nucleoli and the moderate quantities of cytoplasm (H & E, X 80).

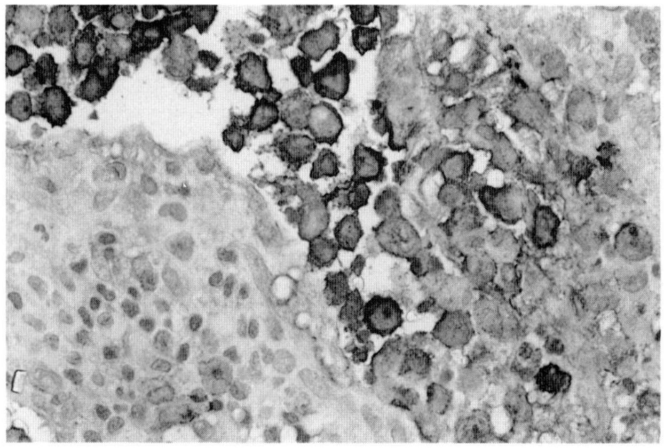

Fig. 2.2B. The tumour cells show distinct membranous and faint cytoplasmic staining for EMA (anti-EMA, X 160).

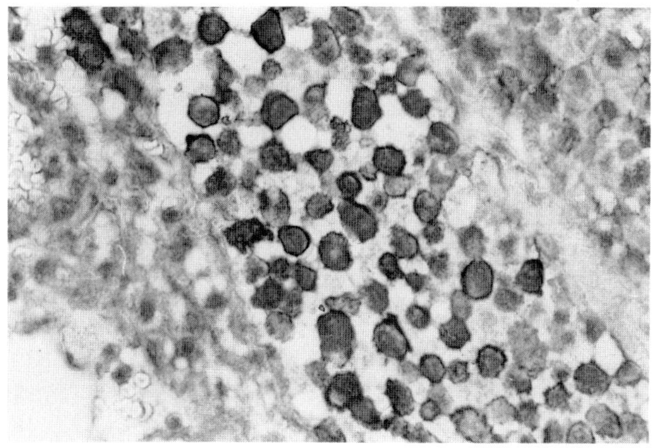

Fig. 2.2C. The tumour cells also show membranous staining for Ki-1 (CD 30) (anti-BERH2, X 160).

Having identified the tumour as lymphoid in origin, other antibodies may be employed for lineage typing. However, it should be remembered that the expression of LCA is the most reliable marker of lymphoid lineage and, in its absence, perhaps with the exception of Hodgkin's disease and Ki-1-anaplastic large cell lymphoma, the diagnosis of a lymphoid neoplasm should be viewed with circumspect. The demonstration of monotypic immunoglobulin expression by the tumour cells is indicative of a neoplastic population of B lymphocytes, however, the interpretation of paraffin section immunoglobulin staining is difficult and must be correlated with other pathological and clinical parameters (Warnke and Rouse, 1985). Immunoglobulin staining in paraffin sections, therefore, cannot be employed as the sole means of identifying a lymphoma. Immunoglobulin staining is best performed on cell suspensions or on frozen sections (Forbes and Leong, 1987). Other lymphocyte markers also do not provide definitive evidence of lymphoid differentiation. For example, MB2 (no CD) and LN1 (CDw75) characteristically react with various benign and neoplastic epithelial cells (Epstein et al., 1984; Hall et al., 1987; Poppema et al., 1987) so that in the absence of staining for LCA, cannot be used to identify lymphoid neoplasms.

Anaplastic carcinoma

The demonstration of cytokeratin intermediate filament proteins in the cytoplasm of tumour cells is the most specific immunohistochemical marker for epithelial differentiation in an anaplastic tumour. The cytokeratins are one of the five classes of intermediate filament proteins found in eukaryotic cells and monoclonal antibodies to this group of intermediate filaments have shown high sensitivity and specificity for epithelial cells in both neoplastic and non-neoplastic tissues.

Intermediate filaments form part of the cytoskeleton of cells. They are of 7–10 nm diameter, intermediate in size between the other cytoskeletal filaments, namely actin at 6 nm, and the larger filaments, myosin at 15 nm and tubulin at 25 nm. The five classes of intermediate filaments are largely indistinguishable at ultrastructural level, but they are biochemically and immunologically distinct, each displaying characteristic tissue specificities. Thus, intermediate filament analysis has become an important generic marker for tumour identification and classification. In humans, the expression of the five major classes of intermediate filaments corresponds to specific tissue types, viz., cytokeratins are expressed by epithelial cells, vimentin by mesenchymal cells, desmin by myogenic cells, glial fibrillary acidic protein by glial cells and neurofilaments by neurons and certain other cells of the peripheral neuroendocrine system. More importantly, intermediate filament protein expression is conserved in neoplastic cells, so that malignant cells, even when poorly differentiated, retain this same class restriction of intermediate filament expression in that carcinomas express cytokeratins, sarcomas express vimentin, myogenic tumours express desmin, and glial tumours express glial fibrillary acidic protein.

The cytokeratins, characteristic of epithelial cells and their tumours, are a multigene-coded family of water-insoluble intracellular filamentous polypeptides which are clearly the most complex among the five classes of intermediate filament proteins. There was some confusion caused by the earlier use of the terms 'cytokeratins' and 'prekeratins' to designate the keratins present in cells that are not traditionally associated with keratinization, such as those of simple epithelia. However, there has been no convincing evidence for this distinction and the generic term 'cytokeratins' is now used for this family of intermediate filament proteins. Moll et al. (1982) catalogued cytokeratin polypeptides on the basis of their molecular weight using numbers 1–19, with cytokeratin 1 corresponding to the heaviest member (68 kD) and cytokeratin 19 to the lightest (40 kD). It appears that the various keratin polypeptides are coded individually and are not degradation products of larger keratin molecules and the isolation and sequencing of the gene coding for some members of the cytokeratin family have also been achieved (Magin et al., 1983; Franke et al., 1984).

Two-dimensional gel electrophoresis has provided some insights into the expression of cytokeratins in epithelial cells and has revealed some empirical 'rules' or patterns of cytokeratin expression (Sun et al., 1983; Cooper et al., 1985). For example, it has been found that cytokeratin proteins are typically expressed as pairs, consisting of one acidic and one basic molecule, with the basic member of a pair 8 kD larger than the acidic component. Usually, a subset of up to 10 of the 19 cytokeratins copolymerizes *in vivo* to form the intermediate filament protein. The composition of the subset can vary depending not only on the cell type, but also on the stage of embryonic development and factors such as the presence or absence of various disease states, the growth environment, and the degree of cellular differentiation (Tseng et al., 1982; Sun et al., 1984; Romano et al., 1986). Comparison of different types of epithelia has revealed that the exact pattern of cytokeratin expression is markedly different from one cell type to another (Tseng et al., 1982). Hepatocytes, for example, regularly express cytokeratins 8 and 18, whereas, epidermal keratinocytes typically contain a more complex mixture which includes cytokeratins 1, 2, 5, 10, and 14. Given the large number of cytokeratin proteins that have been identified, it is remarkable that only a limited number of combinations of cytokeratins occur in epithelia and their tumours. As a rule, these patterns of cytokeratin expression are constant in a given tissue or tumour type, a property which allows categorization of epithelia on the basis of their cytokeratin profiles.

The lowest molecular weight cytokeratin (40 kD, Moll 19) is characteristic of simple epithelia and is the first to appear during embryonic life. This member of the cytokeratin family is also common in neoplastic epithelial cells. The higher molecular weight cytokeratins may have evolved from the simpler, low molecular weight cytokeratins. This hypothesis is supported by the fact that within each cytokeratin subfamily, members with increasing sizes are associated with structures of greater complexity, from simple to stratified squamous epithelia. The terms 'high' and 'low' molecular weight have been used generically to describe the subfamilies of cytokeratin proteins. Although biologically inexact, these terms are useful as points of reference for diagnostic purposes.

Cytokeratin immunophenotyping potentially has an important role in the classification of epithelial neoplasms, although, to date, this has not come into fruition. It has been suggested that the use of just one or two cytokeratin antibodies allows subdivision of carcinomas with respect to their histogenetic origins (Raemakers et al., 1983; Debus et al., 1984). The patterns of cytokeratin expression in tumours are limited and separation of carcinomas into diagnostically important groups is potentially possible with monoclonal antibodies directed at individual proteins or subsets of proteins. The immunohistochemical cytokeratin profiles of individual tumour types remains generally constant in both primary and metastatic neoplasms so that selected cytokeratin antibodies that react with diagnostically useful subsets of normal and neoplastic epithelium maybe strategically and selectively employed in diagnostic surgical pathology. A growing list of antibodies that recognise non-shared cytokeratin epitopes, as determined by their immunoreactivity on gel electrophoresis or enriched cytoskeletal preparations, is commercially available. While their immunochemical behaviour on gel electrophoresis does not necessary imply that the reagent can be applied successfully in histological sections, some reagents have shown a potential to discriminate between different epithelial neoplasms, however, the results are currently not sufficiently reliable for diagnostic application and some overlap in the expression by glandular and non-glandular carcinomas has been demonstrated (Visscher et al., 1988).

Immunostaining for cytokeratins provides a highly sensitive method for the identification of carcinomas from non-epithelial neoplasms such as lymphomas and melanomas (Osborn and Weber, 1983) as cytokeratins are expressed even in very poorly differentiated carcinomas, including those that show inconclusive evidence of epithelial differentiation upon ultrastructural examination. In practice, the detection of cytokeratins is most conveniently performed by employing monoclonal antibodies with broad specificity for cytokeratins.

Broad spectrum antisera prepared against cytokeratins from both human and from several species of animals, as well as antisera with limited specificity are commercially available. Similarly, monoclonal antibodies which are broadly reactive, recognizing an epitope shared by many members of the cytokeratin family, as well as a selective group which recognizes an epitope restricted to fewer members, or even to a single keratin, are also available. Monoclonal antibodies have clearly been demonstrated to be of greater sensitivity and specificity compared to heterologous antisera (Battifora, 1987). Heterologous antisera are a mixture of antibodies directed against antigenic sites present in many different keratin molecules as well as some epitopes that may be shared by non-keratin intermediate filaments. Heterologous antisera thus have an increased risk of non-specific reactions, especially when very sensitive techniques of immunostaining are employed.

Monoclonal antibodies are also available as a mixture or 'cocktails'. By using a combination of various monoclonal antibodies which have different sensitivities and specificities, a broader range of specificity and perhaps sensitivity can be obtained. Such mixtures can be prepared by combining several monoclonal antibodies of proven sensitivity and specificity, employing each at their optimal concentrations as determined by prior titration of the individual reagents. Two such cocktails of monoclonal antibodies to cytokeratins are currently available commercially (AE1/3, Boehringer Mannheim, Sydney, Australia; MAK-6, Triton Biosciences Inc., California, USA). Table 2.2 provides a list of various anti-cytokeratin reagents used in our laboratory, their sources and their specificities.

In our practice, the detection of cytokeratins is performed in two ways. We do not prepare our own antibody cocktails, but, instead, use single reagents with broad specificity for cytokeratins. We employ the monoclonal antibodies AE1/3 which is a mixture of the two antibodies AE1 and AE3 (Boehringer Mannheim, Sydney), or the polyclonal reagent, anti-bovine keratin (Dakopatts, California, USA). These two reagents function efficiently as screening reagents for the detection of cytokeratins in anaplastic tumours. A second approach is to use two or more antibodies with different reactivities.

Table 2.2. Specificities† of selected cytokeratin antibodies

Mol wt (Kd)	**AE1**	**AE3**	**CAM 5.2**	**35βH11**	**34βE12**	***Anti-callus ker**	***Anti-bovine ker**
39			+				
45			+				
48							+
50	+				+		
51							+
52							+
52.5			+	+			
54							
56						+	+
56.5	+				+		
57							
58		+			+		+
60							+
64						+	
65		+					
66		+					
67		+					
68					+		

Sources: AE1, AE3 (available as AE1/3 cocktail) (Boehringer, Sydney, Australia); Cam5.2 (Becton Dickinson, California, USA); Anti-callus keratin, Anti-bovine keratin (Dako Corporation, California, USA); 35βH11 and 34βE12 (Dako Corporation, California, USA)
*polyclonal antisera
†specificities as supplied by manufacturers

which, in combination, recognize a broad spectrum of cytokeratins. This approach has the added advantage in that it may also yield additional diagnostic information as high molecular weight cytokeratins are associated with structures of increasing complexity such as stratified epithelium. For example, the use of monoclonal antibodies to high molecular weight cytokeratins such as 34βE12 against Moll cytokeratins 1, 5, 10 and 14 (68, 58, 56.5 and 50 kD) (Gown and Vogel, 1984; Gown and Vogel, 1985) and to low molecular weight cytokeratins such as 35βH11 against Moll cytokeratin 8 (52.5 kD) may be employed. Similarly, Cam5.2 (Becton–Dickinson, California, USA) may be used to detect low molecular weight cytokeratins of 39, 45 and 52.5 kD and we employ the polyclonal antibody to callus keratin, raised against cytokeratins of 56 and 64 kD, for the detection of high molecular weight cytokeratins.

In summary, the identification of an anaplastic carcinoma from malignant lymphoma and malignant melanoma is based on the demonstration of cytokeratin intermediate filaments within the tumour cells. This can be achieved by employing monoclonal antibodies with broad specificity to cytokeratins or by employing two reagents with more narrow specificities to low molecular weight and to high molecular weight cytokeratins. Having established the epithelial nature of the anaplastic neoplasm, further characterization of the tumour by the identification of tissue-associated antigens may be conducted and this is illustrated in the case examples below.

CASE 2.3: Metastatic, poorly differentiated carcinoma in cervical lymph node

An enlarged anterior cervical lymph node was removed from a 62 year-old man who had a malignant melanoma excised from the face, 6 years previously. He also had two squamous cell carcinomas excised from the skin, 4 and 2 years previously.

The lymph node contained a diffuse infiltrate of large polygonal cells which were poorly cohesive. They showed large vesicular nuclei and prominent eosinophilic nucleoli and displayed moderate to abundant amounts of pale cytoplasm. No epithelial pearls or intercellular bridges were noted and no pigment was seen in the tumour (Fig. 2.3A).

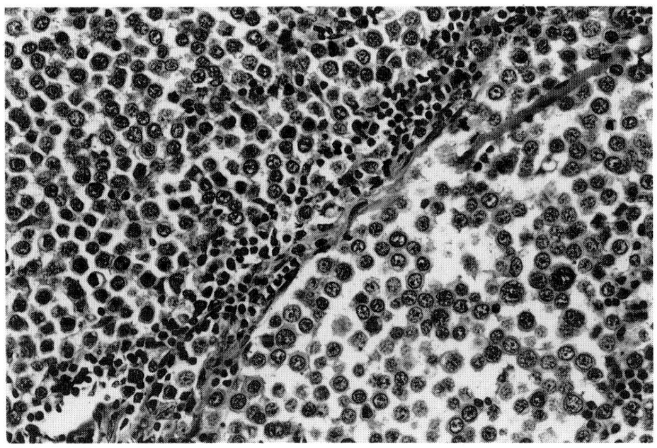

Fig. 2.3A. Metastatic round cell tumour in the cervical lymph node composed of pleomorphic, poorly cohesive cells with vesicular nuclei, prominent nucleoli and moderate to abundant amounts of pale cytoplasm. No evidence of differentiation or pigment is seen (H & E, X 80).

The differential diagnoses in this case were those of metastatic amelanotic melanoma and metastatic poorly differentiated squamous cell carcinoma. The panel of antibodies employed in this instance is shown in Table 2.3 as are the results of staining. The tumour cells were strongly positive for cytokeratins as revealed by AE1/3, a cocktail of two monoclonal antibodies to a broad spectrum of cytokeratins (Fig. 2.3B). Staining for vimentin, S100 protein and melanoma-specific antibody HMB45 were negative.

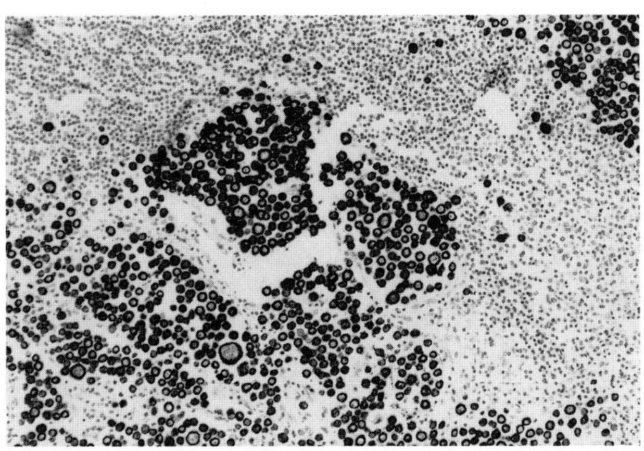

Fig. 2.3B. The tumour cells are strongly positive for cytokeratin (AE1/3, X 40).

Table 2.3. Immunostaining results in example of metastatic anaplastic carcinoma

Antibody	AE1/3	VIM	S100	HMB45
Melanoma	–	+	+	+
Carcinoma	+	–/+	–/+	–
Case 2.3	+	–	–	–

Notes AE1/3: cocktail of monoclonal antibodies to a broad spectrum of cytokeratins; VIM = vimentin; S100 = S100 protein; HMB45 = melanoma-specific antibody

CASE 2.4: Metastatic, prostatic mucinous adenocarcinoma in the pelvic bone

A 77 year-old man was referred for bone pain in the region of the sacro-iliac joint which was shown to be due to lytic metastatic deposits. Biopsy revealed a mucinous adenocarcinoma which large pools of mucin containing small clusters of epithelial tumour cells, sometimes showing glandular formation (Fig. 2.4A). Endoscopy and colonoscopy revealed no tumour. The kidneys were not enlarged and manual examination of the prostate suggested no abnormality. Staining for prostate-specific antigen and prostatic acid phosphatase, however, showed strong positivity for both markers (Fig. 2.4B), suggesting

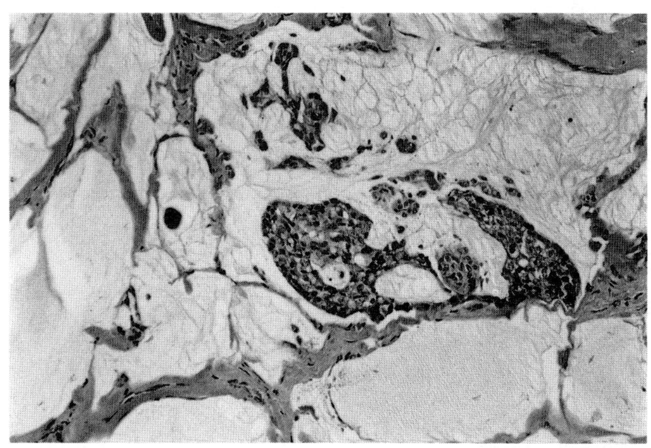

Fig. 2.4A. Metastatic mucinous adenocarcinoma in the pelvis. Large pools of mucin are seen with small groups of epithelial tumour cells, sometimes showing glandular differentiation (H & E, X 40).

the prostate gland as a source of the metastatic tumour. A needle biopsy of the prostate confirmed the presence of a moderately differentiated mucinous adenocarcinoma, an uncommon subtype of prostatic carcinoma.

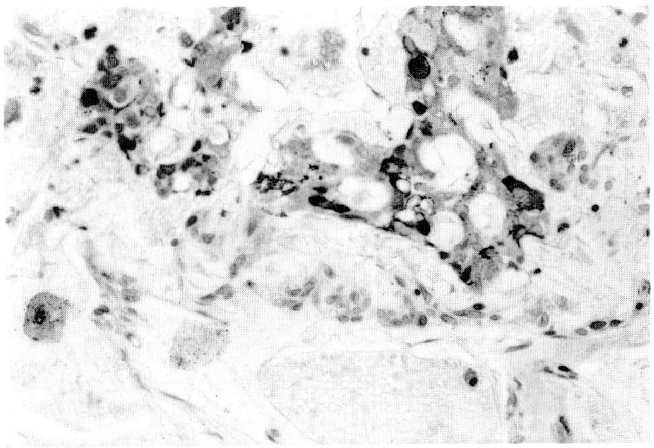

Fig. 2.4B. There is strong positivity for prostate-specific antigen in the tumour cells which lie in pools of mucous (anti-PSA, X 80).

Malignant melanoma

The identification of melanin and melanin-producing cells is traditionally dependent on reducing methods such as the Schmorl and Masson–Fontana silver stains or by the demonstration of Dopa-oxidase in frozen sections. More rapid techniques such as the recently described microwave-stimulated colloidal silver nitrate method may be employed (Leong and Gilham, 1989b). A significant number of melanomas, however, do not show detectable melanin and it is in such cases of amelanotic tumours that immunostaining is particularly helpful. Unlike the preceding entities of malignant lymphoma and anaplastic carcinoma in which sensitive markers allow their specific immunohistochemical identification, the recognition of amelanotic melanoma is based on the demonstration of certain cellular antigens as well as the exclusion of other antigens, a good illustration of the need to employ a panel of antibodies in tumour identification.

The mainstay of immunohistochemical markers for melanoma in paraffin-embedded tissues has been the demonstration of S100 protein. This protein was so named because of its solubility in 100 per cent ammonium sulphate solution at neutral pH. S100 occurs in three biochemically distinct forms, each a protein dimer composed of the α and β subunits. The three naturally occurring dimers are α-α, α-β and β-β. While originally thought to be nervous system specific, S100 has now been described in diverse cell types and among many animal species. It displays variation in the amount and distribution of the subunits in human brain and peripheral nervous system, as well as normal and neoplastic extraneural tissues. The latter groups include melanocytes, Langerhans' histiocytes, adipocytes, eccrine sweat glands, interdigitating reticulum cells, salivary glands, myoepithelial cells, sustentacular cells of phaeochromocytoma, and a variety of carcinomas, including carcinomas of the breast, lung, sweat glands, salivary glands, pancreas and some tumours of the genito-urinary tract (Drier et al., 1987; Schmitt and Bacchi, 1989).

Both subunits of S100 protein are known to code for the calcium binding sites of the calmodulin proteins which have a role in cation diffusion (Perumal et al., 1976; Baudier et al., 1986; Leung et al., 1986) S100 protein appears to have several other biological roles which are not fully understood, but they seem to be sufficiently important for the conservation of this protein in nature and for its presence within cells of all three germ layers in humans. Despite its widespread occurrence, it is clear that S100 protein is not distributed randomly, since it has not been detected in a large number of other non-neurogenic tumours and non-neural cell types (Kahn et al., 1983).

The usefulness of S100 protein as a marker for melanoma is well established (Kahn et al., 1983; Springall et al., 1983; Michetti et al., 1983). In our hands, S100 protein expression is a highly sensitive marker for melanomas fixed either by microwave irradiation or in buffered formalin. Unlike most other tissue antigens, the preservation of S100 protein in formalin-fixed tissues was as good as that fixed by microwave irradiation (Leong et al., 1988). S100 protein is highly resistant to aldehyde fixation and may be present even after weeks of exposure to formaldehyde (Leong and Gilham, 1989a). Aldehyde fixation may serve to prevent diffusion of the antigen and preserve architectural immunolocalization patterns. In contrast, the use of fresh tissue for S100 immunostaining may yield non-specific results. For example, it has been reported that immunostaining of fresh frozen tissue with a monoclonal anti-S100 antibody resulted in granular staining of virtually every cell type (Gatter et al., 1984).

S100 protein is localized not only to the cytoplasm of melanoma cells but may also be present in their nuclei. While being a marker of low specificity, S100 is a highly sensitive marker for melanoma cells, being expressed in as many as 99 per cent of melanomas (Leong and Milios, 1989). It is therefore, not only of use in identifying amelanotic melanomas, but also in the separation of melanoma cells from other intraepidermal lesions such as Paget's disease and Bowen's disease. S100 staining can be used to identify otherwise inconspicuous melanoma cells in metastatic sites such as lymph nodes as well as to delineate the extent of the tumour, particularly its depth of invasion. The intensity of S100 staining has been suggested to be of prognostic relevance with more intense reactivity in metastatic lesions and in those primary tumours that had early metastasis (Rode and Dillon, 1984), however, this latter application of S100 staining awaits confirmation.

HMB45 is a monoclonal antibody recently produced by Gown et al. (1986) which appears to be specific for malignant melanomas and some subpopulations of melanocytes. Gown et al. (1986) show positive staining in 60 of 62 melanomas, whereas none of the 168 non-melanocytic tumours tested were decorated by the antibody, indicating a specificity of 100 per cent. The antigen is sensitive to prolonged fixation in formaldehyde and in our study of 73 cases of melanomas fixed by microwave irradiation, 86 per cent were labelled for HMB45, whereas only four out of 21 formalin-fixed tumours were immunostained (Leong and Milios, 1989).

Four of 200 examples of non-melanocytic tumours stained positive with HMB45, two being cases of mammary carcinoma. Bonetti et al. (1989) also observed immunostaining for HMB45 in two of 100 breast carcinomas; in addition, normal breast lobules and ducts were occasionally positive in six of 100 cases. It has been suggested that these examples of false positive staining may be the result of impurities in the commercial reagent (Gown, personal communication).

Neuron-specific enolase (NSE) is a dimeric enzyme which has been reported to be specifically detected in neurons and neuroendocrine cells. In addition, NSE has been demonstrated in non-neoplastic cells including those of the pituitary, peptide-secreting cells, pinealocytes, neuroendocrine cells of the lung, thyroid, parafollicular cells, cells of the adrenal medulla, islets of Langerhans, Merkel cells of the skin as well as in melanocytes. NSE is also positive in normal striated muscle and liver cells and to a lesser extent in smooth muscle (Wick et al., 1983; Venores et al., 1984; Tsokos et al., 1984). Although NSE has been shown to be useful in the identification of malignant melanomas (Dhillon and Rode, 1982), and we have found it to be positive in 97 per cent of melanomas (Leong and Milios, 1989), the major problem with most commercially distributed anti-NSE preparations is the high rate of unwanted cross-reactivities in such hetero-antisera. It is, therefore, essential not to perform NSE immunostaining in isolation and interpretation done only in the context of other immunostaining results.

Several other melanoma-associated antigens have been described, many directed against determinants in the same molecule, and not preserved in formalin-fixed paraffin embedded tissues (Hersey, 1985). NK1/C3 is one exception which reacts preferentially with melanoma and naevo-melanocytic lesions in formalin-fixed tissues (van Duinen et al., 1984). However, the antibody is not melanoma-specific and labels a variety of carcinomas and sarcomas (Palmer et al., 1985). NK1/beteb is reported to be melanocyte and melanoma-specific but its reactivity in formalin-fixed tissue is weak (Vennegor et al., 1988).

CASE 2.5: Metastatic amelanotic melanoma in upper left cervical lymph node

A 44 year-old female presented with a 15 mm diameter left upper cervical lymph node of two months duration. The biopsy showed an enlarged lymph node with prominent germinal centre hyperplasia and small, interfollicular collections of large mononuclear cells which appeared to merge with the surrounding lymphocytes (Fig. 2.5A). Immunohistochemical stains were performed to separate the entities of metastatic carcinoma, metastatic melanoma and large cell lymphoma. The results of immunostaining are shown in Table 2.4.

Table 2.4. Immunostaining results in an example of metastatic melanoma

Antibody	VIM	CK	LCA	S100	HMB45
Lymphoma	+/−	−	+	−	−
Carcinoma	−/+	+	−	−	−
Melanoma	+	−	−	+	+
Case 2.5	+	−	−	+	+

The tumour cells stained strongly positive for vimentin (Fig. 2.5B), S100 (Fig. 2.5C) and HMB45 (Fig.2.5D), while staining for cytokeratins and LCA were negative. With the confirmation of the diagnosis of metastatic melanoma, further questioning of the patient revealed previous biopsies of several pigmented lesions in the skin which had been labelled 'benign', however, none of these were available for review.

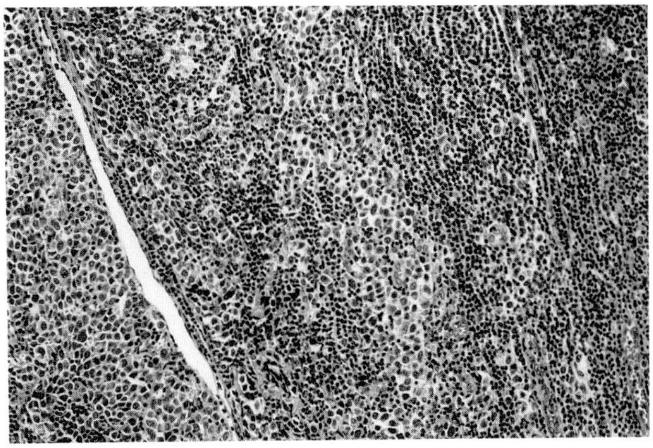

Fig. 2.5A. The tumour in the cervical lymph node is represented by small, interfollicular clusters of large mononuclear cells which appear to merge with the surrounding lymphoid tissue. Also seen, in the rest of the lymph node, were enlarged germinal centres (H & E, X 40).

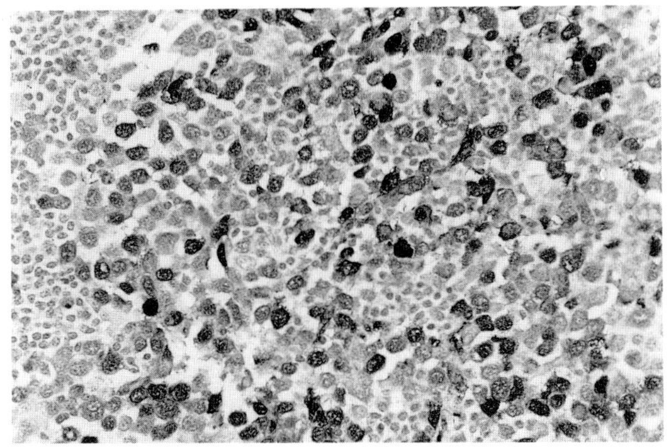

Fig. 2.5C. There is diffuse cytoplasmic and some nuclear staining for S100 protein within the tumour cells (anti-S100, X 80).

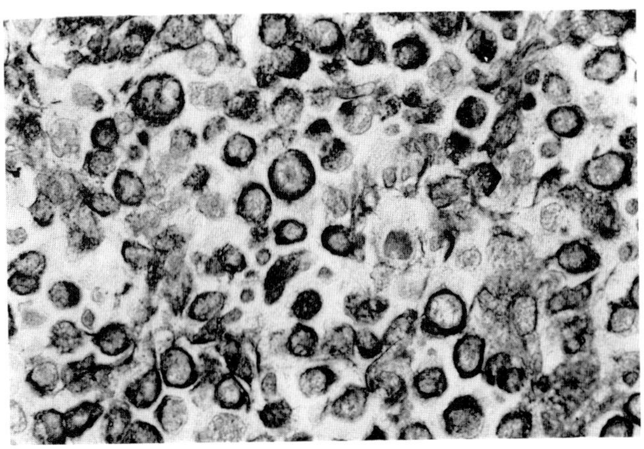

Fig. 2.5B. Staining for vimentin reveals filamentous cytoplasmic positivity in the tumour cells (anti-vimentin, X 160).

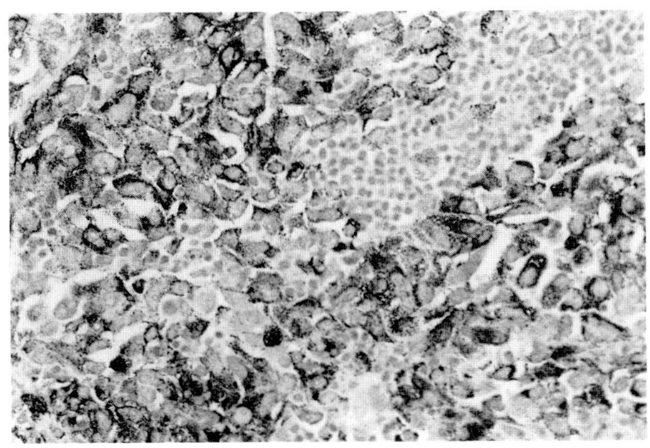

Fig. 2.5D. Diffuse cytoplasmic staining for HMB45, a melanoma-specific antigen, is seen within the tumour (HMB45, X 80).

Epithelioid sarcoma

Epithelioid sarcoma is a rare soft tissue tumour which involves the distal extremities and occurs as nodules within the dermis, subcutis, fascia and tendons. Enzinger (1970) first drew attention to the existence of this tumour, coining the term 'epithelioid sarcoma' because of its epithelioid features had frequently resulted in the incorrect diagnosis of squamous cell carcinoma or granulomatous inflammation. The tumour shows two cellular components – epithelioid cells with oval nuclei and abundant eosinophilic, refractile cytoplasm, and spindle cells with oval, irregular or notched nuclei and inconspicuous cytoplasm, the two often merging imperceptibly at the periphery of the nodules. Necrosis is frequent and multinucleated giant cells are occasionally present. Nucleoli are easily identifiable but are usually not prominent in the tumour cells. Other differential diagnoses for epithelioid sarcoma include malignant melanoma, angiosarcoma, synovial sarcoma, and even metastatic signet-ring adenocarcinoma, the latter being excluded by positive staining for mucin.

Epithelioid sarcoma cells coexpress cytokeratins and vimentin. Cytokeratin expression is seen consistently in the epithelioid cells and occasionally in the spindle cells. Low molecular weight cytokeratins are present more frequently and the tumour cells label with antibodies such as CAM5.2 or with those to a broad spectrum of cytokeratins, such as the polyclonal anti-bovine keratin or the cocktail of monoclonal antibodies, AE1/3. Occasionally, the epithelioid cells may express high molecular weight cytokeratins such as those labelled by polyclonal anti-callus keratin (Manivel et al., 1987; Meis et al., 1988; Fisher, 1988; Papas-Corden et al., 1989). Staining for cytokeratin often accentuates the nodularity of the lesions especially in some of the atypical cases, providing a better definition of the histological appearances than apparent in H & E stained sections (Meis et al., 1988). In addition, there is often staining of the spindle cell component for low molecular weight cytokeratins and coexpression of vimentin is seen in both the epithelioid as well as spindle tumour cells. Staining for cytokeratin occasionally demonstrates distinct 'buttons' or nodular aggregates of the intermediate filaments in a paranuclear or juxtanuclear location. Both epithelial and spindle cells stain for epithelial membrane antigen (Fisher, 1988), while staining for desmin, muscle specific actin, smooth muscle actin and the endothelial cell antigens, such as factor VIII-related protein, are negative, allowing a separation from myogenic tumours and vascular tumours. Staining for basal lamina components such as laminin and collagen type IV fails to identify investing basal lamina, a finding which allows distinction from synovial sarcoma (Ordonez et al., 1990).

CASE 2.6: Epithelioid sarcoma in the right thigh with probable cerebral metastases

A 36 year-old man presented with 'fits' and CT (computerized tomographic) scan of the head revealed probable cerebral metastases. He was also found to have a 2 cm diameter subcutaneous tumour in the right thigh which had been present for some months.

Excisional biopsy of the subcutaneous tumour revealed a cellular tumour composed of nodular aggregates of epithelioid cells with large vesicular nuclei, prominent eosinophilic nucleoli and moderate amounts of eosinophilic cytoplasm. Small areas of necrosis were present in the centre of some of the nodular aggregates, while in the periphery, the tumour cells showed a more spindled appearance. Some of the larger epithelioid cells contained globular, eosinophilic cytoplasmic inclusions, sometimes indenting the nucleus (Fig. 2.6A). Immunohistochemical staining revealed diffuse cytoplasmic labelling for vimentin (Fig. 2.6B) while staining

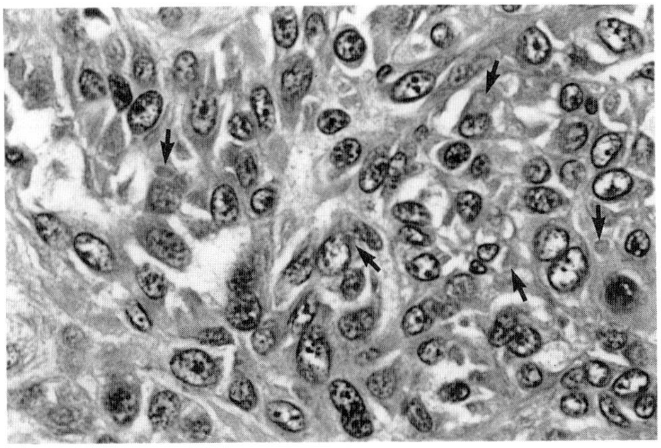

Fig. 2.6A. The tumour cells are large and epithelioid in appearance with vesicular nuclei and prominent nucleoli. Also observed are globular cytoplasmic inclusions which are eosinophilic and glassy in nature (arrows) (H & E, X 250).

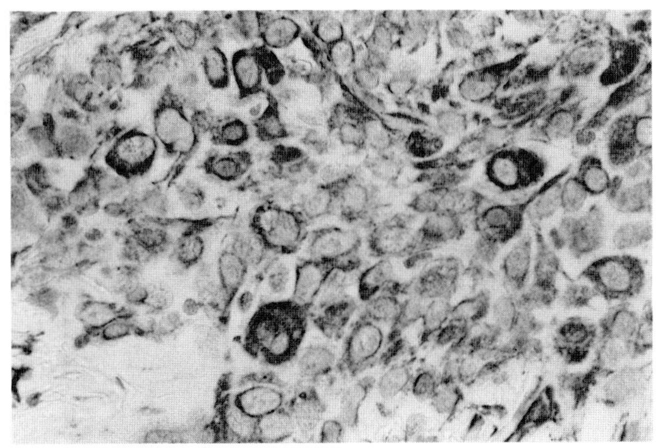

Fig. 2.6B. There is diffuse cytoplasmic labelling for vimentin intermediate filaments (anti-vimentin, X 250).

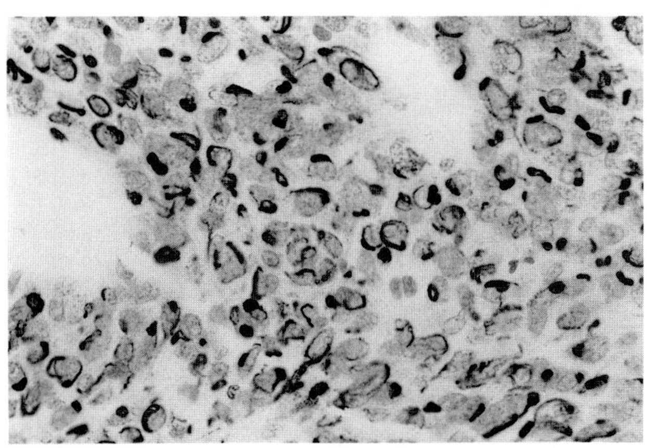

Fig. 2.6C. Staining for low molecular weight cytokeratin reveals globular inclusions of cytokeratin corresponding to the eosinophilic inclusions seen on H & E staining (CAM5.2, X 160).

for low molecular weight cytokeratin (CAM5.2) showed cytoplasmic labelling which was often distinctively globular and corresponded to the glassy eosinophilic inclusions seen on H & E stains (Fig. 2.6C). There was occasional expression of high molecular weight cytokeratin but staining for desmin, muscle-specific actin and alpha smooth muscle actin was negative. Ultrastructural examination confirmed the presence of globular aggregates of intermediate filaments in a juxta-nuclear location and the tumour cells showed readily identified cell junctions but no distinct desmosomes. The tumour cells were not invested by basal lamina.

Rhabdoid tumour

The rhabdoid tumour was first described as a rare, highly malignant neoplasm which develops principally in the kidneys of infants under the age of two years (Haas et al., 1981), but since has been described in a number of extrarenal sites (Gonzalez-Crussi et al., 1982) and in older children as well as adults (Dervan et al., 1987). The tumour is characterized by diffuse sheets of non-cohesive, moderately pleomorphic oval cells with moderate to abundant amounts of cytoplasm that shows distinctive large, round, eosinophilic inclusions, imparting a rhabdoid appearance. Their nuclei, which may be compressed or displaced by the cytoplasmic inclusions, contain prominent, darkly staining and usually single nucleoli. The cytoplasmic inclusions correspond to striking whorls of intermediate filament by electron microscopy and show immunoreactivity for both vimentin and cytokeratin. The tumour cells may express epithelial membrane antigen but fail to stain for desmin and S100 protein (Vogel et al., 1984; Parham et al., 1988; Gansler et al., 1991).

Recently, Tsuneyoshi et al. (1985) described the presence of rhabdoid cells in a variety of other soft tissue sarcomas including epithelioid sarcoma, synovial sarcoma, extra-skeletal myxoid chondrosarcoma and malignant mesothelioma. If other tumours which show prominent ultrastructural aggregates of whorled filamentous cytoplasmic inclusions are considered, this list can be expanded to include neuroendocrine tumours such as Merkel cell carcinoma (Leong et al., 1986), signet-ring cell melanoma, anaplastic thyroid carcinoma, and poorly differentiated endometrial carcinoma (Perrone et al., 1989). More recently, rhabdomyosarcoma has also been described to show the same eosinophilic globular cytoplasmic inclusions of intermediate filaments (Kodet et al., 1991).

Epithelioid smooth muscle tumour

Smooth muscle tumours are not generally included among the differential diagnoses of round cell tumours except in the uncommon situation when they occur in sheets and nodules rather than fascicles and comprise epithelioid cells with polygonal shapes and prominent cell borders, mimicking the features of epithelial neoplasms. Such epithelioid smooth muscle tumours show abundant cytoplasm which may be amphophilic, clear or vacuolated; short, spindled forms may also be present. These tumours have also been accorded the term 'leiomyoblastoma' and may be benign or malignant. While classic leiomyosarcomas, in general, show immunoreactivity for desmin and vimentin, staining for these antigens has been reported to be weak or absent in epithelioid smooth muscle tumours (Miettinen et al., 1982a; Enzinger and Weiss, 1988). Anti-desmin antibodies may fail to label some cases and we have found anti-smooth muscle actin to be a more sensitive marker. Perhaps the inability to demonstrate desmin intermediate filaments in some cases corroborates electron microscopy reports that myofilaments seem to be less well represented in such lesions compared to conventional smooth muscle tumours. When demonstrated, myofilaments are sparsely distributed at the periphery of the cytoplasm (Enzinger and Weiss, 1988). Compounding these difficulties of identification is the recent recognition that smooth muscle tumours, including the epithelioid variants, may sometimes express low molecular weight cytokeratins (Gown et al., 1988). Cytokeratins have also been described in human myocardium and myometrium (Huitfeldt and Brandtzaeg, 1985). The immunoreactivity was confined to the perinuclear regions, a pattern which we have observed in epithelioid leiomyosarcomas (James and Leong, 1989). It was initially suggested that staining may have resulted from cross-reacting epitopes or cross-reactivity with non-keratin proteins but staining with a wide variety of monoclonal and polyclonal antibodies and the demonstration of cytokeratins by immunoblotting techniques would argue against this suggestion. The distinction from carcinoma can be made by employing a panel of antibodies which includes not only antibodies to cytokeratins and desmin, but also those to muscle specific actins and vimentin.

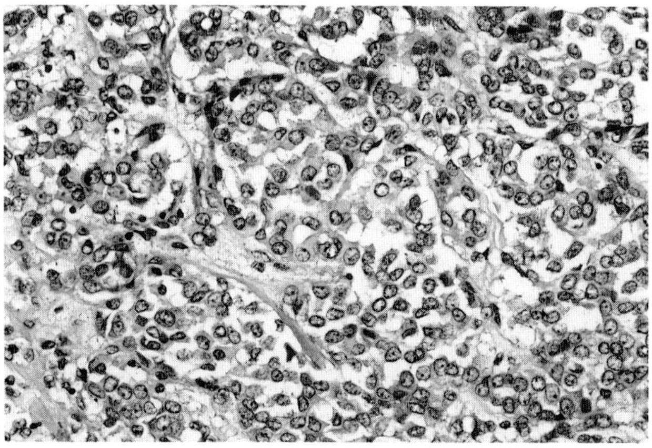

Fig. 2.7A. The densely cellular tumour is composed of sheets of intermediate sized cells with moderate amounts of cytoplasm and an epithelioid appearance (H & E, X 80).

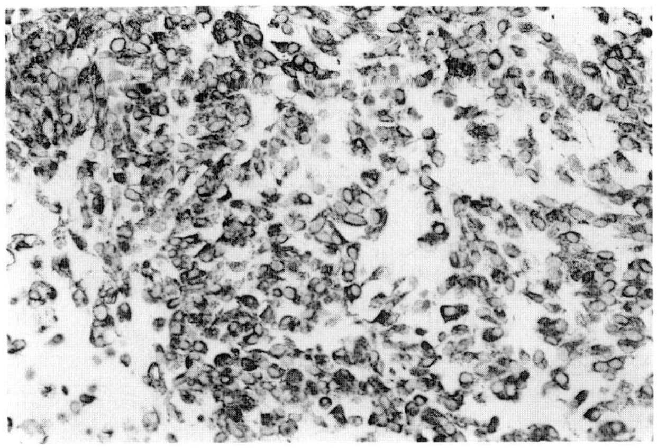

Fig. 2.7B. The tumour cells stain distinctly positive for vimentin which highlights long cytoplasmic processes in occasional cells (anti-vimentin, X 80).

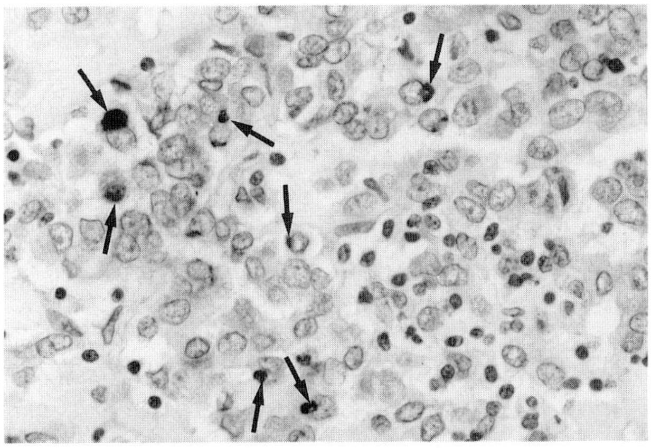

Fig. 2.7C. Juxtanuclear globular masses of desmin filaments are seen in scattered tumours cells (arrows) (anti-desmin, X 160).

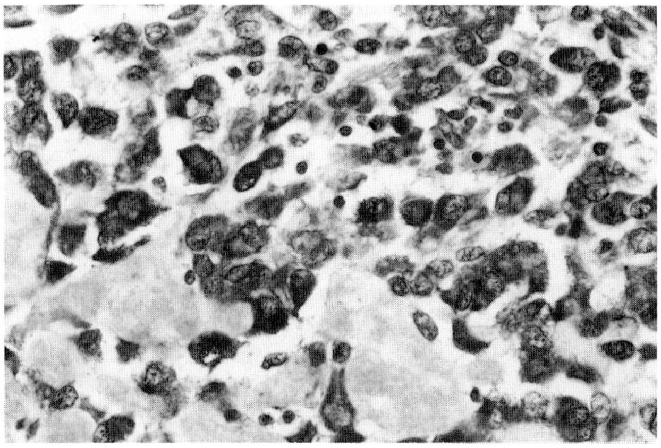

Fig. 2.7D. Distinct positivity for alpha smooth muscle actin is observed in the tumour (anti-alpha smooth muscle actin, X 160).

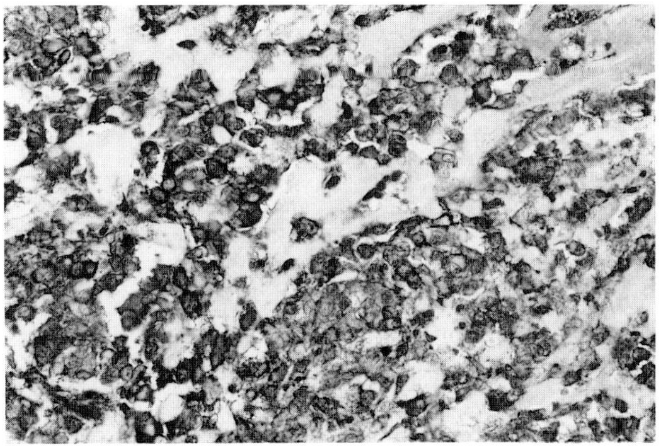

Fig. 2.7E. There is diffuse cytoplasmic positivity for muscle-specific actin (anti-muscle specific actin, X 160).

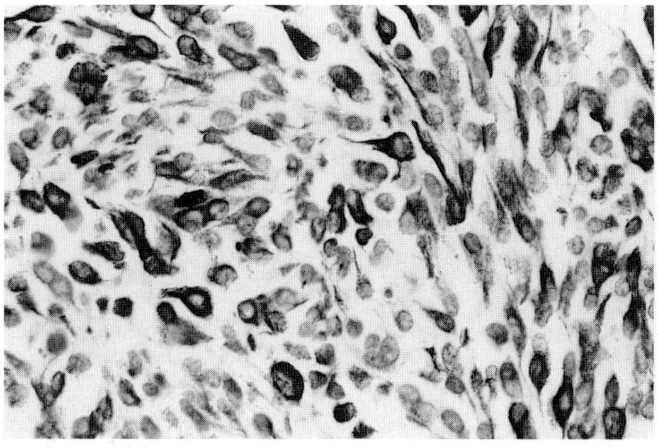

Fig. 2.7F. There is distinct cytoplasmic positivity for low molecular weight cytokeratin in both the epithelioid as well as spindle cells (CAM5.2, X 160).

CASE 2.7: Epithelioid leiomyosarcoma of the transverse mesocolon, coexpressing desmin, vimentin and low molecular weight cytokeratin

A 60 year-old man presented with a large abdominal tumour and vague abdominal pain. At laparotomy, a multinodular mass, 25 × 20 × 20 cm, was found in the transverse mesocolon, with the colon stretched over it but distinctly separate and uninvolved by the mass. There were multiple peritoneal deposits present, varying up to 1 cm in diameter. No para-aortic lymphadenopathy was present. The liver, spleen and pancreas were normal. The excised tumour showed areas of solid and cystic change, with varying consistency and a cream/tan appearance. No obvious areas of necrosis were present.

The tumour showed varying degrees of cellularity with numerous areas of myxoid degeneration and cystic change. In most areas, the tumour cells were of intermediate size with mainly oval nuclei and scanty amounts of cytoplasm, imparting an epithelioid appearance (Fig. 2.7A). In a few areas the tumour nuclei were more fusiform and bipolar cytoplasmic processes could be discerned, these were highlighted by staining for vimentin (Fig. 2.7B). The myogenic nature of the tumour was confirmed by focal but distinct positivity for desmin (Fig. 2.7C), and alpha smooth muscle actin (Fig. 2.7D). There was diffuse cytoplasmic staining for muscle-specific actin (Fig. 2.7E). The tumour cells were also positive for low molecular weight cytokeratin as revealed by staining for CAM5.2 (Fig. 2.7F).

Glomus tumour

Glomus tumours are readily identified by their histological appearance, with nests of characteristic uniform, polygonal to round epithelioid cells which surround narrow vascular lumina. They only rarely enter into the differential diagnoses of round cell tumours, when they are malignant (Aiba et al., 1988) or when only small or squashed fragments of the tumour are available for examination. Based on the ultrastructural presence of intermediate filaments, dense bodies and pinocytotic vesicles, glomus tumours are currently thought to be derived from smooth muscle cells and not from pericytes (Goodman and Abele, 1971; Tsuneyoshi and Enjoji, 1982; Aiba et al., 1988). Immunohistochemical investigations have demonstrated the presence of vimentin and muscle specific actin in almost all such tumours, and the presence of desmin is found in as many as 70 per cent of cases, although varying in extent and intensity of staining (Nuovo et al., 1990). Staining for cytokeratins and S100 protein is negative (Dervan et al., 1989). By contrast, haemangiopericytomas show only vimentin intermediate filaments and are not immunoreactive for muscle-specific actin, smooth muscle actin or desmin.

Epithelioid malignant schwannoma

It has been estimated that about 5 per cent of all malignant schwannomas show epithelioid features and need to be distinguished from melanoma and carcinoma (Lodding et al., 1986; Enzinger and Weiss, 1988). Spindle cell areas, more characteristic of the conventional malignant schwannoma, may be present and involvement of a major nerve allows the correct diagnosis to be made. In the remaining cases, immunohistochemical staining may be helpful in making the correct diagnosis. The few reported immunohistochemical studies of epithelioid malignant schwannoma suggest that the staining characteristics of this tumour are not different to that of conventional malignant schwannomas (Morgan and Gray, 1985; Lodding et al., 1986). The tumours are invariably positive for vimentin, and S100 protein has been reported in up to two-thirds of malignant schwannomas (Diamaru et al., 1985; Wick et al., 1987; Johnson et al., 1991). Except for areas of distinct glandular differentiation in malignant schwannomas, malignant epithelioid schwannomas have not shown immunoreactivity for cytokeratin, EMA or CEA; (Lodding et al., 1986; Wick et al, 1987; Axiotis et al., 1990; Johnson et al., 1991) the only exception being a case reported by Axiotis et al. (1990) where S100, cytokeratin and EMA positivity was demonstrated in a purely epithelioid malignant peripheral nerve sheath tumour which showed ultrastructural evidence of schwannian, perineural and squamous differentiation. Experience with other antigens associated with schwann cell tumours such as Leu7 (CD57), glial fibrillary acidic protein (GFAP) and myelin basic protein has not been reported. The recent demonstration of nerve growth factor receptor in 100 per cent of 25 peripheral nerve sheath tumours (Thompson et al., 1989) suggests that this may be a useful marker for epithelioid schwannoma. A more recent paper describing 26 examples of such tumours showed that 80 per cent of cases expressed S100 protein and NSE, but all lacked cytokeratin and HMB45 (Laskin et al., 1991).

Epithelioid angiosarcoma

The large endothelial cells with abundant cytoplasm which line the vascular spaces of epithelioid haemangioma, epithelioid haemangioendothelioma and epithelioid angiosarcoma may mimic the appearance of epithelial cells. It is unlikely that epithelioid haemangioma and epithelioid haemangioendothelioma would pose diagnostic difficulties, but, in the case of epithelioid angiosarcoma, the atypical large polygonal endothelial cells may result in an erroneous diagnosis of carcinoma. This may be particularly the case when the tumour cells stain positive for cytokeratin, as has been demonstrated with some cases of epithelioid vascular neoplasms (Gray et al., 1990; van Haelst et al., 1990). Keratin expression by vascular tumours is not altogether surprising since non-neoplastic endothelial cells have been reported to express cytokeratins (Lothar et al., 1987). The endothelial nature of these tumours is clearly revealed by positive labelling for factor VIII-related protein and with *Ulex europaeus* agglutinin-1 lectin (Weiss and Enzinger, 1982; Angervall et al., 1985; Gray et al., 1990). Other endothelial cell associated antibodies such as QBEnd/10 (Sankey et al., 1990) and JC70 (Parums et al., 1990) may also be used in paraffin-embedded tissues, and anti-vimentin uniformly reacts with endothelial cells.

Other round cell tumours

Two other round cell tumours in adults need to be briefly discussed. Both have distinctive morphological appearances on H & E stained sections and would seldom pose a problem in the differential diagnosis of the anaplastic round cell tumour. The interest in these lesions is more related to histogenesis and differentiation rather than diagnosis.

Granular cell tumour

The granular cell tumour and the so-called granular cell myoblastoma are composed of plump polygonal cells with distinctive PAS positive-diastase resistant granules. Several cell types have been proposed as the possible origin of the tumour cells and these include skeletal muscle, fibroblasts, undifferentiated mesenchymal cells, histiocytes and neural or Schwann cells. The demonstration of S100 and NSE positivity has provided supportive evidence of a neural origin (Rode et al., 1982; Stefansson et al., 1982; Armin et al., 1983), furthermore, some tumours also express myelin basic protein and Leu7 (CD57) (Mazur et al., 1990). Less commonly, these tumours have stained for CEA (Ingram et al., 1984) and laminin (Nathrath and Remberger, 1986). It is possible that not all granular cell tumours are of Schwann cell derivation as some have been described to show myofilaments and other ultrastructural evidence of smooth muscle differentiation (Christ and Ozzello, 1971; Zarbo et al., 1983). Furthermore, granular degeneration of appendiceal smooth muscle has also been observed (Sobel et al., 1971) and rare cases of congenital granular cell epulis in the gingiva have not stained for S100 protein (Lifschitz et al., 1984).

Alveolar soft part sarcoma

Alveolar soft part sarcoma is a rare tumour of soft tissue which characteristically shows sharply defined masses of tumour cells that are compartmentalized by thin-walled vascular channels. The individual tumour cells are large, rounded and somewhat uniform in appearance, displaying vesicular nuclei with small nucleoli and abundant eosinophilic, sometimes vacuolated cytoplasm. Cytoplasmic glycogen is a prominent feature of the tumour and PAS staining also reveals diastase resistant needle-like intracytoplasmic crystals, a diagnostic feature of the tumour. Lesions with a similar histologic appearance have been misdiagnosed as either malignant granular cell myoblastoma or malignant non-chromaffin paraganglioma. The tumour cells do not stain for cytokeratin, EMA, S100 protein, NSE, myelin basic protein or actin. Although stains for myoglobin have been consistently negative, Mukai et al. (1986a) demonstrated the presence of desmin, vimentin, actin and Z-protein in the tumour cells, features which support the myogenic character of this tumour. Similarly, Denk et al. (1983) demonstrated the presence of vimentin and desmin positivity with fluorescent methods and, more recently, muscle specific actin and smooth muscle actin have also been found in these tumours (Hirose et al., 1990). Miettinen and Ekfors (1990) have also demonstrated both desmin and muscle specific actin in alveolar soft part sarcomas, however, they also showed positivity for S100 protein and NK1/C3, a monoclonal antibody which consistently stains melanomas. HMB45, a melanoma-specific marker, was negative in all cases. The immunohistochemical presence of renin has been reported in four cases of alveolar soft part sarcoma, prompting the authors to name it 'malignant angioreninoma' (DeSchryver-Kecskemeti et al., 1982) but this finding has not been repeated.

Childhood small round cell tumours

The group of small round cell tumours in childhood includes rhabdomyosarcoma, neuroblastoma, malignant lymphoma, skeletal and extraskeletal Ewing's sarcoma and peripheral primitive neuroectodermal tumours (PNETs). As in the case of adult anaplastic round cell tumours, it is equally important from a therapeutic standpoint to distinguish these entities. The introduction of multimodality treatment regimens has resulted in substantial improvements in survival rates among children with malignant diseases. Today some tumours are curable, while many others can be put into long term remission. The selection of the appropriate treatment regime is primarily determined by the histological diagnosis and stage of the disease. Given optimal morphologic preservation, the separation of this group of small round cell tumours can often be made on conventional histological examination, but the less differentiated forms can test the diagnostic acumen of even the most experienced pathologist. While the clinical features and the site of the tumour are paramount considerations in arriving at a diagnosis, immunohistochemical analysis and ultrastructural examination have proven to be useful adjuncts to the histological distinction of these entities.

(The illustrative cases discussed in this section of 'childhood round cell tumours' were chosen because the ages were slightly more than would conventionally be regarded as 'childhood' and hence posed further problems in diagnostic considerations).

Rhabdomyosarcoma

Rhabdomyosarcoma is the commonest soft tissue sarcoma in childhood. Its microscopic diagnosis depends on pattern recognition, and particularly on evidence of skeletal muscle differentiation such as the presence of rhabdomyoblasts and cytoplasmic cross striations. The latter, however, occurs in less than 50 per cent of tumours and rhabdomyoblasts with abundant eosinophilic, slightly granular cytoplasm without demonstrable cross-striations have become acceptable as diagnostic of this tumour (Enzinger and Weiss, 1988).

Rhabdomyosarcomas consistently express vimentin, a reflection of their mesenchymal origin. In our experience, desmin is the most reliable marker of rhabdomyosarcoma, being present in all 18 tumours examined (Leong et al., 1989). Molenaar et al. (1985) reported vimentin to be present in 21 cases of rhabdomyosarcoma examined but failed to demonstrate desmin in three cases which they graded as poorly differentiated rhabdomyosarcomas. As these cases were composed entirely of primitive mesenchymal cells which lacked myogenic characteristics at both light and electron microscopic levels, the absence of desmin raises doubts as to whether this group of tumours truly represented rhabdomyosarcomas. Two other cases of rhabdomyosarcoma have been reported to be desmin-negative, but both expressed fast myosin, and one of these became desmin-positive in a recurrent tumour (Carter et al., 1990). This discrepancy is interesting although the inability to stain for desmin in the primary tumour may well be accounted for by suboptimal preservation of the antigen. The presence of desmin immunoreactivity in a broad span of differentiating tumour cells, particularly in optimally preserved tissues, makes it a reliable marker for rhabdomyosarcomas (Molenaar et al., 1985; Altmannsberger et al., 1985; Leong et al., 1989). Desmin is present in both striated as well as smooth muscle tumours, but the latter are uncommon in childhood and should not pose a problem in diagnosis. Desmin has also been demonstrated rarely in non-myogenous tumours such as malignant fibrous histiocytoma (Miettinen et al., 1982a), presumably representing myofibroblastic differentiation, in fibromatosis (Miettinen, 1988a), again reflecting myofibroblastic differentiation, in glomus tumours (Brooks et al., 1987), and in benign mesothelial cells (van Muijen et al., 1987). Desmin has also been reported in some cases of squamous and small cell carcinomas of the lung (Gatter et al., 1986) and in scattered cells in very rare examples of epithelioid sarcomas (Manivel et al., 1987).

Cytoplasmic actins vary in amino acid sequences and can be separated by electrophoresis into six different isotopes, all having the same molecular weight of 42 kD. Alpha actins are present in muscle cells, beta actins in non-muscle cells, whereas some gamma actins are found in both muscle as well as non-muscle cells. Both striated and smooth muscle cells differ in their expression of actin types and this has formed a basis for the generation of antibodies directed at muscle-specific actin subtypes. HHF35, is an antibody produced to muscle-specific actins and selectively reacts with alpha and gamma actins of muscles (Tsukada et al., 1987a, 1987b). HHF35 stains both smooth and skeletal muscle cells as well as pericytes, myoepithelial cells and myofibroblasts, all of which are often desmin-negative. The antibody reacted with 29 out of 30 cases of rhabdomyosarcoma and showed no reactivity with neuroblastoma, retinoblastoma or Ewing's sarcoma (Schmidt et al., 1988).

Myoglobin, the oxygen carrier haemoprotein, is a specific marker for striated muscle cells. Unfortunately, a sizeable number of rhabdomyosarcomas, particularly the poorly differentiated ones, exhibit no staining. Myoglobin expression appears to be linked to the differentiation of rhabdomyosarcoma cells. In our experience, morphologically recognizable rhabdomyoblasts show staining for myoglobin, whereas the poorly differentiated tumours fail to stain so that myoglobin staining is not helpful when rhabdomyoblasts are not present (Leong et al., 1989).

Other markers which have been used for the identification of rhabdomyosarcoma include skeletal muscle myosin, creatinine kinase, alpha-actinin and tropomyosin, but these markers are absent from a fair number of poorly differentiated rhabdomyosarcomas, reducing their value as diagnostic agents (Eusebi et al., 1986; Tsokos, 1986; Scupham et al., 1986). It is of interest to note that a variable number of rhabdomyosarcomas have been reported to express cytokeratin (Coindre et al., 1988; Miettinen and Rapola, 1989; Carter et al., 1990). This observation may reflect the finding of cytokeratins in fetal striated muscle tissues of the heart and tongue during some phases of embryonic development (van Muijen et al., 1987). Although reported to vary between 8 and 44 per cent, the expression is probably not consistent and was not found in our series of 18 cases, when a monoclonal antibody to low molecular weight cytokeratin and broad spectrum anti-cytokeratin antisera were employed (Leong et al., 1989).

CASE 2.8: Embryonal rhabdomyosarcoma arising in the right side of the neck

A 19 year-old female presented with a large painful mass on the right side of the neck. There was associated ulceration of the overlying skin and the mass was attached to underlying structures. While being investigated, she developed jaundice and was found to have liver metastases. CAT scan revealed no other deposits in the thorax or abdomen.

An incisional biopsy revealed a small round cell tumour with hyperchromatic nuclei and small nucleoli. The tumour cells formed sheets and displayed small quantities of ill-defined cytoplasm. Mitotic figures and apoptotic bodies were frequent. No rhabdomyoblasts or ganglion cells were seen (Fig. 2.8A). The tumour cells extended up to the papillary dermis and into the area of ulceration. There was strong immunolabelling for vimentin (VIM) and for desmin (DES) (Fig. 2.8B) while staining for neurofilaments (NF), cytokeratin (CK) and LCA were negative. The panel of antibodies employed and the immunophenotype of the tumour is shown in Table 2.5.

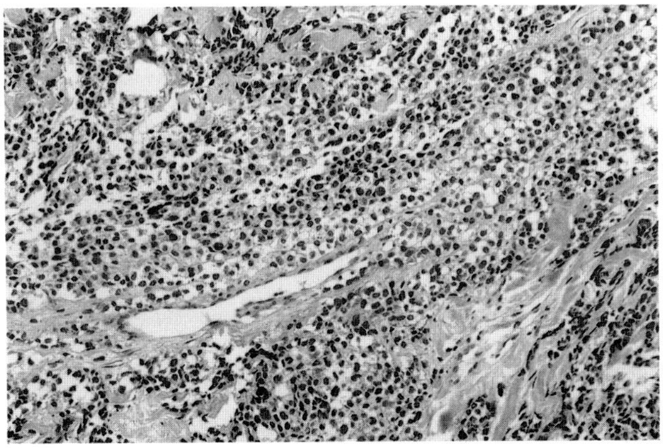

Fig. 2.8A. A small round cell tumour with hyperchromatic nuclei, small nucleoli and varying quantities of ill-defined cytoplasm is seen infiltrating the dermis. No features of differentiation are present (H & E, X 40).

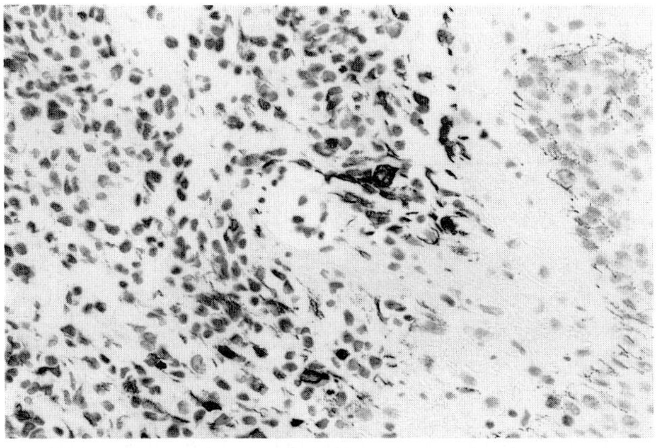

Fig. 2.8B. There is strong cytoplasmic filamentous staining for desmin in scattered tumour cells, particularly in those with moderate amounts of cytoplasm (anti-desmin, X 80).

Table 2.5. Immunostaining results in an example of rhabdomyosarcoma

Antibody	VIM	CK	LCA	DES	NF
Lymphoma	+/−	−	+	−	−
Neuroblastoma	−/+	−	−	−	+
Rhabdomyosarcoma	+	−	−	+	−
Case 2.8	+	−	−	+	−

Neuroblastoma

Neuroblastoma is the third commonest solid malignant tumour of infancy and childhood, being superseded only by lymphoid neoplasms and cerebral tumours. The adrenal gland is the most common site of the tumour, accounting for about 25 per cent of cases. In order of decreasing frequency, the remaining tumours occur mainly along the sympathetic chain and in variety of paraspinal locations including the retroperitoneum, posterior mediastinum and cervical area. While this tumour may often show progressive neurogenesis with differentiation to produce the spectrum of neuroblastoma, ganglioneuroblastoma and ganglioneuroma, the undifferentiated neuroblastoma with its structureless array of small round hyperchromatic cells may be difficult to identify on H & E sections alone.

Neuron-specific enolase (NSE) is a useful marker for neuroblastoma, being present in 10 out of 10 cases examined in one series (Leong et al., 1989). NSE initially held great promise as a marker of tumours of neural origin and the gamma-gamma isoenzyme was considered specific for neurons and neuroendocrine cells. However, it has since been found in non-neural tissues such as the liver and skeletal muscle (Haimoto et al., 1985). The polyclonal antiserum to NSE also produces varying degrees of background staining which may sometimes interfere with interpretation, although the monoclonal antibody (Dako, California, USA) appears to show greater sensitivity. Protein gene product (PGP 9.5) (Jackson and Thompson, 1981) is a neuronal protein of unknown function, isolated from human brain and shows a distribution very similar to that of NSE, with neuronal and neuroendocrine specificity (Rode et al., 1985). This reagent shows a clearer staining pattern with less non-specific background staining than with NSE and appears to be an equally sensitive marker for neuroblastoma (Carter et al., 1990). It is relevant to note that NSE occurs in skeletal muscle cells and immunoreactivity for the enzyme has been observed in rhabdomyoblasts (Tsokos et al., 1984; Leong et al., 1989; Osborn et al., 1986; Schmechel, 1985), reducing its usefulness as a discriminatory marker.

Anti-chromogranin A has been employed for the identification of neuroblastoma, staining all six cases examined in one series, and synaptophysin has been reported to stain neuroblastomas weakly (Chang et al., 1989). Neurofilaments have been demonstrated in neuroblastomas with varying degrees of frequency. Osborn et al. (1982), working on fresh frozen material, were able to show positivity for neurofilaments in all 29 neuroblastomas examined, however, fixation and paraffin-embedding appeared to destroy the epitopes recognized by the monoclonal antibody employed. Using a cocktail of antibodies to the 68, 150 and 200 kD subcomponents, we were able to demonstrate positivity in four out of 10 cases of neuroblastoma, corresponding to the presence of ganglion cell differentiation (Leong et al., 1989). Mukai et al. (1986b) suggested that neuroblastomas reacted largely with antibody to the 68 kD subunit, whereas ganglioneuromas and ganglioneuroblastomas contain cells that reacted with antibodies to all three components of neurofilaments. Immunostaining with anti-neurofilaments not only labelled the neuronal bodies but also the neural processes or nerves within the tumours (Virtanen et al., 1983; Osborn et al., 1986; Leong et al., 1989).

GFAP is generally expressed only in the central nervous system and in earlier studies, with the exception of teratomas with foci of glial differentiation, GFAP immunoreactivity was not observed outside the central nervous system (Trojanowski et al., 1984). In our series, GFAP positivity was seen in neurons and ganglion-like cells and their cytoplasmic process in two out of 10 cases of neuroblastoma. The immunoreactivity was initially considered to represent cross-reactivity as it has been suggested that the GFAP molecule shows important similarities with neurofilaments (Goldman et al., 1978; Leong et al., 1989). GFAP has since been consistently documented with both polyclonal and monoclonal antibodies in peripheral nerve sheath cells and their tumours (Memoli et al., 1984; Fields and Yen, 1985; Gould et al., 1986; Johnson, 1991) as well as in non-neuronal tissues such as the parotid gland and pleomorphic adenomas (Achtstatter et al., 1986), mixed Mullerian tumours (Liao and Choi, 1986) and benign cartilage (Viale et al., 1988), chordomas and bone (Kasantikul and Shuangshoti, 1989).

Positivity for S100 protein has been demonstrated in the sustentacular cells and in Schwann cells in the differentiated forms of neuroblastoma (Carlie et al., 1984; Shimada et al., 1985).

CASE 2.9: Poorly differentiated neuroblastoma in the pelvis

This biopsy is from a 4 year-old boy who presented with a 6 cm diameter pelvic tumour which obstructed the right ureter and displaced the bladder. Urine catecholamine levels were not raised. At laparotomy,

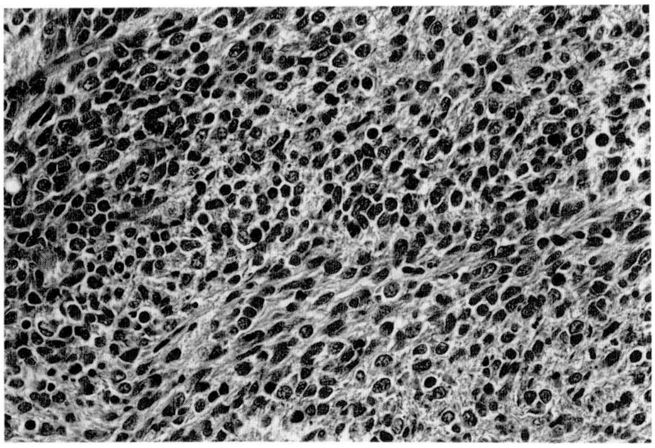

Fig. 2.9A. The pelvic tumour is composed of sheets and clusters of small round cells with hyperchromatic nuclei and scant cytoplasm. Very occasional foci suggest a fibrillary background (H & E, X 80).

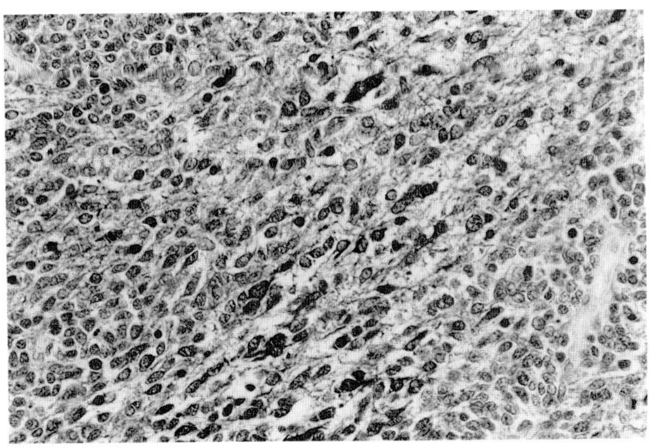

Fig. 2.9B. There is diffuse cytoplasmic and occasional nuclear staining for NSE (anti-NSE, X 80).

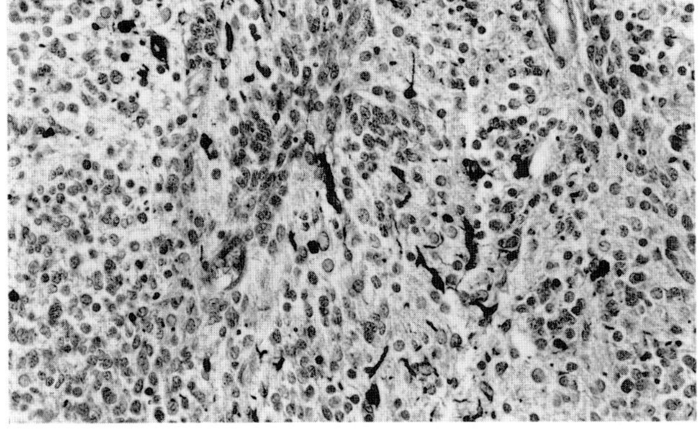

Fig. 2.9C. Occasional nerve sheath cells and cytoplasmic processes show labelling for GFAP (anti-GFAP, X 80).

the pelvic mass was firm and immobile and appeared to arise between the bladder and the rectum. Incisional biopsies revealed large clusters and sheets of round to oval tumour cells with scanty amounts of cytoplasm. Very occasional cells appear to show slightly more basophilic cytoplasm and there was a suggestion of a focal fibrillary background. Rosettes and pseudo-rosettes were not observed (Fig. 2.9A). Immunostaining revealed diffuse cytoplasmic and scattered nuclear positivity for NSE (Fig. 2.9B) and very occasional cells and cell processes were positive for GFAP (Fig. 2.9C). Antibodies to all three components of neurofilaments failed to label the tumour cells which were also negative for cytokeratin, desmin and vimentin.

Leukaemia/lymphoma

Non-Hodgkin's lymphoma in childhood differs from that in adults in so far as they are predominantly extranodal and rarely nodular. They are often leukaemic and rapidly proliferative and the majority fall into four major histological categories, namely, lymphoblastic lymphoma, Burkitt's lymphoma, undifferentiated lymphoma and large cell lymphoma (Callihan and Coston, 1982; Kjeldsberg et al., 1983). The immunohistochemical diagnosis of non-Hodgkin's lymphoma in childhood is no different to that in the adult. LCA is the most reliable marker of its lymphoid origin and when used in conjunction with other markers to exclude entities considered in differential diagnosis, LCA shows 100 per cent specificity (Andres and Kadin, 1983; Mierau et al., 1985; Leong et al., 1989; Chang et al., 1989). Burkitt's lymphoma and undifferentiated lymphoma are largely of B-cell lineage and may be identified in paraffin sections with B-cell markers such as L26 (CD20) and LN2 (CD74), whereas lymphoblastic lymphoma is largely of T-cell origin and labels with T-cell markers such as UCHL1 (CD45RO) and MT1 (CD43). The repertoire of lineage-associated markers is much larger in frozen tissue. Vimentin expression is observed in optimally fixed tissues.

Large cell lymphoma is heterogenous, with the majority being derived from B-cells and a smaller proportion from T-cells. True histiocytic lymphomas are uncommon.

Granulocytic sarcoma (chloroma) is uncommon and is associated with or frequently precedes the onset of leukaemia, usually of the acute myeloid type. Bone, soft tissue, lymph node, orbit and skin are common sites and such lesions may be labelled by myelomonocytic markers such as LeuM1 (CD15) and KP1 (CD68).

Ewing's sarcoma (skeletal and extra-skeletal types)

When James Ewing first described the primary malignant tumour of bone which came to bear his name, he suggested a derivation from vascular endothelium (Ewing, 1921). The histogenesis of this tumour is still a matter of controversy and among the many suggestions are an origin from primitive mesenchyme and from myelogenous tissue. Initial immunohistochemical studies showed the tumour to be largely only reactive for vimentin and staining for desmin, muscle-specific actin, chromogranin and LCA were all negative (Leong et al., 1989; Chang et al., 1989; Carter et al., 1990). It was believed that Ewing's sarcoma is a primary tumour of bone and the occurrence of neuroblastoma in bone was invariably conceived to be metastatic. More recent ultrastructural studies have suggested that skeletal Ewing's sarcoma has a wide spectrum of differentiation that overlaps with neuroblastoma. Schmidt et al. (1982) described four cases of Ewing's sarcoma of bone which showed elongated cell processes, microtubules and some neurosecretory granules by electron microscopy. Additional bone tumours of similar appearance have been published under the terms 'neuroectodermal tumour' and 'peripheral neuroepithelioma' (Jaffe et al., 1984; Cavazzana et al., 1987; Steiner et al., 1988). Most of these lesions were clinically, radiologically and morphologically consistent with skeletal Ewing's sarcoma, however, evidence of neural differentiation was demonstrated by electron microscopy and/or by the presence of a positive reaction to NSE (Kawaguchi and Koike, 1986). Similarly, a case of adult neuroblastoma of bone has been reported to show typical rosette formation and positivity for NSE (Mackay and Ordonez, 1987). Long-term cell cultures from three tumours which conformed to the clinical, radiologic and biopsy diagnosis of skeletal Ewing's sarcoma showed cells with moderately long, beaded cell processes and the presence of tumour rosettes and cytoplasmic microtubules as well as rare neurosecretory granules (Jaffe et al., 1984). Another study (Cavazzana et al., 1987) of five Ewing's sarcoma tumour cell lines revealed pronounced morphological evidence of neural differentiation following treatment with either cyclic AMP or TPA. The cultured cells developed elongate processes with filaments, microtubules and uraniffin-positive dense core granules. Three neural markers, NSE, neurofilaments and cholinesterase became abundant in the treated cells. Examination of 11 cases of classic skeletal and extraskeletal Ewing's sarcomas using immunofluorescence, immunoelectron microscopy as well as gel electrophoresis, revealed the presence of desmoplakin-labelled desmosomes in all cases, scattered cells with simple epithelium-type cytokeratins 18 and 8 in nine cases and neurofilaments in three suggesting that Ewing's sarcoma in bone and soft tissue may be derived from a primitive, pluri-potential cell that differentiates in variable proportions into cells with mesenchymal, epithelial and even neural characteristics (Moll et al., 1987). Other reports have confirmed the presence of NSE, HNK-1 (CD57) and neurofilament triplet proteins in cell lines from classic Ewing's sarcoma showing the 11:22 translocation (Lizard-Nacol et al., 1989) as well as the presence of cytokeratin proteins and tonofilaments (Greco et al., 1988). PGP 9.5 has also been observed in these tumours (Carter et al., 1990).

CASE 2.10: Skeletal Ewing's sarcoma in the right tibia with extension into the overlying soft tissue

A 26 year-old, unemployed man presented to casualty for a gun-shot injury to the head, having attempted suicide because of excruciating pain in the right ankle. X-ray examination revealed an expansile lytic tumour in the lower tibia with extension of the tumour into the overlying soft tissue. A biopsy revealed diffuse sheets of round cells with hyperchromatic nuclei and negligible, ill-defined cytoplasm (Fig. 2.10A). The tumour cells were strongly positive for glycogen (Fig. 2.10B) and immunostaining revealed cytoplasmic vimentin (Fig. 2.10C). The tumour cells were not immunoreactive for desmin, neuron-specific enolase, cytokeratin or Leu7 (CD57).

Peripheral neuroectodermal tumours (PNETs)

The term *primitive neuroectodermal tumour* has been employed in the literature for a group of small, round cell tumours which occur largely in childhood and adolescence, in the central nervous system as well as the sympathetic nervous system and soft tissues. More recently, the term peripheral neuroectodermal tumour (PNET) has

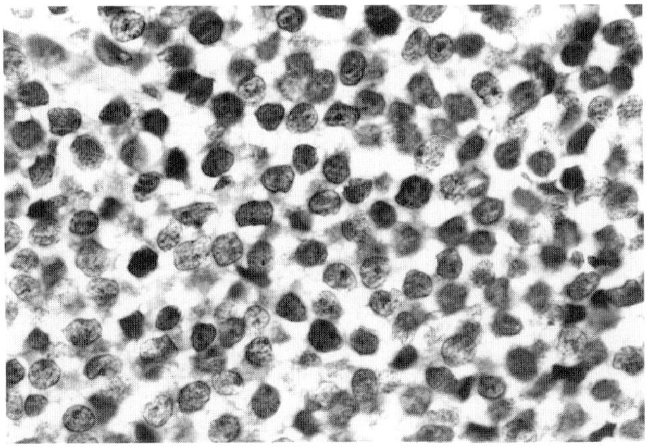

Fig. 2.10A. Light microscopic appearance of the small round cell tumour which show hyperchromatic nuclei and negligible amounts of ill-defined cytoplasm. No discernible pattern is observed (H & E, X 250).

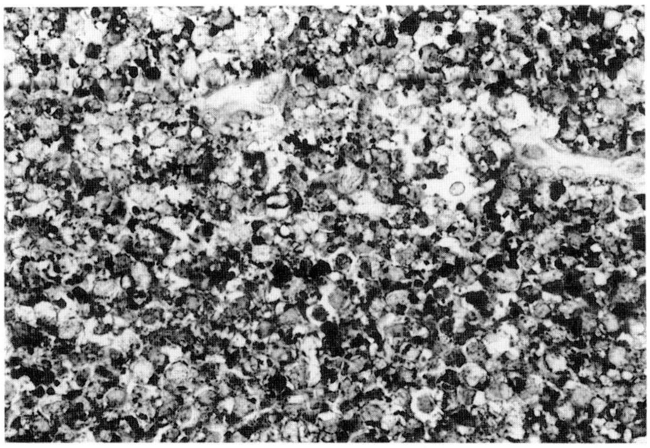

Fig. 2.10B. There is prominent cytoplasmic glycogen in the tumour (PAS, X 160).

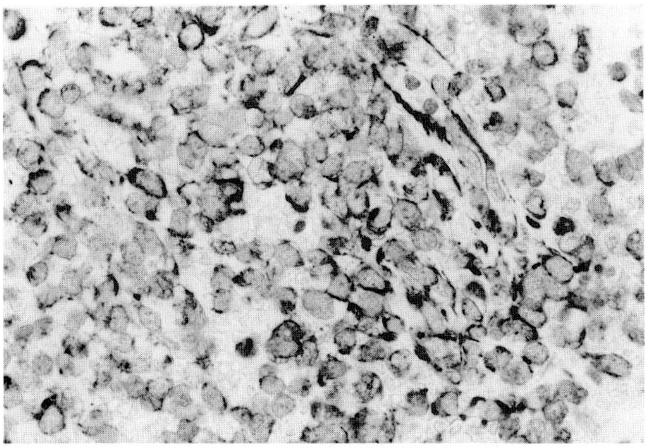

Fig. 2.10C. The tumour is immunoreactive for vimentin intermediate filaments (anti-vimentin, X 160).

been used for the latter group of tumours which occurs outside of the central nervous system. It incorporates neoplasms of probable neural crest derivation including the peripheral neuroepithelioma, malignant small cell tumour of thoracopulmonary origin ('Askin's tumour'), and pigmented neuroectodermal tumour of infancy or melanotic progonoma (Dehner, 1986). The classic neuroblastoma is the prototype of a PNET and is the most common, but shows a degree of differentiation which is different from that of other PNETs. Neuroblastomas occur in children, often under the age of 6 years, as solid abdominal or retroperitoneal tumours with specific localization to the adrenal gland or other sympathetic nervous system-related sites. These lesions may show varying degrees of ganglion-cell differentiation and often have elevated catecholamine values (Dehner, 1986). The morphological and immunohistochemical similarity of other PNETs to neuroblastoma has been recently recognized. By light and electron microscopy, PNETs are composed or monotonous small round cells with or without rosettes and pseudorosettes, and have dense core neurosecretory-like granules, microtubules, and complex interdigitating cytoplasmic processes similar to that of neuroblastomas except in a lesser degree. Cytoplasmic glycogen is invariably present in these tumours. Indeed, it has been suggested that PNETs are probably derived from the neural crest like the classic neuroblastoma, but do not differentiate along the lines of the sympathetic nervous system as in the latter case (Dehner, 1986). PNETs are typically immunoreactive for NSE, PGP 9.5, HNK-1 (CD57), and have also been variably reported to be positive for neurofilaments, S100 protein and chromogranin, vimentin and GFAP (Saski et al., 1985; Mierau, 1985; Schmidt et al., 1985; Llombart-Bosch et al., 1989; Harris et al., 1990). Recently, Gould and associates (1990a,b) have shown that central nervous system PNETs may express synaptophysin, neuropeptides as well as all the five classes of intermediate filament protein. These findings add further support to the suggestion of derivation from a pluri-potential cell and fuel Gould's argument that as newer technological advancements provide refined and subtle characteristics of tumour cells, 'it may prove useful to classify certain groups of neoplasms on the basis of what they in fact are, as defined by a series of appropriate phenotypic-differentiation marker expressions, rather than on the basis of questionable assumptions about their origins' (Gould, 1986).

CASE 2.11: Peripheral neuroectodermal tumour (PNET) in the pelvis

A 16 year-old female presented with multiple pelvic peritoneal deposits of tumour which appear to encase both ovaries. Incisional biopsy revealed sheets of small round cells with finely stippled chromatin and small nucleoli. Cytoplasm was scanty and mitotic figures and apoptosis were frequent (Fig. 2.11A). No discernible pattern was observed. Immunolabelling showed positivity for NSE and PGP 9.5 (Fig. 2.11B) and there was focal but distinct positivity for vimentin (Fig. 2.11C), cytokeratin (Fig. 2.11D) and Leu7 (CD 57) (Fig. 2.11E). Stains for desmin, neurofilaments, chromogranin and synaptophysin were negative.

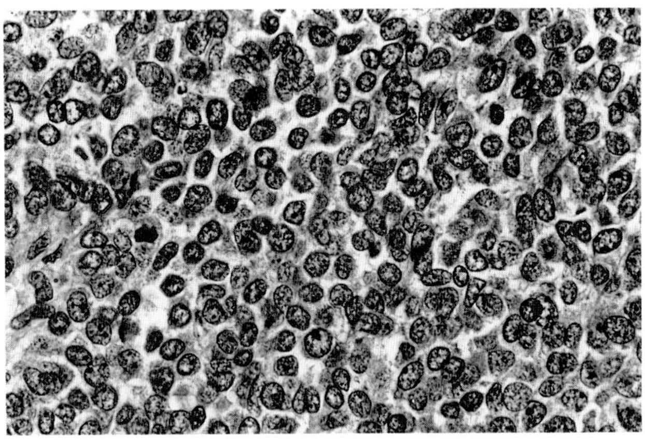

Fig. 2.11A. The pelvic peripheral neuroectodermal tumour comprises sheets of small round cells with stippled chromatin and small nucleoli. No discernible pattern is observed (H & E, X 160).

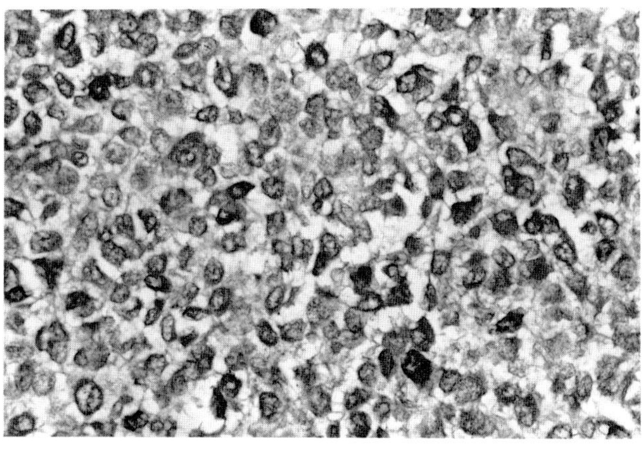

Fig. 2.11B. Antisera to PGP9.5 labels the tumour cells (anti-PGP9.5, X 160).

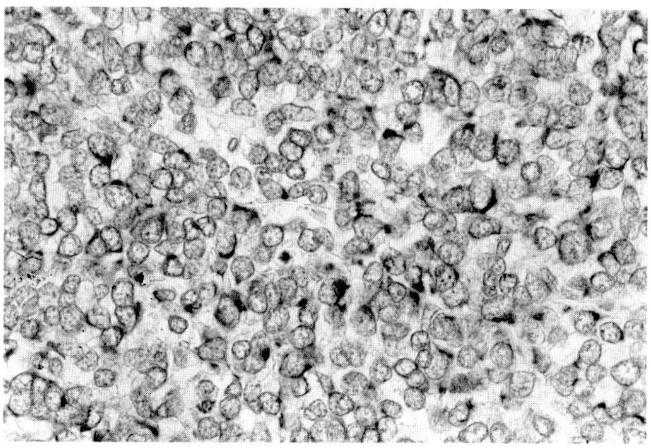

Fig. 2.11C. The tumour cells show distinct expression of vimentin intermediate filaments (anti-vimentin, X 160).

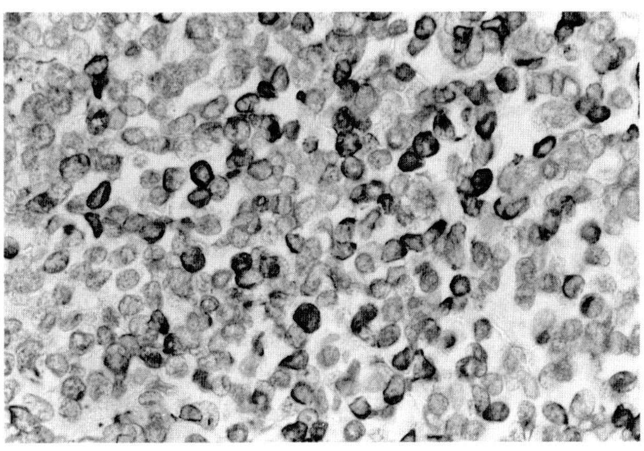

Fig. 2.11D. There is distinct cytoplasmic labelling for cytokeratins (AE1/3, X 160).

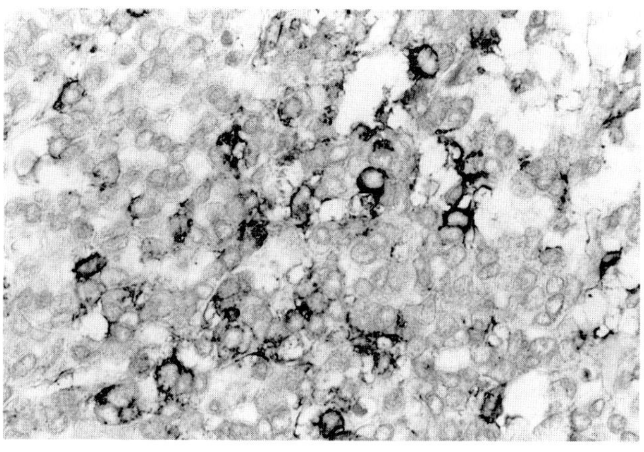

Fig. 2.11E. The tumour cells label for CD 57 (Leu7, X 160).

Adult spindle cell tumours

The differential diagnosis of a poorly differentiated spindle cell tumour can be extensive. While subtle features in haematoxylin-eosin stained sections may provide clues to the diagnosis, it is often necessary to resort to ancilliary techniques such as immunostaining and/or electron microscopy to make the distinction.

Leiomyosarcoma

Leiomyosarcomas account for about 7 per cent of soft tissue sarcomas (Russell et al., 1977; Hashimoto et al., 1986a). While most commonly seen in the uterus and gastrointestinal tract, soft tissue leiomyosarcomas can arise from the great vessels, in the retroperitoneum, subcutis and bone, among other sites. While the more well-differentiated spindle cell variants, with a classic alternating bundle pattern, are not difficult to recognize, leiomyosarcoma can also present as a myxoid tumour, or a pleomorphic spindle or even epithelioid neoplasm. The differential diagnosis of leiomyosarcoma usually includes other spindle cell sarcomas such as fibrosarcoma, malignant schwannoma, malignant fibrous histiocytoma, as well as spindle cell carcinoma and desmoplastic melanoma. Fortunately, in recent years, a set of highly sensitive and specific markers of muscle, and particularly smooth muscle, differentiation have become available and can reliably discriminate even poorly differentiated leiomyosarcomas from other non-muscle sarcomas. Furthermore, the overall immunophenotype, including a range of expected and unexpected markers, present in leiomyosarcoma has become apparent.

It is useful to divide markers of leiomyosarcoma into 'expected' and 'unexpected' subgroups: in the 'expected' group are muscle proteins such as desmin, actin and the basement membrane associated protein, type IV collagen, in the 'unexpected' group are markers more traditionally associated with epithelial differentiation, e.g. epithelial membrane antigen and low MW cytokeratins.

'Expected' markers of leiomyosarcoma

Not surprisingly, virtually all leiomyosarcomas – and all other sarcomas – express vimentin, the mesenchyme-associated intermediate filament protein. While expression of vimentin is therefore not of differential diagnostic significance, it can serve as a barometer of antigenic preservation, which can aid in the assessment of other antibody studies (Battifora, 1991).

Desmin is one of the five classes of intermediate filament proteins, and the only one associated with muscle differentiation. Its expression in normal tissues is restricted a subset of mesenchymal cells, specifically those demonstrating skeletal, smooth, and cardiac muscle cell differentiation. As might be expected, desmin expression is characteristic of tumours demonstrating muscle differentiation, e.g. rhabdomyosarcomas and leiomyosarcomas (Truong et al., 1990). A plethora of reports, reviewed by Truong et al. (1990), have documented the frequency of expression of desmin by leiomyosarcomas ranging from 0 to 85 per cent; the frequency of positivity is a function of fixation, degree of tumour differentiation, and tumour site. In optimally fixed tissue, our experience suggests that, overall, approximately 80 per cent of leiomyosarcomas are desmin-positive. Less certain from the literature are numbers regarding specificity of desmin for muscle tumours. While there are scattered reports of desmin expression in a small fraction of non-muscle sarcomas, e.g., malignant fibrous histiocytoma (Hirose et al., 1989) or malignant nerve sheath tumour (Wick et al., 1987), our experience has been that, when examined in optimally fixed (e.g. methacarn-fixed) tissue where intermediate filament protein immunoreactivity is maximally retained (Mitchell et al., 1985), desmin expression is completely restricted to sarcomas manifesting smooth or skeletal muscle differentiation.

The intermediate filament proteins are not the only members of the cytoskeleton which display tissue-restricted expression. At least six different isoforms of actin have been described, four of which are largely restricted in their expression to cells manifesting a muscle phenotype (Vanderkerckhove and Weber, 1978). Furthermore, unlike desmin, there is restriction on a finer basis, e.g. one that can distinguish smooth from skeletal muscle differentiation. Despite the fact that a change in only a few amino acids within a protein of a molecular weight of 43,000 distinguish them, it has nevertheless recently become possible to generate monoclonal antibodies specific to both subgroups of actin isoforms as well as individual actins. Monoclonal antibody HHF35 (Tsukada et al., 1987a, b) identifies all four muscle-specific actin isoforms; unlike desmin, however, muscle actin expression is not restricted to 'pure' muscle cells, but can also be found in cells displaying a 'partial' muscle phenotype, such as myoepithelium and myofibroblasts.

Not surprisingly, muscle actin expression can be found not only in leiomyosarcoma and rhabdomyosarcoma, but also in tumours manifesting myofibroblastic and myoepitheliomatous differentiation (Tsukada et al., 1987a, b). Antibodies such as CGA7 (Gown et al., 1985), asm-1 or 1A4 (Skalli et al., 1986; Schurch et al., 1987) specifically identify smooth muscle actin isoforms; in the case of the latter, only the single alpha smooth muscle isoform is identified. These latter antibodies are thus the most specific and sensitive markers currently available to identify leiomyosarcomas. None the less, the pathologist must be aware that expression of smooth muscle actins is also characteristic of myofibroblasts, which can appear in fibromatoses (Jones et al., 1990) and in reactive and stromal components of many tumours including sarcomas. Finally, in the hands of most investigators, antibodies to muscle actins and smooth muscle actins are more sensitive than antibodies to desmin in identifying smooth muscle differentiation in sarcomas (Miettinen, 1988a; Jones et al., 1990), although some have found comparable sensitivity of the two markers (Rangdaeng and Truong, 1991). In our experience, greater than 90 per cent of leiomyosarcomas are HHF35-positive, although there will be the rare leiomyosarcoma that is desmin-positive and muscle actin-negative. It may be prudent to employ both markers in a screen of spindle cell lesions.

Based largely upon ultrastructural evidence, it has been recognized that a subset of soft tissue tumours have the capacity of synthesizing basement membrane (Stern, 1981). Antibodies to two protein components of the basement membrane, laminin and type IV collagen, have been demonstrated to identify a subset of soft tissue sarcomas, particularly those demonstrating smooth muscle or Schwann cell or endothelial differentiation (Ogawa K et al., 1986; Miettinen et al., 1983a). In our experience, antibodies to type IV collagen can assist in the identification of leiomyosarcomas, in particular distinguishing them from the non-basal lamina producing sarcomas such as malignant fibrous histiocytoma (Hoffman and Dichersin, 1983), when used in conjunction with antibodies to the muscle-specific proteins discussed above.

'Unexpected' markers of leiomyosarcoma

Frozen sections of the smooth muscle cell-rich myometrium of the uterus (along with myocardial cells) were first reported to 'react with' various anti-cytokeratin antibodies by Huitfeldt and Bradtzaeg (1985). Documentation of true 'anomalous' (i.e. non-epithelium-associated) cytokeratin (CK8 and CK18) expression by smooth muscle cells was presented by Gown et al. (1988), in which immunostaining was corroborated by Western blots and further documented by two-colour immunofluorescence in myometrial smooth muscle cells grown in culture. In addition, 8 of 19 cases of leiomyosarcoma were found to be positive with the anti-cytokeratin 8 antibody 35βH11. This 'anomalous cytokeratin expression' in smooth muscle and smooth muscle tumours must be recognized, and should not pose a diagnostic problem if the panel of antibodies is wide enough to include antibodies to muscle-specific proteins such as desmin and/or muscle actins. Expression of cytokeratin, as well as epithelial membrane antigen, another epithelial-associated antigen, in a significant subset of leiomyosarcomas has been confirmed by other investigators (Miettinen, 1988b).

Other antigens expressed by leiomyosarcoma

Finally, it should be recognized that a minority of leiomyosarcomas can express some antigens associated primarily with non-muscle tumours. Leu7, which in the context of spindle cell tumours has been recognized as a marker of nerve sheath tumours, has also been shown to be expressed in approximately 25 per cent of leiomyosarcomas (Swanson et al., 1987).

CASE 2.12: Leiomyosarcoma primary to lung

A 34 year-old male with no previous medical history presented with a 5 x 2 x 2 cm haemorrhagic, soft, fleshy tumour mass in the right lung. Histologic examination of the tumour (Fig. 2.12) revealed a relatively low grade spindle cell tumour with scattered mitotic figures and no necrosis. The differential diagnosis in this case includes a variety of soft tissue sarcomas, including low grade malignant nerve sheath tumour (e.g. malignant Schwannoma), leiomyosarcoma, and spindle cell carcinoma. The results of immunostaining with a panel of antibodies are shown in Table 2.6; the cells were strongly positive for vimentin (Fig. 2.12B) and two different muscle-specific proteins, desmin (Fig. 2.12E), muscle actins (Fig. 2.12C), and, in addition, they expressed the basement membrane protein, type IV collagen (Fig. 2.12D), pointing rather unequivocally to the diagnosis of a smooth muscle tumour. Markers of nerve sheath differentiation (e.g. S100 protein, Fig. 2.12F) were negative, as were markers of epithelial differentiation (low MW cytokeratin).

Table 2.6. Immunostaining results in leiomyosarcoma of lung

	Vim	MA	Des	Col IV	S100	LMCK
MNST	+	–	–	+	+	–
SCCa	+	–	–	–	–	+
LMS	+	+	+	+	–	–
Case 2.12	+	+	+	+	–	–

Notes: Vim = vimentin
MA = muscle actins
Des = desmin
Col IV = collagen type IV
S100 = S100 protein
LMCK = low molecular cytokeratin
MNST = malignant nerve sheath tumour
SCCa = squamous cell carcinoma
LMS = leiomyosarcoma

Malignant nerve sheath tumour

Sarcomas of nerve sheath cells have been given a variety of names, including *malignant schwannomas, neurofibrosarcomas, neurogenic sarcomas*, etc. As each of these terms possesses its own shortcomings (e.g. Schwann cells are not the only cell type present in the nerve sheath, and these sarcomas do not 'form nerves'), the more generic yet less mellifluous term, malignant nerve sheath tumour (MNST), is preferred. However, owing to the lack of agreement over nomenclature and diagnostic criteria for these tumours, it is difficult to find consensus views on their clinical and immunohistochemical characteristics. It would appear that approximately one-half of these tumours arise in patients with von Recklinghausen's disease; only a small minority of such patients will develop MNST, often in the setting of multiple benign neurofibromas, and usually after a long latent period of 10–20 years. The diagnosis of MNST is most critically made in non-von Recklinghausen's disease patients, and in clinical situations where the relationship to peripheral nerves is not apparent at surgery or upon gross inspection.

There are a number of markers which can assist the pathologist in rendering the diagnosis of MNST, although it is important to understand the limitations of the markers involved. One must also approach the published literature with caution, given the lack of agreement on diagnostic criteria, as outlined above. The intermediate filament composition of these tumours is much as might be theoretically predicted: vimentin, the 'mesenchymal' intermediate filament, was demonstrated to be present in all MNST in the study of Gould et al. (1986), and in 58/62 cases in the study of Wick et al. (1987); neither of these investigators found

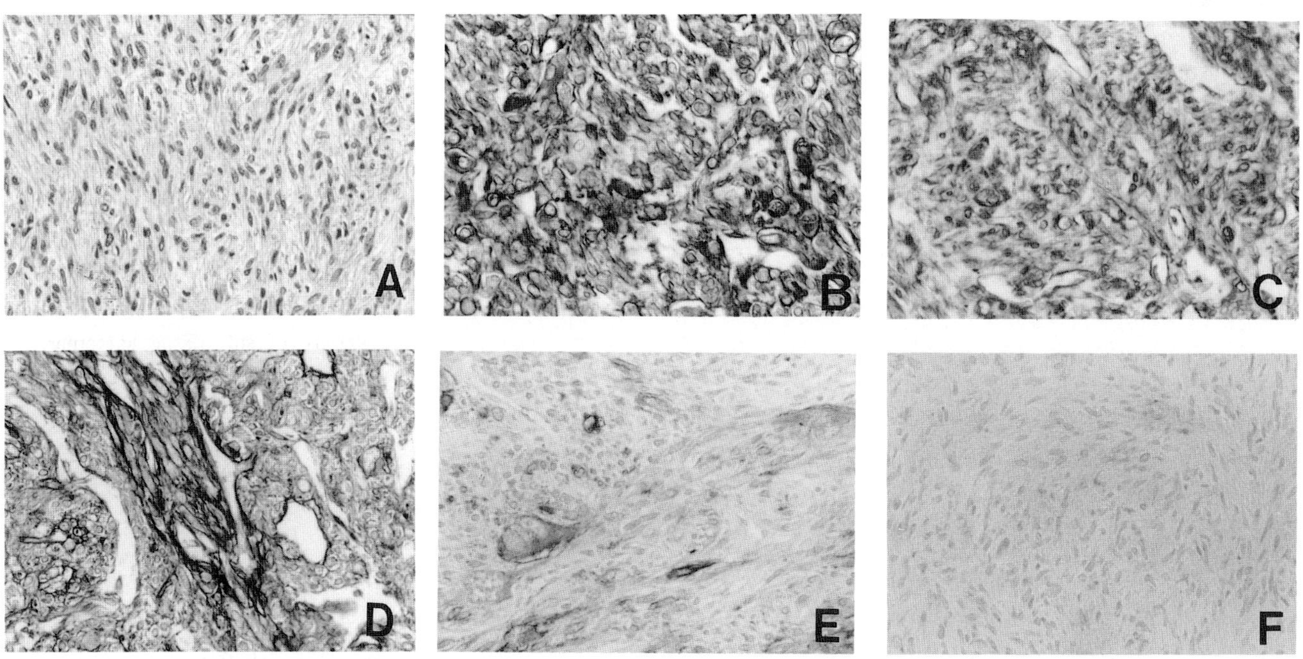

Fig. 2.12A–F. The low grade spindle cell tumour displays scattered mitotic figures and no necrosis (a). There is strong staining for vimentin (B), desmin (E) and muscle actins (C). Type IV collagen is shown to invest the tumour cells (D) whereas markers for nerve sheath differentiation such as S100 protein (f) are negative, as were markers of epithelial differentiation. (We thank Carlos E. Bacchi, MD, for taking the photographs.)

evidence of expression of other intermediate filament proteins. However, reports of a small fraction of MNST expressing GFAP (less than 10 per cent, in studies of Gray et al. (1989) and Giangaspero et al. (1989) have not been confirmed by at least two different investigators (Yasuda et al., 1991; Gould et al., 1986). Such expression might not be totally surprising, given the documented existence of 'glial-like' Schwann cells in the peripheral nervous system which do express GFAP, a property shared by a subset of benign Schwann cell tumours (Gray et al., 1989). Most investigators have not found cytokeratin expression in MNST (Gould et al., 1986; Wick et al., 1987), although Miettinen (1991) recently reported widespread cytokeratin 8 and 18 expression in his study of sarcomas using acetone-fixed frozen sections, including 5/5 MNST. Biochemical confirmation of this finding has not yet been presented, as it has in the case of leiomyosarcomas (see above). However, one must distinguish here the rare variant of MNST which contains heterologous cytokeratin-positive glandular differentiation (Christensen et al., 1988).

Specific markers of nerve sheath differentiation do not exist. However, a number of markers have been successfully employed in the identification of MNST, usually in conjunction with a panel of markers, and recognizing the limitations of the specificity of many of the individual markers. S100 protein is present in 50–90 per cent of MNST; in the large series of Wick et al. (1987) slightly over one-half MNST were S100-positive, and in the more recent studies of Gray et al. (1989), and Giangaspero et al. (1989), 40 per cent and 63 per cent, respectively, of MNST expressed S100 protein. MNST, in contrast to their normal Schwann cell counterparts, also alter their subunit composition of S100 protein; in the study of Hayashi et al. (1987), all MNST lacked the S100 beta component. Lack of expression of this differentiation marker may be explained both by the 'partial' differentiation phenotype encountered in many malignant tumours, but also by the heterogeneous nature of the cell types found in peripheral nerves, which may correspond the range of phenotypes displayed by MNSTs. For example, in the correlative immunocytochemical and ultrastructural study of Hirose et al. (1988), a subset of S100-negative MNST corresponded to tumours manifesting apparent perineural, rather than Schwann cell, differentiation. Regardless of the explanation, the relative insensitivity of S100 as a marker of MNST has encouraged the development of additional markers. The specificity of S100 protein for tumours manifesting nerve sheath differentiation is also not great; S100 protein is expressed in many other spindle cell neoplasms, including a subset of liposarcomas, leiomyosarcomas, spindle cell carcinomas, spindle cell melanomas, etc. (Barwick, 1990), and thus it is unwise and improper to use antibodies to S100 protein as a single putative marker of nerve sheath differentiation.

CD57 (Leu7), was originally defined as a marker of 'natural killer cells', a unique subset of bone-marrow-derived cells, but the epitope recognized by antibody HNK-1, the most frequently used antibody, is shared by several other molecules, including a member of the neural cell adhesion molecule (N-CAM) family and a 100 kD myelin-associated glycoprotein (Kruse et al., 1984). The latter cross-reactivity accounts for the utility of antibodies to CD57 in the identification of nerve sheath tumours. In two studies by Swanson et al. (1987) and Giangaspero et al. (1989) 75 per cent of MNST were CD57-positive, although in the study of Swanson et al, the marker was also expressed by a limited number of other non-nerve sheath sarcomas (e.g. leiomyosarcomas). Myelin basic protein (MBP) has also been employed by several investigators as a marker of nerve sheath differentiation, with disparate results: Wick et al. (1987), found MBP expression by approximately 40 per cent, whereas Giangaspero et al. (1989), found MBP expression in 0 per cent in their respective MNST series. Nerve growth factor receptor is a more recently described marker of nerve sheath differentiation, and has been found in an overwhelming majority of MNST (78 and 100 per cent) in the two studies published to date (Perosio and Brooks, 1988; Thompson et al., 1989). None of the above markers, however, shows absolute specificity for MNST among other soft tissue sarcomas; nerve growth factor receptor, for example, is also expressed by other sarcomas such as synovial sarcoma and hemangiopericytoma. As discussed by Wick et al. (1987), it is wisest to employ a combination of antibodies, including those to the markers discussed above, and search for 'conjoint' expression of these markers, to improve sensitivity and specificity for identification of MNST.

CASE 2.13: Malignant nerve sheath tumour of thigh

A 46 year-old female presented with an 8 cm mass in her distal thigh just above the knee. Biopsy revealed the presence of a low-to-intermediate grade spindle cell sarcoma (Fig. 2.13A) with the differential diagnosis including leiomyosarcoma, malignant nerve sheath tumour, and synovial sarcoma, among others. The results of immunostaining with a panel of antibodies are shown in Table 2.7. Markers of muscle differentiation (desmin, muscle actins) were negative, with good internal control immunostaining of vascular smooth muscle cells (Fig. 2.13E), although the tumour cells did strongly express the basement membrane-related protein, type IV collagen (Fig. 2.13C). However, the diagnosis of malignant nerve sheath tumour was confirmed by the expression of two independent markers of nerve sheath differentiation: S100 protein (Fig. 2.13B) and the nerve growth factor receptor (Fig. 2.13D).

Table 2.7. Immunostaining Results in Malignant Nerve Sheath Tumour

	LMCK	Vim	MA	Des	Col IV	S100	NGF
LMS	–	+	+	+	+	–	–
SS	+	+	–	–	+	–	–
MNST	–	+	–	–	+	+	+
Case 2.13	–	+	–	–	+	+	+

Notes:
LMCK = low molecular cytokeratin
Vim = vimentin
MA = muscle actins (HHF35)
Des = desmin
Col IV = collagen type IV
S100 = S100 protein
NGF = nerve growth factor receptor
MNST = malignant nerve sheath tumour
SS = synovial sarcoma
LMS = leiomyosarcoma

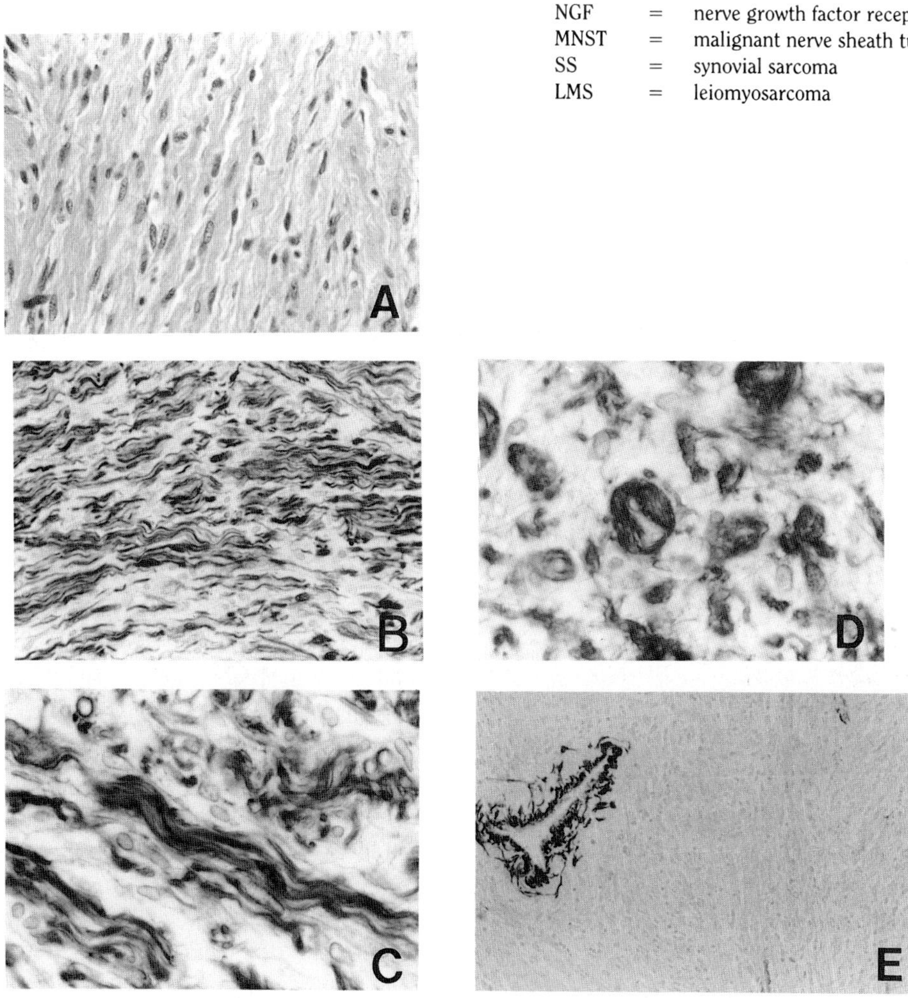

Fig. 2.13A–E. The tumour is a low- to intermediate-grade spindle cell sarcoma (A) and the differential diagnoses included leiomyosarcoma, malignant nerve sheath tumour and synovial sarcoma, among others. Staining for markers of muscle differentiation including desmin and muscle actins were negative, with good internal control immunostaining of vascular smooth muscle cells (E), although the tumour cells strongly express the basement membrane-related protein, type IV collagen (C). The diagnosis of malignant nerve sheath tumour is confirmed by the expression of two independent markers of nerve sheath differentiation, namely S100 protein (B), and the nerve growth factor receptor (D). (We thank Carlos E. Bacchi, MD, for taking the photographs.)

Malignant fibrous histiocytoma

Malignant fibrous histiocytoma (MFH) is the most common variant of soft tissue sarcoma of late adult life (Weiss and Enzinger, 1978), occurring most frequently in the lower extremity and characterized by a protean histologic appearance which has led to several sub-classifications (Enzinger and Weiss, 1988). There has been considerable controversy regarding the histogenesis of this tumour; based upon the morphologic heterogeneity of this tumour and early tissue culture reports, it was suspected that this was a unique tumour manifesting a bifurcated differentiation pathway, i.e. one of fibroblasts and histiocytes (hence the nomenclature, 'fibrous histiocytoma'). Evidence for the latter included the presence of ultrastructurally confirmed histiocyte-like cells, and descriptions of expression, by the tumour cells, of putative 'histiocytic' markers such as alpha-1-antitrypsin (Soini and Miettinen, 1989). The application of immunocytochemical studies to the issue of specific mesenchymal differentiation has, unfortunately, not clarified the issue. It is useful, however, to distinguish two separate issues in studies of differentiation in MFH: (1) Is there a characteristic or specific pathway of mesenchymal differentiation; (2) What is the relationship of histiocytic differentiation to the mesenchymal cells? Early studies had suggested that, based upon expression of intermediate filament proteins, MFH cells were manifesting non-specific mesenchymal differentiation, sometimes characterized as 'fibroblastic' differentiation (Miettinen et al., 1982a), as evidenced by expression of vimentin as the only intermediate filament protein. Lawson et al. (1987), found uniform vimentin expression in a series of 10 tumours, but also described focal reactivity with antibodies to neurofilaments and desmin in a subset of the tumours, and concluded that MFH may represent a tumour with a 'propensity to differentiate in several different directions'. In a larger series of 34 tumours, Hirose et al. (1989) also found evidence for anti-neurofilament, anti-cytokeratin, and anti-desmin positivity in a varying subset of these tumours, which were virtually all vimentin-positive. However, considerable variation in 'expression' of these other intermediate filaments resulted from the use of different antibodies to the same intermediate filament. Miettinen and Soini (1989), in an attempt to resolve some of the concerns regarding the effect of tissue fixation and processing, studied 10 cases of MFH in frozen sections, and found no evidence of desmin expression, but did, in a small minority of cases, find evidence of cytokeratin or neurofilament expression. Miettinen and Soini concluded that there is no 'universal' pattern of IF expression that defines MFH. Xenograft studies by Roholl et al. (1985a, b), in which smooth muscle or nerve sheath differentiation were manifested, would appear to confirm this assessment. Our preliminary studies of over 40 cases of MFH in optimally fixed (methacarn-fixed), deparaffinized tissue fail to confirm the presence of either neurofilament, desmin, or cytokeratin expression in these tumours. Whether reports of these anomalous intermediate filament coexpression represent true expression or false-positive immunostaining must await the completion of larger studies with biochemical confirmation. However, the great morphologic heterogeneity in this class of tumours, and the fact that some consider it a 'wastebasket' term overlapping with other sarcoma types, will continue to obfuscate the issue of differentiation in MFH.

The relationship between the histiocytic and mesenchymal cells in MFH is better understood, although still controversial. Rather than representing a tumour manifesting simultaneous differentiation, MFH probably represents a tumour containing abundant infiltrating (i.e. reactive) blood-borne macrophages, as evidenced by the latter's expression of CD45, as evidence of their origin in the bone marrow, as well as macrophage-specific markers such as KP-1, other anti-CD68 antibodies, and the HAM56-defined antigen. None the less, there is still controversy as to whether these macrophage antigens are associated with the infiltrating macrophages alone or the malignant population of cells, too (Enzinger and Weiss, 1988; Soini and Miettinen, 1989). Our experience has been that the degree of infiltrating macrophages can be marked, occasionally obscuring the underlying malignant population; certainly, the giant cell population so prevalent in this tumour can be composed either macrophage or non-macrophage cells. Significantly, however, it has been reported that cell proliferation, as defined by immunoreactivity with the antibody Ki67, occurs in the mesenchymal, and not the reactive, histiocytic, subpopulation of the tumour (Roessner et al., 1987). This would appear to support the notion that the 'histiocytic' population of cells are the 'passengers' with the proliferating, malignant population of as yet undefined mesenchymal cells.

CASE 2.14: Malignant fibrous histiocytoma

A 64 year-old male presented with a 4 cm mass within the skeletal muscle of the left forearm. The tumour, upon examination of the H & E-stained sections (Fig. 2.14A), proved to be a cellular spindle cell tumour with a fairly high mitotic rate. Differential diagnosis of this intermediate-to-high grade tumour included sarcomas such as a malignant nerve sheath tumour, leiomyosarcoma, and malignant fibrous histiocytoma, or metastatic melanoma. The results of immunostaining with a panel of antibodies are shown in Table 2.8. The tumour expressed vimentin (Fig. 2.14B) but not cytokeratin, and did not express any muscle markers (desmin, muscle actin) or nerve sheath (S100 protein) or melanoma (HMB45-defined antigen) markers. Type IV collagen was not expressed by the tumour cells, while it was present in the 'internal controls', i.e. the vascular smooth muscle cells and endothelium (Fig. 2.14E, F). Monoclonal antibodies to macrophages (HAM56) revealed the presence of an admixed population of the latter along with the spindle cell tumour population (Fig. 2.14D); in some areas, the number of macrophages was so large as to obscure the background malignant population (Fig. 2.14C). The absence of specific connective tissue differentiation and the abundance of accompanying macrophages, in this histologic context, points to the diagnosis of malignant fibrous histiocytoma.

Table 2.8. Immunostaining results in malignant fibrous histiocytoma

	Vim	MA	Des	Col IV	S100	HMB45	HAM56
MNST	+	–	–	+	+	–	–
LMS	+	+	+	+	–	–	–
MM	+	–	–	–	+	+	–
MFH	+	–	–	–	–	–	–*
Case 2.14	+	–	–	–	–	–	–*

Notes: *accompanying cells positive (tumour cells negative)
Vim = vimentin
MA = muscle actins (HHF35)
Des = desmin
Col IV = collagen type IV
S100 = S100 protein
HMB45 = melanoma antigen; HAM56 = macrophage antigen
MNST = malignant nerve sheath tumour; LMS = leiomyosarcoma
MM = malignant melanoma
MFH = malignant fibrous histiocytoma

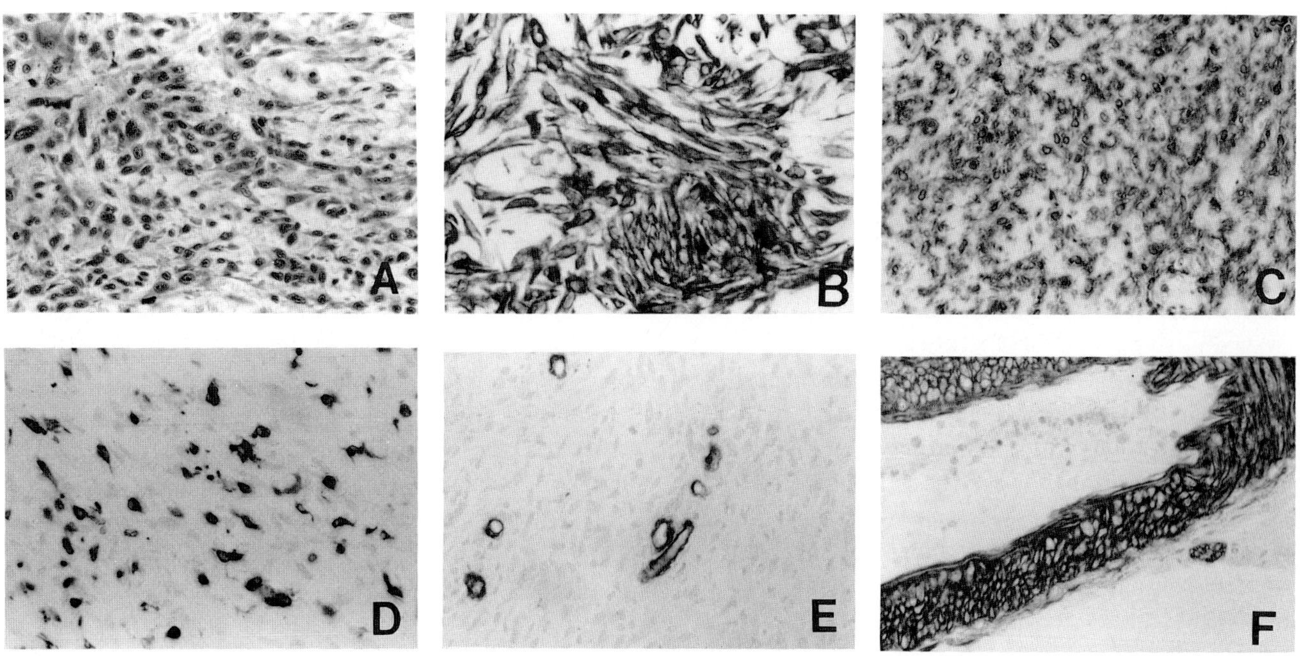

Fig. 2.14A–F. The H & E section reveals a cellular spindle cell tumour with a fairly high mitotic rate (A). The tumour expresses vimentin (B) but not cytokeratin, and did not express any muscle markers (desmin, muscle actin) or nerve sheath markers (S100 protein) or melanoma markers (HMB45). Type IV collagen is not expressed while it is present in the 'internal controls' such as vascular smooth muscle cells and endothelium (E,F). Monoclonal antibodies to macrophages (HAM56) shows scattered macrophages among the spindle tumour cells (D), in some areas so abundant as to obscure the background malignant population (C). (We thank Carlos E. Bacchi, MD, for taking the photographs.)

Angiosarcoma

Angiosarcomas are one of the first tumours successfully identified using cell-specific antibodies in immunohistochemical studies. Beginning with the studies of Mukai et al. (1980) and Burgdorf et al. (1981), antibodies to factor VIII-related antigen, previously identified as an endothelial-specific marker, were employed to identify neoplastic endothelial cells in a variety of benign and malignant tumours; these authors made the seminal observation that the cells of benign endothelial tumours (angiomas) were more consistently positive than were the cells of malignant endothelial tumours (angiosarcomas), probably as consequence of variable loss of this differentiated phenotypic marker with malignant transformation. The other principal marker of endothelial cells which, in the context of mesenchymal tumours, appears to be endothelial-specific, is the binding of the Ulex europaeus lectin. While the latter identifies the sugars which constitute the 'O' blood group, this epitope is accessible apparently independently of blood type of a given individual. Furthermore, several studies (e.g. Little et al., 1986; Walker, 1985; Ordonez and Batsakis, 1984; Miettinen et al., 1983b) have indicated that the Ulex lectin is a more sensitive marker of endothelial differentiation (i.e. is positive in a greater fraction of angiosarcomas) than are anti-Factor VIII related antigen (von Willebrand's factor) antibodies. A number of other monoclonal antibody-defined endothelial-specific markers (e.g. the antibody PAL-E; Schlingemann et al., 1985), have been described, but none have the combination of sensitivity and specificity as the Ulex lectin and antibodies to Factor VIII related antigen. Most recently, interest has been generated in antibodies to the human hematopoietic progenitor cell antigen, CD34, which is also expressed by vascular endothelial cells. This antigen is also coexpressed by a subset of non-endothelial tumours (i.e. anti-CD34 antibodies are not specific for angiosarcomas among malignant tumours), but, like the Ulex europaeus lectin, it is a more sensitive marker of endothelial differentiation than are anti-von Willebrand's factor antibodies (Anthony and Ramani, 1991; Ramani et al., 1990; Traweek et al., 1991).

There are three major classes of vasoformative tumours which can pose diagnostic problems for the pathologist. The first are the class of these tumours of 'intermediate' malignancy, i.e. the haemangioendotheliomas; the second are the spectrum of true angiosarcomas, and the third is the unique form of vasoformative tumour particularly associated with AIDS: Kaposi's sarcoma.

'Haemangioendothelioma' is an empirical term for vascular tumours intermediate in histologic appearance (and clinical behaviour) between haemangiomas and angiosarcoma. The spindle cell variant of this intermediate lesion, first described by Weiss and Enzinger (1986), has a proclivity for occurring in the subcutis or dermis of the distal extremity, often in younger patients (< 25 years of age). The histologic appearance of this tumour can simulate closely that of Kaposi's sarcoma, although one often finds tell-tale foci of 'epithelioid' differentiation, as well as characteristic vacuoles, heralding the presence of intracytoplasmic lumina. Immunocytochemical studies have consistently demonstrated 'incomplete' endothelial differentiation (Fletcher et al., 1991) using a subset of the markers described above.

Angiosarcomas are extremely rare tumours, comprising less than 1 per cent of all sarcomas; in contrast to most other sarcomas, these tumours have a tendency to involve more superficial soft tissue and skin. Poorly differentiated and pleomorphic angiosarcomas may be difficult to distinguish from other sarcomas; several studies have indicated the utility of the anti-endothelial markers discussed above in positively identifying angiosarcomas and distinguishing them from non-vasoformative tumours (Guarda et al., 1982; Alles and Bosslet, 1988).

The vasoformative tumour which can pose the greatest diagnostic dilemma, however, is Kaposi's sarcoma (KS). The incidence of this tumour, originally defined as an unusual tumour affecting the skin of the lower extremity in elderly patients (Kaposi, 1872), has increased dramatically owing to its association with AIDS, the acquired immunodeficiency syndrome associated with the human immunodeficiency virus (HIV). There has been considerable controversy regarding the expression of endothelial markers in the cells of KS, and hence the utility of the antibodies described above in identifying the various phases of this tumour. As with more 'traditional' angiosarcomas, Ulex europaeus lectin and anti-von Willebrand's factor antibodies (Millard and Heryet, 1985; Guarda et al., 1981; Nadji et al., 1981) have had mixed success, especially in identifying the spindle cell population of cells thought to constitute the more undifferentiated component of the process. Some have claimed, on the basis of detailed histochemistry and/or immunohistochemistry using additional endothelial markers on frozen sections (permitting a wider range of antibodies), that the KS cells are 'related' to vascular rather than lymphatic endothelium (Hashimoto et al., 1987; Rutgers et al., 1986), but others have arrived at the opposite conclusion (Beckstead et al., 1985). As suggested in a recent review by Holden (1989), the consensus of most of the voluminous literature regarding the nature of KS cells is that they are lesions arising from undifferentiated stem cells that proliferate with varying degrees of differentiation toward blood vessel endothelium. It is also not clear how, from a histogenetic point of view, KS differs from 'garden variety' angiosarcomas, although in one report by Sankey et al. (1990), it was claimed that anti-CD34 antibodies identified many of the spindle cell population of KS but not other vascular tumours. Confounding the problem, however, in manner analogous to that in MFH, are the presence of many accompanying, and probably non-neoplastic, cells which comprise a significant subset of the 'spindle cell' population, and which mark as macrophages or dermal dendrocytes with appropriate markers (Nickoloff and Griffiths, 1989; Gray et al., 1991).

CASE 2.15: Angiosarcoma

A 77 year-old female presented with a 3 cm pericardial tumour which on biopsy proved to be composed of spindle cells with some papillary features (Fig. 2.15A). The principal differential diagnoses considered were angiosarcoma, metastatic carcinoma, and mesothelioma. The results of immunostaining are summarized in Table 2.9. Either metastatic carcinoma or mesothelioma would be expected to strongly express cytokeratins, but this tumour was negative with several different anti-cytokeratin antibodies. However, the tumour was positive with antibodies to vimentin as well as type IV collagen, which was present in a unique distribution around individual cells (Fig. 2.15B). Two different probes of endothelial differentiation, antibodies to von Willebrand's factor (factor VIII-related antigen) and the Ulex lectin, which identifies the 'H' blood group antigen, were both positive on the tumour cell population (Fig. 2.15C,D), confirming the diagnosis of angiosarcoma.

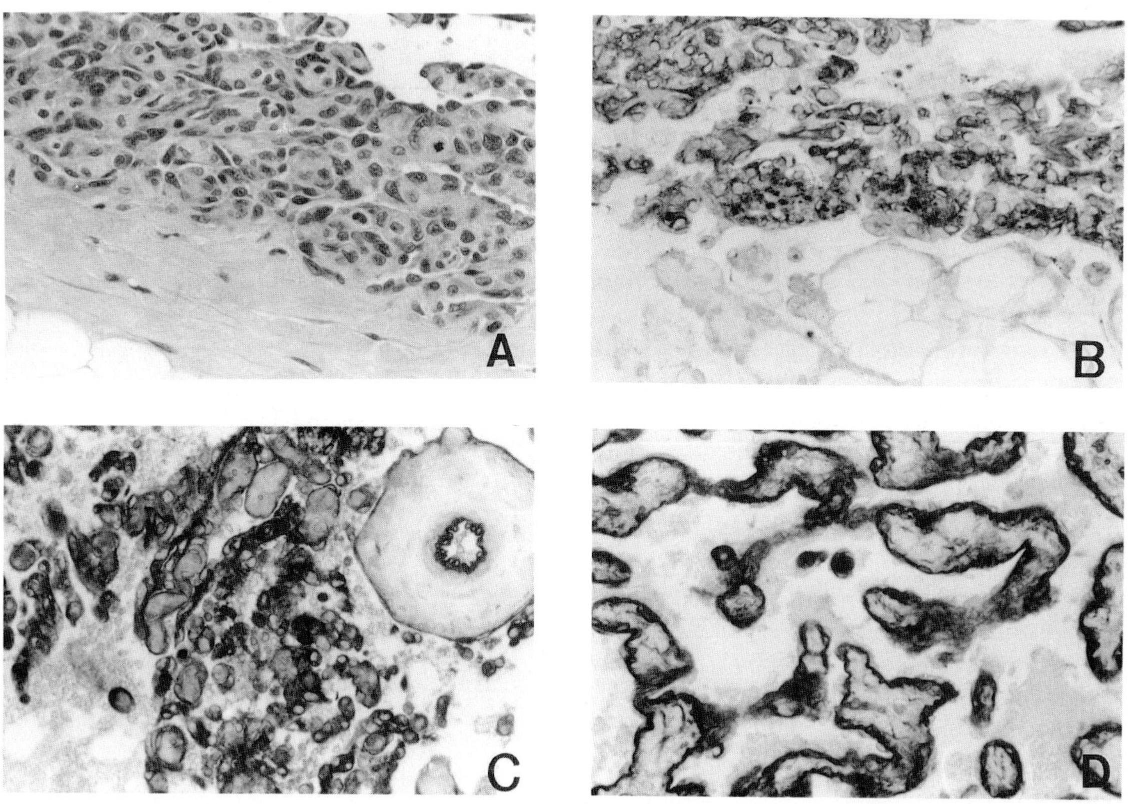

Fig. 2.15A–D. The histologic appearances of the spindle cell tumour with some papillary features is shown in Fig. 2.15A. The tumour cells are positive for vimentin as well as type IV collagen, the latter present in a unique distribution around individual cells (B). Two markers of endothelial differentiation, namely antibodies to von Willebrand's factor or factor VIII related antigen (C) and Ulex lectin, which identifies the 'H' blood group antigen (D) are both positive on the tumour cell population. (We thank Carlos E. Bacchi, MD, for taking the photographs.)

Table 2.9. Immunostaining results in angiosarcoma

	Vim	LMCK	Col IV	FVIII	UEA
Ca	–	+	–	–	+/–
Mesoth	+	+	–	–	–/+
AgSa	+	–	+	+	+
Case 2.15	+	–	+	+	+

Notes: Vim = vimentin
Col IV = collagen type IV
LMCK = low molecular cytokeratin
FVIII = Factor VIII-related antigen
UEA = Ulex lectin
Ca = carcinoma
Mesoth = mesothelioma
AgSa = angiosarcoma

Synovial sarcoma

Synovial sarcoma is a clinicopathologic entity most prevalent in adolescents and young adults (15–40 years old) that typically occurs in the para-articular regions; it is, however, uncommon in joint cavities, its moniker notwithstanding. Knox (1936) is credited with the nomenclature of this tumour, which is, as has been established many times over (Miettinen et al., 1982b; Corson et al., 1984; Miettinen and Lehto et al., 1984; Salisbury and Isaacson, 1985), a misnomer on all counts: the tumour is neither a sarcoma, nor related to normal synovium! Synovial sarcomas are easily identified when presenting microscopically in the so-called 'biphasic' pattern, i.e. with both carcinoma and fibrosarcoma-like areas intermingling. More challenging, however, is the microscopic presentation where little, if any, epithelial differentiation is present, i.e. a 'monophasic' pattern which can be morphologically confused with other sarcomas, including MFH, hemangiopericytoma, and other sarcomas with 'myxoid' features. Immunocytochemical studies, however, have demonstrated the presence of epithelial differentiation, as evidenced by low MW cytokeratin expression, even in synovial sarcomas manifesting a 'monophasic' histologic pattern (Tsujimoto et al., 1987; Sumitomo et al., 1989), although the level of expression and the number of CK-positive cells in a given tumour is generally less. Other epithelial markers, such as EMA, CEA, Ulex agglutinin, and basement membrane proteins such as type IV collagen, are present in a significant subset of synovial sarcomas, although neither of these markers are as sensitive as CK for identifying this subtype of sarcoma (Ordonez et al., 1990). Furthermore, the presence of other markers of true epithelial differentiation, such as the desmoplakins and cytokeratin 13, confirm the rather unique nature of synovial sarcoma among tumours categorized as sarcomas (Miettinen, 1991).

CASE 2.16: Synovial sarcoma

A 30 year-old male presented with a 3 cm retropharyngeal mass; biopsy revealed it to be a moderately cellular spindle cell (Fig. 2.16). Differential diagnoses included spindle cell carcinoma, fibrosarcoma, leiomyosarcoma, nerve sheath tumour, and synovial sarcoma (which can occur in the head and neck region). Results of the immunostaining panel are summarized in Table 2.10. The tumour displayed uniform expression of vimentin (Fig. 2.16B) and a characteristic, patchy expression of low MW cytokeratin (Fig. 2.16C) and epithelial membrane antigen (Fig. 2.16D), pointing to the diagnosis of a spindle cell tumour showing patchy epithelial differentiation, i.e. synovial sarcoma. The tumour cells also uniformly expressed type IV collagen (Fig. 2.16E). Markers of smooth muscle differentiation (desmin, muscle actins) were negative, with good internal controls on the blood vessels in the tumour (Fig. 2.16F).

Table 2.10. Immunostaining results in synovial sarcoma

	Vim	MA	Des	Col IV	LMCK	EMA
SCCa	+/–	–	–	–	+	+
FSa	+	–	–	–	–	–
LMS	+	+	+	+	–/+	–
MNST	+	–	–	+	–	–
SS	+	–	–	+	+	+
Case 2.16	+	–	–	+	+	+

Notes: Vim = vimentin
MA = muscle actins (HHF35)
Des = desmin
Col IV = collagen type IV
LMCK = low molecular cytokeratin
EMA = epithelial membrane antigen
SCCa = squamous cell carcinoma
FSA = fibrosarcoma
LMS = leiomyosarcoma
MNST = malignant nerve sheath tumour
SS = synovial sarcoma

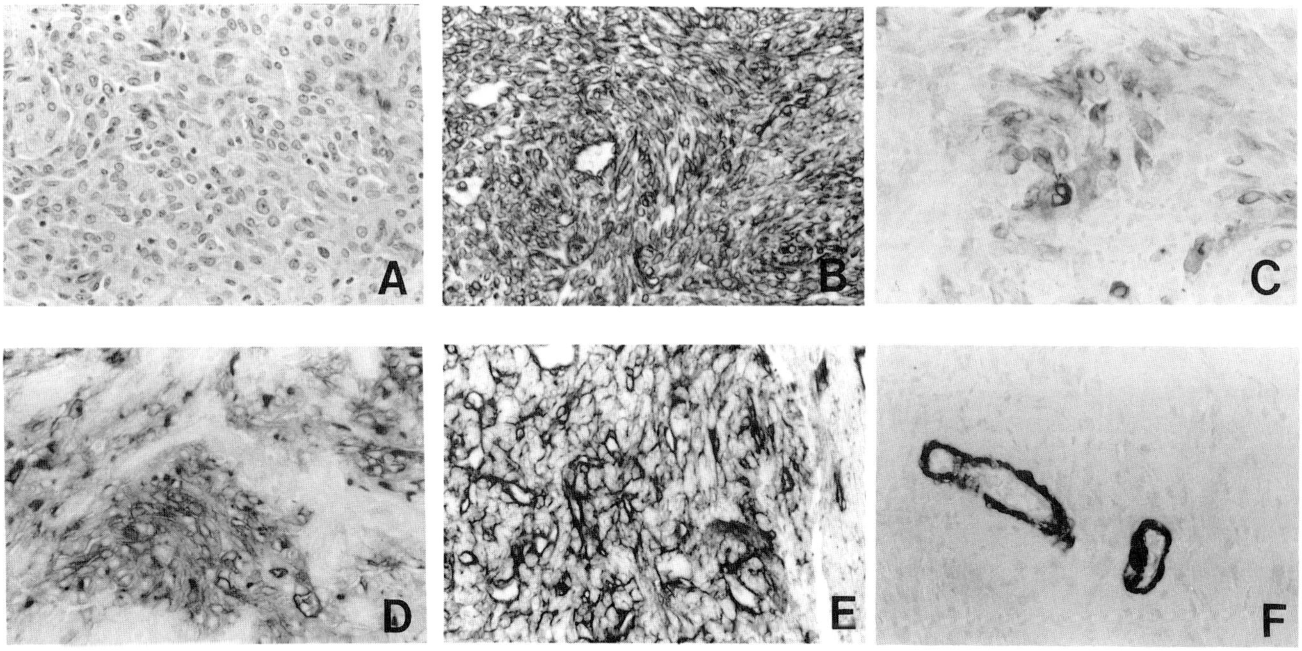

Fig. 2.16A-F. The cellular spindle cell tumour is shown in Fig. 2.16A. The tumour displays uniform expression of vimentin (B) and a characteristic, patchy expression of low molecular weight cytokeratin (C) and epithelial membrane antigen (D). There is also uniform expression of type IV collagen (E) while markers of smooth muscle differentiation were negative with good internal controls on the blood vessels within the tumour (F). (We thank Carlos E Bacchi, MD, for taking the photographs.)

Mesothelioma

This section concerns the differential diagnosis of the sarcomatoid mesothelioma and its morphological mimics. The differential diagnosis of epithelial mesothelioma, mixed mesothelioma, mesothelial hyperplasia and metastatic carcinoma is discussed in Chapter 3.

Serosal tissue is composed of at least two cell types: a surface mesothelial layer, as well as a more inapparent 'submesothelial stromal cell, which has been referred to by some as a 'multipotential subserosal cell' (MSC) (Bolen et al., 1986). In normal or resting serosal tissue, the surface mesothelium is strongly reactive with antibodies to low MW cytokeratin, and the MSC express only the intermediate filament protein, vimentin. However, in reactive mesothelium, e.g. following injury, in addition to the development of enlarged, more epithelial-looking, cytokeratin-positive mesothelial surface cells, there is a marked proliferation of the MSC, which acquire a unique phenotype of coexpression of both vimentin and low MW cytokeratins (Bolen et al., 1987). The latter authors hypothesize that the spectrum of cell appearances and phenotypes seen in mesotheliomas recapitulates this spectrum of cell phenotypes seen in normal and reactive mesothelium. Specifically, epithelial mesotheliomas resemble the surface mesothelium, and so-called 'mixed' and 'transitional' mesotheliomas resemble a combination of the surface mesothelium and the MSC (Bolen et al., 1987). There is a group of spindle cell tumours of the pleura, however, which can be characterized as 'sarcomatoid mesothelioma', and which may represent the malignant counterpart of the MSC. And while most mesotheliomas classically present with diffuse involvement of the pleura, some mesotheliomas present as pleural or diaphragmatic masses and invade the adjacent lung or mediastinum in pattern reminiscent of sarcoma. When the diagnosis of a purely spindle cell, or sarcomatoid, mesothelioma is being entertained, other potential spindle cell tumours involving the pleura must also be considered. Principal among this latter group are true sarcomas involving the pleura, spindle cell carcinomas, and the localized fibrous tumour of the pleura. Most investigators have found uniform coexpression of cytokeratin (predominantly low MW, e.g. cytokeratin 8) and vimentin in sarcomatoid mesotheliomas (Carter and Otis, 1988; Montag et al., 1988; Cagle, et al., 1989), generally in the absence of high MW cytokeratins, which are expressed in mesotheliomas manifesting epithelial differentiation. In contrast, sarcomas involving the pleura, e.g. malignant fibrous histiocytoma, angiosarcoma, fibrosarcoma etc., express only the intermediate filament protein, vimentin. While there are some primary sarcomas, e.g. leiomyosarcomas, which can coexpress vimentin and cytokeratin (see section above), a pattern of uniform, strong cytokeratin expression in a spindle cell tumour involving the pleura strongly favours the diagnosis of a mesothelial tumour. Less easily ruled out, however, is the alternative diagnosis of a spindle cell carcinoma, e.g. spindle cell squamous cell carcinoma of lung origin, or a metastasis from a carcinoma with a proclivity for coexpressing vimentin and cytokeratin and displaying a sarcomatoid phenotype (i.e. metastatic spindle cell carcinoma). No single, or even multiple, immunocytochemical studies can presently make this distinction with certainty; it is thus prudent to always consider the alternative diagnosis of metastatic spindle cell carcinoma in this context, which can often be ruled out on clinical grounds. Finally, the solitary fibrous tumour of the pleura, usually distinguished from sarcomatoid mesothelioma by the former's more benign appearance and localized behaviour, expresses only the intermediate filament, vimentin (Carter and Otis, 1988), and hence may be completely unrelated to the MSC. Caution should be exercised in interpreting all tumours, spindle or otherwise, involving the pleura, as reactive MSC can be present in abundance, sometimes obscuring the malignant cell population; as indicated above, these can be expected to be cytokeratin-positive (Bolen et al., 1987).

CASE 2.17: Spindle cell mesothelioma

A 72 year-old male with a long history of smoking and a distant history of asbestos exposure in conjunction with work at a naval shipyard 25 years earlier, presented with shortness of breath and a peripheral lung mass adjacent to, and involving, the pleura. The histology was that of a predominantly spindle cell tumour with marked cellular pleomorphism and individual tumour cells characterized by relatively abundant, highly eosinophilic cytoplasm (Fig. 2.17A). The principal differential diagnoses include spindle cell carcinoma, mesothelioma, and primary lung sarcoma such as malignant nerve sheath tumour.

The immunostaining profile is summarized in Table 2.11. The tumour cells uniformly expressed vimentin (Fig. 2.17B), and fairly uniformly expressed low MW cytokeratin (Fig. 2.17C), while only focally expressing high MW cytokeratin (Fig. 2.17D). There was no expression of muscle or nerve sheath markers (e.g. muscle actins, with good internal controls in the submesothelial stromal cell population (Fig. 2.17E), and the tumour cells did not express markers associated with adenocarcinoma such as carcinoembryonic antigen (CEA; Fig. 2.17F). These results strongly support the diagnosis of mesothelioma, spindle cell variant.

Table 2.11. Immunostaining results in spindle cell mesothelioma

	Vim	LMCK	HMCK	MA	Des	CEA	S100	NGF
SCCa	+/−	+	+/−	−	−	+/−	−	−
MNST	+	−	−	−	−	−	+	+
LMS	+	−/+	−	+	+	−	−	−
SCM	+	+	+/−	−	−	−	−	−
Case 2.17	+	+	+	−	−	−	−	−

Notes:
Vim = vimentin
MA = muscle actins (HHF35)
Des = desmin
LMCK = low molecular cytokeratin
CEA = carcinoembryonic antigen
S100 = S100 protein
HMCK = high molecular cytokeratin
NGF = nerve growth factor
SCCa = squamous cell carcinoma
LMS = leiomyosarcoma
MNST = malignant nerve sheath tumour
SCM = spindle cell mesothelioma

Carcinosarcoma

Carcinosarcoma, defined as a tumour containing both carcinomatous and sarcomatous elements, is best exemplified in the uterus, where it has a unique appellation: mixed Mullerian tumour (MMT). In its classical presentation, it is a high grade malignant tumour with a 'biphasic' histologic pattern (i.e. both epithelial and 'stromal' malignant components), one of which usually predominates. However, the relationship of these two different parts of the tumour to one another is not yet clear, despite many years of study. While originally there

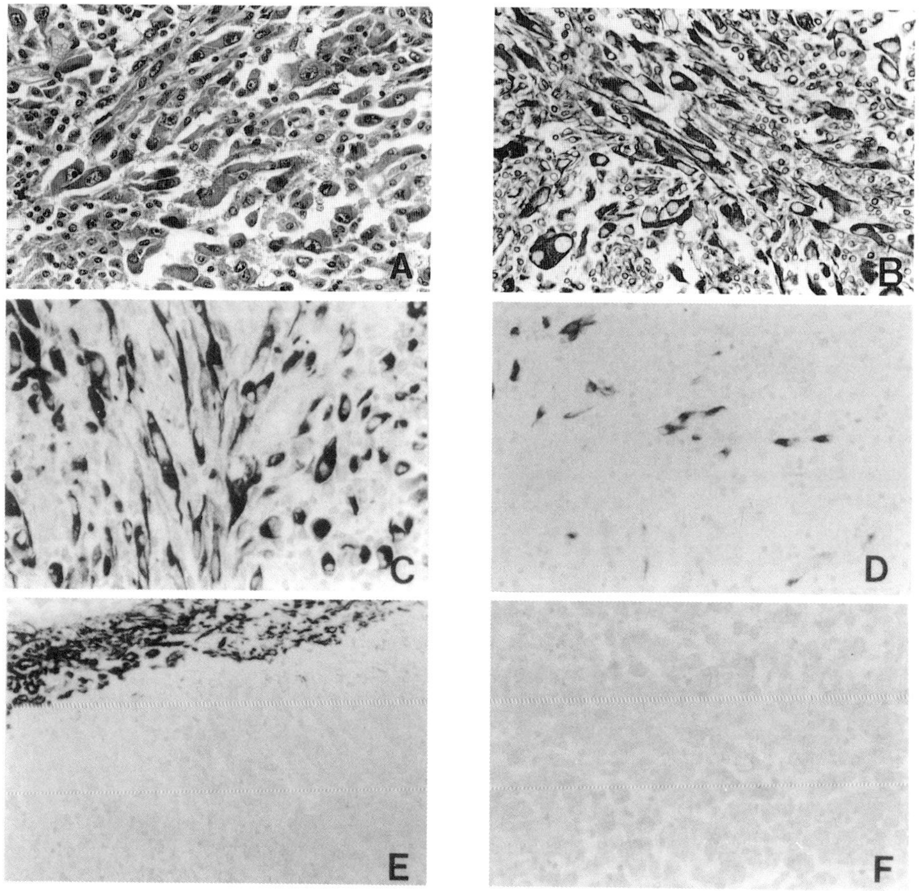

Fig. 2.17A-F. The spindle cell tumour shows marked cellular pleomorphism and relatively abundant, highly eosinophilic cytoplasm (A). There is uniform expression of vimentin (B), and fairly uniform expression of low molecular weight cytokeratin (C), while only focal expression of high molecular weight cytokeratin is seen (D). Staining for muscle and nerve sheath markers are negative and there are good internal controls in the submesothelial stromal cell population (E). The tumour cells are negative for carcinoembryonic antigen (F). (We thank Carlos E Bacchi, MD, for taking the photographs.)

was great attention focused onto the 'stromal' component, i.e. whether there was or was not heterologous differentiation, more recent studies have suggested that this plays no rule in determining clinical outcome (Costa et al., 1991). Furthermore, most recent studies have suggested that epithelial differentiation, as evidenced by expression of cytokeratin and/or epithelial membrane antigen, can be detected in the 'stromal' component of the tumour in virtually all cases (Costa et al., 1991; George et al., 1991). Many have thus concluded that the carcinomatous and sarcomatous components of MMT actually share a common origin, and it becomes problematic whether to consider MMT is a true 'carcinosarcoma' or merely a spindle cell, or metaplastic, carcinoma (Costa et al., 1991). Indeed, the clinical behaviour of MMT is more like that of a high grade carcinoma than a true uterine sarcoma (Zaludek and Norris, 1987). However, unlike 'metaplastic carcinomas', there do appear to be histologically distinct, and non-merging, components of the MMT, and there is the curious presence of 'heterologous differentiation' seen within the sarcomatous component in approximately one-third of the cases. This latter is most frequently skeletal muscle and can thus be identified using antibodies to muscle actin or desmin (Costa et al., 1991), although other types of sarcomas can be mimicked by this 'heterologous' zone, including malignant nerve sheath tumour (George et al., 1991), malignant fibrous histiocytoma (Auerbach et al., 1988), chondrosarcoma (George et al., 1991), etc. To further confuse the picture, coexpression of vimentin and cytokeratin is a feature both of the 'carcinomatous' and 'sarcomatous' components of the tumour. Thus the role of immunohistochemistry in identifying MMT is somewhat vague: while antibodies to low MW cytokeratin and vimentin can highlight the (probably) interrelated sarcomatous and carcinomatous areas, the same panel of antibodies useful in identifying specific sarcoma differentiation can be applied to identify, and study the nature of, the heterologous (sarcomatous) differentiation, although the clinical utility of such an exercise is questionable.

Carcinosarcomas have also been reported in other organs, e.g. the uterus, bladder, breast, lung, cervix, and larynx. In many of these tumours, e.g. carcinosarcoma of the lung, markers of epithelial differentiation (e.g. cytokeratin, CEA, or epithelial membrane antigen) are often (but not always) lacking from the sarcomatous areas (Ishida et al., 1990). In a recent study of prostatic carcinosarcomas, immunocytochemical evidence for epithelial differentiation within the sarcomatous component was absent from both studied cases (Wick et al., 1989). However, absolute discrimination between the possibility that this sarcomatous differentiation represents 'dedifferentiation' of the epithelial component versus an independent malignant component, cannot be ascertained by immunocytochemical studies of cellular differentiation, and must await molecular or chromosomal analyses.

Nodular fasciitis

Nodular fasciitis (NF) is a rapidly developing self-limited mesenchymal process that histologically can simulate the appearance of a sarcoma, owing to its cellularity and presence of mitotic figures. The nature of the cell population comprising this common process was first suggested to be myofibroblasts (Konwaler et al., 1955) with ultrastructural evidence to support this presented by Wirman (1976). Indeed, while there have been few published immunocytochemical studies, our unpublished data suggest that the distinctive feature of NF is the presence of a 'partial' smooth muscle phenotype characteristic of myofibroblasts (muscle and smooth muscle actin-positive, desmin-negative, with characteristic peripheral actin condensations in individual cells). A recent study of Montgomery and Meis (1991) confirmed the expression of muscle actin in 49/53 cases of MF, although these authors did not appreciate the characteristic pattern of actin expression which is so typical of this lesion, as well as other lesions composed of myofibroblasts, such as fibromatoses (Tsukada et al., 1987b).

CASE 2.18: Nodular Fasciitis

A 27 year-old male presented with a rapidly growing 1 cm subcutaneous mass on the back of his hand. Histologic examination of the tumour revealed a cellular spindle cell tumour with interlacing bundles of plump fibroblast-like cells in a somewhat myxoid stroma (Fig. 2.18A). The differential diagnosis includes fibrosarcoma, malignant fibrous histiocytoma, and nodular fasciitis. Results of the immunostaining panel are indicated in Table 2.12. The diagnostic hallmark of this tumour is the expression of a 'partial' smooth muscle phenotype, i.e. that of a myofibroblast, which includes the uniform expression of vimentin (Fig. 2.18B) and a characteristic expression of muscle actin at the periphery of the cells, yielding a 'tram track' appearance (Fig. 2.18C,D). Other markers of 'true' smooth muscle differentiation, e.g. desmin, were negative (Fig. 2.18E).

Table 2.12. Immunostaining results in nodular fasciitis

Antibodies to	Results
Vimentin	+
Muscle actins (HHF35)	+*
Desmin	−

Note: *with characteristic 'myofibroblast' pattern

Liposarcoma

After malignant fibrous histiocytoma, liposarcomas are the most common soft tissue tumours that occur in adults, with a proclivity for such sites as the inguinal region, thigh, and retroperitoneum. Of greatest potential confusion to pathologists is the protean histologic appearance of liposarcomas, ranging from a benign lipoma-like histology to a myxoid appearance not unlike other myxoid sarcomas, to a pleomorphic appearance not unlike that of MFH. Classically, four major histologic types of liposarcoma occur: the 'well-differentiated group', which includes the lipoma-like, sclerosing, inflammatory, and the 'dedifferentiated' subgroups; the myxoid liposarcoma; the round cell liposarcoma; and the pleomorphic liposarcoma. The myxoid liposarcoma displays a histologic pattern which might initially be confused with such other myxoid tumours as myxoma, myxoid MFH, and others,

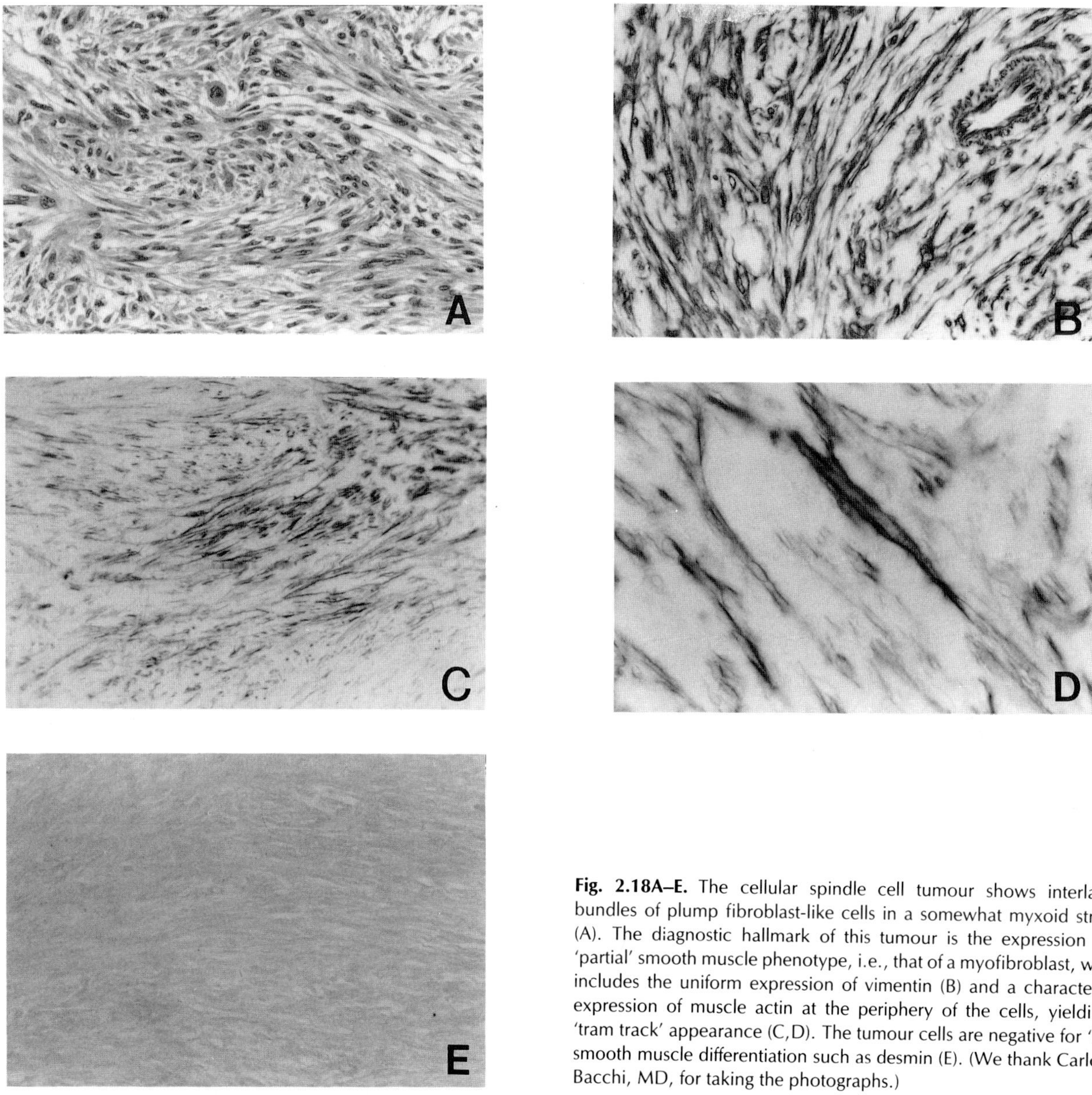

Fig. 2.18A–E. The cellular spindle cell tumour shows interlacing bundles of plump fibroblast-like cells in a somewhat myxoid stroma (A). The diagnostic hallmark of this tumour is the expression of a 'partial' smooth muscle phenotype, i.e., that of a myofibroblast, which includes the uniform expression of vimentin (B) and a characteristic expression of muscle actin at the periphery of the cells, yielding a 'tram track' appearance (C,D). The tumour cells are negative for 'true' smooth muscle differentiation such as desmin (E). (We thank Carlos E. Bacchi, MD, for taking the photographs.)

although it is usually characterized by the presence of lipoblasts, usually of the 'signet ring' variety. The identification of lipoblasts, however, can be problematic, and unfortunately these cells do not possess a characteristic or diagnostic immunophenotype. While several studies (Hashimoto et al., 1984; Andrion et al., 1991; Lopez-Gines et al., 1989) have suggested the utility of antibodies to S100 protein as a diagnostic aid in the identification of lipoblasts and liposarcoma, S100 is a widely expressed calcium binding protein, and can also be expressed by melanomas, chondrosarcomas, and malignant nerve sheath tumours, among others (Barwick, 1990). There may be more limited contexts, however, in which S100 expression may be helpful in rendering a diagnosis of myxoid liposarcoma, such as its distinction from two other 'myxoid' tumours: the myxoid variant of malignant fibrous histiocytoma (Hashimoto et al., 1984), and myxoma (Hashimoto et al., 1986b). However, the relationship between malignant fibrous histiocytoma and liposarcoma may be complex one, as evidenced by the so-called 'dedifferentiated' variant of liposarcoma, which can be histologically and immunocytochemically (Chan et al., 1987) indistinguishable from MFH. Furthermore, Iwasaki et al. (1987) generated monoclonal antibodies to MFH cells and recovered two, designated FU3 and FU4, which cross react, among soft tissue sarcomas tested, only with MFH and liposarcoma. None the less, there are few reports of liposarcoma-specific and -associated markers. Dekmezian et al. (1987) found apolipoprotein B in all 27 liposarcomas examined, but also in a small but significant subset of MFH, rhabdomyosarcomas, and MNST. Weiss et al. (1986), using biochemical as well as a relatively outmoded fluorescein-labelled steroid method of determination of estrogen receptor expression, found that, liposarcoma, among other soft tissue sarcomas, were receptor positive. None the less, there are no more recent studies using anti-ER antibodies, which might provide additional information. Preliminary studies in our laboratory also confirm that, along with malignant tumours of smooth muscle and nerve sheath, liposarcomas possess the ability to express the basement membrane protein, type IV collagen, which should not be surprising given the fact that adult adipocytes, along with Schwann cells and smooth muscle cells, are invested with a basal lamina (Greenwood and Johnson, 1983).

CASE 2.19: Myxoid liposarcoma

A 55 year-old female presented with a large (12 cm) retroperitoneal mass. Biopsy of the mass revealed a mildly pleomorphic, spindle cell tumour with a marked myxoid background (Fig. 2.19A). Mitotic figure count was 5 per 10 high powered fields. The differential diagnosis of myxoid spindle cell tumours can be large, and includes such processes as myxoma and myxoid variants of other sarcomas (e.g., MFH, leiomyosarcoma, chondrosarcoma, nerve sheath tumour, liposarcoma, etc.). No lipoblasts were evident upon initial examination of the tumour, and antibody studies were performed to look for specific differentiation. Results of these studies are summarized in Table 2.13. While 'generic' markers, such as antibodies to vimentin, were uniformly positive on the tumour cells, markers of smooth muscle, muscle actins (Fig. 2.19C), desmin or cartilaginous or nerve sheath (S100, nerve growth factor receptor) were negative. In addition, the tumour cells (along with the prominent vascular endothelium) did express the basement membrane protein, type IV collagen (Fig. 2.19B). Thus, the only distinguishing feature of this sarcoma is the expression of type IV collagen in the absence of muscle or nerve sheath differentiation; in this histologic context, these results favour the interpretation of this as a liposarcoma. Careful examination of other areas of the tumour revealed the presence of lipoblasts, supporting this diagnosis.

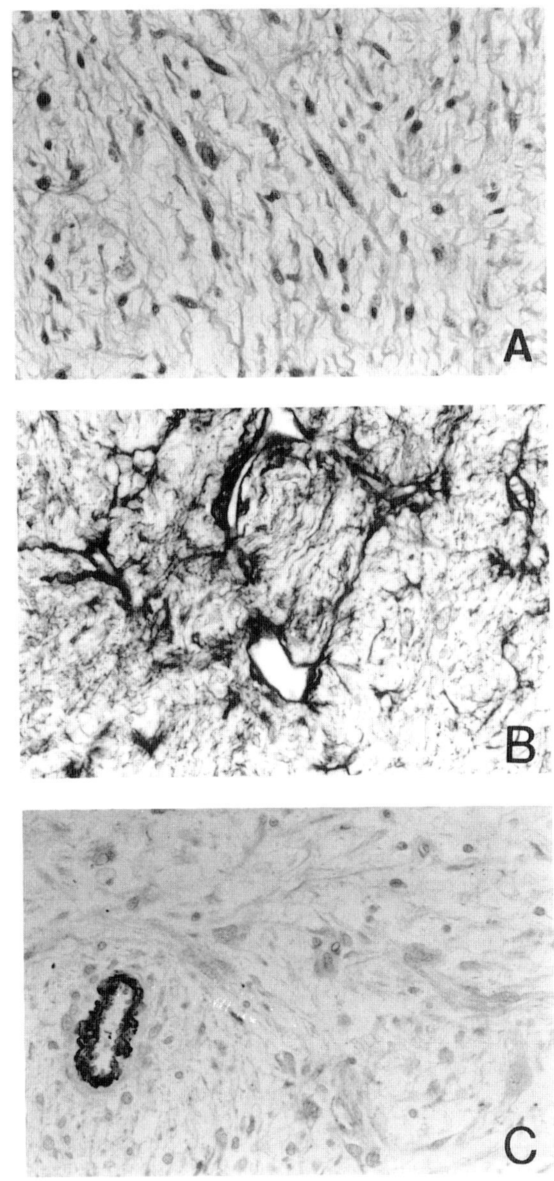

Fig. 2.19A–C. The mildly pleomorphic, spindle cell tumour shows a marked myxoid background with a mitotic count of 5 per 10 high power fields (A). 'Generic' markers such as antibodies to vimentin were uniformly positive on the tumour cells, whereas markers of smooth muscle such as desmin (C), cartilaginous or nerve sheath (S100, nerve growth factor receptor) were negative. The tumour cells express the basement membrane protein, type IV collagen (B). Careful examination of other areas of the tumour revealed the presence of lipoblasts supporting the diagnosis of myxoid liposarcoma. (We thank Carlos E. Bacchi, MD, for taking the photographs.)

Table 2.13. Immunostaining results in myxoid liposarcoma

	Vim	MA	S100	Des	NGF	Col IV
MNST	+	–	+	–	+	+
LMS	+	+	–	+	–	+
MLS	+	–	–	–	–	+
Case 2.19	+	–	–	–	–	+

Notes: Vim = vimentin
MA = muscle actins (HHF35)
Des = desmin
Col IV = collagen type IV
S100 = S100 protein
NGF = nerve growth factor
LMS = leiomyosarcoma
MNST = malignant nerve sheath tumour
MLS = myxoid liposarcoma

References

Achtstatter, T., Moll, R. and Anderson, A. (1986). Expression of glial filament protein (GFP) in nerve sheath and non-neural cells re-examined using monoclonal antibodies, with special emphasis on the coexpression GFP and cytokeratins in epithelial cells of human salivary gland and pleomorphic adenomas. *Differentiation* **31**, 206–77.

Aiba, M., Hirayama, A. and Kuramochi, S. (1988). Glomangiosarcoma in a glomus tumour: An immunohistochemical and ultrastructural study. *Cancer* **61**, 1467–71.

Alles, J.U., Bosslet, K. (1988). Immunocytochemistry of angiosarcomas. A study of 19 cases with special emphasis on the applicability of endothelial specific markers to routinely prepared tissues. *American Journal of Clinical Pathology* **89**, 463–71.

Altmannsberger, M., Weber, K. and Droste, R. (1985). Desmin is a specific marker for rhabdomyosarcomas of human and rat origin. *American Journal of Pathology* **111**, 85–95.

Andres, T.L. and Kadin, M.E. (1983). Immunologic markers in the differential diagnosis of small round cell tumours from lymphocytic lymphoma and leukaemia. *American Journal of Clinical Pathology* **79**, 546–52.

Andrion, A., Gaglio, A., Dogliani, N., Bosco, E. and Mazzucco, G. (1991). Liposarcoma of the thyroid gland. Fine needle aspiration cytology, immunohistology, and ultrastructure. *American Journal of Clinical Pathology* **95**, 675–9.

Angervall, L., Kindblom, L.G. and Karlsson, K. (1985). Atypical haemangio-endothelioma of venous origin. A clinicopathologic, angiographic, immunohistochemical, and ultrastructural study of two endothelial tumours within the concept of histiocytoid haemangioma. *American Journal of Surgical Pathology* **9**, 504–16.

Anthony, P.P. and Ramani, P. (1991). Endothelial markers in malignant vascular tumors of the liver: superiority of QB-END/10 over von Willebrand factor and Ulex europaeus agglutinin 1. *Journal of Clinical Pathology* **44**, 29–32.

Armin, A., Connelly, E.M. and Rowden, G. (1983). An immunoperoxidase investigation of S100 protein in granular cell myoblastomas: Evidence for Schwann cell derivation. *American Journal of Clinical Pathology* **79**, 37–44.

Auerbach, H.E., LiVolsi, V.A. and Merino, M.J. (1988). Malignant mixed Mullerian tumors of the uterus: an immunohistochemical study. *International Journal of Gynecology and Pathology* **7**, 123–30.

Axiotis, C.A., Merino, M.J. and Tsokos, M. (1990). Epithelioid malignant peripheral nerve sheath tumour with squamous differentiation: A light microscopic, ultrastructural, and immunohistochemical study. *Surgical Pathology* **3**, 301–8.

Barwick, K.W. (1990) S-100 protein. In True, L.D. (ed.) *Atlas of Diagnostic Immunohistopathology*, J.B. Lippincott, Philadelphia, pp. 12.1–12.20.

Battifora, H. (1987). Diagnostic uses of antibodies to keratins. A review and immunohistochemical comparison of seven monoclonal and three polyclonal antibodies. In Fenoglio, C., Wolff, M. and Rilke, F.E. (eds) *Progress in Surgical Pathology*, Masson Publishing, New York, pp. 1–17.

Battifora, H. (1991) Assessment of antigen damage in immunohistochemistry. The vimentin internal control. *American Journal of Clinical Pathology* **96**, 669–71.

Baudier, J., Glasser, N. and Gerard, D. (1986). Ions binding to S100 proteins. *Journal of Biology and Chemistry* **261**, 8192–203.

Bonetti, F., Colombari, R. and Manfrin, E. (1989). Breast carcinoma with positive results for melanoma marker (HMB-45). HMB-45 immunoreactivity in normal and neoplastic breast. *American Journal of Clinical Pathology* **92**, 491–5.

Beckstead, J.H., Wood, G.S. and Fletcher, V. (1985). Evidence for the origin of Kaposi's sarcoma from lymphatic endothelium. *American Journal of Pathology* **119**, 294–300.

Bolen, J.W., Hammar, S.P. and McNutt, M.A. (1986). Reactive and neoplastic serosal tissue. A light microscopic, ultrastructural, and immunocytochemical study. *American Journal of Surgical Pathology* **10**, 34–47.

Bolen, J.W., Hammar, S.P. and McNutt, M.A. (1987). Serosal tissue: reactive tissue as a model for understanding mesotheliomas. *Ultrastructural Pathology* **11**, 251–262.

Borowitz, M.J., Stevanovic, G. and Gottfried, M. (1984). Differential diagnosis of undifferentiated malignant tumours with monoclonal antibody T29/33. *Human Pathology* **15**, 928–34.

Brooks, J.J., Miettinen, M. and Virtanen, I. (1987). Desmin immunoreactivity in glomus tumours. *American Journal of Clinical Pathology* **82**, 292–3.

Burgdorf, W.H., Mukai, K. and Rosai, J. (1981). Immunohistochemical identification of factor VIII-related antigen in endothelial cells of cutaneous lesions of alleged vascular nature. *American Journal of Clinical Pathology* **75**, 167–71.

Cagle, P.T., Truong, L.D. and Roggli, V.L. (1989). Immunohistochemical differentiation of sarcomatoid mesotheliomas from other spindle cell neoplasms. *American Journal of Clinical Pathology* **92**, 566–71.

Callihan, T.R. and Coston, W.B. (1982). Childhood non-Hodgkin's lymphomas in current histological perspectives. *Perspectives in Paediatric Pathology* **7**, 259–77.

Carlie, F., Polak, J.M. and Ceccamea, A. (1984). Neuronal and glial markers in tumours of neuroblastic origin. *Virchows Archives (Pathologic Anatomy)* **404**, 313–24.

Carter, D. and Otis, C.N. (1988). Three types of spindle cell tumors of the pleura. Fibroma, sarcoma, and sarcomatoid mesothelioma. *American Journal of Surgical Pathology* **12**, 747–53.

Carter, R.L., Jameson, C.F. and Philp, E.R. (1990). Comparative phenotypes in rhabdomyosarcomas and developing skeletal muscle. *Histopathology* **17**, 301–09.

Cavazzana, A.O., Miser, J.S. and Jefferson, J. (1987). Experimental evidence for a neural origin of Ewing's sarcoma of bone. *American Journal of Pathology* **127**, 507–18.

Chan, Y.F., Yuen, M.Y. and Ma, L.T. (1987). Recurrent dedifferentiated liposarcoma of the spermatic cord simulating malignant fibrous histiocytoma: an immunohistochemical and ultrastructural study. *Pathology* **19**, 99–102.

Chang, T., Li, C. and Smithson, W.A. (1989). Immunocytochemical study of small round cell tumours in routinely processed specimens. *Archives of Pathology and Laboratory Medicine* **113**, 1343–8.

Chott, A., Kaserer, K. and Augustin, I. (1990). Ki-1-positive large cell lymphoma. A clinicopathologic study of 41 cases. *American Journal of Surgical Pathology* **14**, 439–48.

Christ, M.L. and Ozzello, L. (1971). Myogenous origin of a granular cell tumour of the urinary bladder. *American Journal of Clinical Pathology* **56**, 736–49.

Christensen, W.N., Strong, E.W. and Bains, M.S. (1988). Neuroendocrine differentiation in the glandular peripheral nerve sheath tumor. Pathologic distinction from the biphasic synovial sarcoma with glands. *American Journal of Surgical Pathology* **12**, 417–26.

Coindre, J.-M., DeMascarel, A. and Trojani, M. (1988). Immunohistochemical study of rhabdomyosarcoma. Unexpected staining with S100 protein and cytokeratin. *Journal of Pathology* **155**, 127–32.

Cooper, D., Schermer, A. and Sun, T.T. (1985). Classification of human epithelia and their neoplasms using monoclonal antibodies to keratins: Strategies, applications and limitation. *Laboratory Investigation* **52**, 243–56.

Corson, J.M., Weiss, L.M. and Banks-Schlegel, S.P. (1984). Keratin proteins and carcinoembryonic antigen in synovial sarcomas: an immunohistochemical study of 24 cases. *Human Pathology* **15**, 615–21.

Costa, M.J., Khan, R. and Judd, R. (1991). Carcinosarcoma (malignant mixed mullerian [mesodermal] tumor) of the uterus and ovary: correlation of clinical, pathologic, and immunohistochemical features in 29 cases. *Archives of Pathologic Laboratory Medicine* **115**, 583–90.

de Mascavel, I., Trojani, M. and Eghbali, H. (1990). Prognostic value of phenotyping by BERH2, Leu-M1, EMA in Hodgkin's disease. *Archives of Pathology and Laboratory Medicine* **114**, 953–5.

Debus, E., Moll, R. and Franke, W.W. (1984). Immunohistochemical distinction of human carcinomas by cytokeratin typing with monoclonal antibodies. *American Journal of Pathology* **114**, 121–30.

Dehner, L.P. (1986). Peripheral and central primitive neuroectodermal tumours. A nosologic concept seeking a consensus. *Archives of Pathology and Laboratory Medicine* **110**, 997–1005.

Dekmezian, R., Zaatari, G.S., Austin, G.E. (1987). Immunohistochemical staining for apolipoprotein B in human sarcomas. *Archives of Pathology and Laboratory Medicine* **111**, 433–5.

Denk, H., Krepler, R. and Artlieb, U. (1983). Proteins of intermediate filaments – an immunohistochemical and biochemical approach to the classification of soft tissue tumours. *American Journal of Pathology* **110**, 193–208.

Dervan, P.A., Cahalane, S.F. and Kneafsey, P. (1987). Malignant rhabdoid tumour of soft tissue. An ultrastructural and immunohistochemical study of a pelvic tumour. *Histopathology* **11**, 183–90.

Dervan, P.A., Tobbia, I.N. and Casey, M. (1989). Glomus tumours: an immunohistochemical profile of 11 cases. *Histopathology* **14**, 483–91.

DeSchryver-Kecskemeti, K., Kraus, F.T. and Engleman, W. (1982). Alveolar soft part sarcoma – a malignant angioreninoma. Histochemical, immunocytochemical, and electron microscopic study of four cases. *American Journal of Surgical Pathology* **6**, 5–18.

DeVita, V.T., Hubbard, S. and Young, R.C. (1988). The role of chemotherapy in diffuse aggressive lymphomas. *Seminars in Haematology* **25**(Suppl. 2), 2–10.

Dhillon, A.P. and Rode, J. (1982). Patterns of staining for neuron-specific enolase in benign and malignant melanocytic lesions of the skin. *Diagnostic Histopathology*, **5**, 169–74.

Diamaru, Y., Hashimoto, H. and Enjoji, M. (1985). Malignant peripheral nerve sheath tumours (malignant schwannomas). An immunohistochemical study of 29 cases. *American Journal of Surgical Pathology* **9**, 434–44.

Drier, J.K., Swanson, P.E. and Cherwitz, D.L. (1987). S100 protein immunoreactivity in poorly differentiated carcinomas: Immunohistochemical comparison with malignant melanoma. *Archives of Pathology and Laboratory Medicine* **111**, 447–52.

Enzinger, F.M. (1970). Epithelioid sarcoma. A sarcoma simulating a granuloma or a carcinoma. *Cancer* **26**, 1029–41.

Enzinger, F.M. and Weiss, S.W. (1988). *Soft Tissue Tumors*, C.V. Mosby, St Louis, pp. 269–300, 422–32.

Epstein, A.L., Marder, R.J. and Winter, J.N. (1984). Two new monoclonal antibodies (LN1, LN2) reactive in B5 formalin-fixed, paraffin-embedded tissues with follicular centre and mantle zone human B lymphocytes and derived tumours. *Journal of Immunology* **133**, 1028–34.

Eusebi, V., Ceccarelli, C. and Gorza, L. (1986). Immunohistochemistry of rhabdomyosarcoma. The use of four different markers. *American Journal of Surgical Pathology* **10**, 293–9.

Ewing, J. (1921). Diffuse endothelioma of bone. *Proceedings of New York Pathology Society* **21**, 17–24.

Fields, K.L. and Yen, S.H. (1985). A subset of Schwann cells in peripheral nerves contained in 50-Kilodalton protein antigenically related to astrocyte intermediate filaments. *Journal of Neural Immunology* **8**, 311–30.

Fisher, C. (1988). Epithelioid sarcoma: The spectrum of ultrastructural differentiation in seven immunohistochemically defined cases. *Human Pathology* **19**, 265–75.

Fletcher, C.D., Beham, A. and Schmidt, C. (1991). Spindle cell haemangioendothelioma: A clinicopathological and immunohistochemical study indicative of a non-neoplastic lesion. *Histopathology* **18**, 291–301.

Forbes, I.J. and Leong, A.S-Y. (1987) *Essential Oncology of the Lymphocyte* Springer-Verlag, London.

Franke, W.W., Schmid, E. and Mittmacht, S. (1984). Integration of different keratins into the same filament system after micro-injection of mRNA for epidermal keratins into kidney epithelial cells. *Journal Cell* **36**, 813–25.

Gansler, T., Gerald, W. and Anderson, G. (1991). Characterization of a cell line derived from rhabdoid tumour of kidney. *Human Pathology* **22**, 259–66.

Gatter, K.C., Alcock, C. and Heryet, A. (1984). The differential diagnosis of routinely processed anaplastic tumours using monoclonal antibodies. *American Journal of Clinical Pathology* **82**, 33–43.

Gatter, K.C., Dunhill, M.S. and van Murjen, G.N.P. (1986). Human lung tumours may coexpress different classes of intermediate filaments. *Journal of Clinical Pathology* **39**, 950–56.

George, E., Manivel, J.C. and Dehner, L.P. (1991). Malignant mixed mullerian tumors: an immunohistochemical study of 47 cases, with histogenetic considerations and clinical correlation. *Human Pathology* **22**, 215–23.

Giangaspero, F., Fratamico, F.C. and Ceccarelli, C. (1989). Malignant peripheral nerve sheath tumors and spindle cell sarcomas: an immunohistochemical analysis of multiple markers. *Applied Pathology* **7**, 134–44.

Goldman, J.E., Shaumberg, H.H. and Norton, W.T. (1978). Isolation and characterization of glial filaments from human brain. *Journal of Cell Biology* **78**, 426–40.

Gonzalez-Crussi, F., Goldsmidt, R.A. and Hsueh, W. (1982). Infantile sarcoma with intracytoplasmic filamentous inclusions. *Cancer* **49**, 2365–75.

Goodman, T.F. and Abele, D.C. (1971). Multiple glomus tumours: A clinical and electron microscopic study. *Archives of Dermatology* **103**, 11–23.

Gould, V.E. (1986). Histogenesis and differentiation. A reevaluation of these concepts as criteria for the classification of tumours. *Human Pathology* **17**, 212–17.

Gould, V.E., Moll, R. and Moll, I. (1986). The intermediate filament complement of the spectrum of nerve sheath neoplasms. *Laboratory Investigation* **55**, 463–74.

Gould, V.E., Jansson, D.S. and Molenaar, W.M. (1990a). Primitive neuroectodermal tumours of the central nervous system. Patterns of expression of neuroendocrine markers, and all classes of intermediate filament proteins. *Laboratory Investigation* **62**, 498–509.

Gould, V.E., Rorke, L.B. and Jansson, D.S. (1990b). Primitive neuroectodermal tumours of the central nervous system express neuroendocrine markers and may express all classes of intermediate filaments. *Human Pathology* **21**, 245–52.

Gown, A.M. and Vogel, A.M. (1984). Monoclonal antibodies to human intermediate filament proteins. II. Distribution of filament proteins in normal human tissues. *American Journal of Pathology* **114**, 309–21.

Gown, A.M. and Vogel, A.M. (1985). Monoclonal antibodies to human intermediate filament proteins. III. Analysis of tumours. *American Journal of Clinical Pathology* **84**, 413–24.

Gown, A.M., Vogel, A.M. and Gordon, D. (1985). A smooth muscle-specific monoclonal antibody recognizes smooth muscle actin isoenzyme. *Journal of Cell Biology* **100**, 807–13.

Gown, A.M., Vogel, A.M. and Hoak, D. (1986). Monoclonal antibodies specific for melanocytic tumours distinguish subpopulations of melanocytes. *American Journal of Pathology* **123**, 195–203.

Gown, A.M., Boyd, H.C. and Chang, Y. (1988). Smooth muscle cells can express cytokeratins of 'simple' epithelium: immunocytochemical and biochemical studies in vitro and in vivo. *American Journal of Pathology* **132**, 223–32.

Gray, M.H., Rosenberg, A.E. and Dickersin, G.R. (1989). Glial fibrillary acidic protein and keratin expression by benign and malignant nerve sheath tumors. *Human Pathology* **20**, 1089–96.

Gray, M.H., Rosenberg, A.E. and Dickersin, G.R. (1990).

Cytokeratin expression in epithelioid vascular neoplasms. *Human Pathology* **21**, 212–17.

Gray, M.H., Trimble, C.L. and Zim, J. (1991). Relationship of factor XIIIa-positive dermal dendrocytes to Kaposi's sarcoma. *Archives of Pathologic Laboratory Medicine* **115**, 791–6.

Greco, M.A., Steiner, G.C. and Fazzini, E. (1988). Ewing's sarcoma with epithelial differentiation: Fine structural and immunocytochemical study. *Ultrastructural Pathology* **12**, 317–26.

Greenwood, M.R.C. and Johnson, P.R. (1983). The adipose tissue. In Weiss, L. (ed.), *Histology: Cell and Tissue Biology*, Elsevier Biomedical, New York, pp. 178–199.

Guarda, L.G., Silva, E.G. and Ordonez, N.G. (1981). Factor VIII in Kaposi's sarcoma. *American Journal of Clinical Pathology* **76**, 197–200.

Guarda, L.A., Ordonez, N.G. and Smith, J.L. (1982). Immunoperoxidase localization of factor VIII in angiosarcomas. *Archives of Pathology and Laboratory Medicine* **106**, 515–16.

Haas, J.E., Palmer, N.F. and Weinberg, A.G. (1981). Ultrastructure of malignant rhabdoid tumour of the kidney. *Human Pathology* **12**, 646–57.

Haimoto, H., Takahashi, Y. and Koshikawa, T. (1985). Immunohistochemical localization of gamma-enolase in normal human tissues of non-nervous and non-neuroendocrine systems. *Laboratory Investigation* **52**, 257–61.

Hall, P.A., D'Ardenne, A.J. and Butler, M.G. (1987). New marker of B lymphocytes. MB2: Comparison with other lymphocyte subset markers active in conventional processed tissue sections. *Journal of Clinical Pathology* **49**, 151–6.

Harris, M.D., Moore, I.E. and Stewart, P.V. (1990). Protein gene product (PGP) 9.5 as a reliable marker in primitive neuroectodermal tumours – an immunohistochemical study of 21 childhood cases. *Histopathology* **16**, 271–7.

Hashimoto, H., Daimaru, Y. and Enjoji, M. (1984). S-100 protein distribution in liposarcoma. An immunoperoxidase study with special references to the distinction of liposarcoma from myxoid malignant fibrous histiocytoma. *Virchows Archives [A]* **405**, 1–10.

Hashimoto, H., Daimaru, Y. and Tsuneyoshi, M. (1986a). Leiomyosarcoma of the external soft tissues. *Cancer* **57**, 2077.

Hashimoto, H., Tsuneyoshi, M. and Daimaru, Y. (1986b). Enjoji M, Shinohara N. Intramusclear myxoma. A clinicopathologic, immunohistochemical, and electron microscopic study. *Cancer* **58**, 740–47.

Hashimoto, H., Mueller, H. and Falk, S. (1987). Histogenesis of Kaposi's sarcoma associated with AIDS: a histologic, immunohistochemical and enzyme histochemical study. *Pathologic Research and Practice* **182**, 658–68.

Hayashi, K., Takahashi, K. and Sonobe, H. (1987). The distribution of alpha and beta subunits of S-100 protein in malignant schwnnomas arising from neurofibromatosis of von Recklinghausen's disease. *Virchows Archives (A)* **411**, 515–21.

Hersey, P. (1985). Review of melanoma antigens recognised by monoclonal antibodies. Their functional significance and applications in diagnosis and treatment of melanoma. *Pathology* **17**, 346–54.

Hirose, T., Sano, T. and Hizawa, K. (1988). Heterogeneity of malignant schwannomas. *Ultrastructural Pathology* **12**, 107–16.

Hirose, T., Kudo, E. and Hasegawa, T. (1989). Expression of intermediate filament proteins in malignant fibrous histiocytomas. *Human Pathology* **20**, 871–77.

Hirose, T., Kudo, E. and Hasegawa, T. (1990). Cytoskeletal properties of alveolar soft part sarcoma. *Human Pathology* **21**, 204–11.

Hoffman, M.A. and Dickersin, G.R. (1983). Malignant fibrous histiocytoma: an ultrastructural study. *Human Pathology* **14**, 913–22.

Holden, C.A. (1989). Histogenesis of Kaposi's sarcoma and angiosarcoma of the face and the scalp. *Journal of Investigative Dermatology* **93** (Suppl 2), 119S–24S.

Hsu, S.M. and Jaffe, E.S. (1984). LeuM1 and peanut agglutinin stain the neoplastic cells of Hodgkin's disease. *American Journal of Clinical Pathology* **82**, 29–32.

Huitfeldt, H.S. and Brandtzaeg, P. (1985). Various keratin antibodies produce immunohistochemical staining of human myocardium and myometrium. *Histochemistry* **83**, 381–89.

Ingram, D.I., Mossler, J.A. and Snowhite, J. (1984). Granular cell tumours of the breast. Steroid receptor analysis and localization of carcino-embryonic antigen, myoglobin and S100 protein. *Archives of Pathology and Laboratory Medicine* **108**, 897–901.

Ishida, T., Tateishi, M. and Kaneko, S. (1990). Carcinosarcoma and spindle cell carcinoma of the lung: clinicopathologic and immunohistochemical studies. *Journal of Thoracic and Cardiovascular Surgery* **100**, 844–52.

Iwasaki, H., Isayama, T., Johzaki, H. and Kikuchi, M. (1987). Malignant fibrous histiocytoma. Evidence of perivascular mesenchymal cell origin immunocytochemical studies with monoclonal anti-MFH antibodies. *American Journal of Pathology* **128**, 528–37.

Jackson, P. and Thompson, R.J. (1981). The demonstration of new human brain-specific proteins by high resolution two-dimensional polyacrimide gel electrophoresis. *Journal of Neurological Science* **49**, 429–38.

Jaffe, R., Santamaria, M. and Yunis, E.J. (1984). The neuroectodermal tumour of bone. *American Journal of Surgical Pathology* **8**, 885–98.

James, C.L. and Leong, A.S-Y. (1989). Epithelioid leiomyosarcoma of the left atrium: Immunohistochemical and ultrastructural findings. *Pathology* **21**, 308–13.

Johnson, T.L., Lee, M.W. and Meis, J.M. (1991). Immunohistochemical characterization of malignant peripheral nerve sheath tumours. *Surgical Pathology* **4**, 121–35.

Jones, H., Steart, P.V. and du Bouley, C.E.H. (1990) Alpha smooth muscle actin as a marker for soft tissue tumours: a comparison with desmin. *Journal of Pathology* **162**, 29–33.

Kahn, H.J., Marks, A. and Thom, H. (1983). Role of antibody to S100 protein in diagnostic pathology. *American Journal of Clinical Pathology* **79**, 341–7.

Kaposi, M. (1872). Idiopathisches multiples Pigmentsarkom der Haut. *Archives of Dermatology and Syphilis* **4**, 265.

Kasantikul, V. and Shuangshoti, S. (1989). Positivity to glial fibrillary acetic protein in bone, cartilage, and chordoma. *Journal of Surgical Oncology* **41**, 22–6.

Kawaguchi, K. and Koike, M. (1986). Neuron-specific enolase and Leu7 immunoreactive small round cell neoplasm. The relationship to Ewing's sarcoma in bone and soft tissue. *American Journal of Clinical Pathology* **86**, 79–83.

Kjeldsberg, C.R., Wilson, J.F. and Berard, C.W. (1983). Non-Hodgkin's lymphoma in children. *Human Pathology* **14**, 612–27.

Knox, L.C. (1936). Synovial sarcoma: Report of three cases. *American Journal of Cancer* **28**, 461.

Kodet, R., Newton, W.A. and Hamoudi, A.B. (1991). Rhabdomyosarcomas with intermediate filament inclusions and features of rhabdoid tumours. Light microscopic and immunohistochemical study. *American Journal of Surgical Pathology* **15**, 257–67.

Konwaler, B.E., Keasbey, L. and Kaplan, L. (1955). Subcutaneous pseudosarcomatous fibromatosis (fasciitis). Report of 8 cases. *American Journal of Clinical Pathology* **25**, 241.

Kruse, J., Mailhammer, R. and Wernecke, H., (1984). Neural cell adhesion molecules and myelin-associated glycoprotein share a common carbohydrate moiety recognized by monoclonal antibodies L2 and HNK-1. *Nature* **311**, 153–5.

Kurtin, P.J. and Pinkus, G.S. (1985). Leucocyte common antigen – a diagnostic discriminant between haematopoietic and non-haematopoietic neoplasms in paraffin sections using monoclonal antibodies. *Human Pathology* **16**, 353–8.

Laskin, W.B., Weiss, S.W. and Bratthauer, G.L. (1991). Epithelioid variant of malignant peripheral nerve sheath tumour (malignant epithelioid schwannoma). *American Journal of Surgical Pathology* **15**, 1136–45.

Lawson, C. W., Fisher, C. and Gatter, K.C. (1987). An immunohistochemical study of differentiation in malignant fibrous histiocytoma. *Histopathology* **11**, 375–83.

Leong, A.S-Y., Phillips, G.E. and Pieterse, A.S. (1986). Criteria for the diagnosis of primary endocrine carcinoma of the skin (Merkel cell carcinoma). A histological, immunohistochemical and ultrastructural study of 13 cases. *Pathology* **18**, 393–9.

Leong, A.S-Y. and Wright, J. (1987). The contributions of immunohistochemical staining in tumour diagnosis. *Histopathology* **11**, 1295–305.

Leong, A.S-Y. and Milios, J. (1989). An assessment of a melanoma-specific antibody (HMB45) and other immunohistochemical markers of malignant melanoma in paraffin-embedded tissues. *Surgical Pathology* **2**, 137–45.

Leong, A.S-Y., Milios, J. and Duncis, C.G. (1988). Antigen preservation in microwave-irradiated tissues. A comparison with routine formalin fixation. *Journal of Pathology* **156**, 275–82.

Leong, A.S-Y. and Gilham, P.N. (1989a). The effects of progressive formaldehyde fixation on the preservation of tissue antigens. *Pathology* **21**, 266–8.

Leong, A.S-Y. and Gilham, P.N. (1989b). A new, rapid, microwave-stimulated method of staining melanocytic lesions. *Stain Technology* **64**, 81–5.

Leong, A.S-Y., Kan, A.E. and Milios, J. (1989). Small round cell tumours in childhood: Immunohistochemical studies in rhabdomyosarcoma, neuroblastoma, Ewing's sarcoma, and lymphoblastic lymphoma. *Surgical Pathology* **2**, 5–17.

Leong, A.S-Y. and Wannakrairot, P. (1992). A retrospective analysis of immunohistochemical staining in identification of anaplastic round cell and spindle cell tumours – results, reagents and costs. *Pathology*, **24** (5), 254–60.

Leung, I.K., Mani, R.S. and Kay, C.M. (1986). Isolation, characterization and metal-ion-binding properties of the alpha subunit from S100a protein. *Biochemical Journal* **237**, 757–64.

Liao, S.Y. and Choi, B.H. (1986). Expression of glial fibrillary acetic protein by neoplastic cells or Müllerian origin. *Virchows Archives (B)* **52**, 185–93.

Lifschitz, M.S., Flotte, T.J. and Greco, A. (1984). Congenital granular cell epulis. Immunohistochemical and ultrastructural observations. *Cancer*, **53**, 1845–8.

Little, D., Said, J.W. and Siegel, R.J. (1986). Endothelial cell markers in vascular neoplasms: an immunohistochemical study comparing factor VIII-related antigen, blood group specific antigens, 6-keto-PGF1 alpha, and Ulex europaeus 1 lection. *Journal of Pathology* **149**, 89–95.

Lizard-Nacol, S., Lizard, G. and Justrabo, E. (1989). Immunologic characterization of Ewing's sarcoma using mesenchymal and neural markers. *American Journal of Pathology* **135**, 847–55.

Llombart-Bosch, A., Terrier-Lacombe, M.J. and Peydro-Olaya, A. (1989). Peripheral neuroectodermal sarcoma of soft tissue (peripheral neuroepithelioma): A pathologic study of 10 cases with differential diagnosis regarding other small, round-cell sarcomas. *Human Pathology* **20**, 273–80.

Lodding, P., Kindblom, L. and Angervall, L. (1986). Epithelioid malignant schwannoma. A study of 14 cases. *Virchows Archives (Pathologic Anatomy)* 433–51.

Lopez-Gines, C., Navarro, S. and Peydro-Olaya, A. (1989). Malignant myxoid liposarcoma: an immunohistochemical, electron-microscopical and cytogenetical analysis. *Applied Pathology* **7**, 285–93.

Lothar, J., Fouquet, B. and Rohe, K. (1987). Cytokeratins in certain endothelial and smooth muscle cells of two taxonomically distant vertebrate species, xenopus laevis and man. *Differentiation* **36**, 234–54.

Mackay, B. and Ordonez, N.G. (1987). Adult neuroblastoma of bone. A case report. *Ultrastructural Pathology* **11**, 455–64.

Magin, T.M., Jorcano, J.I. and Franke, W.W. (1983). Translation products of mRNA coding for non-epidermal cytokeratins. *EMBO 2*, 1387–92.

Manivel, J.C., Wick, M.R. and Dehner, L.P. (1987). Epithelioid sarcoma: An immunohistochemical study. *American Journal of Clinical Pathology* **87**, 319–26.

Mazur, M.T., Shultz, J.J. and Myers, J.L. (1990). Granular cell tumour – immunohistochemical analysis of 21 benign and one malignant tumours. *Archives of Pathology and Laboratory Medicine* **114**, 692–6.

Meis, J.M., Mackay, B. and Ordonez, N.G. (1988). Epithelioid sarcoma: An immunohistochemical and ultrastructural study. *Surgical Pathology* **1**, 13–31.

Memoli, V.A., Brown, E.F. and Gould, V.E. (1984). Glial fibrillary acetic protein (GFAP) immunoreactivity in peripheral nerve sheath tumours. *Ultrastructural Pathology* **7**, 269–75.

Michetti, F., Levene, A. and Levene, M.M. (1983). The value of S100 immunostaining as a diagnostic tool in human malignant melanomas: A comparative study using S100 and neuron-specific enolase antibodies. *Virchows Archives (Pathology and Anatomy)* **400**, 331–46.

Mierau, G.W. (1985). Extraskeletal Ewing's sarcoma (peripheral neuroepithelioma). *Ultrastructural Pathology* **9**, 91–8.

Mierau, G.W., Berry, P.J. and Orsini, E.N. (1985). Small round cell neoplasms: Can electron microscopy and immunohistochemical studies accurately classify them? *Ultrastructural Pathology* **9**, 99–111.

Miettinen, M. (1988a). Antibody specific to muscle actins in the diagnosis and classification of soft tissue tumors. *American Journal of Pathology* **130**, 205–15.

Miettinen, M. (1988b). Immunoreactivity for cytokeratin and epithelial membrane antigen in leiomyosarcoma. *Archives of Pathologic Laboratory and Medicine* **112**, 637–40.

Miettinen, M. (1991). Keratin subsets in spindle cell sarcomas. Keratins are widespread but synovial sarcoma contains a distinctive keratin polypeptide pattern and desmoplakins. *American Journal of Pathology* **138**, 505–13.

Miettinen, M., Lehto, V.P. and Badley, R.A. (1982a). Expression of intermediate filaments in soft-tissue sarcomas. *International Journal of Cancer* **30**, 541–6.

Miettinen, M., Lehto, V.P. and Virtanen, I. (1982b). Keratin in the epithelial-like cells of classical biphasic synovial sarcoma. *Virchows Archives (B)* **40**, 157.

Miettinen, M., Foidart, J.-M. and Ekblom, P. (1983a). Immunohistochemical demonstration of laminin, the major glycoprotein of basement membranes, as an aid in the diagnosis of soft tissue tumors. *American Journal of Clinical Pathology* **79**, 306–11.

Miettinen, M., Holhofer, H. and Lehto, V.-P. (1983b). Ulex europaeus I lectin as a marker for tumors derived from endothelial cells. *American Journal of Clinical Pathology* **79**, 32–6.

Miettinen, M. and Lehto, V.P. (1984). Synovial sarcoma – a misnomer. *American Journal of Pathology* **117**, 18.

Miettinen, M. and Rapola, J. (1989). Immunohistochemical spectrum of rhabdomyosarcoma and rhabdomyosarcoma-like tumours. Expression of cytokeratin and the 68-Kd neurofilament protein. *American Journal of Surgical Pathology* **13**, 120–32.

Miettinen, M. and Soini, Y. (1989). Malignant fibrous histiocytoma. Heterogeneous patterns of intermediate filaments by immunohistochemistry. *Archives of Pathology and Laboratory Medicine* **113**, 1363–6.

Miettinen, M. and Ekfors, T. (1990). Alveolar soft part sarcoma. Immunohistochemical evidence for muscle cell differentiation. *American Journal of Clinical Pathology* **93**, 32–8.

Millard, P.R. and Heryet, A.R. (1985). An immunohistological study of factor VIII related antigen and Kaposi's sarcoma using polyclonal and monoclonal antibodies. *Journal of Pathology* **146**, 31–8.

Mitchell, D., Ibrahim, S. and Gusterson, B.A. (1985). Improved immunohistochemical localization of tissue antigens using modified methacarn fixation. *Journal of Histochemistry and Cytochemistry* **33**, 491–5.

Molenaar, W.M., Oosterhuis, J.W. and Oosterhuis, A.M. (1985). Mesenchymal and muscle-specific intermediate filaments (vimentin and desmin) in relation to differentiation in childhood rhabdomyosarcomas. *Human Pathology* **16**, 838–43.

Moll, R., Franke, F.F. and Schiller, D.L. (1982). The catalogue of human cytokeratins: Patterns of expression in normal epithelia, tumours and cultured cells. *Cell* **31**, 11–24.

Moll, R., Lee, I. and Gould, V.E. (1987). Immunocytochemical analysis of Ewing's tumours. Patterns of expression of intermediate filaments and desmosomal proteins indicate cell type heterogeneity and pluri-potential differentiation. *American Journal of Pathology* **127**, 288–304.

Montag, A.G., Pinkus, G.S. and Corson, J.M. (1988). Keratin protein immunoreactivity of sarcomatoid and mixed types of diffuse malignant mesothelioma: An immunoperoxidase study of 30 cases. *Human Pathology* **19**, 336–42.

Montgomery, E.A. and Meis, J.M. (1991). Nodular fasciitis. Its morphologic spectrum and immunohistochemical profile. *American Journal of Surgical Pathology* **15**, 942–8.

Morgan, K.G. and Gray, C. (1985). Malignant epithelioid schwannoma of superficial soft tissue? A case report with immunohistology and electron microscopy. *Histopathology* **9**, 765–75.

Mukai, K., Rosai, J. and Brugdorf, W.H.C. (1980). Localization of factor VIII-related antigen in vascular endothelial cells using an immunoperoxidase method. *American Journal of Surgical Pathology* **4**, 273–6.

Mukai, M., Torikata, C. and Iri, H. (1986a). Histogenesis of alveolar soft part sarcoma. An immunohistochemical and biochemical study. *American Journal of Surgical Pathology* **10**, 212–18.

Mukai, M., Torikata, C. and Iri, H. (1986b). Expression of neurofilament triplet proteins in human neural tumours. An immunohistochemical study of paraganglioma, ganglioneuroma, ganglioneuroblastoma and neuroblastoma. *American Journal of Pathology* **122**, 28–35.

Nadji, M., Morales, A.R. and Ziegles-Weissman, J. (1981). Kaposi's sarcoma: immunohistologic evidence for an endothelial origin. *Archives of Pathology and Laboratory Medicine* **105**, 274–5.

Nathrath, W.B.J. and Remberger, K. (1986). Immunohistochemical study of granular cell tumours. Demonstration of neuron-specific enolase, S100 protein, laminin and alpha-1-antichymotrypsin. *Virchows Archives (Pathologic Anatomy)* **408**, 421–34.

Nickoloff, B.J. and Griffiths, C.E. (1989). The spindle-shaped cells in cutaneous Kaposi's sarcoma. Histologic simulators include factor XIIIa dermal dendrocytes. *American Journal of Pathology* **135**, 793–800.

Nuovo, M.A., Grimes, M.M. and Knowles, D.M. (1990). Glomus tumours: A clinico-pathologic and immunohistochemical analysis of 40 cases. *Surgical Pathology* **3**, 31–45.

Ogawa, K., Oguchi, M., Yamabe, H., Nakashima, Y and Hamashima, Y. (1986). Distribution of collagen type IV in soft tissue tumors. *Cancer* **58**, 269–77.

Omary, M.B., Trowbridge, I.S. and Battifora, H.A. (1980). Human homologue of murine T200 glycoprotein. *Journal of Experimental Medicine* **152**, 842–52.

Ordonez, N.G. and Batsakis, J.G. (1984). Comparison of Ulex europaeus I lectin and factor VIII-related antigen in vascular lesions. *Archives of Pathology and Laboratory Medicine* **108**, 129–32.

Ordonez, N.G., Mahfouz, S.M. and Mackay. B. (1990). Synovial sarcoma: an immunohistochemical and ultrastructural study. *Human Pathology* **21**, 733–49.

Osborn, M., Altmannsberger, M. and Shaw, G. (1982). Various sympathetic derived human tumours differ in neurofilament expression. Use in diagnosis of neuroblastoma, ganglioneuroblastoma, and pheochromocytoma. *Virchows Archives (Cellular Pathology)* **40**, 141–56.

Osborn, M. and Weber, K. (1983). Tumour diagnosis by intermediate filament typing: A novel tool of surgical pathology. *Laboratory Investigation* **48**, 372–94.

Osborn, M., Dirk, T. and Kaser, H. (1986). Immunohistochemical localisation of neurofilaments and neuron-specific enolase in 29 cases of neuroblastoma. *American Journal of Pathology* **122**, 433–42.

Palmer, A.A., Hall, B.E. and Lew, M. (1985). A comparison of some methods of identifying amelanotic and oligomelanotic melanoma metastases in paraffin sections. *Pathology* **19**, 335–9.

Papas-Corden, P., Zarbo, R.J. and Gown, A.M. (1989). Immunohistochemical characterization of synovial, epithelioid, and clear cell sarcomas. *Surgical Pathology* **2**, 43–58.

Parham, D.M., Piper, S.C. and Robicheaux, G. (1988). Malignant rhabdoid tumour of the liver. Evidence for epithelial differentiation. *Archives of Pathology and Laboratory Medicine* **112**, 61–4.

Parums, D.V., Cordell, J.L. and Micklem, K. (1990). JC70: A new monoclonal antibody that detects vascular endothelium associated antigen on routinely processed tissue sections. *Journal of Clinical Pathology* **43**, 752–7.

Perosio, P.M. and Brooks, J.J. (1988). Expression of nerve growth factor receptor in paraffin-embedded soft tissue tumors. *American Journal of Pathology* **132**, 152–60.

Perrone, T., Swanson, P.E. and Twiggs, L. (1989). Malignant rhabdoid tumour of the vulva: Is a distinction from epithelioid sarcoma possible? A pathologic and immunohistochemical study. *American Journal of Surgical Pathology* **13**, 848–58.

Perumal, A.S., Mahadik, S.P. and Rapport, M.M. (1976). Mechanism of interaction of myelin basic protein in S100 protein: Metal binding and fluorescence studies. *Journal of Neurochemistry* **27**, 173–7.

Pizzolo, G., Sloane, J. and Beverley, P. (1980). Differential diagnosis of malignant lymphomas and non-lymphoid tumours using monoclonal antileucocyte antibody. *Cancer* **46**, 2640–7.

Poppema, S., Hollema, H. and Visser, L. (1987). Monoclonal antibodies (MT1, MT2, MB1, MB2, MB3) reactive with leucocyte subsets in paraffin-embedded tissue sections. *American Journal of Pathology* **127**, 418–29.

Raemakers, F., Huysmans, A. and Moesker, O. (1983). Monoclonal antibody to keratin filaments, specific for glandular epithelia and their tumours. Use in surgical pathology. *Laboratory Investigation* **49**, 353–61.

Ramani, P., Bradley, N.J. and Fletcher, C.D. (1990). QBEND/10, a new monoclonal antibody to endothelium: assessment of its diagnostic utility in paraffin sections. *Histopathology* **17**, 237–42.

Rangdaeng, S. and Truong, L.D. (1991). Comparative immunohistochemical staining for desmin and muscle-specific actin: a study of 576 cases. *American Journal of Clinical Pathology* **96**, 32–45.

Rode, J. and Dhillon, A.P. (1984). Neuron specific enolase and S100 protein as possible prognostic indicators in melanoma. *Histopathology* **8**, 1041–52.

Rode, J., Dhillon, A.P. and Jackson, P. (1985). PGP 9.5, a new marker for human neuroendocrine tumours. *Histopathology* **9**, 147–58.

Rode, J., Dhillon, A.P. and Papadaki, L. (1982). Immunohistochemical staining of granular cell tumours for neuron-specific enolase: Evidence in support of neural origin. *Diagnostic Histopathology* **5**, 205–11.

Roessner, A., Vassallo, J. and Vollmer, E., (1987) Biological characterization of human bone tumors. X. The proliferation behaviour of macrophages as compared to fibroblastic cells in malignant fibrous histiocytoma and giant cell tumor of bone. *Journal of Cancer Research and Clinical Oncology* **113**, 559–62.

Roholl, P.J., Kleijne J. and van Basten, C.D. (1985a). A study to analyze the origin of tumor cells in malignant fibrous histiocytomas. A multiparametric characterization. *Cancer* **56**, 2809–15.

Roholl, P.J.M., Kleyne, J. and van Unnik, J.A.M. (1985b). Characterization of tumor cells in malignant fibrous histiocytoma. *American Journal of Pathology* **121**, 269–74.

Romano, V., Hatzfeld, M. and Magin, T.M. (1986). Cytokeratin expression in simple epithelia. I. Identification of mRNA coding for human cytokeratin 18 by a cDNA clone. *Differentiation* **30**, 244–53.

Russel, W.O., Cohen, J. and Enzinger, E.M. (1977). A clinical and pathological staging system for soft tissue sarcomas. *Cancer* **40**, 1562–8.

Rutgers, J.L., Wieczorek, R. and Bonetti, F. (1986). The expression of endothelial cell surface antigens by AIDS-associated Kaposi's sarcoma. Evidence for a vascular endothelial cell origin. *American Journal of Pathology* 122, 493–9.

Salisbury, J.R. and Isaacson, P.G. (1985). Synovial sarcoma: an immnohistochemical study. *Journal of Pathology* **147**, 49–57.

Salter, D.M., Krajewski, A.S. and Dewar, A.E. (1985). Immunohistochemical staining of non-Hodgkin's lymphoma with monoclonal antibodies specific for the glucocyte common antigen. *Journal of Pathology* **146**, 345–53.

Sankey, E.A., More, L. and Dhillon, A.P. (1990). QBEnd/10: a new immunostain for the routine diagnosis of Kaposi's sarcoma. *Journal of Pathology* **161**, 267–71.

Saski, A., Ogawa, A. and Nakazato, Y. (1985). Distribution of neurofilament protein and neuron-specific enolase in peripheral neural tumours. *Virchows Archives (Pathologic Anatomy)* **407**, 33–41.

Schmechel, D.E. (1985). Gamma-subunit of the glycolytic enzyme enolase: Non-specific or neuro-specific? *Laboratory Investigation* **52**, 239–42.

Schlingemann, R.O., Dingjan, G.M. and Emeis, J.J. (1985). Monoclonal antibody PAL-E specific for endothelium. *Laboratory Investigation* **52**, 71–6.

Schmitt, F.C. and Bacchi, C.E. (1989). S100 protein: Is it useful as a tumour marker in diagnostic immunohistochemistry? *Histopathology* **15**, 281–8.

Schmidt, R.A., Cone, R. and Haas, J.E. (1988). Diagnosis of rhabdomyosarcomas with HHF35, a monoclonal antibody directed against muscle actins. *American Journal of Pathology* **131**, 19–28.

Schmidt, D., Harms, D. and Burdach, S. (1985). Malignant peripheral neuroectodermal tumours of childhood and adolescence. *Virchows Archives (Pathologic Anatomy)* **406**, 351–65.

Schmidt, D., Mackay, B. and Ayala, A.G. (1982). Ewing's sarcoma with neuroblastoma-like features. *Ultrastructural Pathology* **3**, 143–51.

Scupham, R., Gilbert, E.F. and Wild, E.J. (1986). Immunohistochemistry of rhabdomyosarcoma. *Archives of Pathology and Laboratory Medicine* **110**, 818–21.

Schurch, W., Skalli, O. and Seemayer, T. (1987). Intermediate filament proteins and actin isoforms as markers for soft tissue differentiation and origin. I. Smooth muscle tumors. *American Journal of Pathology* **128**, 91–103.

Soini, Y. and Miettinen, M. (1989). Alpha-1-antitrypsin and lysozyme. Their limited significance in fibrohistocytic tumors. *American Journal of Clinical Pathology* **91**, 515–21.

Sheibani, K., Battifora, H. and Burke, J.S. (1986). LeuM1 antigen in human neoplasms. An immunohistologic study of 400 cases. *American Journal of Surgical Pathology* **10**, 227–36.

Shimada, H., Aoyama, C. and Chiba, T. (1985). Prognostic subgroups for undifferentiated neuroblastoma. Immunohistochemical study with S100 protein antibody. *Human Pathology* **16**, 471–6.

Simon, R., Durrleman, S. and Hoppe, R.T. (1988). The non-Hodgkin lymphoma pathologic classification project. Long-term follow-up of 1153 patients with non-Hodgkin's lymphomas. *Annals of Internal Medicine* **109**, 939–45.

Skalli, O., Ropraz, P. and Trzeciak, A. (1986). A monoclonal antibody against alpha smooth muscle actin: a new probe for smooth muscle differentiation. *Journal of Cell Biology* **103**, 2787–96.

Sobel, H.J., Marquet, E. and Schwartz, R. (1971). Granular degeneration of appendiceal smooth muscle. *Archives of Pathology* **92**, 427–32.

Springall, D.R., Gu, J. and Cocchia, D. (1983). The value of S100 immunostaining as a diagnostic tool in human malignant melanoma. *Virchows Archives (Pathologic Anatomy)* **400**, 331–43.

Stefansson, K., Wollmann, R. and Jerkovic, M. (1982). S100 protein in soft tissue tumours derived from Schwann cells and melanocytes. *American Journal of Pathology* **106**, 261–8.

Stein, H., Gerdes, J. and Schwab, U. (1982). Identification of Hodgkin's and Steinberg-Reed cells as a unique cell type derived from a newly-detected small cell population. *International Journal of Cancer* **30**, 445–59.

Steiner, G.C., Graham, S. and Lewis, M.M. (1988). Malignant

round cell tumour of bone with neural differentiation (neuroectodermal tumour). *Ultrastructural Pathology* **12**, 505–12.

Stern, R. (1981). Current concepts in the diagnosis of human soft tissue sarcomas. *Human Pathology* **12**, 777–81.

Sumitomo, M., Hirose, T. and Kudo, E. (1989). Epithelial differentiation in synovial sarcoma. Correlation with histology and immunophenotypic expression. *Acta Pathologica Japonica* **39**, 381–7.

Sun, T.T., Eichner, R. and Nelson, W.B. (1983). Keratin classes: Molecular markers for different types epithelial differentiation. *Investigative Dermatology* **80**, 109s–15s.

Sun, T.T., Eichner, R. and Schermer, A. (1984). Classification, expression and possible mechanisms of evolution of mammalian epithelial keratins: A unifying model. Cancer Cells. I. The transformed phenotype. *Cold Spring Harbor Laboratory*, 169–76.

Swanson, P.E., Manivel, J.C. and Wick, M.R. (1987). Immunoreactivity for Leu-7 in neurofibrosarcoma and other spindle cell sarcomas of soft tissue. *American Journal of Pathology* **126**, 546–60.

Thomas, M.L. (1989). The leukocyte common antigen family. *Annual Reviews Immunology* **7**, 339–69.

Thompson, S.J., Schatteman, G.C. and Gown, A.M. (1989). A monoclonal antibody against nerve growth factor receptor. Immunohistochemical analysis of normal and neoplastic human tissue. *American Journal of Clinical Pathology* **92**, 415–23.

Trojanowski, J.Q., Lee, V.M.-Y. and Schlaepfer, W.W. (1984). An immunohistochemical study of human central and peripheral nervous system tumours using monoclonal antibodies against neurofilaments and glial filaments. *Human Pathology* **50**, 248–57.

Traweek, S.T., Kandalaft, P.L. and Mehta, P (1991). The human hematopoietic progenitor cell antigen (CD34) in vascular neoplasia. *American Journal of Clinical Pathology* **96**, 25–31.

Truong, L.D., Rangdaeng, S. and Cagle, P. (1990). The diagnostic utility of desmin. *American Journal of Clinical Pathology* **93**, 305–14.

Tseng, S.C.G., Jarvinen, M.J. and Nelson, W.G. (1982). Correlation of specific keratins with different types of epithelial differentiation: Monoclonal antibody studies. *Cell* **30**, 361–72.

Tsokos, M., Linnoila, R.I. and Chandra, R.S. (1984). Neuron-specific enolase in the diagnosis of neuroblastoma and other small, round-cell tumours in children. *Human Pathology* **15**, 575–84.

Tsokos, M. (1986). The role of immunohistochemistry in the diagnosis of rhabdomyosarcoma. *Archives of Pathology and Laboratory Medicine* **111**, 776–8.

Tsujimoto, M., Ueda, T. and Nakamisha, H. (1987). Monophasic and biphasic synovial sarcoma. An immunohistochemical study. *Acta Pathologica Japonica* **37**, 597–604.

Tsukada, T., McNutt, M.A. and Ross, R. (1987a). HHF35, a muscle-actin-specific monoclonal antibody: II. Reactivity in normal, reactive, and neoplastic human tissues. *American Journal of Pathology* **127**, 389–402.

Tsukada, T., Tippens, D. and Gordon, D. (1987b). HHF35, a muscle-actin-specific monoclonal antibody: I. Immunocytochemical and biochemical characterization. *American Journal of Pathology* **126**, 51–60.

Tsuneyoshi, M., Diamaru, Y. and Hashimoto, H. (1985). Malignant soft tissue neoplasms with the histologic features of renal rhabdoid tumours. *Human Pathology* **16**, 1235–42.

Tsuneyoshi, M. and Enjoji, M. (1982). Glomus tumour: A clinico-pathologic and electron microscopic study. *Cancer* **50**, 1601–07.

van Muijen, G.N.P., Ruiter, D.J. and Warnaar, S.O. (1987). Coexpression of intermediate filament polypeptides in human, fetal and adult tissues. *Laboratory Investigation* **57**, 359–69.

van Haelst, U.J.G.M., Pruszezynski, M. and Ten Cate, L.N. (1990). Ultrastructural and immunohistochemical study of epithelioid haemangio-endothelioma of bone: Coexpression of epithelial and endothelial markers. *Ultrastructural Pathology* **14**, 141–9.

van Duinen, S.G., Ruiter, D.J. and Hageman, P. (1984). Immunohistochemical and histochemical tools in the diagnosis of amelanotic melanoma. *Cancer* **53**, 1566–73.

Vandekerckhove, J. and Weber, K. (1978). At least six different actins are expressed in a higher mammal. An analysis based on the amino acid sequence of the amino-terminal tryptic peptide. *Journal of Molecular Biology* **126**, 783–802.

Vennegor, C., Hageman, P. and van Noehuijs, H. (1988). A monoclonal antibody specific for cells of the melanocyte lineage. *American Journal of Pathology* **130**, 179–92.

Venores, S.A., Bonnin, J.M. and Rubinstein, L.F. (1984). Immunohistochemical demonstration of NSE in neoplasms of the CNS and other tissues. *Archives of Pathology and Laboratory Medicine* **108**, 536–40.

Viale, G., Doglioni, C. and Dellorto, P. (1988). Glial fibrillary acetic protein immunoreactivity in human respiratory tract cartilages and pulmonary chondromatous hamartomas. *American Journal of Pathology* **133**, 363–73.

Virtanen, I., Rapola, J. and Lehto, V.-P. (1983). Neurofilaments in childhood neuroblastoma. *Pathology, Research and Practice* **178**, 171–7.

Visscher, D., Zarbo, R.J. and Crissman, J.D. (1988). Application of monoclonal antibodies to high and low molecular weight cytokeratins in the differential diagnosis of human carcinomas. *Surgical Pathology* **1**, 407–16.

Vogel, A.M., Gown, A.M. and Caughlan, J. (1984). Rhabdoid tumours of the kidney contain mesenchymal specific and epithelial specific intermediate filament proteins. *Laboratory Investigation* **50**, 232–8.

Warnke, R.A., Gatter, K.C. and Falini, B. (1983). Diagnosis of human lymphoma with monoclonal antileucocyte antibodies. *New England Journal of Medicine* **309**, 1275–81.

Walker, R.A. (1985). Ulex europeus I–peroxidase as a marker of vascular endothelium: its application in routine histopathology. *Journal of Pathology* **146**, 123–7.

Warnke, R.A. and Rouse, R.V. (1985). Limitations encountered in the application of tissue section immunodiagnosis to the study of lymphomas and related disorders. *Human Pathology* **16**, 326–31.

Weiss, S.W. and Enzinger, F.M. (1978). Malignant fibrous histiocytoma: an analysis of 200 cases. *Cancer* **41**, 2250.

Weiss, S.W. and Enzinger, F.M. (1982). Epithelioid haemangioendothelioma. A vascular tumour often mistaken for a carcinoma. *Cancer* **50**, 970–81.

Weiss, S.W. and Enzinger, F.M. (1986). Spindle cell haemangioendothelioma: a low grade angiosarcoma resembling cavernous haemangioma and Kaposi's sarcoma. *American Journal of Surgical Pathology* **10**, 521.

Weiss, S.W., Langloss, J.M., Shmookler, B.M., Malawer, M.M., D'Avis, J., Enzinger, F.M. and Stanton, R. (1986). Estrogen receptor protein in bone and soft tissue tumors. *Laboratory Investigation* **54**, 689–94.

Wick, M.R., Scheithauer, B.W. and Kovacs, E. (1983). NSE in neuroendocrine tumours of the thymus, bronchus and skin. *American Journal of Clinical Pathology* **29**, 703–7.

Wick, M.R., Swanson, P.E. and Scheithauer, B.W. (1987). Malignant peripheral nerve sheath tumour. An immunohistochemical study of 62 cases. *American Journal of Clinical Pathology* **87**, 425–33.

Wick, M,R,, Young, R.H. and Malvesta, R. (1989). Prostatic carcinosarcoma: Clinical, histologic, and immunohistochemical data on two cases, with a review of the literature. *American Journal of Clinical Pathology* **92**, 131–9.

Wirman, J.A. (1976). Nodular fasciitis, a lesion of myofibroblasts. An ultrastructural study. *Cancer* **38**, 2378.

Wood, G.S., Link, M. and Warnke, R.A. (1984). Pan-leucocyte monoclonal antibody L3B12. Characterisation and application to research and diagnostic problems. *American Journal of Clinical Pathology* **81**, 176–83.

Yasuda, T., Sobue, G. and Ito, T. (1991). Human peripheral nerve sheath neoplasm: expression of Schwann cell-related markers and their relation to malignant transformation. *Muscle and Nerve* **14**, 812–19.

Zaludek, C. and Norris, H.J. (1987). Mesenchymal tumors of the uterus. In Kurman, R.J. *Blaustein's Pathology of the Female Genital Tract*, Springer-Verlag, New York, pp. 373–408.

Zarbo, R.J., Lloyd, R.V., Beals, T.F. and McClatchey, K.D. (1983). Congenital gingival granular cell tumour with smooth muscle cytodifferentiation. *Oral Surgery, Oral Medicine, Oral Pathology* **56**, 512–20.

3 ◆ *Immunohistochemistry of 'solid' tumours: poorly differentiated round cell and spindle cell tumours II*

Allen M. Gown and Anthony S-Y. Leong

Introduction

In the preceding chapter, we have discussed our immunohistochemical approach to the diagnosis of undifferentiated or poorly differentiated tumours by employing a judiciously selected panel of antibodies directed at a narrow list of differential diagnoses derived from the clinical and pathological features of the tumour. In addition to the use of antibodies for the identification of specific antigenic determinants which will enable characterization of the tumour, it is also necessary to employ other antibodies which are not expressed by the tumour, but whose absence would make a contribution by exclusion. A substantial list of common diagnostic entities has been covered through the broad morphological categorization into groups of round cell tumours and spindle cell tumours. This chapter will be devoted to the application of immunohistochemical analyses in specific diagnostic situations. Also, the prognostic relevance of immunohistochemical stains and the use of proliferation markers will be discussed.

Selected categories of tumours

Mesothelioma, reactive mesothelial cells and metastatic carcinoma

Thoracotomy examination and open biopsy is a widely accepted means of making the definitive diagnosis of malignant mesothelioma, although it seems not too long ago when the diagnosis was rendered only after exclusion of an extrapleural primary tumour at autopsy. Greater familiarity with the range of histological appearances of malignant mesotheliomas has given pathologists more confidence in diagnosing the tumour from closed pleural biopsies. Malignant mesothelioma has to be distinguished from both benign, proliferating mesothelial cells, as well as carcinoma growing in the serous cavity. Fibrous mesothelioma resembles fibrosarcoma, schwannoma and malignant fibrous histiocytoma, and biphasic mesothelioma can resemble synovial sarcoma. The recognition of fibrous mesothelioma from its histological mimics is discussed in the preceding chapter. Papillary serous adenocarcinoma of the ovary requires distinction from peritoneal malignant mesothelioma, and macrophages and histiocytes may also mimic mesothelial cells in cytological preparations. In many instances, the distinction of malignant mesothelioma from these entities is greatly aided by immunohistochemistry and ultrastructural examination, indeed, the adjunctive application of these two techniques increases the diagnostic yield considerably (Leong et al., 1992). The presence of neutral mucins as stained by the periodic acid Schiff reaction and diastase digestion, excludes the diagnosis of mesothelioma; however, a negative stain is not helpful as up to 61 per cent in one series of adenocarcinomas were negative with PAS-diastase (Roggli et al., 1987). The presence of hyaluronic acid within the cell cytoplasm or lumina is a marker of mesothelial cells, however, heavy stromal staining for hyaluronic acid may make interpretation difficult, reducing its value as a diagnostic discriminator.

Antibodies employed in the separation of mesothelioma from carcinoma fall into four categories; namely, the intermediate filaments cytokeratin and vimentin; cell surface glycoproteins such as carcinoembryonic antigen (CEA), B72.3 and epithelial membrane antigen (EMA), blood group isoantigens and human milk fat globule protein-2 (HMFG-2); oncofetoplacental antigens such as alpha-fetoprotein, pregnancy-specific glycoprotein, human chorionic gonadotrophin, human placental lactogen, and placental alkaline phosphatase; and the myelomonocytic antigens such as LeuM1 (CD15), LN1 (CD w75), LN2 (CD74) and MAC387. Table 3.1 shows the immunophenotype of malignant mesothelioma and carcinoma by employing a panel of antibodies representative of these four categories of markers. Cells of normal surface mesothelium express both low and high molecular weight cytokeratins. Submesothelial cells are decorated only by antibodies to vimentin. Reactive, non-neoplastic submesothelial cells such as those in peritonitis or adjacent to neoplastic deposits coexpress both low molecular weight cytokeratin and vimentin, and demonstrate the ability for surface differentiation during which they acquire high molecular weight cytokeratins and lose vimentin (Bolen et al., 1986). Corresponding to this maturation sequence, epithelial mesotheliomas express both high and low molecular weight cytokeratins and less frequently, vimentin (Fig. 3.1); whereas, spindle forms of mesothelioma express vimentin and low molecular weight cytokeratins. Cytokeratin may be demonstrated in a perinuclear distribution corresponding to the location of tonofilaments seen at ultrastructural level, and they may also be peripheral, immediately beneath the plasmalemmal membrane (Fig. 3.2). The coexpression of low molecular weight cytokeratin and vimentin, until

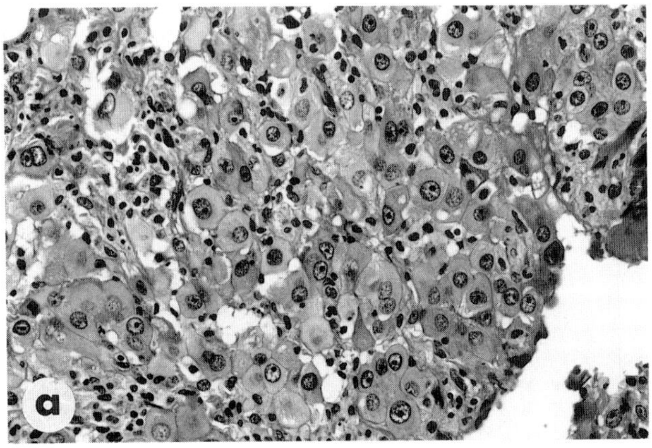

Fig. 3.1a. Epithelial mesothelioma of pleura (H & E, X80).

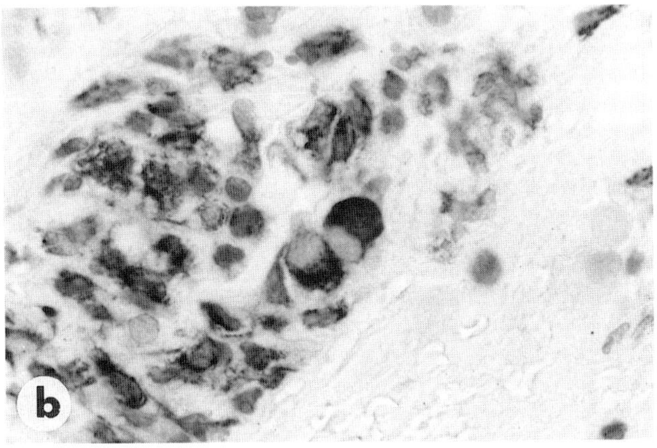

Fig. 3.1b. Same tumour showing vimentin expression in tumour cells (anti-vimentin, X250).

Table 3.1. Immunophenotyping of malignant mesothelioma and adenocarcinoma

	LMCK	HMCK	VIM	CEA	LeuM1	EMA
Mesothelioma	+	+	+/−	−	−	+(M)
Adenocarcinoma	+	−	−/+	+	+	+(C)

Notes:
LMCK = low molecular weight cytokeratin
HMCK = high molecular weight cytokeratin
VIM = vimentin
CEA = carcinoembryonic antigen
LeuM1 = CD 15
EMA(M) = membranous staining in mesothelioma highlight long microvilli
EMA(C) = cytoplasmic staining in adenocarcinoma

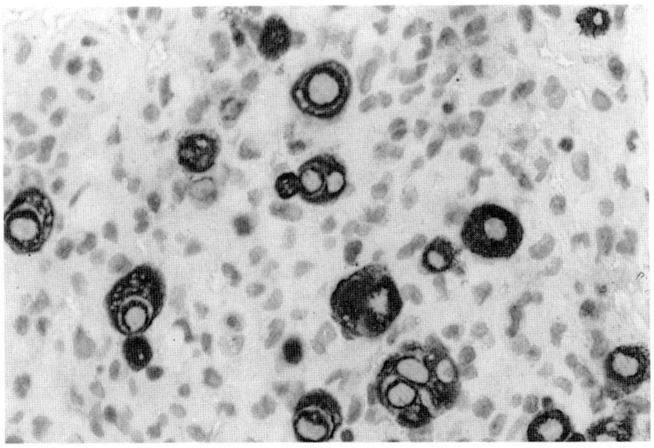

Fig. 3.2. Cytokeratin intermediate filaments are present in both perinuclear as well as subplasmalemmal locations in the tumour cells (anti-bovine keratin, X160).

recently, was thought to be a discriminator for mesothelioma. However, it is now recognized that carcinoma cells growing in serous cavities may acquire vimentin expression so that this marker is no longer a definite diagnostic discriminator (Leong, 1992).

Among the various markers which may be employed for the distinction of malignant mesothelioma from carcinoma, CEA is probably the most useful marker of carcinoma. As many as 90 per cent of metastatic carcinomas are labelled by antibodies to CEA. In contrast, mesotheliomas are only infrequently positive and when so, only focally and faintly staining (Whitaker et al., 1982; Cibas et al., 1987; Strickler et al., 1987; Ordonez, 1989). Other oncofetal placental antigens such as alpha-fetoprotein, pregnancy-specific glycoprotein and human placental lactogen may be expressed by adenocarcinomas, but these are less reliable markers than the expression of CEA. Myelomonocytic antigens are expressed in varying frequencies by adenocarcinomas involving the serosal surfaces, and they may also rarely be detected in malignant mesotheliomas. Wick et al. (1990a,b) found LeuM1 (CD15) to be the most reliable discriminator, being expressed in 38 out of 43 adenocarcinomas. Three out of 41 malignant mesotheliomas expressed this antigen and only in minute foci. Similarly, LN2 (CD74) was found in 39 out of 43 adenocarcinomas, whereas only four cases of mesotheliomas were immunoreactive for this antigen.

Reports of staining for EMA in malignant mesotheliomas have been conflicting. Part of the problem may be attributed to the use of different anti-EMA antibodies. Initial work with HMFG-2, a monoclonal antibody to delipidated milk fat globules, suggested that it was a useful discriminant, staining as many as 85 per cent of adenocarcinomas but not labelling mesotheliomas (Battifora and Kopinski, 1985). However, other workers using HMFG-2 antibody of an identical clone from the same commercial source, have reported contradictory results, with staining in the majority of mesotheliomas as well as adenocarcinomas (Marshall et al., 1984; Bolen et al., 1986; Cibas et al., 1987; Strickler et al., 1987). It has been suggested that the pattern of staining with HMFG-2 may be useful in that the antibodies produced membranous staining in mesotheliomas with weak cytoplasmic staining, in contrast to the diffuse cytoplasmic staining obtained in adenocarcinomas (Tron et al., 1987). A subsequent report of a two-institution study concluded that 'MFG (HMFG-2) was apparently specific for adenocarcinoma, but the findings were difficult to interpret' (Otis et al., 1987).

In a recent study employing a monoclonal antibody to EMA, immunostaining of 13 cases of epithelial mesotheliomas revealed a distinctive pattern of membranous staining with labelling of the periphery of malignant mesothelial cell clusters and circumferentially around individual cells in cytologic preparations, cell blocks, as well as tissue sections. EMA staining displayed 'thick' cell membranes representing the long microvillous processes seen in cases of malignant mesothelioma (Fig. 3.3). Intracellular and intercellular acini were also outlined by anti-EMA, and complex intraluminal microvillous projections were demonstrated (Fig. 3.4). While there was also membranous staining of adenocarcinoma, spiky projections were never seen. Furthermore, mesothelial cells showed only weak cytoplasmic staining in contrast to the strong and diffuse cytoplasmic immunoreactivity in adenocarcinomas from a wide variety of organs (Leong et al., 1989). The immunohistochemical demonstration of thick and spiky membranes circumferentially disposed around individual cells corresponds to the aberrant and long, complex microvilli characteristic of malignant mesothelial cells and provides an important diagnostic clue in the differentiation of malignant mesothelioma from adenocarcinoma (Leong et al., 1989). The monoclonal antibodies employed in the study (clone E29) were raised against human milk fat globule membranes and were of the IgG class. They are closely related to HMFG-2 (Heyderman et al., 1985) and in another study utilizing both antibodies, they have been reported to produce very similar patterns and intensities of staining (Strickler et al., 1987). An immunoelectron microscopic study employing the same anti-EMA antibody (clone E29) showed selective

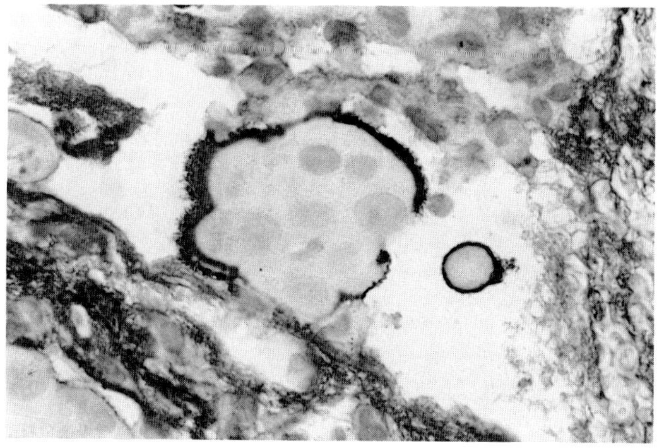

Fig. 3.3. Long microvilli are revealed in the periphery of clusters of mesothelioma cells by immunostaining for EMA (mouse anti-EMA, X400).

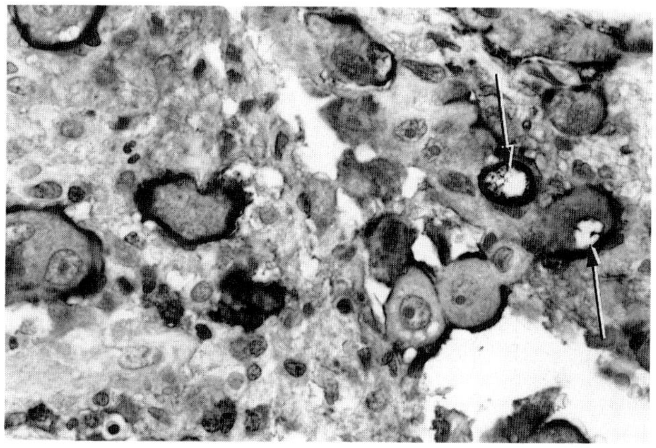

Fig. 3.4. Besides circumferentially dispersed long microvilli, intracellular and intercellular acini with microvilli (arrows) are labelled by anti-EMA antibodies (mouse anti-EMA, X160).

labelling of the surfaces of the microvilli of malignant mesothelial cells. The non-villous flat surfaces were largely EMA-negative and there was virtually no cytoplasmic labelling (van der Kwast et al., 1987). These findings clearly correlate with our immunohistochemical results at light microscopic level. Furthermore, the demonstration of microvilli dispersed circumferentially around the cell membrane indicates the presence of aberrant microvilli, a feature which enables the identification of invasive or malignant mesothelial cells. This contrasts with benign mesothelial cells in which microvilli are present only on the luminal surface. This light microscopic feature, highlighted by staining with anti-EMA, corresponds to the intrastromal projection of microvilli from the abluminal surfaces of mesothelial cells (Fig. 3.5) and the inter-digitation of microvilli with collagen fibres through deficiencies in the basal lamina, ultrastructural features which have recently been recognized to be characteristic of malignant mesothelioma (Dewar et al., 1987). Thus, immunohistochemical stains not only distinguish between malignant mesothelioma and carcinoma but also between malignant mesothelioma and reactive mesothelial cells.

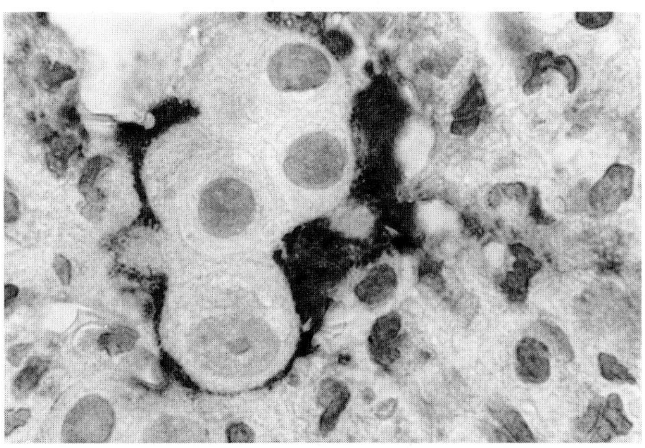

Fig. 3.5. The circumferentially dispersed microvilli represent aberrant microvilli indicative of neoplastic mesothelial cells (mouse anti-EMA, X400).

Chondroid tumours, chordoma and chondroid chordoma

Chondrosarcoma, chondroblastoma, mesenchymal chondrosarcoma and chordoma are discussed briefly as a group, not so much because they mimic poorly differentiated round cell tumours but mainly because they can sometimes be difficult to separate from one another. While chordomas and chondroblastomas have been described almost exclusively in bone, myxoid chondrosarcoma and mesenchymal chondrosarcoma may also occur in extraskeletal sites. Immunohistochemical stains are not overly useful in distinguishing these lesions. Vimentin is expressed by all members of this group of tumours. Cytokeratin is expressed by chondroblastoma (Semmelink et al., 1990), chordomas (Miettinen et al., 1983; Abenoza and Sibley, 1986), and chondroid chordoma (Salisbury, 1987), as is EMA. Both of these antigens are not expressed by chondrosarcoma and mesenchymal chondrosarcoma (Swanson et al., 1990). S100 protein is uniformly found in all tumours in this group (Weiss et al., 1983; Abenoza et al., 1985). In mesenchymal chondrosarcoma, S100 protein expression is present in the lacunar cells and in polygonal cells in cartilaginous transition zones, but usually not in the undifferentiated small cells. NSE is expressed in both lacunar cells as well as undifferentiated cells, whereas Leu7 is occasionally coexpressed in the small transitional cells and lacunar cells (Swanson et al., 1990).

It is of interest that the concept of chondroid chordomas as a distinct entity has recently been challenged by Brooks et al. (1987) who suggested that chondroid chordomas may be simply low-grade chondrosarcomas. Their hypothesis was based on their inability to demonstrate a mixed epithelial-mesenchymal immunophenotype in these neoplasms and the absence of well documented cases of chondroid chordomas outside of the spheno-occipital region. Both these arguments have now been dispensed with. Chu (1987) and Hruban et al. (1990) have each reported one case of chondroid chordoma in the lumbo-sacral region and were able to establish the dual epithelial-mesenchymal nature of the tumours with immunohistochemical stains. A similar example is illustrated in Fig. 3.6.

Neuroendocrine carcinomas

The neuroendocrine (NE) cell population is composed not only of classic 'organs' such as the pituitary or the endocrine pancreas, but a scattered NE cell population found in most major organs. The concept of this diffuse neuroendocrine system has borrowed heavily from the Feyrter's concept of paracrine cells (1969) and Pearse's notion of an APUD (amine precursor uptake and decarboxylation) system of cells (1974). While the unifying concept

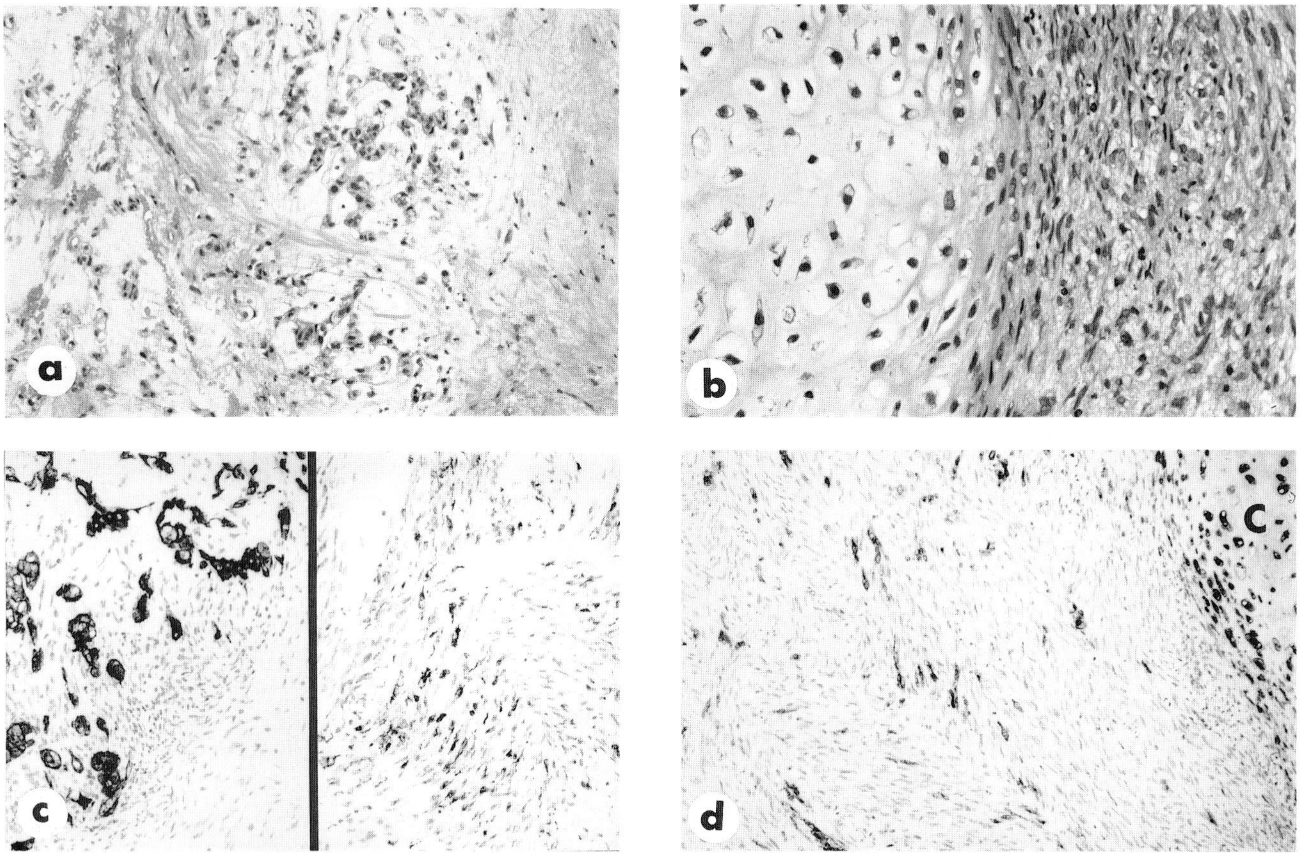

Fig. 3.6a–d. Chondroid chordoma originating in the spheno-occipital region in which an epithelial-mesenchymal immunophenotype is clearly demonstrable. (a) An area typical of chordoma with chords of physaliphorous cells (H & E, X40). (b) Chondroid area surrounded by mildly atypical spindle cells (H & E, X80). (c) Composite photomicrograph of the tumour showing labelling for low molecular weight cytokeratin in both physaliphorous cells and spindle cells (Cam5.2, X40). A similar pattern of staining was observed for EMA. (d) Staining for S100 protein shows positivity in chondrocytes (c) as well as scattered spindle cells. Chordoma areas were negative (anti-S100, X40).

of neural crest derivation is no longer tenable (Le Douarin et al., 1982), a series of immunocytochemistry studies performed over the years has confirmed the presence of common neuroendocrine antigens in a widespread population of cells that can give rise to similar tumours in disparate organs. The spectrum of neuroendocrine tumours ranges from the benign carcinoid tumour to the highly aggressive small cell carcinoma, or 'poorly differentiated neuroendocrine carcinoma'. In the middle of this spectrum are a group of 'intermediate cell' NE carcinomas, including tumours referred to by some as 'well differentiated neuroendocrine carcinomas' and/or 'atypical carcinoids' (Gould et al., 1988). However, there is little agreement in terminology among the various investigators in this area (Travis et al., 1991).

Clinical situations where identification of neuroendocrine differentiation is important

Pulmonary small cell carcinoma

The major important discrimination to be made by the pathologist in lung cancer is between small cell and non-small cell carcinoma (Gazdar, 1989). To the degree that the former is synonymous with 'poorly differentiated neuroendocrine carcinoma', immunocytochemical studies, employing a panel of antibodies to neuroendocrine markers (see below, page 79) would be of great value. However, the WHO classification of lung tumours is based purely on morphology, upon which determination of treatment protocols is generally made, is not always coincident with a classification system based upon immunocytochemically determined neuroendocrine differentiation (Travis et al., 1991). However, there are preliminary data suggesting that the neuroendocrine differentiation per se may be the key factor in predicting response to chemotherapy (Linnoila et al., 1988a; Skov et al., 1991). Indeed, as a small, but significant fraction of non-small cell lung carcinomas can be demonstrated to express any or all of the neuroendocrine markers listed below (Linnoila et al., 1988b), further studies will be required to determine whether morphology or immunocytochemistry will prove to be the more important in predicting clinical outcome.

Extra-pulmonary small cell carcinomas

Tumours bearing a histologic resemblance to pulmonary small cell carcinomas have long been recognized, and, in most cases, these tumours, like their lung counterparts, are associated with an aggressive clinical course and grave prognosis, and occasionally with paraneoplastic syndromes (Silva et al., 1984; Moisa, 1991; Ferlito and Friedmann, 1991). In contrast to their pulmonary counterparts, however, these tumours tend to be rare. In the larynx, both a large and small cell variants of neuroendocrine carcinoma have been recognized (Moisa, 1991), although most of the literature defining these entities are in the form of case reports. Immunocytochemistry can be most helpful in distinguishing these tumours from other poorly differentiated tumours, e.g. squamous cell carcinoma. In the mediastinum, positive identification of neuroendocrine differentiation in poorly differentiated tumours has led to the recognition of the existence of thymic carcinoids and neuroendocrine carcinomas as distinct from thymomas (Wick and Rosai, 1991); there is considerable histologic and immunocytochemical overlap with pulmonary neuroendocrine carcinomas, and the latter must be excluded before the diagnosis of primary thymic neuroendocrine carcinoma can be made. Small cell carcinomas, as corroborated by immunocytochemical demonstration of neuroendocrine markers, have also be identified as a bona fide subset of bladder carcinomas (Blomjous et al., 1988).

The above examples notwithstanding, the concept of 'neuroendocrine carcinomas' in some organs remains poorly defined. For example, in the breast, where a 'resident' neuroendocrine cell population has not been demonstrated, there exist a subset of carcinomas which manifest a 'carcinoid-like' appearance and appear to express several neuroendocrine markers, including chromogranin A. Unlike the small cell neuroendocrine carcinomas described above, these tumours do not necessarily display histologic features or biological behaviour at all distinct from 'garden variety' breast carcinomas (Papotti et al., 1989). Similarly, in the prostate, in addition to a rare, aggressive, small cell carcinoma variant, many non-small cell adenocarcinomas have been demonstrated to contain significant numbers of chromogranin A-positive cells; the significance of this neuroendocrine differentiation is uncertain (Di Sant'Agnese, 1992). Finally, there is incomplete evidence that a subset of primary hepatic carcinomas, especially among the fibrolamellar variant, represent tumours with considerable neuroendocrine differentiation (Wang et al., 1991). This seeming paradox of putative neuroendocrine carcinomas in 'unexpected' locations or within non-traditional histologic contexts is, in part, explained by the fact that one need not invoke a neuroendocrine 'cell of origin' in order to 'explain' the existence of neuroendocrine differentiation within tumours; carcinomas, independent of their 'cell of origin' may manifest neuroendocrine differentiation independent of, or in association with, glandular (or other) differentiation. Pathologists should therefore be wary of overinterpreting the presence of a minor component of neuroendocrine differentiation in carcinomas.

Markers of neuroendocrine differentiation

A panel of antibodies can clearly distinguish small cell carcinoma from potential 'look alike' tumours such as lymphoma, given the expression of CD45 by the latter and cytokeratin by the former. However, there are a number of markers that have, in recent years, been used to specifically identify neuroendocrine carcinomas. Antibody markers of neuroendocrine differentiation range from the very sensitive (with limited specificity) to the very specific (but with limited specificity). While most reports in the literature have focused on the pulmonary neuroendocrine carcinomas, clearly the same markers are expressed in their extrapulmonary counterparts (Springall et al., 1986). The most frequently encountered markers of neuroendocrine differentiation, in increasing order of specificity, are the following:

1. *Low MW cytokeratins:* while cytokeratins are markers of epithelial, and not specifically neuroendocrine, differentiation, in some cases immunocytochemical

identification of specific cytokeratins, or cytokeratins in characteristic patterns of expression, can be instrumental in rendering a specific diagnosis. For example, most small cell carcinomas, in our experience, express low MW cytokeratins (e.g. those identified by such antibodies as CAM5.2 or 35βH11) in a characteristic, albeit not pathognomonic, perinuclear 'dot-like' pattern. Furthermore, Merkel cell tumours of the skin, in contrast to pulmonary small cell carcinomas, express the newly-described cytokeratin 20 (Moll and Franke, 1985).

2. *Neuron specific enolase*, or the gamma subunit of a family of enolase isozymes, when occurring as a homodimer (gamma-gamma) is 'neuron-specific'; unfortunately, the gamma subunit can also exist as a heterodimer with the alpha or beta subunit in non-neural tissues (Kato, 1982). Thus, in practice, while NSE can be more 'nonspecific' than 'neuron-specific', it is most assuredly a very sensitive marker of neuroendocrine differentiation (Lloyd and Warner, 1984). Unfortunately, its sensitivity is not matched by specificity; in practice, antibodies to NSE alone are not useful in discriminating, e.g. neuroendocrine from non-neuroendocrine carcinomas of the lung (Bergh J. et al., 1985).
3. *Leu 7 [CD57]*, identified most readily by the monoclonal antibody HNK-1, was originally defined by its presence in natural killer (NK) cells, a subset of circulating lymphocytes (Abo and Balch, 1981), is also expressed by neuroendocrine cells and tumours in a sensitive fashion (Tsutsumi, 1984). However, Leu7 is also expressed by a number of non-neuroendocrine cells, including the glandular cells of the prostate (Wahab and Wright, 1985) and cells of the nerve sheath (McGarry et al., 1983).
4 *Chromogranin A* was the first truly specific neuroendocrine marker; it is one of a family of acidic, highly sulfated proteins that represent major protein constituents of the neuroendocrine granular matrix (O'Connor and Frigon, 1984). An important feature, therefore, of antibodies to chromogranin A, of which LK2H10 is perhaps the best known (Wilson and Lloyd, 1984), is their recognition of the biochemical analog of the ultrastructurally defined 'dense core granule'. Perhaps not surprisingly, therefore, in tumours in which neuroendocrine differentiation is minimal, e.g. in which there are few 'dense core granules' in the tumour cell population (e.g. small cell carcinoma of the lung), chromogranin A is not a very sensitive marker (averaging about 30 per cent) (de Bruine and Bosman, 1990).
5. *Synaptophysin* (p38) is another intrinsic granule protein, albeit from a different type of granule, the 'presynaptic vesicle', which is present not only in neuroendocrine cells but also in neurons throughout the central and peripheral nervous system (Jahn et al, 1985). In the context of epithelium and epithelial tumours, it is a highly specific, if not the most sensitive, marker of neuroendocrine differentiation (Gould et al., 1987; Kayser et al., 1988). From a practical standpoint, however, synaptophysin is a protein somewhat labile to prolonged formalin fixation (Hoog, 1988), making its use in the routine laboratory somewhat problematic. Furthermore, the pathologist should be cautioned that in poorly differentiated neuroendocrine carcinomas, immunolocalization of markers such as synaptophysin and chromogranin A may be present in a patchy or even focal distribution, making careful scrutiny of the immunocytochemistry slide preparations mandatory.
6. *Other markers*: while the above are those most frequently employed, this list does not exhaust the useful markers of neuroendocrine differentiation. There has been more limited, albeit enthusiastic, use of antibodies to the protein gene product (PGP) 9.5 (Rode et al., 1985), as well as gastrin releasing peptide (bombesin) (Hamid et al., 1987) in the identification of neuroendocrine carcinomas, particularly those in the lung. In addition, antibodies to other specific neuropeptides such as ACTH, VIP, calcitonin, and serotonin have been demonstrated to identify neuroendocrine tumours of the lung (Gould et al., 1988) as well as other neuroendocrine carcinomas. The pathologist would be wise, however, given the incomplete sensitivity and specificity of all of the above markers, to approach the immunocytochemical diagnosis of a neuroendocrine carcinoma with the use of panel of several of antibodies, incorporating those from the more specific and more sensitive categories.

CASE 3.1. Merkel cell tumour of skin

A 79 year-old male with a history of prostatic carcinoma presented with a small chest wall subcutaneous tumour; histologic examination of the H & E-stained sections revealed that the tumour displayed a somewhat trabecular growth pattern (Fig. 3.7A), raising the possi-

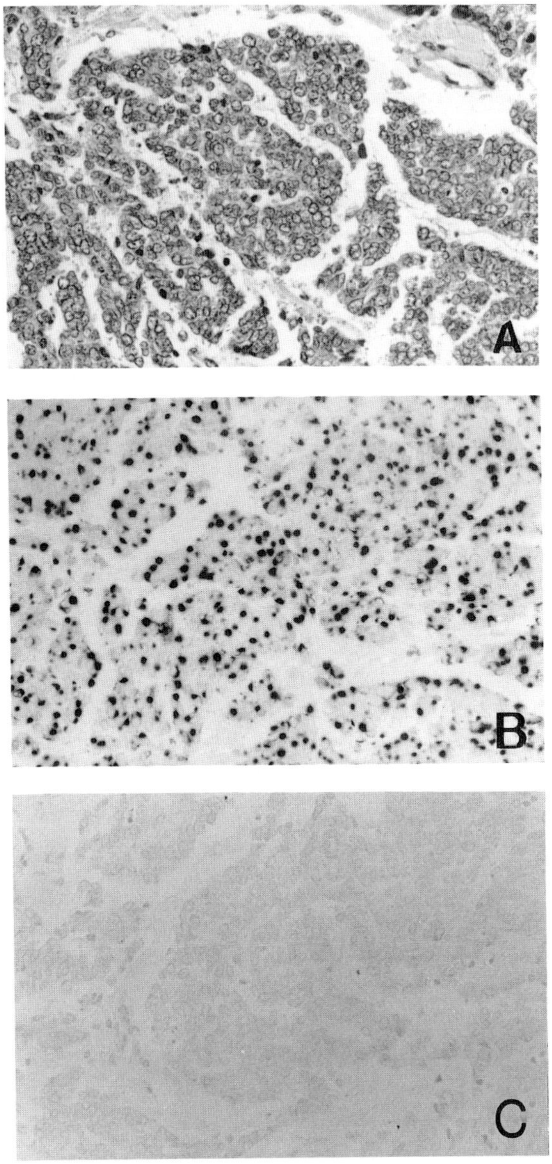

Fig. 3.7A-C. The H & E stained section reveals a round cell tumour with a somewhat trabecular growth pattern (A). Low molecular weight cytokeratin staining reveals uniform positivity with a paranuclear 'dot-like' pattern which is characteristic of neuroendocrine carcinomas (B) and other markers of neuroendocrine differentiation, namely chromogranin A, synaptophysin, were focally present in the tumour. In addition, the tumour cells coexpress neurofilaments in a pattern very similar to that of low molecular weight cytokeratin, but did not express prostate specific antigen (C). (We thank Carlos E Bacchi, MD for taking the photographs.)

bility of the diagnosis of a Merkel cell tumour; other diagnostic considerations included a metastatic carcinoma, including a metastatic prostate adenocarcinoma. The immunophenotype of this tumour is summarized in Table 3.2. Markers of epithelial differentiation (low MW cytokeratin) were uniformly positive, and in a paranuclear 'dot-like' pattern that is characteristic of neuroendocrine carcinomas (Fig. 3.7B). Other markers of neuroendocrine differentiation (chromogranin A, synaptophysin) were focally present in the tumour cell population; in addition, the tumour cells coexpressed neurofilaments in a pattern very similar to that of low MW cytokeratin, but did not express prostate specific antigen (Fig. 3.7C). These studies all confirmed the diagnosis of Merkel cell tumour.

Table 3.2: Immunostaining results in Merkel cell tumour

Antibodies to	Results
Low MW cytokeratin	+
Synaptophysin	+/−
Chromogranin A	+/−
Neurofilaments	+

Germ cell tumours

The nomenclature of germ cell tumours can be somewhat confusing, given the existence of competing British and American 'criteria' for diagnosis, the latter being largely based upon a World Health Organization classification scheme. Immunohistochemistry can be most helpful in identifying particular types of differentiation pathways, some (but not all) of which correspond to histologically defined cell types. Inasmuch as the identification of the latter can lead to the diagnosis of a specific germ cell tumour (or component within a larger tumour), there is an important role to be played by immunohistochemistry in confirming the diagnosis of specific germ cell tumours and components. The tumours/cell types most readily identified are summarized in Table 3.3, which identifies those antibodies most useful in analyses of this group of tumours.

Antibodies to cytokeratin can play an important, albeit contributory, role in the identification of particular germ cell tumours or components. Cytokeratin-positive tumours correspond to those manifesting epithelial differentiation, which include embryonal carcinoma, choriocarcinoma, and yolk sac tumour (Table 3.3). While earlier studies suggested that seminomas could be distinguished from other germ cell tumours by the former's absence of cytokeratin expression (Battifora et al., 1984), it had

Table 3.3. Immunophenotype of germ cell tumours

	Seminoma	Embryonal carcinoma	Yolk Sac tumour	Chorio-carcinoma
Placental alkaline phosphatase	+	+	+/−	+/−
Alpha fetoprotein	−	+/−	+	−
Chorionic gonadotropin	−*	−	−	+
CD 30	−	+	−	−
Cytokeratin	−*	+	+	+

Note: *Scattered trophoblast cells can be found that are cytokeratin-positive and hCG-positive

also been recognized that a subset of seminomas contained scattered cytokeratin-positive cells, some of which were multinucleated (Miettinen et. al., 1985b). These scattered cells which, by virtue of their expression of chorionic gonadotropin appear to represent trophoblast elements, can be found in both 'pure' seminomas as well as those in which seminoma is but one component. The significance of these trophoblastic elements is uncertain (von Hochstetter et al., 1985), although some earlier studies had suggested that the presence of trophoblast cells, as identified by immunohistochemistry, predicts a more aggressive clinical course (Butcher et. al., 1985). More recent studies of seminoma have indicated that even the non-trophoblastic elements may express cytokeratins, although the frequency of this finding may be low (Denk et al., 1987), and it may require the use of frozen sections be detected (Fogel et al., 1990). It cannot be excluded, furthermore, that the cytokeratin expression found in some seminomas implies the existence of 'transitional forms' between seminoma and embryonal carcinoma (Denk et al., 1987). From a practical standpoint, however, with the use of deparaffinized, formalin fixed tissue, seminomas can be characterized as cytokeratin-negative tumours, in contradistinction to other germ cell tumours. Furthermore, expression of particular cytokeratins, e.g. cytokeratin 7, may support the diagnosis of trophoblastic differentiation (Damjanov et al., 1990).

Antibodies to placental alkaline phosphatase (PLAP), which identify one of the several organ specific isotypes of this enzyme, are most useful in identifying seminoma. While antibodies to PLAP are by no means specific for the latter tumour, as they react with a substantial fraction of most non-seminoma germ cell tumours (Burke and Mostofi, 1988a, b; (Table 3.3), anti-PLAP antibodies can help distinguish seminoma from other non-germ cell tumours with which seminoma can sometimes be confused on the basis of morphologic criteria alone, e.g. lymphoma and non-germ cell carcinomas; anti-PLAP antibodies are also useful in identifying seminoma cells which can sometimes be obscured by infiltrating and/or reactive lymphocytes. Recently, it has been demonstrated that the cells of intratubular germ cell neoplasia, which represent 'seminoma-*in situ*', can be distinguished from normal spermatogonia (Burke and Mostofi, 1988a, b) by the former's expression of PLAP. While it can have an indolent course, isolated intratubular germ cell neoplasia shows a high rate of progression to invasive disease, and the positive identification of intratubular germ cell neoplasia can be important to patient management.

Antibodies to alpha fetoprotein (AFP) play a more limited role. AFP expression, while the hallmark of yolk sac tumours (YST), can be seen in a wide range of germ cell tumours, including embryonal carcinoma and many non-embryonal carcinomas. The principal utility of antibodies to AFP is in the distinction of YST (AFP-positive) from seminoma or choriocarcinoma (AFP-negative) (Eglin and Ulbright, 1987).

CD30, the lymphocyte activation associated antigen associated with Hodgkin's disease and anaplastic large cell lymphoma, has recently been demonstrated to be a very specific marker for embryonal carcinoma, with antibodies to CD30 not reacting with other germ cell tumours, including seminoma (Pallesen and Hamilton-Dutoit, 1988). Indeed, CD30 expression, throughout the entire spectrum of human malignancies, appears restricted to these three tumours.

Antibodies to the trophoblast-associated proteins, chorionic gonadotropin (hCG) and placental lactogen (hPL), have their major utility in identifying choriocarcinoma, in detecting trophoblastic differentiation in mixed tumours, and, as discussed above, in seminomas. hCG is generally associated with syncytiotrophoblast differentiation;

although mononuclear trophoblast cells can also express hCG, most of the latter may correspond to so-called intermediate trophoblasts (Kurman et al., 1984). Intermediate trophoblast cells, as well as their malignant counterparts, may also be marked with antibodies to hPL, and may be found in pure choriocarcinomas as well as in germ cell tumours manifesting focal trophoblast differentiation (Manivel et al., 1987). Given the difficulties in identifying intermediate trophoblasts by morphologic criteria alone, the pathologist should not be surprised to find discordances between histologic and immunohistochemical evidence of trophoblast differentiation in germ cell tumours. Indeed, focal trophoblastic differentiation within mixed germ cell tumours is not uncommon, in contrast to 'pure' choriocarcinoma, which is relatively rare.

In summary, the judicious use of the panel of antibodies outlined above can be of great utility in the analysis of germ cell tumours, as long as the interrelationships of the various tumour subtypes, and the limitations of specificity of some of the antibodies are understood.

Carcinomas of unknown primary

Determination of site of origin of a carcinoma presenting as a metastasis can be made in many cases with the judicious use of antibody probes. The types of antibodies that can be of assistance can be divided into several groups:

Antibodies to intermediate filament proteins

The constellation of cytokeratin proteins expressed by a particular tumour is usually more indicative of a particular tissue rather than organ, e.g. squamous cell carcinomas of various site (e.g. skin, lung, cervix) tend to resemble one another in their expression of 'high molecular weight' cytokeratins such as CK5, CK14, CK1, and CK10, i.e. those cytokeratins identified by the antibody 34βE12 (Gown and Vogel, 1985). While carcinomas of different sites can be subdivided into broad groups by their patterns of cytokeratin expression (Quinlan et al., 1985), such an approach is of limited utility in many clinical situations, and must be supplemented by using other markers such as those suggested below. Quite recently, however, it has been demonstrated that the newest member of the cytokeratin family, CK20, has an organ-restricted distribution that can be of clinical utility. CK20 is expressed predominantly be epithelial cells of the gastro-intestinal (GI) tract; in the context of primary and metastatic adenocarcinomas, it is expressed almost universally by colorectal adenocarcinomas, in a larger fraction of pancreatic carcinomas and urothelial carcinomas, in a small fraction of mucinous ovarian adenocarcinomas, but not to any significant degree by adenocarcinomas of the breast or lung (Moll et al., 1992). Thus, the antibody can be of significant assistance in the differential diagnosis of metastatic adenocarcinomas. It had previously been demonstrated, too, that CK20 was expressed in Merkel cell tumours of the skin, but not in metastatic small cell carcinomas, e.g. from the lung (Moll et al., 1992). Coexpression of other intermediate filaments, e.g. neurofilaments, vimentin, or GFAP, is characteristic of carcinomas of specific organs as described in a subsequent section.

Antibodies to CEA and villin

CEA, or carcinoembryonic antigen, was originally described in the human digestive system as a tumour-associated antigen. Although it is now known that CEA can be demonstrated, with sensitive probes and methodologies, even in normal gastrointestinal epithelium and in reactive situations, antibodies to CEA continue to have the diagnostic use, especially when combined with other antibodies in the context of a larger antibody panel. In one sense, antibodies to CEA may be considered a 'poor man's' anti-cytokeratin antibody, in that CEA expression, in a very crude sense, correlates with epithelial differentiation; expression of CEA is never seen in non-epithelial tumours (Zimmerman, 1988). None the less, there is a restricted expression of CEA within the set of epithelial tumours which can be exploited when coupled with site or origin of metastatic tumours. Unlike the intermediate filament proteins, CEA expression may be directly proportional to the degree of cellular differentiation, i.e. more poorly differentiated tumours of a given cell type tend to express less CEA than well-differentiated tumours with the same type. Furthermore, the issue is complicated by the large range of anti-CEA antibodies which are available, and differential reactivity of these antibodies with specimens fixed in aldehyde fixatives versus alcohol-based fixatives. As with the intermediate filament proteins, carcinoembryonic antigen is better demonstrated, and more reliably demonstrated, in the latter. Differences in the cellular distribution of the antigen are also evident when the same tissues are fixed differently; cytoplasmic immunoreactivity is generally emphasized in the alcohol-fixed tissue, making it more visible to the eye.

CEA is actually a family of high molecular weight glycoproteins (all of which are, in turn, part of a 'superfamily' of proteins which include the immunoglobulins, certain cell adhesion molecules, etc.) (True, 1990). The CEA family includes 'true' CEA, along with 'non-specific' cross-reacting antigen (NCA), biliary glycoprotein (BGP), and others. It has been well-established that antisera prepared by conventional immunization with CEA contains several antibodies of different specificities, i.e. such antisera cross react with NCA and BGP (von Kleist, 1979). Although, in the past, there have been recommendations for the absorption of commercially obtained anti-CEA antisera, with a mixture of major blood group erythrocytes, much of the problems with the earlier antibodies to CEA can be avoided through the use of recently-available monoclonal preparations. Most anti-CEA polyclonal antibodies and some monoclonal anti-CEA antibodies react with both CEA and NCA, and hence will identify polymorphonuclear leucocytes in tissue sections. This can have positive as well as negative consequences: while these latter cells serve as good 'built-in' controls, necrotic tumours of any type will often manifest CEA positivity as a consequence of this NCA cross-reactivity. New antibodies are becoming available which do not show this cross-reactivity and can be used in place of, or in conjunction with, the cross-reacting clones. In general, carcinomas can be divided into three groups. In group 1 are carcinomas which are characterized by strong expression of CEA in a very high (greater than 90 per cent) fraction of cases. These include adenocarcinomas primary to the gastrointestinal tract (i.e. colon) and lung (Pascal et al., 1977). The second diagnostically useful group includes those in which CEA expression is almost never seen. This includes adenocarcinomas of the kidney (renal cell carcinomas), prostate, and mesotheliomas of all sites. A larger intermediate group is composed of those tumours in which CEA expression is variable, and of questionable diagnostic significance; this includes adenocarcinomas of the endometrium (generally, but not always CEA negative), epidermoid carcinomas of the endocervix (van Nagell and Goldenberg, 1980), adenocarcinomas of the ovary, transitional cell carcinomas of the urothelium, and others.

Villin is a GI-associated cytoskeletal protein related to microvilli, expression of which characteristic of adenocarcinomas of the GI tract but absent in adenocarcinomas of the lung and breast. Recently, it has been demonstrated that anti-villin antibodies can be useful in detecting the site of origin of metastatic carcinomas. Existing anti-villin antibodies, however, can only be used on alcohol (e.g. methacarn) fixed, and not formalin fixed, tissues (Bacchi and Gown, 1990).

Antibodies to tissue-specific proteins

There are, unfortunately, relatively few tissue-or organ-specific markers that can be exploited in the analysis of metastatic carcinomas, but those that exist have been well characterized and are most helpful in many clinical settings.

Prostate

By far and away the most useful organ-specific markers are those of the prostate gland: PSA (prostatic specific antigen) and PAP (prostatic acid phosphatase). Antibodies to PAP have one of the longest 'track records' of any antibodies in the diagnostic armamentarium; while the high sensitivity of these antibodies for carcinomas (primary or metastatic) of prostatic origin is well known, less well known are the exceptions, i.e. the existence of non-prostatic carcinomas expressing PAP. Best characterized in this regard are a subset of pancreatic islet cell tumours and hindgut-derived carcinoid tumours; recent biochemical (Western blot) studies have confirmed expression of PAP by hindgut-derived, but not foregut- or midgut-derived neuroendocrine tumours (Azumi et al., 1991). This seemingly anomalous PAP expression may be related to the shared cloacal derivation of both the rectum and the prostate. In contrast, expression of PSA, a 34 kd glycoprotein thought to serve as a neutral protease active in lysing of seminal coagulum following ejaculation, has not been reported in non-prostate carcinomas (Ford et al., 1985; Nadji et al., 1981, 1982), although this is not to say that PSA is found exclusively within the prostate: recent studies have demonstrated the expression of PSA (as well as PAP) by glandular epithelium in the male periurethral glands (Frazier et al., 1992) as well as in urachal remnants (Golz and Schubert, 1989).

Thyroid

Other tissue-specific markers include antibodies to thyroglobulin, the very large heavily glycosylated protein synthesized by thyroid follicular epithelial cells which provides iodinations sites for the formation of thyroid hormones. Antibodies to thyroglobulin have an extremely high sensitivity for primary and metastatic carcinomas of the thyroid (Albores-Saavedra et al, 1983; Mizukami et al., 1990), including both follicular and papillary histologic variants. Consequently, a major applications of antibodies to thyroglobulin is in the study of metastatic papillary tumours.

Breast

The interest in tumours of this organ notwithstanding, there does not yet exist a marker for breast cancer with comparable specificity and sensitivity as thyroglobulin and PSA for carcinomas of the thyroid and prostate, respectively. Offering perhaps the greatest promise, however, are antibodies to the apocrine marker protein, gross cystic disease fluid protein-15 (GCDFP-15). This protein, one of the four major protein components isolated from breast cyst fluid (Haagensen et al., 1990), is restricted in its expression primarily to cells manifesting apocrine function (Mazoujian et al., 1983), including axillary and perineal glands, Moll's glands of the eyelids, ceruminous glands of the ear canal, prostate glands, a subset of cells in salivary glands and minor bronchial glands. Not only cell type but cell state appears to affect expression of GCDFP-15: normal breast lobules and ducts express very low, and immunocytochemically undetectable, amounts of this protein, whereas hyperplastic and metaplastic breast epithelium is more frequently GCFDP-15-positive. The overall sensitivity of this marker for primary breast carcinoma, in the study of Mazoujian et al. (1989) was 55 per cent, and the sensitivity varied greatly among different histologic types of breast carcinomas: 90 per cent in infiltrating lobular carcinomas manifesting signet-ring differentiation, 70 per cent in intraductal carcinomas, 23 per cent in infiltrating ductal carcinomas without apocrine differentiation, and only 5 per cent in medullary carcinomas. In the large study of primary and metastatic breast carcinomas of Wick et al. (1989), a much higher overall sensitivity for breast carcinoma (94 per cent) was obtained. Other non-breast metastatic carcinomas positive for GCDFP-15 in the latter study included adenocarcinomas of salivary glands, sweat glands, and prostate. Thus, the predictive value of GCDFP-15 in identifying a metastatic carcinoma as being of breast origin can be high, if other possibilities can be excluded on histologic grounds alone (Wick et al., 1989).

The recent development of techniques permitting the use of antibodies to oestrogen and progesterone receptors on deparaffinized tissue has had considerable impact on the diagnosis and management of breast cancer. While there has been interest in probing for these receptors in the context of metastatic carcinomas in which a primary tumour in the breast is suspected clinically, it should be underscored that the expression of oestrogen and progesterone receptors is by no means a specific property of carcinomas of the breast. Recent immunocytochemical studies have demonstrated the expression of oestrogen receptor (ER) and/or progesterone receptor (PR) in a subset of endometrial carcinomas (Segreti et al., 1989), sweat duct carcinomas of the skin (Swanson et al., 1991), thyroid carcinomas (Diaz et al., 1991), pancreatic islet cell carcinomas (Doglioni et al., 1990), smooth muscle tumours (Colley et al., 1989) and meningiomas (Waelti and Markwalder, 1989; Grunberg, 1991). None the less, in the appropriate clinical context, the expression of these receptors can be of diagnostic significance in determining a primary site of a carcinoma. For example, in the clinical context of a tumour arising in the lung of a patient several years out from apparent successful treatment of ER-positive breast carcinoma, expression of oestrogen receptor by the carcinoma cells in the lung would argue persuasively against the diagnosis of a second lung primary and strongly suggest the diagnosis of metastatic breast carcinoma, given the apparent non-existence of ER-positive primary lung carcinomas (Wick, M.R., personal communication; Battifora, H., personal communication).

CASE 3.2: Metastatic colorectal adenocarcinoma to lung

A 55 year-old male with a history of smoking and a previous history of Dukes C colorectal adenocarcinoma presented with a solitary peripheral lung mass picked up on routine chest x-ray. Biopsy of the tumour (Fig. 3.8A) confirmed the presence of adenocarcinoma, with the principal differential diagnosis metastatic colorectal adenocarcinoma versus a new primary lung adenocarcinoma. Immunocytochemical studies were thus performed to determine the site of origin of this tumour; results are summarized in Table 3.4. Antibodies to low MW cytokeratin (Fig. 3.8B) were uniformly positive on the tumour, as were antibodies to carcinoembryonic antigen (Fig. 3.8E); these two studies by themselves would not distinguish these two principal diagnostic possibilities. However, the tumour expressed two GI-associated markers: cytokeratin 20 (Fig. 3.8C) and villin (Fig. 3.8D), neither of which has been reported to be expressed in lung adenocarcinomas, save for the rare bronchoalveolar adenocarcinoma. Thus, these studies confirmed that this represented a metastatic focus rather than a new lung primary.

Table 3.4. Immunostaining results in metastatic colorectal adenocarcinoma

Antibodies to	Results
Low MW cytokeratin [35βH11]	+
Cytokeratin 20	+
Villin	+
Carcinoembryonic antigen	+

Coexpression of intermediate filaments

As originally hypothesized, individual intermediate filament (IF) proteins were associated with tissue types, e.g. cytokeratins with epithelium, desmin with muscle, vimentin with mesenchymal cells, GFAP with glial cells, and neurofilaments with neurons (Gabbiani et al., 1981). This 'dogma' of 'one IF, one tissue type' has fallen under the weight of considerable published data in the past decade which have, in aggregate, demonstrated that selected tissue, cell and tumour types have the capacity of expressing more than one IF protein. The surgical pathologist, however, can turn these 'exceptions' into diagnostic advantages, as coexpression of particular

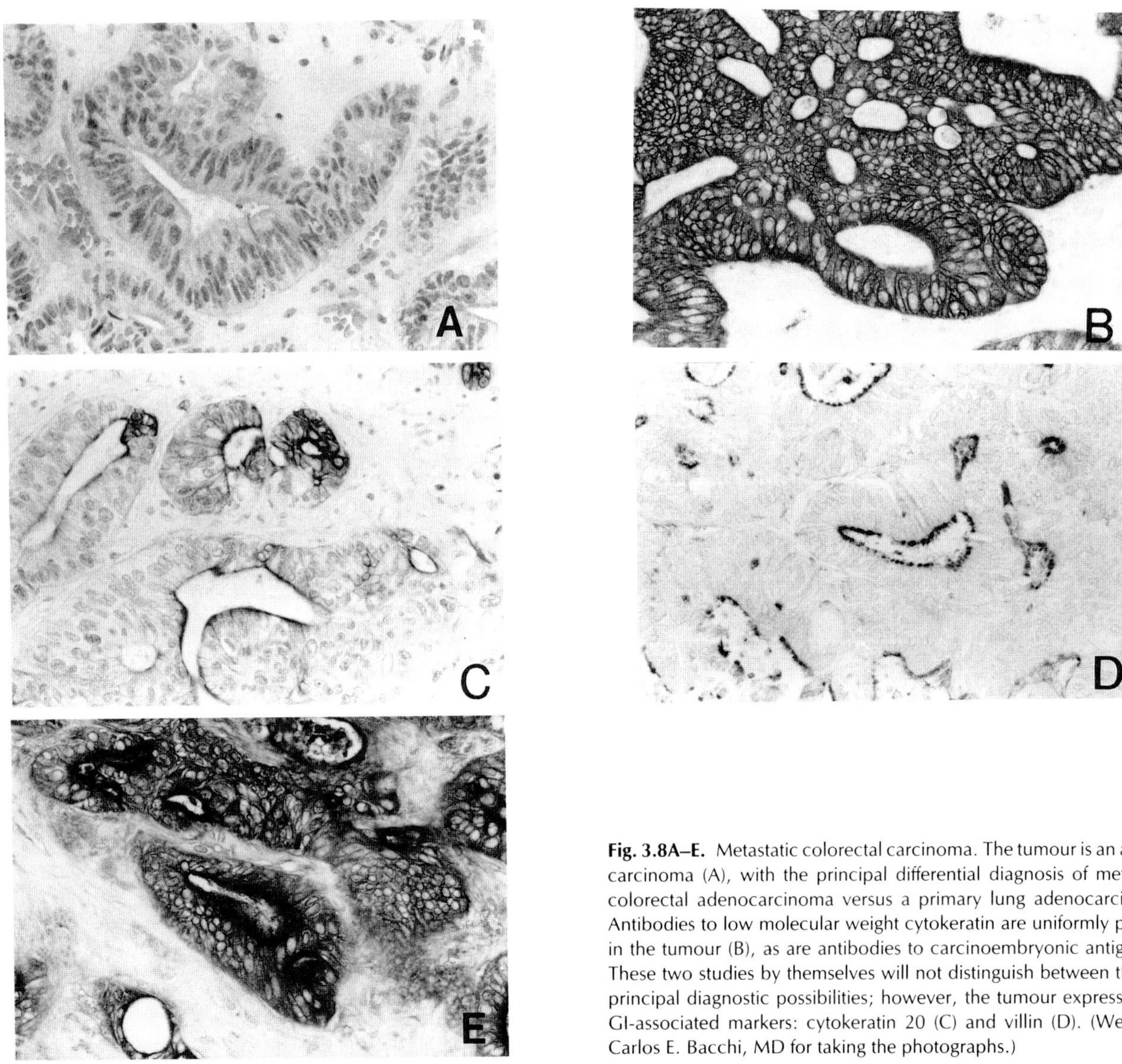

Fig. 3.8A–E. Metastatic colorectal carcinoma. The tumour is an adenocarcinoma (A), with the principal differential diagnosis of metastatic colorectal adenocarcinoma versus a primary lung adenocarcinoma. Antibodies to low molecular weight cytokeratin are uniformly positive in the tumour (B), as are antibodies to carcinoembryonic antigen (E). These two studies by themselves will not distinguish between the two principal diagnostic possibilities; however, the tumour expresses two GI-associated markers: cytokeratin 20 (C) and villin (D). (We thank Carlos E. Bacchi, MD for taking the photographs.)

intermediate filaments can be characteristic of specific tumours, and in some cases can offer specific prognostic information.

Vimentin coexpression in carcinomas

This is the most frequently encountered example of IF coexpression. It should be underscored that cells and tumours in this category express cytokeratins as their primary IF, and that, in almost all cases, this primary IF is the quantitatively dominant IF, which is reflected in tissue immunostaining patterns. Vimentin, as the secondary IF, is often restricted in its expression to a subset of the tumour cell population, and, within individual cells, restricted in its expression to a portion of the cytoplasm. Carcinomas which most reliably coexpress vimentin include: renal cell carcinomas, mesotheliomas, endometrial adenocarcinomas, thyroid carcinomas, and salivary gland tumours (Gown and Vogel, 1985); in some of these cases, the normal cell counterpart, e.g. thyroid (Henzen-Logmans et al., 1987), endometrium (Dabbs et al., 1986), and mesothelium (LaRocca and Rheinwald, 1984) also coexpresses vimentin with cytokeratin. However, it should be noted that a variable frequency of vimentin coexpression has been reported in a wide range of human carcinomas, including those of lung (Gatter et al., 1986), breast (Raymond and Leong, 1989a, 1989b), prostate (Leong et al., 1988), and even carcinoid tumours (Kimura et al., 1989). Thus, while no absolute statements can be made regarding the organ of origin, e.g. of a carcinoma solely on the basis of its coexpression of vimentin, when placed in the context of other markers, useful information about primary site can be derived (Coggi et al., 1989; Leong, 1992). Vimentin coexpression is also a function of morphology: in the case of mesotheliomas, for example, the degree of vimentin coexpression is clearly related to the 'degree' of spindle morphology present in the tumours (Bolen et al., 1986); unattached growth of carcinoma cells within ascitic or pleural fluids may also modulate the phenotype of these cells to express vimentin (Ramaekers et al., 1983). Finally, there is increasing evidence that vimentin coexpression in breast (Raymond and Leong, 1989a, 1989c), lung (Gatter et al., 1987), renal cell carcinoma (Dierick et al., 1991) may be prognostic significance, portending a worse clinical outcome.

Other examples of vimentin coexpression

Vimentin is often coexpressed along with other 'primary' IF expression: in glial cells and tumours, vimentin often accompanies GFAP expression (Yen and Fields, 1981; Dahl et al., 1981; Osborn et al., 1984), and in smooth muscle cells and tumours, vimentin often accompanies desmin expression (Evans et al., 1983). These common findings underscore the necessity of defining IF phenotype of a tumour by employing a panel of anti-IF protein antibodies, not just antibodies to those IFs 'expected' to be present.

Other examples of intermediate filament coexpression

1. *Coexpression of cytokeratin and neurofilaments by neuroendocrine tumours* Reflecting, at least in a teleological sense, their simultaneous epithelial and neural properties, coexpression of the corresponding IF protein, namely cytokeratins and neurofilaments, has been reported in a wide range of neuroendocrine tumours, including carcinoids (Gown and Vogel, 1985; Miettinen et al., 1985a), Merkel cell tumours (Moll et al., 1986), and even small cell carcinomas (Lehto et al., 1983; Blobel et al., 1985).
2. *Coexpression of GFAP by selected carcinomas* While expression of GFAP might logically be expected to be restricted in its distribution to cells and tumours of the central nervous system, GFAP coexpression has been noted to be a highly characteristic feature of pleomorphic adenomas of salivary gland (Caslelitz et al., 1982; Aschtatter et al., 1986); GFAP coexpression has also been documented within the myoepithelial cells of breast tissue, and a limited number of breast cancers (Gould et al., 1990). GFAP is also coexpressed along with vimentin in a subset of Schwann cells and Schwann cell tumours (Aschtatter et al., 1986), and there are reports of GFAP and vimentin coexpression in fetal cartilage and cartilaginous tumours (Orto, 1988; Viale et al., 1988).
3. *Coexpression of cytokeratin by non-epithelial tumours* Expression of cytokeratin by certain sarcomas, e.g. synovial sarcomas (Miettinen et al., 1982) and epithelioid sarcomas (Chase et al., 1984) is reflective of the presence of true epithelial differentiation within what is otherwise considered a mesenchymal tumour. In contrast, 'anomalous cytokeratin coexpression' has been reported (and documented with concurrent biochemical studies) in a number of mesenchymal (i.e. vimentin-positive) cells and tumours without epithelial differentiation, especially smooth muscle (Gown et al., 1988) and

melanomas (Zarbo et al., 1990). It is uncertain, however, whether other recently reported examples of anti-cytokeratin antibody immunostaining in non-epithelial tumours [including angiosarcomas (Gray et al., 1990), malignant fibrous histiocytoma (Weiss et al., 1988), lymphomas (de Mascarel et al., 1989), and gliomas (Ng and Lo, 1989)] represent bone fide examples of 'anomalous cytokeratin coexpression' or, in fact, immunostaining, or other, artefacts (Franke et al., 1991; Bacchi et al., 1990; Swanson, 1991). Miettinen has suggested that 'anomalous coexpression' of particular cytokeratin peptides may be characteristic of sarcoma subtypes (Miettinen, 1991).

Screening of draining lymph nodes for metastatic tumour

In contemporary methods of tumour staging, lymph node metastasis is of paramount importance in the determination of prognosis and choice of therapy. When examining lymph nodes for the presence of metastases, commonly employed methods of sectioning lymph nodes can account for as many as 30 per cent false negative results (Saphir and Amromin, 1948). The failure to identify metastases within a lymph node is related to the size of the node, size of the lesion, number of sections examined, and location of the deposit within the node. Through the application of a mathematical and computer generated model, Wilkinson and Hause (1974), concluded that to increase the probability of detection of metastatic deposits of 1 mm diameter located peripherally or randomly, the node should be cut into at least four 1 mm thick slices along their longest axis and appropriately orientated for sectioning. In a study of occult axillary node metastases in patients with breast cancer, Fisher et al. (1978a, b) employed serial 5 μm sectioning of one block containing one transected half of each axillary node. By assessing every fourth section, these authors detected occult metastases in 24 per cent of cases.

Trojani et al. (1987) found that 14 per cent of lymph nodes originally deemed to be negative for metastases were positive for tumour cells when additional levels were examined with immunohistochemical stains. They found that the presence of micrometastases was a stronger indicator of patient outcome than tumour size, histological type, histological grade, the presence of vascular invasion or oestrogen receptor status.

While the significance of micrometastases in axillary lymph nodes in patients with breast cancer may be controversial (Huvos et al., 1971; Attiyeh et al., 1977; Fisher et al., 1978a; Fisher et al., 1978b; Rosen et al., 1981), the detection of micrometastases in cancer is an area of potential interest to pathologists and oncologists. Serial sectioning and step sectioning, while increasing the yield, are cumbersome and laborious procedures which cannot be performed as a routine service. A handful of studies have employed immunohistochemical techniques to detect axillary node metastases in breast cancer patients. These have largely employed antisera to epithelial membrane antigen (EMA) or to other delipidated human milk-fat-globule membrane antigens. Sloane et al. (1980) employed polyclonal antiserum to EMA to confirm the presence of histologically diagnosed metastatic disease in the liver and in lymph nodes. Wells et al. (1984) demonstrated metastatic tumour in seven of 45 (15 per cent) axillary node-negative cases of breast carcinoma by applying monoclonal antibodies to EMA and KL1 (an anti-cytokeratin antibody). Similarly, other workers employing anti-EMA and anti-HMFG-2 antisera have detected occult metastases in as many as 24 per cent of cases (Bussolati et al., 1986; Trojani et al., 1987). While these immunohistochemical studies have employed predominantly antisera to EMA, EMA is now recognized to be a less sensitive and certainly less specific marker than cytokeratins in the identification of epithelial cells (Pinkus et al., 1986; Thomas and Battifora, 1987). Furthermore, anti-EMA is also reported to decorate plasma cells, lymphocytes, as well as macrophages and non-epithelial tumours (Delsol et al., 1984; Pinkus and Kurtin, 1985). Raymond and Leong (1989d), employing antibodies CAM5.2 and AE1/3, detected occult metastases in seven of 30 cases (23 per cent) of node-negative breast carcinoma and suggested that immunostaining for cytokeratins provided a simple and inexpensive method of detecting metastatic foci which were missed on routine screening of H & E stained sections of lymph nodes (Fig. 3.9).

It would appear from the above that immunostaining offers a sensitive and convenient method of detecting micrometastases of carcinoma in lymph nodes. A study by Cochran et al. (1988) indicated that it may be similarly effective for the detection of occult tumour cells in draining nodes in pathological stage I malignant melanoma. They re-examined 2227 lymph nodes from 100 patients who were pathologically staged as stage I. By employing immunostaining for S100 protein, the authors

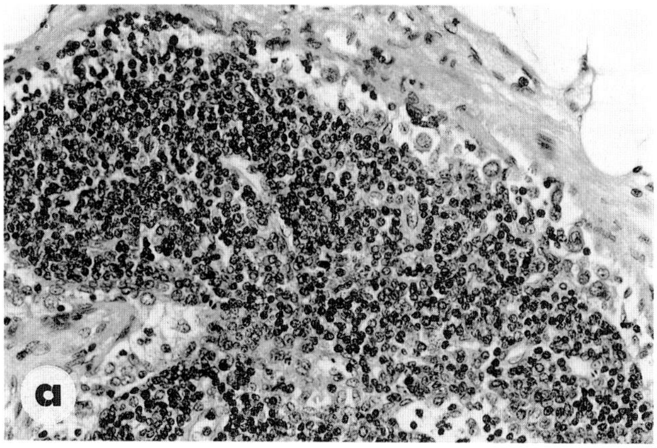

Fig. 3.9a. Axillary lymph node draining a breast with infiltrating duct carcinoma. The node was reported as negative by examination of H & E stained sections. Note the presence of some mononuclear cells in the subcapsular sinus which were interpreted as monocytes (H & E, X80).

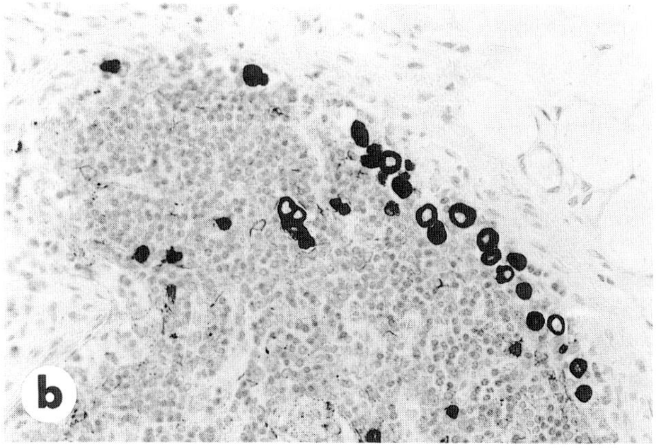

Fig. 3.9b. Consecutive section stained for cytokeratin reveals numerous single metastatic carcinoma cells in the subcapsular sinus as well as infiltrating the lymph node cortex (Cam5.2, X80).

identified melanoma deposits in 16 nodes from 14 patients, confirming the nature of all deposits by reaction with the melanoma-directed monoclonal antibody NKI/C3. The occult deposits appeared to be prognostically significant as 41 per cent died of melanoma compared to 21 per cent of patients without occult nodal deposits.

Detection of metastatic tumour in the bone marrow

As with the detection of occult metastatic carcinoma and melanoma in lymph nodes, the identification of metastatic carcinoma in the bone marrow has been of interest in the prognostication of some tumours. Carcinoma of the breast is an example of a tumour that frequently spreads to bone and bone marrow. Thirty-five to 48 per cent of patients with breast carcinoma, including as many as 24 per cent of patients with no evidence of metastases at the time of diagnosis, develop recurrent disease after primary therapy, suggesting that the tumour may be disseminated very early in the course of the disease. Sedmak et al. (1989) and Sloane et al. (1980), employing immunohistochemistry, evaluated the impact of the presence of bone marrow micrometastases on survival and noted that those patients with better outcome tended to be free of occult metastases compared to a higher percentage of patients with occult metastatic disease among those who subsequently displayed clinically apparent metastases. The detection of tumour in the marrow from patients with apparently early-stage disease could prompt more aggressive adjuvant therapy, stimulating the search for more accurate methods of detecting bone marrow metastases. Earlier methods employed antibodies to EMA on bone marrow smears (Dearnaley et al., 1981). More recently, cocktails of antibodies which included those with specificity for breast carcinoma cells and to cytokeratin have been applied to bone marrow aspirates concentrated on a Ficoll density gradient, using an indirect immunofluorescence technique (Cote et al., 1988). Leslie et al. (1990), employing a cocktail of five monoclonal antibodies to breast cancer antigens and an indirect immunofluorescence technique, were able to detect tumour cells in nine out of 15 normal bone marrows which were contaminated *in vitro* with breast cancer cells from patient effusion samples or from established tumour cell lines. By flow cytometry, the detection rate was one tumour cell among 10,000 marrow precursors in 14 out of 15 instances, however, when both flow cytometry and cytological techniques were combined, it was possible to detect one breast cancer cell among 100,000 normal marrow progenitors (Leslie et al., 1990).

Monoclonal antibodies have also been used to detect occult metastases in the bone marrow of patients with neuroblastoma (Moss et al., 1991; Caillaud et al., 1991), small cell carcinoma of the lung (Bezwoda et al., 1986), prostatic carcinoma (Mansi et al., 1988), and colorectal carcinoma (Schlimok et al., 1990).

While immunohistochemical procedures employing peroxidase as the reporter molecule can be used, the high levels of endogenous peroxidase in the bone marrow results in excessive background staining. The alkaline phosphatase-anti-alkaline phosphatase method with levamisole to block endogenous alkaline phosphatase is a preferable technique (Fig. 3.10) and the procedure is provided in the Appendix.

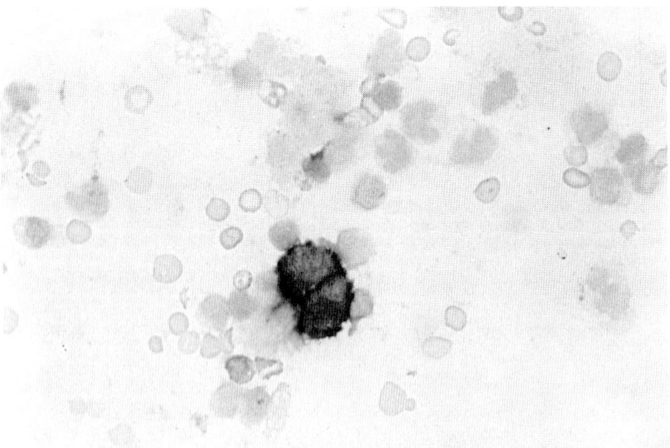

Fig. 3.10. Occult bone marrow micrometastasis in a patient with node-negative, well-differentiated infiltrating carcinoma of the breast (bone marrow aspirate, APAAP technique, Cam5.2, X160).

Basement membrane staining

The basement membrane constitutes a specific compartment of the extracellular matrix and occurs as a sheet-like electron dense structure in close vicinity to adherent epithelial or endothelial cells, or as a complete envelope, especially around mesenchymal cells such as adipocytes, myocytes, and Schwann cells. Besides being responsible for compartmentalization and maintenance of tissue architecture, basement membranes provide anchorage for adjacent cells and stimuli for cell differentiation. They control cell migration and provide a selective filtration barrier such as in the renal glomerulus. The assembly of the basement membrane is the result of intra-molecular, intermolecular, and molecular cell membrane receptor binding although the biochemical mechanisms involved in basement membrane turnover under physiologic conditions remain essentially unknown (Fanguhar et al., 1982; Timpl and Dziadeck, 1986; Abrahamson, 1986).

Four broad categories of diseases are associated with loss of basement membrane integrity, namely, immunological (e.g. immune complex disease), infectious (e.g. trypanosomiasis), metabolic (e.g. diabetes mellitus), and neoplastic. Until recently, basement membranes were studied with histochemical stains, electron microscopy and immunohistochemistry employing immunofluorescence. The more recent availability of sensitive antibodies to type IV collagen and laminin, the two major components of basement membranes, has made it possible to examine basement membranes in paraffin embedded tissue sections. The selective use of proteolytic digestion results in immunostaining patterns with antigen preservation similar to that of frozen tissue sections. Antibodies to fibronectin, a minor basement membrane glycoprotein, have also been made, but immunostaining for this antigen has provided less useful information.

While the synthesis, distribution, and catabolism of basement membrane in various disease states are not well documented, the role of the basement membrane in tumour invasion and metastases is of particular interest to the surgical pathologist (D'Ardenne, 1989). Local invasion by tumour is an early step in the complex multistage process which eventuates in metastatic tumour. After invasion of host tissue barriers adjacent to the primary tumour borders, tumour cells must invade the vascular wall or lymphatic channels in order to disseminate. A number of factors determine the rate of dissemination and these include tumour vascularity, the number of tumour cells entering the circulation, anatomic factors, clumping of tumour cells in the blood stream, and the individual properties of the tumour cell subpopulations (Liotta, 1984). Invasive carcinoma is thought to be preceded by intraepithelial neoplasia that progresses to invasive carcinoma with permeation of the epithelial basement membrane by neoplastic cells. The usefulness of immunohistochemical staining of basement membrane in the diagnosis of breast carcinoma has been demonstrated by several workers (Willebrand et al., 1986; Sakr et al., 1988; Raymond and Leong, 1991; Wetzels et al., 1992). In our experience, enzymic digestion with protease type XXIV (Sigma Chemical Company) at 0.5 mg/ml for one minute at 37°C, resulted in optimal staining for type IV collagen and laminin. Basement membrane stains facilitated identification of small invasive foci through breaks in the basement membrane in cases of pure intraductal carcinoma (Fig. 3.11). Invasive carcinomas including tubular carcinomas were surrounded by variable amounts of abnormal, fragmented and discontinuous basement membrane (Fig. 3.12) which was completely absent in poorly differentiated tumours and in single invasive lobular and ductal carcinoma cells (Raymond and Leong, 1991). Other studies of the basement membrane in neoplasms include rectal adenocarcinoma (Forster et al., 1984), pancreatic adenocar-

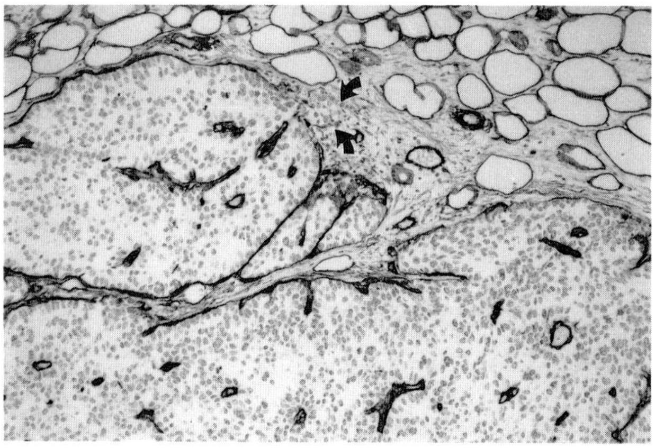

Fig. 3.11. Intraduct carcinoma, comedo type, showing a fragmented basal membrane and a focus of invasion where the basement membrane is deficient (arrows) (anti-type IV collagen, X160).

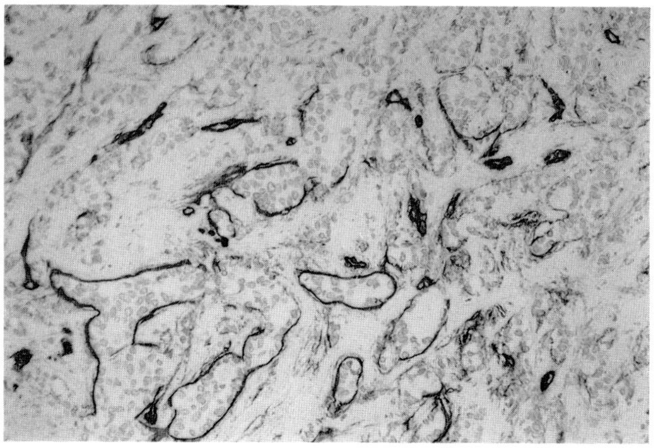

Fig. 3.12. Low-grade infiltrating duct carcinoma stained for laminin. Note the fragmented and focally deficient basal lamina around the infiltrating tubules (anti-laminin, X160).

cinoma (Barsky et al., 1983a), pulmonary adenocarcinoma and squamous cell carcinoma (Barsky et al., 1983a; Albrechtsen et al., 1986), peripheral nerve sheath tumours (Reibel et al., 1985; Ogawa et al., 1986), cutaneous naevi and melanoma (Stenback and Wasenius, 1986), cervical carcinoma (Birembant et al., 1983; Birembant et al., 1985; Stewart and McNicol, 1992; Pitt et al., 1992), bladder carcinoma (Schapers et al., 1990), prostatic carcinoma (Fuchs et al., 1989) and malignant mesothelioma (Kallianpur et al., 1990).

Basement membranes have been studied in a wide variety of cutaneous bullous diseases but only recently have enzyme immunohistochemical techniques been used in place of conventional immunofluorescence stains (Pardo and Penneys, 1990). The presence of basement membrane around blood vessel capillaries has been used to distinguish them from lymphatic capillaries, which, by contrast, uniformly lack immunoreactivity with antibodies to basement membrane components (Barsky et al., 1983b; Otsuki et al., 1990). The presence of subepithelial basement membrane deposition has also been employed to distinguish between choroid plexus neoplasms and ependymomas, being a feature of the former but absent in the latter (Furness et al., 1990).

The identification of selected epitopes of basement membrane adds to our ability to study the genesis of tumour invasion and metastasis. In some instances, it may provide information of prognostic relevance. Subjective quantitation of type IV collagen indicated that as a single variable, it was significantly related to better prognosis in patients with colorectal cancer (Offerhaus et al., 1991) and operable squamous cell carcinoma of the lung (Ten Velde et al., 1991) and carcinoma of the uterine cervix (Pitt et al., 1992). Immunostaining of type IV collagen and laminin has also shown a progressive loss of basement membrane with decreasing differentiation in prostatic carcinoma (Fuchs et al., 1989). Computerized image analysis, employing the SAMBA system, has been applied to breast and endometrial disorders to provide a convenient, accurate and reproducible method of analysing type IV collagen immunostaining (Charpin et al., 1989). With the availability of more specific antibodies to proteoglycans and other minor components of basement membrane such as entactin, nidogen, type VI and type VII collagen, it is anticipated that interest in basement membrane staining will continue to increase (Wetzels et al., 1992).

Receptors for hormones and growth factors

Hormones and growth factors have trophic effects on normal tissues and have been shown to have a similar role in tumours. The presence and quantitation of oestrogen receptor (ER) protein has been demonstrated to be a valuable way of predicting clinical response to endocrine ablative therapy. Patients with ER-positive breast cancer with negative lymph nodes have a better prognosis than those with ER-negative tumours; they are also more likely to respond to endocrine therapy and have longer disease-free intervals than those with ER-negative tumours (Poulsen, 1987; McGuire et al., 1986; Moot et al., 1987).

The progesterone receptor (PR) is induced by the action of oestrogen on ER-positive beast epithelium and is, therefore, a post-receptor marker of ER, its presence indicating an intact oestrogen response pathway (Giri et al., 1988). Patients with both ER-positive and PR-positive tumours have the best chance of responding to hormonal therapy, whereas those with tumours positive for only one receptor have a lower response rate (Benner et al., 1988). It has also been suggested that PR appears to be a more important prognosticator than ER (Clark et al., 1983).

Steroid receptors may also have prognostic significance in other epithelial tumours such as ovarian cancer (Isola et al., 1990) and endometrial cancer (Creasman et al., 1985; Quinn et al., 1985; Carcangui et al., 1990).

Biochemical assays have, until recently, been the main method of measuring hormone receptors but such radioligand-binding assays performed on tumour homogenates have severe limitations and are being superseded by immunohistochemical methods. ER and PR can be demonstrated in the nuclei of approximately 60 per cent of female breast carcinomas by immunohistochemistry with specific monoclonal antibodies. These antibodies recognize an epitope on the receptor that is often impaired by routine formalin fixation and paraffin embedding and the sensitivity of the immunostaining procedure is dependent on whether the tissue is frozen or paraffin-embedded and on other factors such as fixation and specific aspects of the assay itself. Several investigators have reported successful application of the monoclonal H222 anti-ER antibody to formalin-fixed, paraffin-embedded sections. They have employed high concentrations of the antibody (Shimada et al., 1985), or enzymatic pre-treatment of the sections with deoxyribonuclease (Shintaku and Said, 1987), trypsin and deoxyribonuclease (Hiort et al., 1988) or pronase (Cheng et al., 1988). Other workers have used different fixatives such as Bouin's solution and antibodies to different epitopes on the ER (Poulsen, 1987; DeRosa et al., 1989), or a cocktail of monoclonal antibodies (Giri et al., 1988). We have successfully employed the H222 antibody with a standard streptavidin-biotin method to paraffin sections of tissue fixed only for short durations in neutral buffered formalin, following pre-treatment with pronase (Fig. 3.13). The detailed fixation and staining protocol is provided in the Appendix (Raymond and Leong, 1990). A strong concordance between paraffin section and frozen section-determined receptor status and a strong correlation was observed (Raymond and Leong, 1988) and a reverse correlation with tumour growth fraction, histological grade and vimentin expression was demonstrated (Raymond and Leong, 1989b, c). Freeze-dried, paraffin-embedded sections have also been shown to preserve both ER and PR proteins (Onetti-Muda et al., 1991).

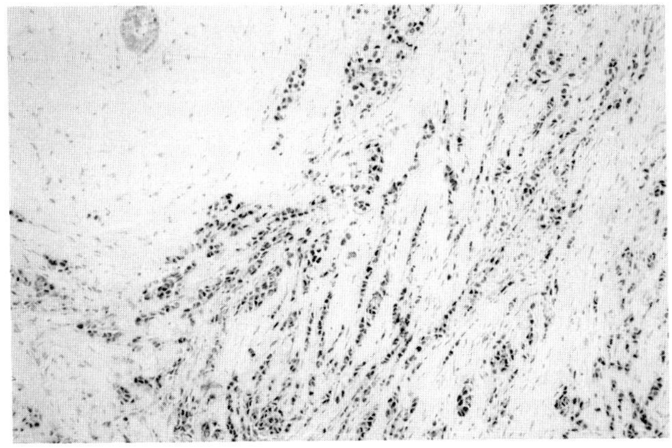

Fig. 3.13. Staining for ER in an infiltrating duct carcinoma of the breast (anti-ER, X40).

The anti-PR antibody (Abbott Laboratories, Chicago, USA) can similarly be employed to paraffin-embedded sections but without the requirement for enzyme pre-treatment (Fig. 3.14).

Steroid hormone receptors can also be analyzed in imprint preparations employing the fluorescent cytochemical method or the immunoperoxidase technique (Raymond and Leong, 1988; DeRosa et al., 1989) with the advantage

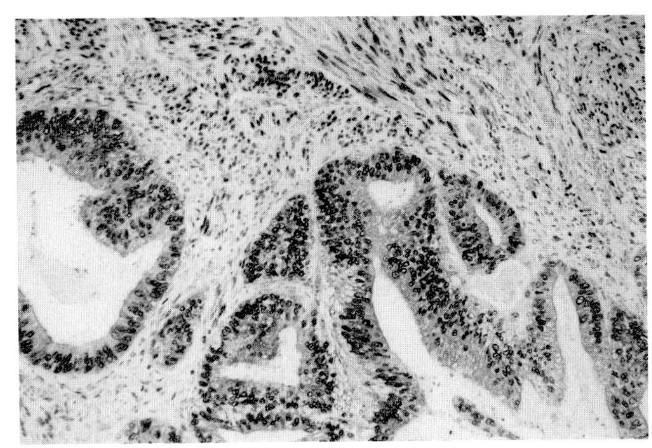

Fig. 3.14. Staining for PR in an endometrial carcinoma. There is strong nuclear staining in both the neoplastic epithelium as well as benign stromal cells. The latter must be taken into account when measuring PR levels in homogenised samples (anti-PR, X160).

that imprint preparations may be particularly useful for small specimens from clinically early or occult breast carcinomas or from small metastatic lesions where there is insufficient material for a separate specimen to be submitted for receptor analysis. It is also useful for the analysis of cells obtained by fine needle aspiration particularly from lesions detected by mammography.

Steroid-regulated proteins

Steroid hormones induce the synthesis of new proteins in receptor-positive cells. The presence of these 'post-receptor markers' are of prognostic relevance because they denote a more favourable response to endocrine therapy. One such marker is cathepsin D which is a lysosomal protease. Like PR, it is oestrogen regulated in ER-positive breast cancer cells and its presence verifies the functional integrity of the receptor pathway. The presence of cathepsin D has been correlated with significantly prolonged survival in patients with ER-positive breast cancer (Henry et al., 1990). Cathepsin D can be demonstrated readily by immunohistochemistry in routine paraffin sections.

Another protein whose synthesis is oestrogen-regulated and is rarely present in ER-negative breast cancers is pS2. It has been shown to be a marker of good prognosis and an indicator of likely response to endocrine therapy (Foekens et al., 1990; Predine et al., 1992). This protein can be readily demonstrated in routine paraffin sections (Fig. 3.15).

Epidermal growth factor receptor

The epidermal growth factor receptor (EGFR) can be demonstrated by immunohistochemical techniques in tissue sections. In breast carcinomas, EGFR expression correlates with poor prognosis and reciprocally with ER expression. In other tumours studied, EGFR expression is a marker for reduced disease-free interval and survival. For example, it can be detected in approximately 50 per cent of bladder carcinoma where it is associated with multiple tumours, recurrences and reduced survival (Neal et al., 1990).

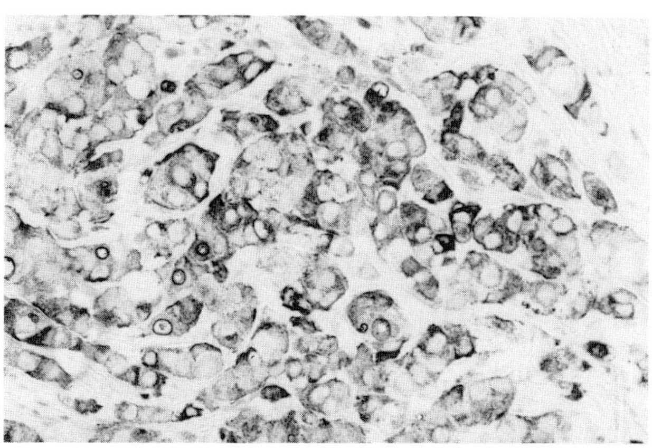

Fig. 3.15. High grade carcinoma of the breast showing strong cytoplasmic staining for pS2, an oestrogen-regulated protein (anti-pS2, X160).

Detection of cell proliferation in tissue sections

In recent years, there have been considerable advances in our ability to obtain qualitative and quantitative information regarding cell proliferation in normal and pathologic processes. Cell proliferation is of interest at two different levels in the malignant process. First, abnormal cell proliferation appears to be a precursor, and perhaps a predictor, of tumourigenesis (Cohen and Ellwein, 1990); secondly, studies of cell proliferation in human tumours, principally through the use of techniques such as flow cytometry, have demonstrated that quantitative aspects of the proliferative activity within a fully developed tumour can predict clinical outcome (Coon et al., 1987).

The oldest, and simplest, method is 'mitosis counting', i.e. the direct assessment of the fraction of cell nuclei in the 'M' phase of the cell cycle by morphological identification. While this technique has been applied to a variety of tumours, it is within the smooth muscle cell tumours of the uterus that the technique has had greatest impact. Indeed, the counting of 'mitoses' is one of the few quantitative exercises undertaken by the diagnostic pathologist, and one which, according to some studies, can be of great importance in distinguishing benign from malignant smooth muscle tumours, i.e. can predict clinical outcome (Kempson and Bari, 1970).

None the less, there are considerable limitations, both theoretical and practical, to the use of 'mitosis counting' as an assessment of cell proliferation. First, as demonstrated by Silverberg (1976), identification of mitotic figures is by no means a reliable exercise, and considerable interobserver disagreement can result. Secondly, in a seminal paper by Evans in 1926 employing experiment mice, it was demonstrated that the number of mitotic figures identified in normal organs such as skin, lymph node, and intestine fell dramatically as a function of post-mortem interval, prior to immersion into fixation. Evans demonstrated that cells in the course of mitosis could continue through the cell cycle even following the death of the animal. A more recent study suggested that the denominator used in most mitotic figure counting exercises, the 'high powered field', can vary in area over a factor of six as a factor of microscope type and lens combinations. Indeed, given these limitations it is surprising that any significance whatsoever has been ascribed to this exercise; at the very least, it suggests that the ability to apply data obtained from one laboratory to another is severely limited.

Our understanding of the process of mitosis has increased dramatically in recent years. In the current state of knowledge, the cell cycle, of which actual mitosis is but one part, has been divided into several 'phases', as represented in Fig. 3.16 below. In different cell types, the actual and relative amount of time spent in a given portion of the cell cycle will vary; in some cells, such as granulocytes and neurons, the cell is permanently 'removed' from the cell cycle.

The 'gold standard' for determination of proliferative activity in tissues has long been the ^{3}H-thymidine method. Thymidine, one of the four DNA bases, is incorporated into the nuclear DNA only during the actual 'S' phase of the cycle, and thus 'thymidine uptake' has become a rigorous indicator of this aspect of cell proliferation. ^{3}H-labelled thymidine is generally administered to an animal or incubated with a tissue for a defined period of time (e.g. 1 h), and can be detected by fixing and embedding the tissue, cutting a standard section, and then overlaying the section with a photographic emulsion

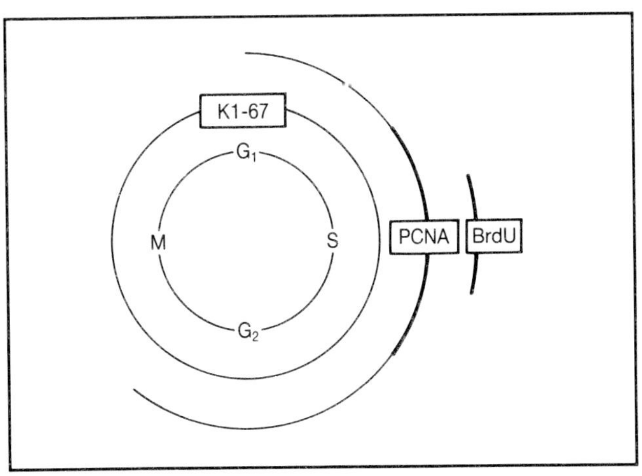

Fig. 3.16. The cell cycle with localization of various markers.

film. In most experimental contexts ^{3}H-thymidine uptake is still a very useful marker of cell proliferation; it also has the advantage that the resulting nuclear silver grains can be detected at both the light microscopic and ultrastructural level. Theoretically, exposing human tumours to ^{3}H-thymidine would provide a precise measurement of cell proliferation in human tumours. There are, however, several features of ^{3}H-thymidine uptake which make it unsuitable for routine work. First, it requires incubation of viable tumour tissue with ^{3}H-thymidine; in the experimental context, this generally entails intravenous injection prior to tumour removal, which is not possible in human specimens. While it is theoretically possible to take freshly isolated human tumour tissue and incubate it with a thymidine-containing buffer, in reality this is a very impractical method, as the uptake of thymidine can be inhibited by loss of tissue viability, physical factors such as density of tumour stroma, etc. Finally, the requirement for days-to-weeks of incubation to expose the photographic emulsion, as well as the problem of working with (and disposing of) radioactive materials severely limits the applicability of this technique to the diagnostic pathology laboratory.

The latter problems can be overcome by replacing ^{3}H-thymidine with a different analog, bromodeoxyuridine (BrdU). The latter retains the S-phase specificity of thymidine uptake, and has the advantage of being able to be recognized with an antibody detection system (e.g. Nagashima et al., 1985). Several different monoclonal anti-BrdU antibodies have been developed, although most require denaturation of the DNA prior to antibody incubation. This can be achieved with incubation of the tissue with 1 M NaOH or 1 M HCl, which can adversely affect tissue histology. Despite the fact that, if an appropriate fixative such as Carnoy's, is employed, the antibody method can be employed on deparaffinized tissue, BrdU shares with ^{3}H-thymidine the requirement of incubation of viable tissue with the analog; this is generally a practical impossibility, although the method lends itself well to the experimental animal, where a single intravenous injection of BrdU can be performed one hour prior to sacrifice to permit a 'snapshot' of S phase activity at that time.

For many years it had been realized that the optimal reagent would be an antibody that could identify proteins, expression of which was restricted to various portions of the cell cycle, and would thus require no tissue preincubation. A number of candidate proteins have emerged that could be useful; they are summarized below.

The Ki-67 defined antigen

Ki-67 is a monoclonal antibody that was generated by Gerdes et al. (1983). It was generated to a Hodgkin's disease cell line, but was determined to identify a nuclear antigen present in most proliferating cells. The antigen recognized by Ki-67, only recently defined as a 345-395 kD protein complex (Gerdes et al., 1991), is expressed during all non-G_0 phases of the cycle, and is thus a useful marker for those cells participating in cell proliferation; antigenic expression in many cells and cell lines appears to increase with cell cycle progression. In many cells, Ki-67 immunostaining appears to localize to the nucleolar or perinucleolar region, although when used on standard frozen sections, a homogenous nuclear immunostaining pattern is generally apparent. Gerdes et al. (1983), in the original description of the antibody, noted that the distribution of Ki-67-positive cells in normal tissues was suggestive of one that correlated with cell kinetic parameters. In a subsequent publication, Gerdes et al. (1984), described a good correlation between ^{3}H-thymidine labelling indices and the number of cells immunostained by antibody Ki-67. None the less, in general, the fraction of cells of a given tissue or tumour which are Ki-67-positive, however, is generally significantly more than that in S-phase, as defined, e.g. by flow cytometric analysis or ^{3}H-thymidine uptake. Several studies have compared Ki-67- and other parameters such as histologic grade in a number of different tumour types; in general, Ki-67 indices correlate with histologic grade and, in selected studies where follow-up has been obtained, can be predictive of clinical outcome (Ueda et al., 1989; Brown and Gatter, 1990). None the less, as the antigen detected by Ki-67 is quite labile to most fixation and embedding protocols, this has proven to be a less than optimal reagent for the routine pathology laboratory, and has limited the applicability of this antibody to prospective studies. However, with the knowledge of the nature of the Ki-67-defined protein now emerging, it may be possible to generate new antibodies which identify formalin-stable epitopes.

PCNA (proliferating cell nuclear antigen; PCNA/cyclin)

PCNA is a protein first described independently by two groups of investigators, and now known to represent a component of DNA polymerase-δ (Bravo and Macdonald-Bravo, 1987). Miyachi et al. (1978) described an antibody present in the sera of selected patients with systemic lupus erythematosus that reacted with a nuclear antigen in proliferating cells, i.e. the sera did not react with nuclei of renal tubular or hepatic parenchymal cells, but did react with the lymphocytes of lymphoid follicles; normal peripheral lymphocytes were negative with the sera, but 20 per cent of the cells became positive upon mitogenic stimulation with phytohaemagglutinin. Working independently, Bravo and Celis (1980), using high resolution two-diensional gel electrophoresis, screened for proteins whose rate of synthesis increased substantially in proliferating, as compared with resting, cells. The protein, which they dubbed *cyclin*, at ca. 36,000 daltons, demonstrated the most striking association with the proliferative rate of cells, i.e. it was present in very small amounts in normal or non-dividing cells but synthesized by normal, proliferating cells; the level of cyclin also manifested a striking increase in the S-phase. Following demonstration of the identify of the two proteins PCNA and cyclin, the appellation PCNA/cyclin was, until recently, used to describe these proteins. With the rapid expansion of knowledge regarding the class of proteins called 'cyclins', which help regulate cell progression to S-phase, the name 'PNCA' has become established.

Ogata et al. (1987) developed the first set of monoclonal antibodies, 19A2 (a murine IgM) and 19F4 (a murine IgG) to PCNA. These antibodies were used to demonstrate (Kurki et al., 1988) that, using appropriate fixation protocols, PCNA immunostaining (using the monoclonal antibodies) increased during the G_1 phase of the cell cycle, reaching a maximum at the S-phase, and declined during the G_2/M phase, suggesting that monoclonal antibodies to PCNA could be used as a handy tool for the detection of cell proliferation. Earlier studies of human tumours by Robbins et al. (1987), using anti-PCNA autoantisera, had suggested that PCNA positivity correlated with mitotic activity and tumour grade. Following work by Thaete et al. (1989), again using the human antisera, who verified that cell proliferation in mouse lung tissue could be reliably quantitated using anti-PCNA immunostaining, Garcia et al. (1989), successfully employed the 19A2 monoclonal antibody of Ogata et al., in a retrospective analysis of methacarn-fixed, deparaffinized human tumour tissue. These latter authors compared the 'proliferative index', as determined by the quartile of tumour cells positive with the antibody, with the flow cytometrically determined S-phase fraction. There was generally an excellent correlation, although there were enough discrepancies to suggest that the slide-based technique might prove more reliable and yield additional information. Others have demonstrated the ability to use 19A2 in formalin fixed, deparaffinized tissue (Kamel et al., 1991), although only with short fixation times (3–10 h). Other antibodies have recently been developed, including PC10, which identifies PCNA epitopes more stable to formalin fixation (Wasseem and Lane, 1990; Hall et al., 1990a), and promise further applications.

None the less, certain caveats apply to the use of anti-PCNA antibodies as markers of cell proliferation in tissues sections. First, as noted by Morris and Mathews (1989), in malignant cell lines such as HeLa, while the PCNA level increases during S-phase, it is not zero during other phases of the cell cycle; indeed, in this cell line the relative amount of PCNA increases by only a factor of 2 or 3. This has important implications for the study of malignancies, as noted by Hall et al. (1990b), in which there was thought to be a 'loss of control' of PCNA expression with respect to the cell cycle. Indeed, as demonstrated by Coltrera and Gown (1991), the relative amounts of PCNA differ in different cell types, and the relationship of immunocytochemically detected PCNA to the phase of the cell cycle, as defined by BrdU uptake, differs in different cell types. Further complicating the situation is the association in the nucleus of at least two forms of PCNA, one associated with the 'replicon' structure and one more loosely associated in the cell nucleus; both forms are retained by formalin fixation, while only the former is retained by alcohol (e.g. methacarn) fixation (Bravo et al., 1987). Thus, the apparent proliferation index using anti-PCNA antibodies will depend upon the cell type identified as well as the fixative type and duration, and it can be expected that such studies will yield 'proliferative indices' discordant with those obtained via flow cytometry or ^{3}H-thymidine incubation.

Other antibody-defined markers

A host of other antibodies defining proliferation-related markers have been presented, although there are very limited data on their utility in human tumour analysis. These include antibodies to: topoisomerase II (Heck and Earnshaw, 1986); the M1 subunit of ribonucleotide reductase (Engstrom et al., 1984); DNA polymerase alpha (Tsutsumi et al., 1990); p105 (Clevinger et al., 1987); 'PAA' (Dubey et al., 1987); and antibodies such as C_5F_{10}, which identifies cells in the 'M' phase of the cell cycle (Lloyd et al., 1985).

H3 and H4 mRNA localization

The most recent innovation in tissue identification of proliferating cells is the use of *in situ* hybridization for the localization of histone H3 and/or H4 mRNA. Histones are highly basic proteins tightly bound to DNA; based on earlier studies suggesting an S-phase dependence of H3 mRNA expression (Artishevsky et al., 1985), Chou, et al. (1990) recently demonstrated the feasibility of using *in situ* hybridization to identify H3 mRNA in tissue sections, and the H3 mRNA-positive cells appear to be those 'expected' to be positive, e.g. basal cells of the skin, crypt cells of the intestine. This method has the advantage of applicability to deparaffinized sections of formalin fixed tissue; none the less, the method has not yet been validated with respect to independent measurements of cell proliferation in studies of human tumours.

Other prognostic tumour markers

Prognostication in oncology is largely dependent on the accurate grading and staging of tumours. Short-term survival is determined mainly by the grade and stage, whereas, long-term survival is more dependent on histologic typing of the tumour. However, the criteria employed for typing, grading, and to some extent, staging, are subjective and prone to observer error. Furthermore, routine histopathological examination may not reveal all possible markers of prognostic relevance and the individual categories of histologic type, grade and stage may overlap as regards clinical outcome. These reasons have accounted for the poor correlation between histopathological assessment and prognosis in many instances and, together with the problems imposed by the diminishing size of biopsy samples, there has been a need for ancillary techniques and new indices to improve accuracy and reproducibility in diagnosis and prognostication.

The development of sensitive immunohistochemical techniques has provided an alternative avenue of assessment which is becoming an invaluable adjunct not only to diagnosis and typing, but also for the identification of new prognostic markers. In the preceding sections, some of these have already been discussed. Immunohistochemical stains aid in the staging of tumours by providing a sensitive method of identifying metastatic deposits in regional lymph nodes and in the bone marrow, as well as identifying invasion of the basal lamina, and vascular and lymphatic spaces. Aberrant phenotypes such as the expression of vimentin filaments in epithelial tumours may be an indicator of aggressive behaviour. Ki-67 and antibodies to PCNA/cyclin allow the assessment of the growth fraction of the tumour. Steroid receptors have been shown to be of relevance in the prediction of outcome in breast carcinoma and also in endometrial and ovarian cancer. Cathepsin D and pS2 are both steroid regulated proteins which, like the progesterone receptor, also serve as post-receptor markers of a functional ER pathway. Both markers have been shown to correlate significantly with prolonged survival in patients with ER-positive breast cancer (Henry et al., 1990; Predine et al., 1992) and can be demonstrated readily by immunohistochemistry in routine paraffin sections. Similarly, epidermal growth factor receptor can be demonstrated in tissue sections, and in most tumours studied, the epidermal growth factor receptor expression is a marker of reduced disease-free interval and survival.

The discovery of oncogenes has lead to a considerable interest in their biological role and their value as markers of neoplastic behaviour. When oncogenes become amplified, undergo mutation or translocation, their inappropriate activity is reflected by increased levels of expression of mRNA and oncoprotein. The alteration at DNA level can presently only be demonstrated by the techniques of molecular biology and *in situ* hybridization can be used to demonstrate the mRNA, but often the signal is weak and the methodology is not reliable for routine application. The oncoprotein often has a short half-life which makes it difficult to detect immunohistochemically, however, the mutant oncoprotein can be detected in several instances. *c-erbB-2, c-myc* and *ras* proteins have been the most widely studied. *c-erbB-2* (HER-2/neu) expression in invasive breast carcinoma (Fig. 3.17) has been shown to be associated with a relatively poor survival (Wright et al., 1989). It correlates with high grade tumours and is positive in intraduct carcinomas of comedo type but not of cribriform type. Amplification of the *c-erbB-2* gene is also found in about 30 per cent of ovarian cancers and it has been suggested that amplification and overexpression might be associated with a poor prognosis in patients with ovarian cancer (Slamon et al., 1989). The *c-myc* oncogene interacts with nuclear

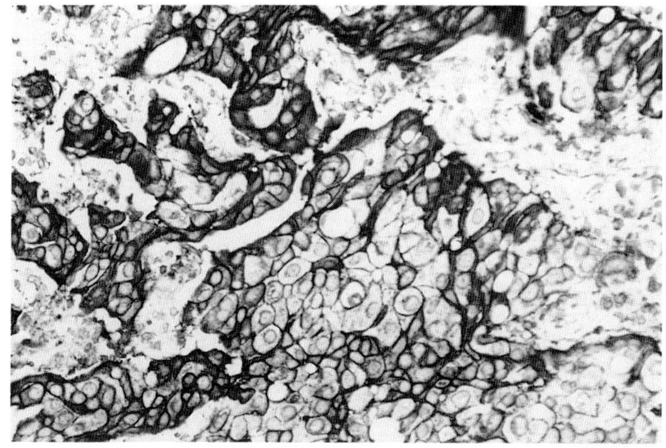

Fig. 3.17. *c-erbB-2* oncoprotein staining in a high grade infiltrating duct carcinoma of the breast showing intense membranous as well as focal cytoplasmic staining (anti-*c-erbB-2*, X 250).

DNA to stimulate DNA synthesis. Inappropriately increased expression may be associated with tumour development and progression. Increased expression of the gene in general, is associated with more aggressive behaviour, a shorter disease-free interval and reduced survival time as in the case of carcinoma of the cervix (Sowani et al., 1989) and small cell carcinoma of the lung (Johnson et al., 1987). p21, a *ras* oncoprotein has been most extensively studied by immunohistochemistry and increased expression as been reported in hepatocellular and colorectal carcinomas. Overexpression has also been found in ovarian carcinomas, although correlations with clinical outcome of these tumours are controversial.

Several tumour suppressor genes have been identified, the three more important ones in human tumours being the retinoblastoma susceptibility gene, deleted in colonic cancer (DCC) gene and p53. The p53 protein binds to specific DNA sequences and appears to be a transcription factor that blocks the progression of cells through the G1 phase of the cell cycle. Mutation in one allele of this tumour-suppressor gene renders a normal cell susceptible to transformation, and subsequent loss of the other allele presumably removes all growth restraints from the tumour cells. Mutated p53 genes have been shown to cooperate with *ras* to transform cells *in vitro*. Compared to wild-type p53 proteins, mutant p53 proteins have much longer half-lives, and their concentration is much higher in cancer cells so that they are detectable by immunohistochemistry (Fig. 3.18). Sporadic mutations of p53 gene are the single most common genetic alteration observed in human cancers, involving 70 per cent of colonic cancers, 30–50 per cent

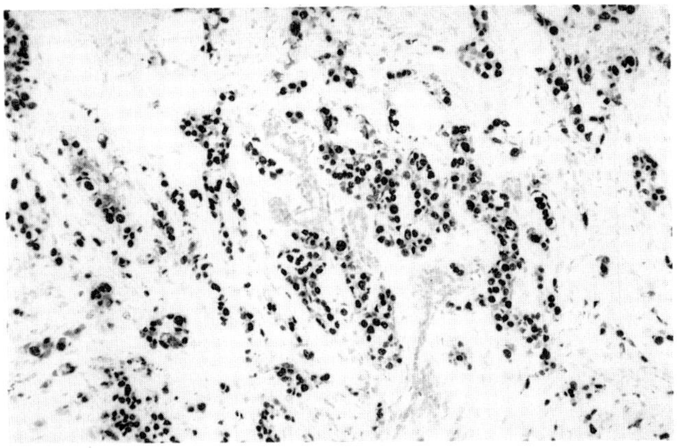

Fig. 3.18. Staining for p53 protein in an intermediate grade infiltrating carcinoma of the breast. There is strong labelling of the nuclear antigen in a high proportion of the neoplastic cells. Note the absence of staining in the benign duct in the centre of the field (anti-p53, X 40).

of breast cancers, 50 per cent of lung cancers, and 100 per cent of small cell lung cancers. Germline mutations in p53 were recently identified in families with the Li–Fraumeni syndrome characterized by a high incidence of soft tissue sarcomas, pre-menopausal breast cancers and other diverse neoplasms. More recent studies indicate that the group of patients with cancer who carry germline mutations of the p53 gene is more diverse than is suggested by the clinical definition of the Li–Fraumeni syndrome (Toguchida et al., 1992; Malkin et al., 1992).

Lastly, markers to monitor therapy have recently become available. It is well recognized that some tumours are characteristically resistant to chemotherapy for various reasons. Intrinsic causes of such resistance include increased activation of the enzymes dihydrofolate reductase or the increased expression of the p-glycoprotein encoded for by the multidrug resistant (MDR) gene. MDR and its presence in a cell correlates with resistance to various drugs (Deuchars and Ling, 1989) and p-glycoprotein can be demonstrated immunohistochemically. Other markers of potential prognostic significance such as p24 protein, heatshock protein and transforming growth factor β can also be studied immunohistochemically as can various adhesion molecules and cytokines which may influence tumour metastasis and behaviour.

Histological assessment of cancers can now provide more precise diagnoses as well as more accurate anatomical staging (Leong and Raymond, 1989). In addition, important prognostic parameters and information concerning pathogenesis can be obtained by assessing a variety of parameters which include steroid receptors, growth fractions, oncogene proteins, cell proliferation markers, lineage-associated antigens and other markers of potential prognostic relevance. Sensitive antibodies to all these markers are commercially available and can be applied through immunohistochemical techniques which have the advantage of being rapid, relatively inexpensive, with the majority reactive in paraffin-embedded tissue, allowing their use in retrospective studies. Such analyses have already contributed significant new insights into cancer histogenesis and the ability to assess for biological parameters accords histopathological examination new power and prestige (Leong, 1990).

References

Abenoza, P. and Sibley, R.K. (1986). Chordoma: An immunohistologic study. *Human Pathology* **17**, 744–7.

Abenoza, P., Sibley, R.K. and Rosai, J. (1985). Immunocytochemistry in the differential diagnosis of chordoma and chondrosarcoma. *Laboratory Investigation* **52**, 1a (abstract).

Abo, T. and Balch, C.M. (1981). A differentiation antigen of human NK and K cells identified by a monoclonal antibody (HNK-1). *Journal of Immunology* **127**, 1024.

Abrahamson, D.R. (1986). Recent studies on the structure and pathology of basement membranes. *Journal of Pathology* **149**, 257–78.

Aschtatter, T., Moll, R. and Anderson, A. (1986). Expression of glial filament protein (GFP) in nerve sheaths and non-neural cells re-examined using monoclonal antibodies, with special emphasis on the coexpression of GFP and cytokeratins in epithelial cells of human salivary gland and pleomorphic adenomas. *Differentiation* **31**, 206–27.

Albores-Saavedra, J., Nadji, M. and Civantos, F. (1983). Thyroglobulin in carcinoma of the thyroid: an immunohistochemical study. *Human Pathology* **14**, 62–6.

Albrechtsen, R., Weber, U.M. and Liotta, L.A. (1986). Basement Membranes in Human Cancer. In Rosen, P.P. and Fechner, R.E. (eds), *Pathology Annual, Part II*, pp. 251–65. Sommers, S.C., Lippincott, New York.

Artishevsky, A., Grafsky, A. and Lee, A.S. (1985). Isolation of a mammalian sequence capable of conferring cell cycle regulation to a heterologous gene. *Science* **230**, 1061–3.

Attiyeh, F.F., Jansen, M., Huvos, A.G. and Fracchia, A. (1977). Axillary micrometastasis and macrometastasis in carcinoma of the breast. *Surgery, Gynecology and Obstetrics* **144**, 839–42.

Azumi, N., Trawseek, S.T. and Batiffora, H. (1991). Prostatic acid phosphatase in carcinoid tumors. Immunohistochemical and immunoblot studies. *American Journal of Surgical Pathology* **15**, 785–90.

Bacchi, C.E., Gown, A.M. and Zarbo, R.J. (1990). Do malignant glioma cells display anomalous low molecular weight cytokeratin expression? *Laboratory Investigation* **62**, 6A.

Barsky, S.H., Siegal, G.P., Jannotta, F. and Liotta, L.A. (1983a). Loss of basement membrane components by invasive tumours but not by their benign counterparts. *Laboratory Investigation* **49**, 140–6.

Barsky, S.H., Baker, A., Siegal, G.P., Togo, S. and Liotta, L.A. (1983b). Use of anti-basement membrane antibodies to distinguish blood vessel capillaries from lymphatic capillaries. *American Journal of Surgical Pathology* **7**, 667–72.

Battifora, H., Sheibani, K. and Tubbs, R.R. (1984). Anikeratin antibodies in tumour diagnosis. Distinction between seminoma and embryonal carcinoma. *Cancer* **54**, 843–8.

Battifora, H. and Kopinski, M. (1985). Distinction of mesothelioma from adenocarcinoma: an immunohistochemical approach. *Cancer* **55**, 1679–85.

Benner, S.E., Clark, G.M. and McGuire, W.L. (1988). Review: steroid receptors, cellular kinetics and lymph node status as prognostic factors in breast cancer. *American Journal of Medical Science* **296**, 59–66.

Bergh, J., Esscher, T. and Steinholtz, L. (1985). Immunocytochemical demonstration of neuron-specific enolase (NSE) in human lung cancers. *American Journal of Clinical Pathology* **84**, 1–7.

Bezwoda, W.R., Lewis D. and Livini, N. (1986). Bone marrow involvement in anaplastic small cell lung cancer. Diagnosis, hematologic features, and prognostic implications. *Cancer* **58**, 1762–5.

Birembant, P., Caron, Y. and Adnet, J.J. (1985). Usefulness of basement membrane markers in tumoral pathology. *Pathology* **145**, 283–90.

Birembant, P., Caron, Y., van Couwenberge, D. and Foidart, J.M. (1983). Distribution of laminin, a basement membrane glycoprotein in epithelial proliferations. A preliminary study of the breast, the lungs and uterine cervix. *Collagen Related Research* **3**, 25–33.

Blobel, G.A., Gould, V.E. and Moll, R. (1985). Coexpression of neuroendocrine markers and epithelial cytoskeletal proteins in brochopulmonary neuroendocrine neoplasms. *Laboratory Investigation* **52**, 39–51.

Blomjous, C.E.M., Thunnissen, B.J.M. and Vos, W. (1988). Small cell neuroendocrine carcinoma of the urinary bladder: an immunohistochemical and ultrastructural evaluation of 3 cases with a review of the literature. *Virchows Archives (Pathology Anatomy A)* **413**, 505–12.

Bolen, J.W., Hammar, S.P. and McNutt, M.A. (1986). Reactive and neoplastic serosal tissue: A light microscopic, ultrastructural and immunocytochemical study. *American Journal of Surgical Pathology* **10**, 34–47.

Bravo, R. and Celis, J.E. (1980). A search for differential polypeptide synthesis throughout the cell cycle of HeLa cells. *Journal of Cell Biology* **84**, 795.

Bravo, R. and Macdonald-Bravo, H. (1987). Existence of two populations of cyclin/proliferating cell nuclear antigen during the cell cycle: Association with DNA replication sites. *Journal of Cell Biology* **105**, 1549–54.

Brooks, J.J., LiVolsi, V.A. and Trojanowski, J.Q. (1987). Does chondroid chordoma exist? *Acta Neuropathologica* **72**, 229–35.

Brown, D.C. and Gatter, K.C. (1990). Monoclonal antibody Ki-67: Its use in histopathology. *Histopathology* **17**, 489–503.

Burke, A.P. and Mostofi, F.K. (1988a). Intratubular malignant germ cells in testicular biopsies: Clinical course and identification by staining for placental alkaline phosphatase. *Modern Pathology* **1**, 475–9.

Burke, A.P. and Mostofi, F.K. (1988b). Placental alkaline phosphatase immunohistochemistry of intratubular malignant germ cells and associated testicular germ cell tumours. *Human Pathology* **19**, 663–70.

Bussolati, G., Gugliotta, P. and Morra, I. (1986). The immunohistochemical detection of lymph node metastases from infiltrating lobular carcinoma of the breast. *British Journal of Cancer* **54**, 631–6.

Butcher, D.N., Gregory, W.M. and Gunter, P.A. (1985). The biological and clinical significance of HCG-containing cells in seminoma. *British Journal of Cancer* **51**, 473–8.

Caillaud, J.M., Martinez-Madrigal, F., Hartmann, O. and Carlu, C. (1991). Immunohistochemical demonstration of neuron-specific enolase in bone marrow infiltrated by neuroblastoma. *Journal of Clinical Pathology* **44**, 309–12.

Carcangui, M.L., Chambers, J.T. and Voynick, I.M. (1990). Immunohistochemical evaluation of estrogen and progesterone receptor content in 183 patients with endometrial carcinoma. Part I: Clinical and histologic correlations. *American Journal of Clinical Pathology* **94**, 247–54.

Caselitz, J., Osborn, M. and Wustrow, J. (1982). The expression of different intermediate-sized filaments in human salivary gland and their tumors. *Pathology Research Practice* **175**, 2265–78.

Charpin, C., Andrac, L. and de Victor, B. (1989). Type IV collagen immunostaining and computerised image analysis (SAMBA) in breast and endometrial disorders. *Histopathology* **14**, 47–60.

Chase, D., Enzinger, F.M. and Weiss, S.W. (1984). Keratin in epithelioid sarcoma: an immunohistochemical study. *American Journal of Surgical Pathology* **5**, 137–51.

Cheng, L., Binder, S.W., Fu, Y.S. and Lewin, K.J. (1988).

Demonstration of oestrogen receptors by monoclonal antibody in formalin-fixed breast tumours. *Laboratory Investigation* **58**, 346–53.

Chou, M.Y., Chang, A.L. and McBride, J. (1990). A rapid method to determine proliferation patterns of normal and malignant tissues by H3 mRNA in situ hybridization. *American Journal of Pathology* **136**, 729–33.

Chu, T.A. (1987). Chondroid chordoma of the sacral coccygeal region. *Archives of Pathology and Laboratory Medicine* **111**, 861–64.

Cibas, E.S., Corson, J.M. and Pinkus, G.S. (1987). The distinction of adenocarcinoma from malignant mesothelioma in cell blocks of effusions: The role of routine mucin histochemistry and immunohistochemical assessment of carcinoembryonic antigen, keratin proteins, epithelial membrane antigen, and milk fat globule-derived antigen. *Human Pathology* **18**, 67–74.

Clark, G.M., McGuire, W.L., Hubray, C.A., Pearson, O.H. and Marshall, J.S. (1983). Progesterone receptors as a prognostic factor in stage II breast cancer. *New England Journal of Medicine* **309**, 1343–7.

Clevinger, C.V., Epstein, A.L. and Bauer, K.D. (1987). Modulation of the nuclear antigen, p105 as a function of cell cycle proliferation. *Journal of Cell Physiology* **130**, 336–43.

Cochran, A.J., Wen, D. and Morton, D.L. (1988). Occult tumour cells in the lymph nodes of patients with pathological stage I malignant melanoma. An immunohistological study. *American Journal of Surgical Pathology* **12**, 612–18.

Coggi, G., Dell'Orto, P., Braidotti, P., Coggi, A. and Viale, G. (1989). Co-expression of intermediate filaments in normal and neoplastic tissue: a reappraisal. *Ultrastructural Pathology* **13**, 501–14.

Cohen, S.M. and Ellwein, L.B. (1990). Cell proliferation in carcinogenesis. *Science* **249**, 1007–11.

Colley, M.H., Geppert, E. and Franklin, W.A. (1989). Immunohistochemical detection of steroid receptors in a case of pulmonary lymphangioleiomyomatosis. *American Journal of Surgical Pathology* **13**, 803–7.

Coltrera, M.D. and Gown, A.M. (1991). PCNA/cyclin and BrdU uptake define different subpopulations in different cell lines. *Journal of Histochemistry and Cytochemistry* **39**, 23–30.

Coon, J.S., Landay, A.L. and Weinstein, R.S. (1987). Biology of disease: advances in flow cytometry for diagnostic pathology. *Laboratory Investigation* **57**, 453–78.

Cote, R.J., Rosen, P.P. and Hakes, T.B. (1988). Monoclonal antibodies detect occult breast carcinoma metastases in the bone marrow of patients with early stage disease. *American Journal of Surgical Pathology* **12**, 333–40.

Creasman, W.T., Soter, J.T., McCarty, K.S.,Jr., McCarty, K.S.,Sn., Henshaw, W. and Clarke-Pearson, D.L. (1985). Influence of cytoplasmic steroid receptor content on prognosis of early stage endometrial carcinoma. *American Journal of Obstetrics and Gynaecology* **151**, 922–32.

D'Ardenne, A.J. (1989). Use of basement membrane markers in tumour diagnosis. *Journal of Clinical Pathology* **42**, 449–57.

Dabbs, D.J., Geisinger, K.R. and Norris, H.T. (1986). Intermediate filaments in endometrial and endocervical carcinomas. The diagnostic utility of vimentin patterns. *American Journal of Surgical Pathology* **10**, 568–76.

Dahl, D., Reuger, D.C. and Bignami, A. (1981). Vimentin, the 57,000 molecular weight protein of fibroblast filaments, is the major cytoskeletal component of immature glia. *European Journal of Cell Biology* **24**, 191–6.

Damjanov, I., Osborn, M. and Miettinen, M. (1990). Keratin 7 is a marker for a subset of trophoblastic cells in human germ cell tumours. *Archives of Pathology and Laboratory Medicine* **114**, 81–3.

de Mascarel, A., Merlio, J.-P. and Coindre, J.-M. (1989). Gastric large cell lymphoma expression cytokeratin but no leukocyte common antigen. *American Journal of Clinical Pathology* **91**, 478–81.

Dearnaley, D.P., Sloane, J.P. and Ormerod, M.G. (1981). Increased detection of mammary carcinoma cells in marrow smears using antisera to epithelial membrane antigen. *British Journal of Cancer* **44**, 85–90.

deBruine, A.P. and Bosman, F.T. (1990). Neuroendocrine tumours in the respiratory tract. *Acta Histochemistry* **38**, S.99–105.

Delsol, G., Gatter, K.C. and Stein, H. (1984). Human lymphoid cells express epithelial membrane antigen. *Lancet* **2**, 1124–8.

Denk, H., Moll, R. and Weybora, W. (1987). Intermediate filaments and desmosomal plaque proteins in testicular seminomas and non-seminomatous germ cell tumours as revealed by immunohistochemistry. *Virchows Archives (Pathology, Anatomy, Histopathology A)* **410**, 295–307.

DeRosa, C.M., Ozzello, L., Habif, D.V., Konrath, J.G. and Greene, G.L. (1989). Immunohistochemical assessment of oestrogen and progesterone receptors in stored imprints and cryostat sections of breast carcinoma. *Annals of Surgery* **212**, 224–8.

Deuchars, K.L. and Ling, V. (1989). P-glycoprotein and multidrug resistance in cancer chemotherapy. *Seminars in Oncology* **16**, 156–69.

Dewar, A., Valente, M., Ring, N.P. and Corrin, B. (1987). Pleural mesothelioma of epithelial type and pulmonary adenocarcinoma: An ultrastructural and cytochemical comparison. *Journal of Pathology* **152**, 309–16.

Di Sant'Agnese, P.A. (1992). Neuroendocrine differentiation in human prostatic carcinoma. *Human Pathology* **23**, 287–96.

Diaz, N.M., Mazoujian, G. and Wick, M.R. (1991). Estrogen receptor protein in thyroid neoplasms. An immunohistochemical analysis of papillary carcinoma, follicular carcinoma, and follicular adenoma. *Archives of Pathology and Laboratory Medicine* **115**, 1203–7.

Dierick, A.M., Praet, M. and Roels, H. (1991). Verbeeck P, Robyns C, Oosterlinck W. Vimentin expression of renal cell carcinoma in relation to DNA content and histologic grading: a combined light microscopic, immunocytochemical and cytophotometrical analysis. *Histopathology* **18**, 315–22.

Doglioni, C., Gambacorta, M. and Zamboni, G. (1990). Immunocytochemical localization of progesterone receptors in endocrine cells of the human pancreas. *American Journal of Pathology* **137**, 999–1005.

Dubey, D.P., Staunton, D.E. and Parekh, A.C. (1987). Unique proliferation-associated marker expressed on activated and transformed human cells defined by monoclonal antibody. *JNCI* **78**, 203–12.

Eglin, D.E. and Ulbright, T.M. (1987). The differential diagnosis of yolk sac tumour and seminoma. Usefulness of cytokeratin, alpha-fetoprotein, and alpha-1–antitrypsin immunoperoxidase reactions. *American Journal of Clinical Pathology* **88**, 328–32.

Engstrom, Y., Rozell, B. and Hansson, H.-A. (1984). Localization of ribonucleotide reductase in mammalian cells. *EMBO Journal* **3**, 863–67.

Evans, D.J., Lampert, I.A. and Jacobs, M. (1983). Intermediate filaments in smooth muscle tumours. *Journal of Clinical Pathology* **36**, 57–61.

Evans, N. (1926). Mitotic figures in malignant tumors as affected by time before fixation of tissues. *Archives of Pathology* **1**, 894–98.

Fanguhar, M.G., Courtoy, P.J., Lemkin, M.C. and Kenmar, Y.S. (1982) Current knowledge of the functional architecture of the glomerular basement membrane. In Kuehn, R., Schoene, H.H. and Timpl, R. (eds), *New Trends in Basement Membrane Research*, Raven Press, New York, pp. 57–69.

Ferlito, A. and Friedmann, I. (1991). Contribution of immunohistochemistry in the diagnosis of neuroendocrine neoplasms of the larynx. *Journal of Otorhinolaryngol Relative Species* **53**, 235–44.

Feyrter, F. (1969). Die Peripheren endokrinen (parakriken) Drusen. In Kauffman-Staemler, H. (ed), *Lehrbuch der Speziellen Pathologischen Anatomie*, vols. 11–12, De Guyrter, Berlin.

Fisher, E.R., Palekar, A. and Rockette, H. (1978a). Pathologic findings from the National Surgical Adjuvant Breast Project (Protocol No. 4). V. Significance of axillary node micro- and macrometastases. *Cancer* **42**, 2032–8.

Fisher, E.R., Swamidoss, S. and Lee, C.H. (1978b). Detection and significance of occult axillary node metastases in patients with invasive breast cancer. *Cancer* **42**, 2025–31.

Foekens, J.A., Rio, M.C. and Seguin, P. (1990). Prediction of relapse and survival in breast cancer patients by pS2 protein status. *Cancer Research* **50**, 3832–7.

Fogel, M., Lifschitz-Mercer, B. and Moll, R. (1990). Heterogeneity of intermediate filament expression in human testicular seminomas. *Differentiation* **45**, 242–9.

Ford, T.F., Butcher, D.M. and Masters, J.R.W. (1985). Immunocytochemical localisation of prostate-specific antigen: specificity and application to clinical practice. *British Journal of Urology* **57**, 50–5.

Forster, S.J., Talbot, I.C. and Critchley, D.R. (1984). Laminin and fibronectin in rectal adenocarcinoma: Relationship to tumour grade, stage and metastasis. *British Journal of Cancer* **50**, 51–8.

Franke, F.E., Schachenmayr, O.M. and Altmannsberger. M. (1991). Unexpected immunoreactivities of intermediate filament antibodies in human brain and brain tumors. *American Journal of Pathology* **139**, 67–79.

Frazier, H.A., Humphrey, P.A. and Burchette, J.L. (1992). Immunoreactive prostatic specific antigen in male periurethral glands. *Journal of Urology* **147**, 246–8.

Fuchs, M.E., Brawer, M.K. and Rennels, M.A. (1989). The relationship of basement membrane to histologic grade of human prostatic carcinoma. *Modern Pathology* **2**, 105–11.

Furness, P.N., Lowe, J. and Tarrant, G.S. (1990). Subepithelial basement membrane deposition and intermediate filament expression in choroid plexus neoplasms and ependymomas. *Histopathology* **16**, 251–5.

Gabbiani, G., Kapanci, Y. and Barazzone, P. (1981). Immunochemical identification of intermediate-sized filaments in tissues and cultures cells. *American Journal of Pathology* **104**, 206–16.

Garcia, R.L., Coltrera, M.D. and Gown, A.M. (1989). Analysis of proliferative grade using anti-PCNA/cyclin monoclonal antibodies in fixed, embedded tissues: comparison with flow cytometric analysis. *American Journal of Pathology* **134**, 733–9.

Gatter, K.C., Dunnill, M.S. and Heryet, A. (1987). Human lung tumors: does intermediate filament coexpression correlate with other morphological or immunocytochemical features? *Histopathology* **11**, 705–14.

Gatter, K.C., Dunnill, M.S. and van Muijen, G.N.P. (1986). Human lung tumors may coexpress different classes of intermediate filaments. *Journal of Clinical Pathology* **39**, 950–4.

Gazdar, A.F. (1989). Advances in the biology of lung cancer: clinical significance of neuroendocrine differentiation. *Chest* **96**, 39S-41S.

Gerdes, J., Lemke, H. and Baisch, H. (1984). Cell cycle analysis of a cell proliferation-associated human nuclear antigen defined by the monoclonal antibody Ki-67. *Journal of Immunology* **133**, 1710–15.

Gerdes, J., Li, L. and Schlueter, D.M (1991). Immunohistochemical and molecular biologic characterization of the cell proliferation-associated nuclear antigen that is defined by monoclonal antibody Ki-67. *American Journal of Pathology* **138**, 867–73.

Gerdes, J., Schwab, U. and Lemke, H. (1983). Production of a mouse monoclonal antibody reactive with a nuclear antigen associated with cell proliferation. *International Journal of Cancer* **31**, 13–20.

Giri, D.D., Goepel, J.R., Rogers, K. and Underwood, J.C.E. (1988). Immunohistological demonstration of progesterone receptor in breast carcinomas: correlation with radioligand-binding assays and oestrogen receptor immunohistology. *Journal of Clinical Pathology* **44**, 444–7.

Golz, R. and Schubert, G.E. (1989). Prostatic specific antigen: immunoreactivity in urachal remnants. *Journal of Urology* **141**, 1480–2.

Gould, V.E., Koukoulis, G.K. and Jansson, D.S. (1990). Coexpression patterns of vimentin and glial filament protein with cytokeratins in the normal, hyperplastic, and neoplastic breast. *American Journal of Pathology* **137**, 1143–55.

Gould, V.E., Lee, I. and Warren, W.H. (1988). Immunohistochemical evaluation of neuroendocrine cells and neoplasms of the lung. *Pathology, Research and Practice* **183**, 200–13.

Gould, V.E., Weidenmann, B., Lee, I.S.K., Dockhorn-Dworniczak, B., Radosevich, J.A., Moll, R. and Franke, W.W. (1987). Synaptophysin expression in neuroendocrine neoplasms as determined by immunohistochemistry. *American Journal of Pathology* **126**, 243–57.

Gown, A.M. and Vogel, A.M. (1985). Monoclonal antibodies to human intermediate filament proteins III. Analysis of tumors. *American Journal of Clinical Pathology* **84**, 413–22.

Gown, A.M., Boyd, H.C. and Chang, Y. (1988). Smooth muscle cells can express cytokeratins of 'simple' epithelium: immunocytochemical and biochemical studies in vitro and in vivo. *American Journal of Pathology* **132**, 223–32.

Gray, M.H., Rosenberg, A.E. and Dickersin, G.R. (1990). Cytokeratin expression in epithelioid vascular neoplasms. *Human Pathology* **21**, 212–17.

Grunberg, S.M. (1991). The role of progesterone receptors in meningioma. *Cancer Treatment and Research* **58**, 127–37.

Haagensen, D.E. Jr., Dilley, W.G. and Mazoujian, G. (1990). Review of GCDFP-15: an apocrine marker protein. *Annals of the New York Academy of Science* **586**, 161–73.

Hall, P.A. and Levison, D.A. (1990a). Review: Assessment of cell proliferation in histological material. *Journal of Clinical Pathology* **43**, 184–92.

Hall, P.A., Levison, P.A. and Woods. A.L. (1990b). Proliferating cell nuclear antigen (PCNA) immunolocalisation in paraffin sections. An index of cell proliferation with evidence of deregulated expression in some neoplasms. *Journal of Pathology* **162**, 285–94.

Hall, P.A., Richards, M.A. and Gregory, W.M. (1988). The prognostic value of Ki-67 immunostaining in non-Hodgkin's lymphoma. *Journal of Pathology* **154**, 223–35.

Hamid, Q.A., Addis, B.J. and Springall, D.R. (1987). Expression of the C-terminal peptide of human pro-bombesin in 361 lung endocrine tumours, a reliable marker and possible prognostic indicator for small cell carcinoma. *Virchows Archives (Pathology Anatomy A)* **411**, 85–92.

Heck, M.M.S. and Earnshaw, W.C. (1986). Topoisomerase II: A specific marker for cell proliferation. *Journal of Cell Biology* **103**, 2569–81.

Henry, J.A., McCarthy, A.L. and Angus, B. (1990). Prognostic significance of the oestrogen-regulated protein, Cathepsin D, in breast cancer: An immunohistochemical study. *Cancer* **65**, 265–71.

Henzen-Logmans, S.C., Mullink, H. and Ramaekers, F.C.S. (1987). Expression of cytokeratins and vimentin in epithelial cells of normal and pathological thyroid tissue. *Virchows Archives (Pathology Anatomy A)* **410**, 347–54.

Heyderman, E., Strudley, I., Powell, G., Rocjardspm. T.C., Cordell, J.L. and Mason, D.Y. (1985). A new monoclonal antibody to epithelial membrane antigen (EMA)–E29. A comparison of its immunocytochemical reactivity with polyclonal anti-EMA antibodies and with another monoclonal antibody, HMFG-2. *British Journal of Cancer* **52**, 355–61.

Hiort, O., Kwan, P.W.L. and de Lellis, R.A. (1988). Immunohistochemistry of oestrogen receptor protein in paraffin sections. Effects of enzymatic pre-treatment and cobalt chloride intensification. *American Journal of Clinical Pathology* **90**, 559–63.

Hoog, A., Gould, V.E. and Grimelius, L. (1988). Tissue fixation methods alter the immunohistochemical demonstrability of synaptophysin. *Ultrastructural Pathology* **12**, 673–8

Hruban, R.H., May, M., Marcov, R.C. and Huvos, A.G. (1990). Lumbosacral chordoma with high-grade malignant cartilaginous and spindle cell components. *American Journal of Surgical Pathology* **14**, 384–9.

Huvos, A.G., Hutter, R.V.P. and Berg, J.W. (1971). Significance of axillary macrometastases and micrometastases in mammary cancer. *Annals of Surgery* **173**, 44–6.

Isola J, Kallioniemi, O-P. and Korte, J-M. (1990). Steroid receptors in Ki-67 reactivity in ovarian cancer and in normal ovary: Correlation with DNA flow cytometry, biochemical receptor assay and patient survival. *Journal of Pathology* **162**, 295–301.

Jahn, R., Schiebler, W., Ouimet, C. and Grengard, P. (1985). A 38,000 dalton membrane protein (p38) present in synaptic vesicles. *Proceedings National Academy of Science USA* **82**, 4137–41.

Johnson, B.E., Ihde, D.C. and Makuch, R.W. (1987). *Myc* family amplification in tumour cell lines established from small cell carcinoma and its relationship to clinical status and course. *Journal of Clinical Investigation* **79**, 1629–34.

Kallianpur, A.R., Carstens, P.H. and Liotta, L.A. (1990). Immunoreactivity in malignant mesotheliomas with antibodies to basement membrane components and their receptors. *Modern Pathology* **3**, 11–18.

Kamel, O.W., LeBrun, D.P. and Davis, R.E. (1991). Growth fraction estimation of malignant lymphomas in formalin fixed paraffin embedded tissue using anti-PCNA/cyclin 19A2. *American Journal of Pathology* **138**, 1471–7.

Kato, K. (1982). Distribution of nervous-system-specific forms of enolase in peripheral tissues. *Brain Research* **237**, 441–8.

Kayser, K., Schmid, W. and Ebert, W. (1988). Expression of neuroendocrine markers (neuron-specific enolase, synaptophysin and bombesin) in carcinoma of the lung. *Pathology, Research and Practice* **183**, 412–17.

Kempson, R.L. and Bari, N. (1970). Uterine sarcomas. Classification, diagnosis and prognosis. *Human Pathology* **1**, 331–49.

Kimura, N., Sasano, N. and Namiki, T. (1989). Coexpression of cytokeratin, neurofilament and vimentin in carcinoid tumors. *Virchows Archives (Pathology Anatomy A)* **415**, 69–77.

Kurki, P., Ogata, K. and Tan, E.M. (1988). Monoclonal antibodies to proliferating cell nuclear antigen (PCNA)/cyclin as probes for proliferating cells by immunofluorescence microscopy and flow cytometry. *Journal of Immunological Methods* **109**, 49–59.

Kurman, R.J., Young, R.H. and Norris, H.J. (1984). Immunocytochemical localization of placental lactogen and chorionic gonadotropin in the normal placenta and trophoblastic tumours, with emphazis on intermediate trophoblast and placental site trophoblastic tumour. *International Journal of Gynecological Pathology* **3**, 101–21.

LaRocca, P.J. and Rheinwald, J.G. (1984). Coexpression of simple epithelial keratins and vimentin by human mesothelium and mesothelioma in vivo and in culture. *Cancer Research* **44**, 2291–9.

Le Douarin, N.M. (1982). *The Neural Crest*. Cambridge University Press, Cambridge, England.

Lehto, V.-P., Stenman, S., Miettinen, M. (1983). Expression of a neural type intermediate filament as a distinguishing feature between oat cell carcinoma and other lung cancers. *American Journal of Pathology* **110**, 113–18.

Leong, A.S-Y. (1990). New Technologies for the surgical pathologist. *Journal of Medical Laboratory Sciences* **4**, 45–8.

Leong, A.S-Y. (1992). The expression of vimentin in epithelial neoplasms. Progress in Surgical Pathology **12**, 31–48.

Leong, A.S.-Y., Gilham, P. and Milios, J. (1988). Cytokeratin and vimentin intermediate filament proteins in benign and neoplastic prostatic epithelium. *Histopathology* **13**, 435–42.

Leong, A.S-Y., Parkinson, R. and Milios, J. (1989). 'Thick' cell membranes revealed by immunocytochemical staining: A clue to the diagnosis of mesothelioma. *Diagnostic Cytopathology* **5**, 58–62.

Leong, A.S-Y. and Raymond, W.A. (1989). Prognostic parameters in breast carcinoma. *Pathology* **21**, 169–75.

Leong, A.S-Y., Stevens, M.W. and Mukherjee, T.M. (1992). Malignant mesothelioma – cytologic diagnosis with histologic, immunohistochemical and ultrastructural correlation. *Seminars in Diagnostic Pathology* **9**, 141–50.

Leslie, D.S., Johnston, W.W. and Daly, L. (1990). Detection of breast carcinoma cells in human bone marrow using fluorescence-activated cell sorting and conventional cytology. *American Journal of Clinical Pathology* **94**, 8–13.

Linnoila, R.I., Jensen, S. and Steinberg, S. (1988a). Neuroendocrine differentiation correlates with favourable response to chemotherapy in patients with non-small cell lung cancer. *Lung Cancer* **4s**, A33.

Linnoila, R.I., Mulshine, J.L. and Steinberg, S.M. (1988b). Neuroendocrine differentiation in endocrine and nonendocrine lung carcinomas. *American Journal of Clinical Pathology* **90**, 641–52.

Liotta, L.A. (1984). Tumour invasion and metastases: Role of the basement membrane. *American Journal of Pathology* **117**, 339–48.

Lloyd, R.V. and Warner, T.F. (1984). Immunohistochemistry of neuron-specific enolase. In DeLellis, R.A. (ed.), *Advances in Immunohistochemistry*, Mason, New York, pp. 127–40.

Lloyd, R.V., Wilson, B.S. and Varani, J. (1985). Immunocytochemical characterization of a monoclonal antibody that recognizes mitosing cells. *American Journal of Pathology* **121**, 275–83.

Malkin, D., Jolly, K.W. and Barbier, N. (1992). Germline mutations of the p53 tumour suppressor gene in children and young adults with second malignant neoplasms. *New England Journal of Medicine* **326**, 1309–15.

Manivel, J.C., Niehans, G., Wick, M.R. and Dehner, L.P. (1987). Intermediate trophoblast in germ cell neoplasms. *American Journal of Surgical Pathology* **11**, 693–701.

Mansi, J.L., Berger, U. and Wilson, P. (1988). Detection of tumour cells in bone marrow of patients with prostatic carcinoma by immunocytochemical techniques. *Journal of Urology* **139**, 545–8.

Marshall, R.J., Herbert, A., Braye, S.G. and Jones, D.B. (1984). Use of antibodies to carcinoembryonic antigen and human milk fat globule to distinguish carcinoma, mesothelioma, and reactive mesothelium. *Journal of Clinical Pathology* **37**, 1215–21.

Mazoujian, G., Bodian, C. and Haagensen, D.E. Jr. (1989). Expression of GCDFP-15 in breast carcinomas. Relationship to pathologic and clinical factors. *Cancer* **63**, 2156–61.

Mazoujian, G., Pinkus, G.S. and Davis, S. (1983). Immunohistochemistry of a breast gross cystic disease fluid protein (GCDFP-15): a marker of apocrine epithelium and breast carcinomas with apocrine features. *American Journal of Pathology* **110**, 105–11.

McGarry, R.C. (1983). Recognition of myelin-associated glycoprotein by the monoclonal antibody HNK-1. *Nature* **306**, 376.

McGuire, W.L., Clark, G.M., Dressler, L.G. and Owens, M.A. (1986). Role of steroid hormone receptors as prognostic factors in primary breast cancer. *National Cancer Institutes Monograph* **1**, 19–24.

McNutt, M., Bolen, J. and Gown, A.M. (1985). Coexpression of intermediate filament proteins in human epithelial neoplasms. *Ultrastructural Pathology* **9**, 35–47.

Miettinen, M. (1991). Keratin subsets in spindle cell sarcomas. *American Journal of Pathology* **138**, 505–13.

Miettinen, M., Lehto, V.-P. and Dahl, D. (1985a). Varying expression of cytokeratin and neurofilaments in neuroendocrine tumors of the gastrointestinal tract. *Laboratory Investigation* **52**, 429–36.

Miettinen, M., Lehto, V., Dahl, D. and Virtanen, I. (1983). Differential diagnosis of chordoma, chondroid, and ependymomal tumours as aided by anti-intermediate filament antibodies. *American Journal of Pathology* **112**, 160–9.

Miettinen, M., Lehto, V.-P. and Virtanen, I. (1982). Keratin in the epithelial-like cells of the classical biphasic synovial sarcoma. Virchows Archives [Cell Pathology B] **40**, 157–62.

Miettinen, M., Virtanen, I. and Talerman, A. (1985b). Intermediate filament proteins in human testis and testicular germ cell tumours. *American Journal of Pathology* **120**, 402–10.

Miyachi, K., Fritzler, M.J. and Tan, E.M. (1978). Autoantibody to a nuclear antigen in proliferating cells. *Journal of Immunology* **121**, 2228–34.

Mizukami, Y., Michigishi, T., Nonomura, A, Hashimoto T, Terahata S, Noguchi M, Hisada, K. and Matsubara, F. (1990). Distant metastases in differentiated thyroid carcinomas: a clinical and pathologic study. *Human Pathology* **21**, 283–90.

Moisa, II. (1991). Neuroendocrine tumors of the larynx. *Head and Neck* **13**, 498–508.

Moll, R. and Franke, W.W. (1985). Cytoskeletal differences between human neuroendocrine tumors: a cytoskeletal protein of molecular weight 46,000 distinguishes cutaneous from pulmonary neuroendocrine neoplasms. *Differentiation* **30**, 165–75.

Moll, R., Osborn, M. and Hartschuh, W. (1986). Variability of expression and arrangement of cytokeratin and neurofilaments in cutaneous neuroendocrine carcinomas (Merkel cell tumors): Immunocytochemical and biochemical analysis of twelve cases. *Ultrastructural Pathology* **10**, 473–95.

Moll, R., Lowe, A. and Laufer, J. (1992). Cytokeratin 20 in human carcinomas. A new histodiagnostic marker detected by monoclonal antibodies. *American Journal of Pathology* **140**, 427–47.

Moot, S.K., Peters, G.N. and Cheek, J.H. (1987). Tumour hormone receptor status and recurrences in pre-menopausal node-negative breast carcinoma. *Cancer* **60**, 382–85.

Morris, G.F. and Mathews, M.B. (1989). Regulation of proliferating cell nuclear antigen during the cell cycle. *Journal of Biology and Chemistry* **264**, 13856–64.

Moss, T.J., Reynolds, C.P. and Sather, H.N. (1991). Prognostic value of immunocytochemical detection of bone marrow metastases in neuroblastoma. *New England Journal of Medicine* **324**, 219–66.

Nadji, M. and Morales, A.R. (1982). Immunohistochemistry of prostatic acid phosphatase. *Annals of the New York Academy of Science* **390**, 133–41.

Nadji, M., Tabei, S.Z. and Castro, A. (1981). Prostatic specific antigen: an immunohistologic marker for prostatic neoplasms. *Cancer* **48**, 1229–32.

Nagashima, T., DeArmond, S.J. and Murovic, J. (1985). Immunohistochemical demonstration of S-phase cells by anti-bromodeoxyuridine monoclonal antibody in human brain tumor tissues. *Acta Neuropathology* **67**, 155–9.

Neal, D.E., Sharples, L. and Smith, K. (1990). The epidermal growth factor receptor and the prognosis of bladder cancer. *Cancer* **65**, 161–25.

Ng, H.-K. and Lo, S.T.H. (1989). Cytokeratin immunoreactivity in gliomas. *Histopathology* **14**, 359–68.

O'Connor, D.T. and Frigon, R.P. (1984). Chromogranin A, the major catecholamine vesicle soluble protein. *Journal of Biologic Chemistry* **259**, 3237–47.

Offerhaus, G.J., Giardiello, F.M., Brunijn, J.A., Stijnen, T., Molyras, E.N. and Fleuren, G.J. (1991). The value of immunohistochemistry of collagen IV expression in colorectal carcinomas. *Cancer* **67**, 99–105.

Ogata, K., Kurki, P., Celis, J.E., Nakamura, R.M and Tan, E.M. (1987). Monoclonal antibodies to a nuclear protein (PCNA/cyclin) associated with DNA replication. *Experimental Cell Research* **168**, 475–86.

Ogawa, K., Oguchi, M., Yamabe, Nakashima, Y. and Hamashima, Y. (1986). Distribution of collagen type IV in soft tissue tumours. An immunohistochemical study. *Cancer* **58**, 269–77.

Olympus Optical Company (1981). *How to Improve Photography through the Microscope*.

Onetti-Muda, A., Crescenzi, A., Pujia, N, Faraggiana, T. and Marinozzi, V. (1991). Demonstration of oestrogen and progesterone receptors in freeze dried, paraffin-embedded sections of breast. *Histopathology* **18**, 511–16.

Ordonez, N.G. (1989). The immunohistochemical diagnosis of mesothelioma. Differentiation of mesothelioma and lung adenocarcinoma. *American Journal of Surgical Pathology* **13**, 276–91.

Orto, P. (1988). Glial fibrillary acidic protein immunoreactivity in human respiratory tract cartilages and pulmonary chondromatous hamartomas. *American Journal of Pathology* **133**, 363–73.

Osborn, M., Debus, E. and Weber, K. (1984). Monoclonal antibody specific for vimentin. *European Journal of Cell Biology* **34**, 137–43.

Otis, C.N., Carter, D., Cole, S. and Battifora, H. (1987). Immunohistochemical evaluation of pleural mesothelioma and pulmonary adenocarcinoma. A bi-institutional study of 47

cases. *American Journal of Surgical Pathology* **11**, 445–56.
Otsuki, Y., Kubo, H. and Magari, S. (1990). Immunohistochemical differentiation between lymphatic vessels and blood vessels – use of anti-basement membrane antibodies and anti-factor VIII-related antigen. *Archives of Histology and Cytology* **53** (Suppl.), 95–105.
Pallesen, G. and Hamilton-Dutoit, S.J. (1988). Ki-1 (CD 30) antigen is regularly expressed by tumour cells of embryonal carcinoma. *American Journal of Pathology* **133**, 446–50.
Papotti, M., Macri, L., Finzi, G., Capella, C., Eusebi, V. and Bussolati, G. (1989). Neuroendocrine differentiation in carcinomas of the breast: A study of 51 cases. *Seminars in Diagnostic Pathology* **6**, 174–88.
Pardo, R.J. and Penneys, N.S. (1990). Location of basement membrane type IV collagen beneath subepidermal bullous diseases. *Journal of Cutaneous Pathology* **17**, 336–41.
Pascal, R.R., Mesa-Tejada, R. and Bennet, S.J. (1977). Carcinoembryonic antigen. Immunohistologic identification in invasive and intraepithelial carcinomas of the lung. *Archives of Pathology and Laboratory Medicine* **101**, 568–71.
Pearse, A.G.E. (1974). The APUD concept and its implications in pathology. *Pathologic Annual* **9**, 27–41.
Pinkus, G.S. and Kurtin, P.J. (1985). Epithelial membrane antigen: A diagnostic discriminant in surgical pathology. *Human Pathology* **16**, 929–40.
Pinkus, G.S., Etheridge, C.L. and O'Connor, E.M. (1986). Are keratin proteins a better tumour marker then epithelial membrane antigen? *American Journal of Clinical Pathology* **85**, 269–77.
Pitt, M.A., Hale, R.J. and Buckley, C.H. (1992). The distribution of type IV collagen in invasive carcinoma of the uterine cervix. *Histopathology* **20**, 139–43.
Poulsen, H. (1987). *In vitro* tests and hormone therapy in breast cancer. *Progress in Surgical Pathology* **12**, 37–66.
Predine, J., Spyratos, F., Prud'homme, J.F., Andrieu, C., Hacene, K., Brunet, M., Pallud, C. and Milgrom, E. (1992). Enzyme-linked immunosorbent assay of pS2 in breast cancers, benign tumours, and normal breast tissues. *Cancer* **69**, 2116–23.
Quinlan, R.A., Schiller, D. L., Hatzfeld, M., Achtstatter, T., Moll, R., Jorcano, J.L., Magin, T.M. and Franke, W.W. (1985). Patterns of expression and organization of cytokeratin intermediate filaments. *Annals of the New York Academy of Sciences* **455**, 282–306.
Quinn, M.A., Cauchi, M. and Fortune, D. (1985). Endometrial carcinoma: Steroid receptors and response to medroxyprogesterone acetate. *Gynaecologic Oncology* **21**, 314–18.
Ramaekers, F.C.S., Haag, D. and Kant, A. (1983). Coexpression of keratin- and vimentin-type intermediate filaments in human metastatic carcinoma cells. *Proceedings of the National Academy of Science USA* **80**, 2618–22.
Raymond, W.A. and Leong, A.S-Y. (1988). An evaluation of potentially suitable fixatives for immunoperoxidase staining of oestrogen receptors in imprints and frozen sections of breast carcinoma. *Pathology* **20**, 320–5.
Raymond, W.A. and Leong, A.S-Y. (1989a). Coexpression of cytokeratin and vimentin intermediate filament proteins in benign and neoplastic breast epithelium. *Journal of Pathology* **157**, 299–306.
Raymond, W.A. and Leong, A.S-Y. (1989b). Vimentin – a new prognostic parameter in breast carcinoma? *Journal of Pathology* **158**, 107–14.
Raymond, W.A. and Leong, A.S-Y. (1989c). Nucleolar organiser regions related to growth fractions in human breast carcinoma. *Human Pathology* **20**, 741–6.
Raymond, W.A. and Leong, A.S-Y. (1989d). Immunoperoxidase staining in the detection of lymph node metastases in Stage I breast cancer. *Pathology* **21**, 11–15.
Raymond, W.A. and Leong, A.S-Y. (1990). Oestrogen receptor staining of paraffin-embedded breast carcinomas following short fixation in formalin: A comparison with cytosolic and frozen section receptor analyses. *Journal of Pathology* **160**, 295–303.
Raymond, W.A. and Leong, A.S-Y. (1991). Assessment of invasion in breast lesions using antibodies to basement membrane components and myoepithelial cells. *Pathology* **23**, 291–7.
Reibel, J., Weber, U. and Albrechtsen, R. (1985). The pattern of laminin in neurogenic tumours, granular cell tumours, and naevi of the oral mucosa. *Acta Pathologica Microbiologica Immunology Scandinavia, Section A* **93**, 41–8.
Rode, J., Dhillon, A.P. and Doran, J.F. (1985). PGP 9.5 – a new marker for human neuroendocrine tumours. *Histopathology* **9**, 147–58.
Robbins, B.A., de la Vega, D. and Ogata, K. (1987). Immunohistochemical detection of proliferating cell nuclear antigen in solid human malignancies. *Archives of Pathology and Laboratory Medicine* **111**, 841–5.
Roggli, V.L., Kolbeck, J. and Sanfilippo, F. (1987). Pathology of human mesothelioma. Etiologic and diagnostic considerations. *Pathology Annual 22 (Part 2)*, 91–131.
Rosen, P.P., Saigo, P.E. and Braun, D.W. (1981). Axillary micro- and macrometastases in breast cancer. *Annals of Surgery* **194**, 585–91.
Sakr, W.A., Zarbo, R.J. and Crissman, J.D. (1988). Immunohistologic distribution of basement membrane in breast neoplasia. *Human Pathology* **18**, 1043–50.
Salisbury, J.R. (1987). Demonstration of cytokeratins and an epithelial membrane antigen in chondroid chordoma. *Journal of Pathology* **153**, 37–40.
Saphir, O. and Amromin, G.D. (1948). Obscure axillary lymph node metastasis in carcinoma of the breast. *Cancer* **1**, 238–41.
Schapers, R.F., Pauwels, R.P. and Havenith, M.G. (1990). Prognostic significance of type IV collagen and laminin

immunoreactivity in urothelial carcinomas of the bladder. *Cancer* **66**, 2583–8.

Schlimok, G., Funke, I. and Bock, B. (1990). Epithelial cells in bone marrow of patients with colorectal cancer: immunocytochemical detection, phenotypic characterisation and prognostic significance. *Journal of Clinical Oncology* **8**, 831–7.

Sedmak, D.D., Meineke, T.A., Knechtges, D.S. and Anderson, J. (1989). Prognostic significance of cytokeratin positive breast cancer metastases. *Modern Pathology* **2**, 516–20.

Segreti, E.M., Novotny, D.B. and Soper, J.T. (1989). Endometrial cancer: histologic correlates of immunohistochemical localization of progesterone receptor and estrogen receptor. *Obstetrics and Gynecology* **73**, 780–5.

Semmelink, H.J.F., Pruszczynski, M. and Tilburg, A.W. (1990). Cytokeratin expression in chondroblastomas. *Histopathology* **16**, 257–63.

Shimada, H., Aoyama, C., Chiba, T. and Newton, W.A.,Jr. (1985). Prognostic subgroups for undifferentiated neuroblastoma. Immunohistochemical study with S100 protein antibody. *Human Pathology* **16**, 471–6.

Shintaku, I.P. and Said, J.W. (1987). Detection of oestrogen receptors with monoclonal antibodies in routinely processed formalin-fixed paraffin sections of breast carcinoma. Use of DNASE pre-treatment to enhance sensitivity of the reaction. *American Journal of Clinical Pathology* **87**, 161–7.

Silva, E.G., Kott, M.M. and Ordonez, N.G. (1984). Endocrine carcinoma intermediate cell type of the uterine cervix. *Cancer* **54**, 1705–13.

Silverberg, S.G. (1976). Reproducability of the mitosis count in the histologic diagnosis of smooth muscle tumors of the uterus. *Human Pathology* **7**, 451–4.

Skov, B.G., Sorensen, J.B. and Hirsch, F.R., (1991). Prognostic impact of histologic demonstration of chromogranin A and neuron specific enolase in pulmonary adenocarcinoma. *Annals of Oncology* **2**, 355–60.

Slamon, D.J., Godolphin, W. and Jones, L.A. (1989). Studies of the HER2/neu proto-oncogene in human breast and ovarian cancer. *Science* **240**, 707–12.

Sloane, J.P., Ormerod, M.G., Imrie, S. and Coombes, R.C. (1980). The use of antisera to epithelial membrane antigen in detecting micrometastases in histological sections. *British Journal of Cancer* **42**, 392–8.

Sowani, A., Ong, G. and Dische, S. (1989). *C-myc* oncogene expression and clinical outcome in carcinoma of the cervix. *Molecular Cell Probes* **3**, 117–23.

Springall, D.R., Ibrahim, N.B.N. and Rode, J. (1986). Endocrine differentiation of extrapulmonary small cell carcinoma demonstrated by immunohistochemistry using antibodies to PGP9.5, neuron-specific enolase and the C-flanking peptide of human pro-bombesin. *Journal of Pathology* **150**, 151–62.

Stenback, F. and Wasenius, V.M. (1986). Occurrence of basement membranes in pigment cell tumours of the skin: Relation to cell type and clinical behaviour. *Journal of Cutaneous Pathology* **13**, 175–81.

Stewart, C.J.R. and McNicol, A.M. (1992). Distribution of type IV collagen immunoreactivity to assess questionable early stromal invasion. *Journal of Clinical Pathology* **45**, 9–15.

Strickler, J.G., Herndier, B.G. and Rouse, R.V. (1987). Immunohistochemical staining in malignant mesotheliomas. *American Journal of Clinical Pathology* **88**, 610–14.

Swanson, P.E., Lillemoe, T.J., Manivell, C. and Wick, M.R. (1990). Mesenchymal chondrosarcoma. An immunohistochemical study. *Archives of Pathology and Laboratory Medicine* **114**, 943–8.

Swanson, P.E. (1991). Heffalumps, jagulars, and cheshire cats. A commentary on cytokeratins and soft tissue sarcomas. *American Journal of Clinical Pathology* **95**(4 Suppl 1), S2–7.

Swanson, P.E., Mazoujian, G. and Mills, S.E. (1991). Immunoreactivity for estrogen receptor protein in sweat gland tumors. *American Journal of Surgical Pathology* **15**, 835–41.

Ten Velde, G.P., Havenith, M.G., Volovics, A. and Bosman, F.T. (1991). Prognostic significance of basement membrane deposition in operable squamous cell carcinomas of the lung. *Cancer* **67**, 3001–5.

Thaete, L.G., Ahnen, D.J. and Makinson, A.M. (1989). Proliferating cell nuclear antigen (PCNA/cyclin) immunocytochemistry as a labelling index in mouse lung tissues. *Cell Tissue Research* **256**, 167–73.

Thomas, P. and Battifora, H. (1987). Keratins versus epithelial membrane antigen in tumour diagnosis: An immunohistochemical comparison of 5 monoclonal antibodies. *Human Pathology* **18**, 728–34.

Timpl, R. and Dziadeck, M. (1986). Structure, development and molecular pathology of basement membranes. *International Review of Experimental Pathology* **29**, 1–112.

Toguchida, J., Yamaguchi, T. and Dayton, S.H. (1992). Prevalence and spectrum of germline mutations of the p53 gene among patients with sarcoma. *New England Journal of Medicine* **326**, 1301–8.

Travis, W.D., Linnoila, R.I. and Tsokos, M.G. (1991). Neuroendocrine tumors of the lung with proposed criteria for large cell neuroendocrine carcinoma. *American Journal of Surgical Pathology* **15**, 529–53.

Trojani, M., de Mascarel, I. and Bonichon, F. (1987). Micrometastases to axillary lymph nodes from carcinoma of breast: Detection by immunohistochemistry and prognostic significance. *British Journal of Cancer* **55**, 303–6.

Tron, V., Wright, J.L. and Schurg, A. (1987). Carcinoembryonic antigen and milk fat globule protein staining of malignant mesothelioma and adenocarcinoma of the lung. *Archives of Pathology and Laboratory Medicine* **111**, 291–3.

True, L.D. (1990). Epithelial membrane antigens. In True, L.D. (ed.), *Atlas of Diagnostic Immunohistopathology*, J.B. Lippincott, Philadelphia, pp. 5.1–5.28.

Tsutsumi, Y., Hori, S. and Onada, N. (1990). DNA polymerase alpha: an immunohistochemical marker for proliferating cells in normal and neoplastic human tissues. *American Journal of Clinical Pathology* **93**, 643–50.

Tsutsumi, Y. (1984). Leu-7 immunoreactivity as histochemical marker of paraffin embedded neuroendocrine tumors. *Acta Histochemistry and Cytochemistry* **17**, 15–22.

Ueda, T., Aozasa, K. and Tsujimoto, M. (1989). Prognostic significance of Ki-67 immunoreactivity in soft tissue sarcomas. *Cancer* **63**, 1607–11.

van der Kwast, T.H., Versnel, M.A., Delahaye, M., de Jong, A., Zondervan, P.E. and Hoogsteden, H. (1987). Expression of epithelial membrane antigen on malignant mesothelial cells. An immunocytochemical and immunoelectron microscopic study. *Acta Cytologica* **32**, 169–74.

van Nagell, J.R. and Goldenberg, D.M. (1980). Carcinoembryonic antigen staining of endometrial and endocervical carcinomas. *Lancet* **1**, 213.

Viale, G., Dodlioni, C. and Cell'Orto, P. (1988). Glial fibrillary acidic protein immunoreactivity in human respiratory tract cartilages and pulmonary chondromatous hamartomas. *American Journal of Pathology* **133**, 363–73.

von Hochstetter, A.R., Sigg, C., Saremaslani, P. and Hedinger, C. (1985). The significance of giant cells in human testicular seminomas. A clinico-pathological study. *Virchows Archives (Pathology, Anatomy, Histopathology A)* **407**, 309–22.

von Kleist, S. (1979). Antigens cross-reacting with CEA. Evaluation of their interrelationship and clinical role. In Lehmann, F.G. (ed.), *Carcinoembryonic Proteins*, Elsevier, Amsterdam, pp. 35–39.

Waelti, E.R. and Markwalder, T.M. (1989) Immunocytochemical evidence of progesterone receptors in human meningiomas. *Surgical Neurology* **31**, 172–6.

Wahab, Z.A. and Wright, G.L. (1985). Monoclonal antibody (anti-Leu7) directed against natural killer cells reacts with normal, benign, and malignant prostate tissues. *Journal of Cancer* **36**, 677–83.

Wang, J., Dhillon, A.P., Sankey, E.A., Wightman, A.K., Lewin, J.F. and Scheuer, P.J. (1991). Neuroendocrine differentiation in primary neoplasms of the liver. *Journal of Pathology* **163**, 61–7.

Wasseem, N.H. and Lane, D.P. (1990). Monoclonal antibody analysis of the proliferating cell nuclear antigen (PCNA). Structural conversion and the detection of a nucleolar form. *Journal of Cell Science* **90**, 121–9.

Weiss, S.W., Bratthouer, G.L. and Morris, P.A. (1988). Post-irradiation malignant fibrous histiocytoma expressing cytokeratin. *American Journal of Surgical Pathology* **12**, 554–8.

Weiss, S.W., Langloss, J.M. and Enzinger, F.M. (1983). Value of S100 protein in the diagnosis of soft tissue tumours with particular reference to benign and malignant Schwann cell tumours. *Laboratory Investigation* **49**, 299–308.

Wells, C.A., Heryet, A. and Brochier, J. (1984). The immunocytochemical detection of axillary micrometastases in breast cancer. *British Journal of Cancer* **50**, 193–7.

Wetzels, R.H.W., Schaafsma, H.E., Leigh, I.M., Lane, E.B., Troyanovsky, S.M., Wagenaar, S.S.C., Vooijs, G.P. and Ramaekers, F.C.S. (1992). Laminin and type VII collagen distribution in different types of human lung carcinoma: correlation with expression of keratins 14, 16, 17 and 18. *Histopathology* **20**, 295–303.

Whitaker, D., Sterrett, G. and Shilkin, K.B. (1982). Detection of CEA-like substance as an aid in the differential diagnosis of malignant mesothelioma. *Pathology* **14**, 255–8.

Wick, M.R., Lillemoe, T.J., Copland, G.T., Swanson, P.E., Manivel, J.C. and Kiang, D.T. (1989). Gross cystic disease fluid protein-15 as a marker for breast cancer: Immunohistochemical analysis of 690 human neoplasms and comparison with alpha-lactalbumin. *Human Pathology* **20**, 281–7.

Wick, M.R., Loy, T., Mills, S.E., Legier, J.F. and Manirel, J.C. (1990a). Malignant epithelioid pleural mesothelioma versus peripheral pulmonary adenocarcinoma: A histochemical, ultrastructural and immunohistologic study of 103 cases. *Human Pathology* **21**, 759–66.

Wick, M.R., Mills, S.E. and Swanson, P.E. (1990b). Expression of 'myelomonocytic' antigens in mesotheliomas and adenocarcinomas involving the serosal surfaces. *American Journal of Clinical Pathology* **94**, 18–26.

Wick, M.R. and Rosai, J. (1991) Neuroendocrine neoplasms of the mediastinum. *Seminars in Diagnostic Pathology* **8**, 35–51.

Wilkinson, E.J. and Hause, L. (1974). Probability in lymph node sectioning. *Cancer* **33**, 1269–74.

Willebrand, D., Bosman, F.T. and De Goeij, A.F.P.M. (1986). Patterns of basement membrane deposition in benign and malignant breast tumours. *Histopathology* **10**, 1231–41.

Wilson, B.S. and Lloyd, R.V. (1984). Detection of chromogranin in neuroendocrine cells with a monoclonal antibody. *American Journal of Pathology* **115**, 458–68.

Wright, C., Nicholson, S. and Angus, B. (1989). Expression of *c-erbB-2* oncoprotein: A prognostic indicator in human breast cancer. *Cancer Research* **49**, 2087–90.

Yen, S-H. and Fields, K.L. (1981). Antibodies to neurofilaments, glial filaments, and fibroblast intermediate filaments proteins bind to different cell types of the nervous system. *Journal of Cell Biology* **80**, 115–26.

Zarbo, R.J., Gown, A.M., Nagle, R.B., Visscher, D.W. and Crissman, J.D. (1990) Anomalous cytokeratin expression in malignant melanoma: one and two dimensional western blot analysis and immunohistochemical survey of 100 melanomas. *Modern Pathology* **3**, 494–501.

Zimmerman, W. (1988). Chromosomal localization of the carcinoembryonic antigen gene family and differential expression in various tumors. *Cancer Research* **48**, 2550–4.

4 • *Lymphoproliferative disorders*

David W. Ellis

Introduction

In recent years, the use of monoclonal antibodies in conjunction with new immunohistochemical techniques has had a profound effect on the diagnostic pathology of lymphoproliferative diseases. This effect has been apparent in four ways.

The first and most significant improvement has been the ability to distinguish lymphoid from non-lymphoid tumours. Before the development of antibodies reactive in fixed tissues against the CD45 leucocyte common antigen, a percentage of patients with potentially curable, but morphologically atypical lymphomas were misdiagnosed as inoperable and incurable sarcomas, carcinomas or melanomas (Gatter et al., 1985).

The second area of diagnostic significance is the determination of tumour lineage. Monoclonal antibodies used in frozen or paraffin-sections accurately indicate whether a tumour is of B-cell, T-cell (Elghetany et al., 1991), myeloid or histiocytic origin (Kurec et al., 1990; Warnke et al., 1989) in all but a small percentage of cases. This ability to distinguish between T-cell and B-cell tumours is fundamental to both the Lukes and Collins, and the revised Kiel classifications (Stansfeld et al., 1988).

Thirdly, reactive and neoplastic lymphoid conditions can now be differentiated using sensitive methods for the detection of immunoglobulin or other immunophenotypic criteria for clonality or neoplasia (Norton and Isaacson, 1987; Picker et al., 1987). Using these techniques, many 'benign' extranodal lymphoid proliferations or 'pseudolymphomas' have been shown to be monoclonal (Isaacson, 1990; Medeiros and Harris, 1990; Wotherspoon et al., 1990) and are now regarded as lymphomas (Knowles et al., 1989).

The most controversial area of lymphoid investigation is that of disease subclassification in which immunophenotype, and more recently genotype, are correlated with morphological subgroup. The assumption has been widely adopted that lymphomas are equivalent in phenotype to normal lymphoid cells arrested at a certain stage of maturation (Mason, 1987; van der Valk and Meijer, 1988). This 'maturation arrest' hypothesis has provided a useful conceptual framework for the understanding and subclassification of lymphomas. Characteristic immunophenotypes are recognized for many of the known lymphoma entities however the correlations are far from absolute and immunophenophenotypic heterogeneity is the rule in some groups (Salter et al., 1989; Schuurman et al., 1987). Although many lymphomas share phenotypic features with normal cells at certain stages of development, novel or 'aberrant' patterns of antigen expression are found in a majority of T-cell, and many B-cell lymphomas (Hastrup et al., 1989; Knowles, 1989; Su et al., 1988) – an observation which is often diagnostically useful (Picker et al., 1987).

Recently, the commercial availability of monoclonal antibodies which are reactive in fixed, paraffin-embedded tissues, has returned the responsibility for lymphoma immunodiagnosis to the routine laboratory. Many pathologists consequently find themselves confronted with the confusing task of trying to integrate essentially morphological classification systems with phenotypic information of variable and unfamiliar specificity. The aim of this chapter is to provide a useful and detailed bibliographic resource for laboratories regularly encountering lymphomas, while at the same time offering a pattern-oriented approach for pathologists who rarely venture into the ever-expanding literature of lymphoproliferative disease.

A brief discussion of lymphocyte ontogeny and architecture of the immune system is followed by a review of currently available antibodies. Special emphasis is placed upon antibodies which are reactive in fixed, paraffin-embedded tissue. A detailed discussion of the immunophenotypic features of different lymphoproliferative diseases follows and is corroborated by an extensive bibliography. Diagnostic applications are then considered with discussion of tissue allocation, interpretation of staining and differentiation of reactive from neoplastic lesions. A 'navigational aid' or pattern-oriented approach to lymphoma diagnosis is outlined in which the morphological pattern encountered suggests a checklist of differential diagnoses and associated immunophenotypic findings. Finally, a minimal panel of antibodies is discussed, together with indications for its use.

The normal immune system

The development of a functional immune system requires, as a first step, the creation of large numbers of mature T- and B-lymphocytes with diverse antigen specificities. This 'antigen independent' phase of programmed lymphocyte development occurs in the primary lymphoid organs and is a feature of fetal development but continues throughout adult life, ensuring replenishment of the virgin lymphocyte pool.

The second stage of lymphocyte development is antigen driven and comprises specific activation, blastic transformation, and proliferation of T or B cells with the formation of effector cells and memory cells. The microarchitecture of secondary lymphoid organs and lymphocyte homing patterns throughout the different body compartments, ensure that the many cellular elements of the immune system are able to interact optimally with foreign antigen, and with each other.

B-cell development and function

The primary function of the B-cell arm of the immune system is the production of specific antibodies against foreign antigens. This is achieved through two phases of development (Fig. 4.1). The first phase takes place in the adult bone marrow independently of antigen and consists of the continuous, programmed production of large numbers of immunocompetent, virgin B-cells in which antigen specificity is determined by immunoglobulin heavy and light chain gene rearrangement. The second phase is antigen driven, takes place largely in secondary lymphoid organs, and consists of the activation, clonal proliferation, and terminal differentiation of B-cells bearing immunoglobulin complimentary to foreign antigen.

Phase 1 – The generation of antibody diversity

Commitment to the first phase of B-cell development begins in the eighth week of gestation, when haemopoietic stem cells migrate from the yolk sac to the embryonic liver (Cooper, 1987). Soon after, haemopoietic stem cells

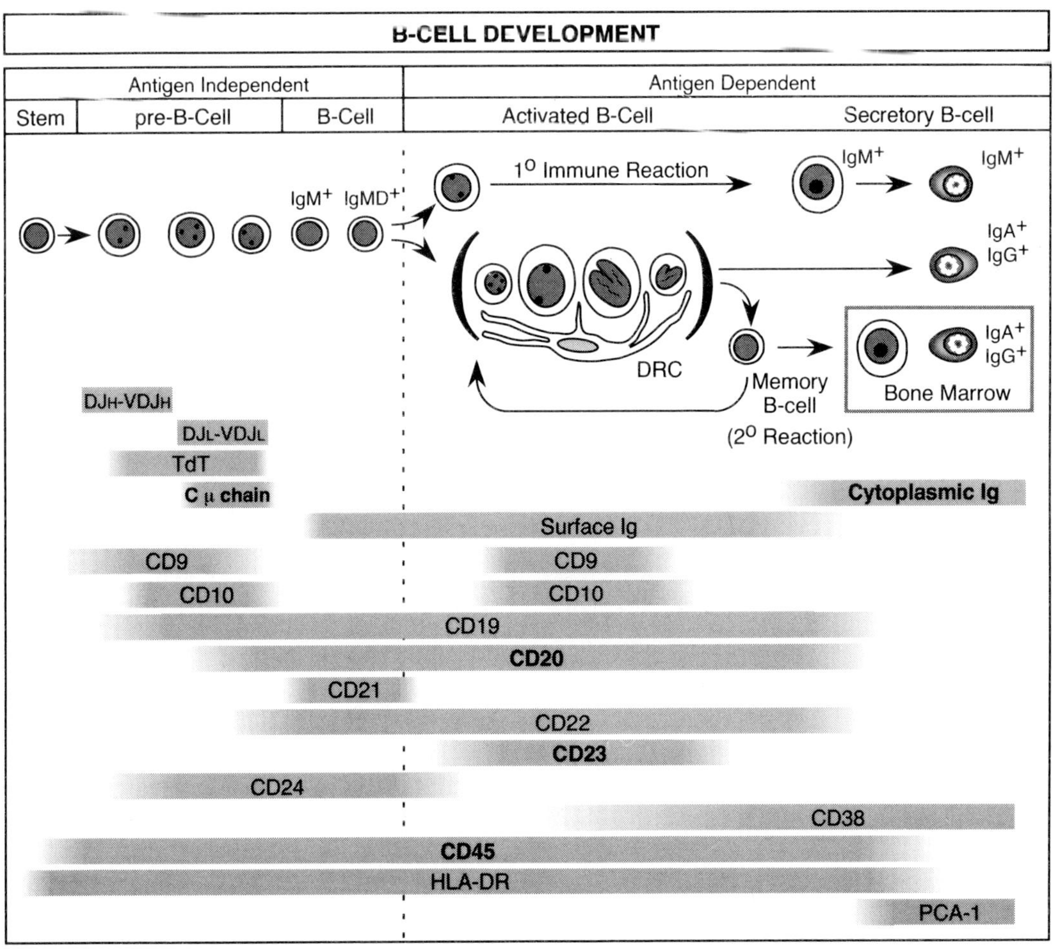

Fig. 4.1 DJH-VDJH and DJL-VDJL refer to immunoglobulin heavy and light chain rearrangements respectively. C μ refers to the cytoplasmic expression of μ heavy chains at the completion of Ig heavy chain gene rearrangement. DRC refers to follicular dendritic reticulum cell.

migrate to the bone marrow which then becomes the major source of B-cell progeny throughout life. Commitment to the B-cell lineage and the generation of antibody diversity begins in large pre-B cells with the first heavy chain gene rearrangement. In this initial DJH translocation, which occurs on both chromosomes, one of 20 or more diversity (D) genes joins one of six joining (JH) genes and the intervening DNA is deleted. Following this, one of 50 or more variable-region (VH) genes on one of the two chromosomes translocates to the DJH region, producing the complete VDJH complex, encoding the complete variable region of the heavy chain. Completion of this translocation process induces active gene transcription which culminates in the cytoplasmic expression of μ heavy chains. VDJH translocation on the other chromosome occurs only if the first is defective.

The resulting small, post-mitotic pre-B cells then undergo light chain gene rearrangement, commencing with the kappa locus on one of the chromosomes 2. This VJk translocation is defective in roughly one third of cases, causing a switch of activity to the lambda locus on one of the chromosomes 22. Successful light chain rearrangement at any stage leads to transcriptional activity and the accumulation of light chains in the endoplasmic reticulum.

Here, heavy and light chains combine to form IgM molecules which are then transported to the cell surface, marking the transition to immature B-cells.

Immature IgM positive B-cells undergo isotype switch by the production of a long nuclear transcript, VDJ-Cμ-Cδ, which is then spliced into VDJ-Cμ and VDJ-Cδ mRNA enabling the coexpression of IgM and IgD at the cell surface. This coexpression coincides with the transition for each B-cell from antigen tolerance to antigen responsiveness (Weisenburger, 1990). Approximately 10^9 virgin B-cells coexpressing IgM and IgD are produced in the marrow daily in this way and migrate via the blood to populate the spleen and other secondary lymphoid organs. Thus, large numbers of virgin B-lymphocytes with roughly 10^6 different antibody specificities are continually distributed throughout the body in readiness for the second, or antigen dependent phase of B-cell development.

Phase 2 – Antigen dependent differentiation

The pattern of response to foreign antigen depends upon prior exposure.

The primary immune response involves surface IgM and IgD-bearing, virgin B-cells, located within primary follicles and within the cortex of lymph nodes. These cells do not recirculate, are constantly replenished from the bone marrow, and are short-lived. Without activation, most die within a few days of reaching the spleen. In the presence of specific antigen, however, cross-linkage of surface immunoglobulin occurs and the resting B-cells undergo activation, enlargement and DNA synthesis. Recently, it has been shown that this activation occurs via a transmembrane signalling complex composed of a heterodimeric molecule analogous to the T-cell receptor complex , and referred to as 'the B-cell receptor' (Reth, 1992; Vannoesel et al., 1992). Following activation, antigen fragments are internalised and reappear on the cell surface in combination with Class II major histocompatibility complex (MHC) molecules. This antigen-presenting role leads to activation of CD4 positive T-helper cells which in turn produce lymphokines leading to proliferation of the B-cell clone and differentiation into IgM-secreting plasma cells.

Antigen-antibody complexes formed as a result of this primary plasma cell reaction, become attached to follicular dendritic reticulum cells (DRCs) in lymph nodes, activating virgin B-cells within primary follicles. Upon activation, these germinal centre B-cells proliferate, lose surface IgD expression and with continued antigenic stimulation, undergo isotype switching, leading to the coexpression of IgM and IgG or IgM and IgA.

Recent evidence suggests that actively dividing B-cells within the follicle centre are programmed to undergo apoptotic cell death unless rescued by cross-linking of surface immunoglobulin or stimulation of their CD40 receptors (Hollowood and Macartney, 1991). The mechanism appears to involve the induction of the bcl-2 proto-oncogene within mitochondrial membranes, which protects against apoptosis (Hockenbery et al., 1991; Liu et al., 1991; Nunez et al., 1991). The resulting competition for antigen provides evolutionary pressure in favour of higher affinity antibodies. This process is accelerated by somatic hypermutation and the rapid rate of proliferation within follicles. The function of germinal centres therefore, includes affinity maturation of antibodies, amplification of clonal proliferation and, under the regulatory influence of T-cells, production of memory B-cells, fundamental to the secondary immune response.

Unlike virgin B-cells, memory B-cells generated by the germinal centre reaction, usually express high affinity IgG or IgA antibodies, are long-lived and constantly recirculate.

In the secondary immune response, foreign antigen, arriving in the cortex and medullary cords of lymph nodes attaches to memory B-cells bearing complimentary immunoglobulin. This leads to blastic transformation and differentiation into IgG and /or IgA secreting plasma cells (secondary plasma cell reaction). The secondary germinal centre reaction ensues.

Immunological memory thus confers the advantage of rapid production of high-affinity antibodies. In addition, however, the circulating pool of memory B-cells is under further evolutionary pressure due to the high frequency of point mutations within the V region genes. Antibodies of greater affinity may therefore become available during the next encounter with antigen. Unlike the primary plasma cell reaction which largely occurs *in situ* within secondary lymphoid organs, the secondary plasma cell reaction involves IgG and IgA committed pre-plasma cells which migrate to the bone marrow before plasmacytic differentiation. In the secondary immune reaction therefore, antibody production is predominantly within the bone marrow.

Follicle morphology

The morphology of the germinal centre reaction has been extensively studied. Although there has been controversy about their order of appearance, there is general agreement that follicle centre B-cells comprise small and large cleaved cells (centrocytes) and small and large non-cleaved cells (centroblasts). There is good evidence from several authors that following activation, germinal centre B-cells undergo the following sequence: small non-cleaved to large non-cleaved to large cleaved to small cleaved cell (Fig. 4.1)(Hollema and Poppema, 1988; Hsu and Jaffe, 1984a; Hsu and Jaffe, 1984b; van der Valk and Meijer, 1988). By the seventh day following antigenic stimulation, dark and light zones become apparent within the follicle centre. Actively proliferating, pyroninophilic centroblasts which constitute the dark zone, lose expression of surface IgD and subsequently show decreased expression of surface IgM. A concomitant increase in cytoplasmic immunoglobulin then occurs as the follicle centre cells migrate to the light zone and mature into paler centrocytes. A significant proportion of B-cells within the follicle centre are Ig negative, an observation of significance as approximately one third of follicular lymphomas similarly do not express detectable surface or cytoplasmic immunoglobulin (Hsu and Jaffe, 1984b). Although most centroblasts within the dark zone express surface IgM or IgD, the majority of cIg-positive cells in the light zone express IgG.

Recently, the structure of lymphoid follicles and their relation to T-cell areas of the lymph node has been reviewed (Van den Oord et al., 1986a). Paracortical T-cell nodules are known to occur in reactive nodes and are frequently found in association with lymphoid follicles. It has been proposed that B-cell follicles and the adjacent T-cells form a functional unit or 'composite nodule' similar to the Malpighian body of the spleen. This comprises an ovoid body in which the peripheral, subcapsular, or B-cell pole of the nodule contains follicle centre B-cells, follicular dendritic reticulum cells and the surrounding mantle zone lymphocytes. The opposite pole of the composite nodule contains post-capillary venules, interdigitating reticulum cells and the elements of the T-cell compartment. The whole structure is surrounded by a rim of high endothelial venules, macrophages and alkaline phosphatase-positive B-cells reminiscent of the splenic marginal zone. Functionally, the close association of B and T-cells within the composite nodule facilitates T-helper induced proliferation and maturation of B-cells.

The marginal zone of B-cell follicles

The marginal zone (MGZ) is best developed in the splenic white pulp where it forms a layer of B-cells surrounding the follicles and T-zone or periarteriolar lymphoid sheath. It is seen in H & E sections as a cuff of more pale-staining, intermediate or medium-sized lymphoid cells with indistinct nucleoli and pale cytoplasm. The MGZ cells appear to be immunologically naive precursors of the primary immune response in which IgM secreting plasma cells develop independently of T-cell cooperation. In addition, splenic MGZ B-cells may migrate into the follicle centres, conveying antigens from the splenic red pulp to dendritic reticulum cells, promoting B-cell proliferation, and probably, creation of memory B-cells. In lymph nodes, the marginal zone is usually not well developed and only occasional alkaline phosphatase positive MGZ cells are seen, scattered amongst the smaller, alkaline phosphatase negative mantle zone B-cells. Proliferation of these cells however, in some reactive states, in normal mesenteric lymph nodes, and in monocytoid B-cell lymphomas, can lead to a well-defined parafollicular or marginal zone pattern. In the gut, cells resembling marginal zone lymphocytes are seen forming a broad zone around the lymphoid follicles of Peyer's patches and extending up into the dome epithelium overlying the lymphoid follicles. In this site, as in the spleen, they may be important both in the primary formation of antibodies, and in the transport of antigens to the DRCs. Marginal zone lymphocytes are heavily implicated in the pathogenesis of mucosal associated lymphoid populations (MALT) and monocytoid B-cell lymphomas as well as splenic marginal zone lymphoma.

Phenotypically, the MGZ lymphocytes express pan B-cell antigens CD19, 20, 22, and 24 and sIgM but not sIgD. The cells are alkaline phosphatase positive and bear C3d (CD21), C3b (CD35), and FcgRII (CDw32) receptors (Schmid et al., 1992; Van Krieken et al., 1989b). CD5, 9, 10 and 23 are negative. Monoclonal antibody UCL4d12, raised against a MALT lymphoma (see below) is characteristically expressed (Smith-Ravin et al., 1990). In comparison, mantle zone lymphocytes are positive for CD5, 23, KiB3, IgD and UCL-3d3 (Table 4.1).

In paraffin sections, the cells are positive for L26 (CD20), CD45RA and IgM, but not KiB3 or IgD (see Table 4.1).

Table 4.1. Immunophenotype of follicle centre, mantle, marginal zone and thymic B-cells

	FCC	MTZ	MGZ	Thymic B-cells
CD5	–	+/–	–	–
CD10	+	–	–	–
CD20	+	+	+	+
CD21	–	+	+	–
CD23	+	–	–	+/–
CDw32	–	+	+	–
CD35	–	+	+	–
IgM	+	+	+/–	+
IgD	–	+	–	+/–
KiB3	+	+	–	
UCL-3d3	–	+	–	
UCL-4d12	–/+	–	+	
ALP	–	+/–	+	

Thymic B-cells

In 1961, Miller first demonstrated the critical importance of thymic function to the immune system (Miller, 1961), and subsequent attention has largely focused upon thymic T-cells. The presence of a distinctive thymic B-cell population has only recently been investigated, mainly as a response to recent descriptions of thymic large cell lymphomas of B-cell type (Isaacson et al., 1987).

B-cells represent only a small subpopulation of thymic lymphocytes, and are present almost entirely within the medulla, where they exhibit an 'asteroid' appearance, and are found clustered around Hassal's corpuscles, in contact with thymocytes (Hofmann et al., 1988; Isaacson et al., 1987). The function of these cells remains uncertain, however their activated state, association with Hassal's corpuscles, and intimate contact with thymocytes suggests that they are involved in negative clonal selection (Spencer et al., 1992).

Thymic B-cells express a distinctive phenotype as follows: $CD1^-$, $CD2^-$, $CD3^-$, $CD5^-$, $CD9^-$, $CD10^-$, $CD19^+$, $CD20^+$, $CD21^-$, $CD22^+$, $CD23^{+/-}$, $CD30^-$, $CDw32^-$, $CD35^-$, $CD37^+$, IgM^+, $IgD^{+/-}$, $IgA^{+/-}$. Many of the cells are also $Ki\text{-}67^+$. In fixed paraffin-embedded tissues, the cells strongly express L26 (CD20), with some staining for IgM and IgD and IgA.

This phenotype is unlike that of other defined B-cell populations (Fig. 4.2). There are some similarities to marginal zone B-cells and monocytoid B-cells, however thymic B-cells differ by being negative for CD21, CDw32, CD35; and variably positive for CD23 and IgD. The distinctive phenotype of normal thymic B-cells is reiterated in large cell B-cell lymphomas of the thymus and mediastinum.

$CD5^+$, 'B-1 cells'

CD5 is generally regarded as a T-cell antigen and is expressed by most mature post-thymic T-cells. It is not T-cell restricted, however, and a small but distinctive population of $CD5^+$ B-cells has been recognised for some time. Recently, these have been designated 'B-1' cells (Bhat et al., 1992; Kantor, 1991). B-1 cells make up a large percentage of circulating B-cells in the fetus and following bone marrow transplantation, and are the major source of autoreactive antibodies and serum immunoglobulin, but represent only a small percentage of the B-lymphocyte population in adults. They are thought to represent a phylogenetically primitive lineage of B-cells (analogous to $\gamma\delta$ T-cells) and are further divided into $CD5^+$ B-1a and $CD5^-$ B-1b subgroups. In lymphoproliferative disease, this B-cell subset is implicated in the pathogenesis of small lymphocytic lymphoma and variants, as well as Castleman's disease.

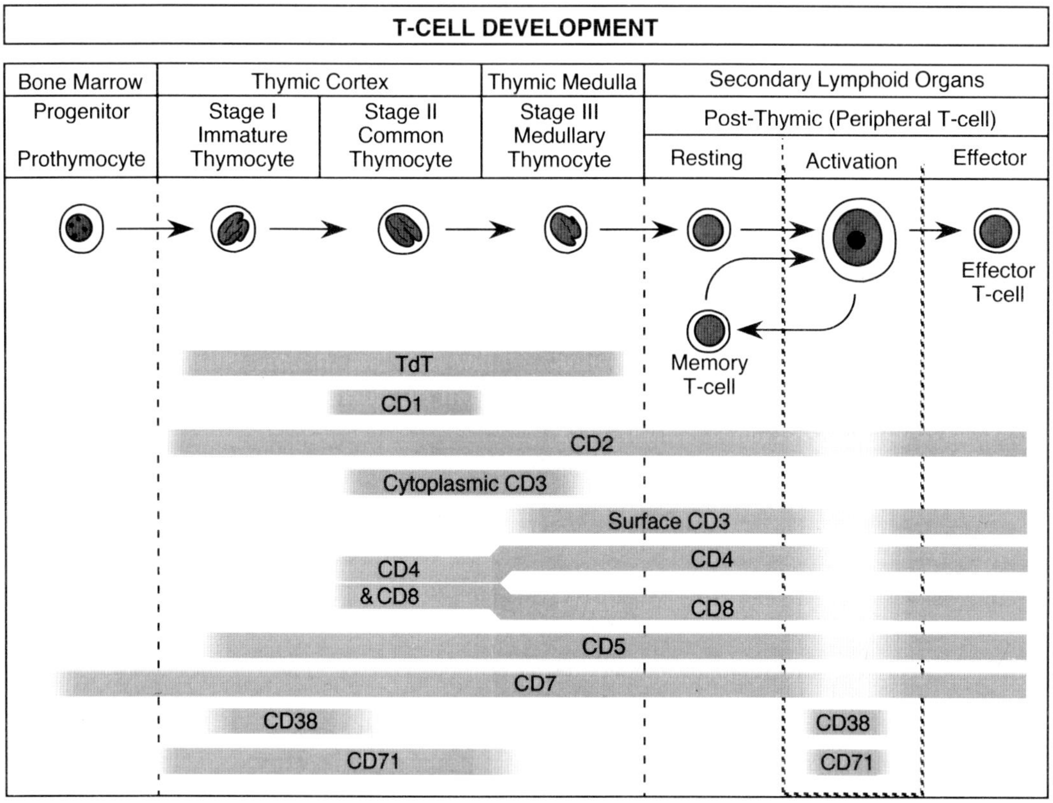

Fig. 4.2. T-cell activation is marked by both the expression of 'activation antigens' and often reduced expression of pan-T antigens.

T-cell development and function

The functions of the T-cell arm of the immune system include both cytotoxicity and immunoregulation. This is usually MHC restricted, meaning that antigen must be presented to the T-cell in association with membrane bound products of the major histocompatibility complex. The process of T-cell development, begining with marrow-based prothymocytes, takes place largely within the thymus and culminates in the production of immunocompetent, circulatory, mature T-cells bearing a complex system of interacting receptors including the TCR/CD3 complex, CD4 or CD8 coreceptors, one or other isoform of the CD45 leucocyte common antigen, CD2 and CD5. Evidence is now accumulating that many of these receptors interact synergistically with each other in the plane of the membrane to modulate transmembrane signalling, thus controlling T-cell activation and function principally via tyrosine kinase, and tyrosine-specific phosphatase activity (Dianzani et al., 1992; Janeway, 1992).

Intra-thymic T-cell ontogeny

The earliest T-cell precursors (prothymocytes), expressing HLA-DR, nuclear terminal deoxynucleotidyl transferase (TdT) and CD7, migrate from the marrow to the thymus (possibly assisted by CD7 acting as a homing receptor). All subsequent intra-thymic developmental stages continue to express nuclear terminal deoxynucleotidyl transferase (TdT), CD2 and CD7. The transferrin receptor (CD71) is expressed by all except the more mature (medullary) thymocytes. CD10 (calla), is generally associated with common (non-T) ALL, but is also expressed by early thymocytes, as are CD9 and CD38 (Hsu and Jaffe, 1985). (See Fig. 4.2.)

Stage 1, thymocyte

The immature or stage 1 thymocyte stage is characterized by the acquisition of surface CD5, transcription of mRNA coding for CD3 subunits, and commencement of TCRβ gene rearrangement (Acuto et al., 1985; Jaffe, 1990; Knowles, 1989; Royer and Reinherz, 1987).

The components of the T-cell receptor complex are all members of the immunoglobulin supergene family, and TCRβ rearrangement occurs via a process similar to that previously described for immunoglobulin genes. Briefly, under the influence of a recombinase enzyme, a D (or diversity) segment (where present) is brought into apposition with a J (or joining) segment and the intervening DNA is deleted to form a DJ segment. Next, a V (or variable) segment is repositioned downstream and placed contiguously 5' to the DJ segment, producing a continuous V-D-J sequence which is separated from the C (or constant) segment by an intervening sequence (Royer and Reinherz, 1987).

Stage 2, intermediate or common thymocyte

The next phase (stage 2 or common cortical thymocyte) is characterized by the appearance of CD1, the coexpression of surface CD4 and CD8 and the cytoplasmic accumulation of CD3 and TCRβ chain, detectable using antibody βF1 (Mori et al., 1990). Rearrangement of the TCRα gene occurs at this stage.

Stage 3 or medullary thymocyte

In the third or final stage of thymic maturation, following transcription and expression of the TCRα subunit, T-cells migrate into the thymic medulla where they finally show surface expression of CD3 in combination with the complete T-cell receptor and the mature pan-T antigens: CD2, CD5 and CD7. At the same time, CD1 and CD71 antigens are lost, and the cells become committed to either CD4 or CD8 co-receptor expression. Further progression from thymocyte to peripheral T-cell is marked by the loss of TdT, cytoplasmic CD3, and the expression of lymphocyte homing receptor detected by antibody Leu8.

T-cell receptor structure

In more than 95 per cent of human T lymphocytes, the T-cell receptor complex consists of the disulphide-linked Ti α-β heterodimer in association with the CD3 γ,δ, and ε subunits. The structure of the Ti α and β subunits is similar to that of immunoglobulin molecules, and is coded for by recombination of variable (V), constant (C), joining (J), and often diversity (D) genomic segments (Royer and Reinherz, 1987). In common with immunoglobulin molecules, this structure provides the vast repertoire of antigen specificities required for immune surveillance.

Both the Ti αβ and CD3 subunits are transmembrane molecules, and while the former provides specificity for antigen-MHC recognition, CD3 appears to function as a signal transducer across the cell membrane.

The effective recognition of antigen-MHC complexes depends critically upon the presence of CD4 or CD8 co-receptors. MHC class 1 molecules bind to peptides derived from endogenously synthesized molecules such as viral proteins, and are recognized by the CD8 co-receptor. MHC class 2 molecules bind to peptides derived from endocytosed antigen and are recognized by the CD4 co-receptor (Springer, 1990). Thus $CD4^+$ helper T-cells recognize antigen-MHC (class 2) complexes on the surface of B-cells whose proliferation they induce, and $CD8^+$ cytotoxic cells recognize antigen-MHC (class 1) complexes on the surface of virally infected cells which they kill.

Recently, attention has also focused on the different CD45 isoforms (CD45RA, CD45RO, CD45RC, CD45RB), and the role they play in modulating TCR function in different stages of T-cell maturation (Dianzani et al., 1992; Janeway, 1992).

T-cells bearing the TCRγδ (γδ T-cells)

Although more than 90 per cent of circulating T-cells in normal humans express the αβ TCR (as detailed above), between 1 and 10 per cent express an alternative TCR heterodimer consisting of gamma and delta rather than alpha and beta subunits (Knowles, 1989; Royer and Reinherz, 1987). The structure of the γδ TCR is similar to the αβ TCR. Productive γ and δ genes arise by rearrangement of V, D, J and C regions, and the γ and δ subunits produced, are non-covalently linked with the CD3 molecule. The ontogeny of γδ T-cells and their relationship with αβ T-cells has not yet been established. It is known that γ and δ genes are rearranged before α and β genes. The δ gene is strategically located on chromosome 14q11, between the V and J regions of the α chain gene. Rearrangement of the α chain gene therefore deletes the δ gene, ensuring that only γδ or αβ TCR subunits are expressed on any one cell (Zutter, 1991). Gamma or delta chains are never expressed on the surface of αβ T-cells, yet recent evidence suggests that all αβ T-cells have none the less rearranged one or both γ chain loci. It is therefore suspected that γδ and αβ T-cells develop from a common linear or branched hierarchy (Alexandre and Lefranc, 1992; Thompson et al., 1991). Although γδ T-cells utilizing the

Vδ1 segment are thought to arise in the thymus along with αβ T-cells, there is some evidence that Vδ2 γδ T-cells may be thymus independent (Editorial, 1991).

Phenotypically, all γδ T-cells express CD2 and CD3, but between 30 and 90 per cent express CD5. Antigen recognition appears to be largely non-MHC-restricted, and therefore most γδ T-cells are subset double-negative ($CD4^-$ and $CD8^-$), with a minority expressing CD8. CD11b, CD56 (Leu7) and CD16 are variably expressed (Inghirami et al., 1990; Zutter, 1991). CD4 may be weakly expressed in thymic γδ T-cells, but is otherwise negative. Although the TCR αβ is not expressed, antibodies to the β chain such as WT31 or βF1 may be weakly positive in some cases, due presumably to sequence homology and/or cross reactivity between β and δ chains (Falini et al., 1989; Inghirami et al., 1990).

Functionally, γδ T-cells exercise MHC-restricted as well as non-restricted cytotoxicity (Zutter, 1991). Preferential expansion of γδ T-cell clones occurs in response to specific antigens including mycobacteria, some forms of leishmaniasis, measles and malaria (Editorial, 1991). γδ T-cells are implicated in some forms of autoimmune disease, and constitute most of the increase in intraepithelial T-cells observed in coeliac disease (Editorial, 1991; Spencer et al., 1989). In the mouse and other animals, γδ T-cells exhibit epithelial tropism, preferentially infiltrating the skin, lungs, intestine and reproductive tract (Dembic, 1991). In humans however, this does not appear to be the case. γδ T-cells are most prevalent in the splenic red pulp cords, where they constitute up to 17 per cent of $CD3^+$ cells (Bordessoule et al., 1990), and in the intestinal crypt epithelium (Vroom et al., 1991). In other tissues and peripheral blood, they represent less than 5 per cent of $CD3^+$ cells, the actual percentage varying according to the individual and in response to specific antigens (Volk et al., 1991). In the thymus, >90 per cent are located within the medulla, and in peripheral lymphoid organs they are found in the interfollicular areas (Inghirami et al., 1990).

Although the precise role of γδ T-cells in the immune system remains uncertain, they are often viewed as a phylogenetically primitive population of T-cells, providing immune surveillance of highly conserved antigens (Bordessoule et al., 1990).

T-cell activation

T-cells express a maximum number of antigen-MHC receptors (approximately 40,000 per cell) in the resting phase (Royer and Reinherz, 1987). Following the triggering of these receptors by the specific antigen-MHC complexes in concert with macrophage derived products such as IL-1, the number of surface receptors rapidly diminishes, and the cells produce both interleukin-2 (IL-2) and interleukin-2 receptors (IL-2R, CD25). The autocrine loop thus established leads to DNA synthesis and cell mitosis. Other surface molecules expressed during activation include HLA-DR, CD38, CD71 and CD30.

Following cessation of stimulation by antigen-MHC complexes, the expression of surface Il-2 receptors diminishes, the Ti/CD3 complex reappears on the cell surface, and the cell returns to a resting phase. This physiological modulation of surface antigen expression may be an important factor contributing to the phenotypic 'aberrancy' found in a majority of T-cell lymphomas.

In addition to MHC-restricted activation via the Ti-CD3 complex, T-cells are also capable of TCR/MHC-independent activation via surface CD2 or CD5 antigens in vitro (Alberolaila et al., 1992; Royer and Reinherz, 1987). The physiological significance of these alternative activation pathways is unknown.

Naive vs memory T-cells

Activation induces long-term phenotypic and functional alterations in T-cells, converting them from 'naive' to 'memory' cells. Upon leaving the thymus, immunocompetent, 'naive' $CD4^+$ T-cells express the high MW form of leucocyte common antigen (CD45RA), recognized by antibodies such as 4B4 and 4KB5. Following activation and conversion to 'memory' T-cells, leucocyte common antigen expression switches to the low MW (CD45RO) form recognized by antibodies such as UCHL1, OPD4 and A6. In neonates therefore, the majority of T-cells are 4KB5 positive and UCHL1 negative; a situation which gradually reverses as T-cells encounter specific antigen and undergo activation. Other long-term phenotypic alterations associated with the conversion to 'memory' status include increased expression of CD2, LFA-1, CD44 and a number of VLA integrins such as CD29, CD49d and CD49f. Expression of CD31 is reduced, and LFA-3, absent from naive cells, appears on the cell surface (Ashman and Aylett, 1991; Clement, 1992; Sanders et al., 1988; Springer, 1990).

Functionally, naive and memory T-cells differ in the following ways:

1. Memory cells respond to much lower doses of antigen than are required to activate naive cells. This may be particularly so for CD2 and CD3-mediated activation (Sanders et al., 1988; Springer, 1990). The coexpression in memory cells of both CD2 and its ligand (LFA-3) may lead to partial activation, or lower the threshold required for antigenic stimulation. Recent evidence indicates that changes in configuration of the CD45 molecule, and its interactions with the CD3-Ti receptor may also play an important role in this modulation of T-cell activation (Dianzani et al., 1992).
2. Naive and memory T-cells differ in the amounts and types of cytokines produced following activation, and further differ in their usage of, and dependence upon CD4 and CD8 co-receptors.
3. $CD4^+$ $CD45RA^+/CD45RO^-$ 'naive' T-cells function as *helper-suppressor* cells, either directly or via the induction of $CD8^+$ T-cell activity. $CD4^+$ $CD45RA^-/CD45RO^+$ 'memory' T-cells on the other hand, function as *helper-inducer* cells, increasing immune cell recruitment and assisting B-cell function (Clement, 1992).
4. Changes in the surface expression of adhesion molecules following activation (including CD2, CD11, and the integrins) appear to be critical in determining subsequent lymphocyte homing patterns (Picker and Butcher, 1992; Springer, 1990).

Homing receptors and lymphocyte circulation

Normal lymphocyte homing patterns throughout the different body compartments, and within the microarchitecture of primary and secondary lymphoid organs, ensure that the many cellular elements of the immune system are able to interact optimally with foreign antigen, and with each other (Butcher, 1990; Springer, 1990).

Adhesion of peripheral blood lymphocytes to the endothelium of specific sites is the fundamental mechanism whereby lymphocytes are able to recirculate from the peripheral blood into the tissues and back again via the thoracic duct. The exquisite specificity of lymphocyte trafficking is determined by complex interactions between lymphocyte surface adhesion molecules and ligands (addressins) expressed on high endothelial venules (HEV) in lymphoid tissues. Further trafficking into specific microcompartments occurs within lymphoid organs and is also mediated by intercellular adhesion molecules expressed by lymphocytes and other cells, such as follicular dendritic reticulum cells (DRCs) (Duijvestijn et al., 1988; Koopman et al., 1991).

Although there may be some unique lymphocyte subsets which leave the thymus or bone marrow already restricted in their homing programme, the majority of immunocompetent, virgin T- and B-cells are able to circulate widely, ensuring that the full repertoire of clonal antigen specificities is available throughout the body. Current evidence suggests that antigenic stimulation, and activation of these cells with conversion to memory lymphocytes, results in reprogramming of surface adhesion molecules, with acquisition of site specific homing. In fact there is evidence that memory lymphocytes preferentially home back to the tissue in which activation first occurred (Picker and Butcher, 1992; Springer, 1990). The peripheral blood therefore, is a common conduit for many different lymphocyte pools, circulating through different organs and tissues of the body. These include relatively short-lived and unprogrammed naive lymphocytes, as well as constantly recirculating, memory B and T-cells, programmed to follow specific homing patterns. The latter include such broad subgroups as mucosal associated lymphoid populations (MALT), and cells of the skin-associated lymphoid tissue (SALT).

Most of the lymphocyte adhesion molecules belong to one of three main families: the immunoglobulin supergene family, the integrin family, and the selectins. Other groups include oligosaccharide ligands for the selectins, and the Hermes antigen (CD44). Much remains to be understood, however certain patterns have emerged. Homing to peripheral lymph nodes for example, appears to be mediated by lymphocyte expression of the selectin molecule LECAM-1, (recognized by antibody Mel-14/Leu8) coupled to HEV expression of the peripheral lymph node addressin molecule (PNAd) recognized by antibody MECA-79. Similarly, homing to cutaneous sites appears to be mediated via expression of the oligosaccharide, cutaneous lymphocyte antigen or CLA (recognized by antibody HECA-452), coupled to the skin vascular addressin ELAM-1.

There is general agreement that normal lymphocyte homing mechanisms may be preserved to a greater or lesser extent, within neoplastic cells (Picker et al., 1988) so accounting for patterns of tumour dissemination and the clinicopathological features of many lymphomas. The study of lymphocyte adhesion molecules and homing receptors promises new avenues for prediction of tumour behaviour and treatment, but to date has no direct application within diagnostic immunohistochemistry. A detailed study of this complex biology is therefore outside the brief for this chapter, and for further information, the reader is directed to one of the recent reviews (Butcher, 1990; Jalkanen, 1991; Pabst, 1991; Picker and Butcher, 1992; Springer, 1990; Thiele, 1991).

Natural killer (NK) cells

Natural killer (NK) cells share a number of antigenic and functional similarities to cytotoxic T-cells but lack the complex array of surface antigen receptors and co-receptors required for specific MHC-restricted recognition. They have been defined as 'CD3-epsilon^{-}, CD16^{+} and/or CD56^{+} lymphocytes that mediate major histocompatibility complex (MHC)-unrestricted cytotoxicity against certain tumours and virus-infected cells' (Lanier and Phillips, 1992; Phillips et al., 1992). Cytotoxicity, independent of MHC recognition is however not limited to NK cells, as CD3^{+} cells such as $\gamma\delta$ T-cells, and lymphokine activated killer (LAK) cells are also capable of MHC-unrestricted, or 'natural' killing function (Dinarello and Mier, 1987; Editorial, 1991).

NK cells differ from T-cells then, in that they do not express CD3, CD4 or CD8, and they do not rearrange or express T-cell receptor $\alpha\beta$ or $\gamma\delta$ genes. The ontogenetic relationship between these two cell types is not clear, however a recent study has shown CD3 δ and ϵ chain transcription in fetal NK cells suggesting the possibility of a common progenitor (Phillips et al., 1992).

NK cells usually express the following phenotype: CD2^{+}, CD3^{-}, CD4^{-}, CD8$^{+/-}$, CD11b^{+}, CD11c^{+}, CD16^{+}, CD56^{+}, CD57$^{+/-}$ (Cattoretti et al., 1990; Chan et al., 1992; Ritz et al., 1988). Although CD11b, CD11c, and CD57 antigens are often grouped as 'NK markers', they are expressed in many other lineages and taken in isolation, have little specificity for NK function or lineage.

In human lymphoproliferative disease, tumours of NK lineage are most frequently encountered in certain forms of Tγ lymphoproliferative disease (Chan et al., 1992). It has also been suggested that a high percentage of angiocentric immunoproliferative lesions of the sinonasal tract are also related to NK cells (Ho et al., 1990; Ng et al., 1988; Ng et al., 1987a; Wong et al., 1992).

The mononuclear phagocytic system

The term mononuclear phagocytic system (MPS) has been used to define that component of the immune system which is derived from monocytes, but does not take into account the important role of antigen presenting cells. Recently, the acronym M-PIRE (mononuclear phagocytic and immunoregulatory effector) system has been proposed somewhat facetiously as being more indicative of the range of functions involved (Foucar and Foucar, 1991). Whereas our knowledge of lymphocyte biology has exploded since the advent of hybridoma technology, we have at present, relatively little knowledge of monocyte ontogeny or function (Komp and Perry, 1991).

It is generally agreed that all components of the MPS or M-PIRE system derive from bone marrow precursors via promonocyte and monocyte stages. Monocytes, released into the blood show some heterogeneity of phenotypic expression but generally express HLA-DR, CD4, CD11b, CD11c, CD13, CD14, CD15, CD21, CD25, CD33, CD45 and CD68. Typically, the cells show diffuse cytoplasmic positivity for the following enzymes: tartrate-sensitive acid phosphatase, fluoride-sensitive non-specific esterase, β-glucuronidase, lysozyme, α1-antitrypsin and α1-antichymotrypsin.

Once in the tissues, the cells of the MPS or M-PIRE system are usually separated into phagocytic and accessory cells compartments, although there is considerable overlap between the two (Favara, 1991).

Phagocytic cells include 'histiocytes', tingible body macrophages, Von Kuppfer cells, alveolar macrophages, osteoclasts, microglia and macrophages of the splenic cords. Phenotypically these cells usually express HLA-DR, CD4, CD11c, CD25, CD45, CD68, and MAC 387, with variable expression of CD11b, CD13, CD14 and CD33. In common with peripheral blood monocytes, acid phosphatase, non-specific esterase, lysozyme, α1-antitrypsin and α1-antichymotrypsin are also expressed (Table 4.2).

Functionally, this component of the immune system is responsible for:

1. phagocytosis of degenerate cells;
2. phagocytosis and killing of microorganisms;
3. secretion of cytokines and coagulation factors;
4. some antigen presentation;
5. tissue remodelling.

The 'epithelioid' histiocyte has long been recognized within the Kiel group, as a particular form of histiocyte with deeply eosinophilic or amphophilic cytoplasm, which has adopted a specialized secretory role. Plasmacytoid monocytes, recently rescued from the misnomer 'plasmacytoid T-cells' (Facchetti et al., 1988; Facchetti et al., 1989; Koo et al., 1990) have been variously suggested to be precursors of epithelioid histiocytes or antigen presenting cells.

Accessory cells include dendritic reticulum cells (DRCs), interdigitating reticulum cells (IRCs), Langerhans cells (LCs) and fibroblastic dendritic cells (FDCs). Phenotypically, all express class 1 or class 2 histocompatibility antigens, IgG Fc receptors, and CD45. S-100 is expressed strongly by LCs, IRCs and weakly by DRCs. CD1 is expressed by LCs, IRCs and some FDCs. ATPase is present in DRCs, IRCs and LCs, while acid phosphatase is expressed by DRCs, and some LCs. Alkaline phosphatase is present in FDCs. The ability to identify DRCs in tissue sections is useful in a number of diagnostic situations and can be achieved using antibodies to CD21 (1F8), CD23 (BU38), CD35 (C3bR) or in frozen sections, anti-DRC antibodies such as Dako-DRC (R4/23).

Functionally, accessory cells are responsible for:

1. antigen processing and presentation to B-cells (DRCs) and T-cells (IRCs);
2. contact hypersensitivity, mediated through LCs;
3. structural integrity through FDCs.

The induction of the foregoing functions, via 'activation' of histiocytes, is typically mediated by Il-2 or γ interferon (Favara, 1991).

The dynamic nature of these two major functional populations of cells is emphasized by the identification of intermediate forms, and the discovery that following immune depletion, the accessory cell population may be replenished from within the phagocytic compartment (Murphy et al., 1986).

CD designations and commercially available antibodies

In the following section, antibodies which are reactive in fixed, paraffin-embedded tissues are emphasized in bold typeface.

CD1: *Antibodies:* T6 (Coulter), OKT6, Leu6 (Becton Dickinson) and NA1/34 (Dako). (Subtypes CD1a, CD1b and CD1c)

CD1 is normally expressed in stage 2, or common cortical thymocytes and Langerhans cells. In lymphoproliferative disease, its expression is confined to Langerhans cell histiocytosis (LCH) and T-lymphoblastic leukaemias and lymphoma. Weak staining has been described in interdigitating reticulum cells (IRCs) and sarcomas thereof.

CD2: *Antibodies:* T11 (Coulter), OKT11, Leu5 (Becton Dickinson), Lyt3

CD2, a specific pan-T antigen, corresponds to the sheep erythrocyte receptor, and is present on all T-cells from

Table 4.2. Markers of histiocytes

	Histiocyte	**IRC**	**DRC**	**LC**
HLA-DR	+	+	+	+
Non-specific esterase	Diffuse +	Focal +/−	Focal +/−	−
Acid Phos	Diffuse +	Focal +/−	Focal +/−	+/−
ATPase	−	+	+	+
Mannosidase	−	+		+
α1-antichymotrypsin	+	−	−	−
CD1	−	+/−	−	+
CD4	+	+	+	+
CD14	+	+	+	+
CD45	+	+	+	+
CD68	+	−	−	−
S100	−	+	+/−	+
Peanut lectin	Diffuse	Dot	Dot	Dot
Birbeck granules	−	−	−	+

the immature thymocyte stage onwards and acts as an alternative receptor for the activation of T-cells (Royer and Reinherz, 1987). LFA-3 (CD58) acts as the receptor ligand. Recent evidence indicates that it is functionally associated with the CD45RO antigen on the T-cell membrane (Dianzani et al., 1992). It is one of the most conserved T-cell antigens in T lymphoma and expressed only on T-cells, NK cells and rare histiocytic tumours.

CD3: *Antibodies:* T3 (Coulter), OKT3, Leu4 (Becton Dickinson), UCHT1 (Dako), polyclonal CD3

The CD3 molecule consists of α, δ, and ϵ subunits, non-covalently bound to the T-cell receptor (Ti) to form the CD3/Ti (TCR) receptor complex . It is thought to have a transmembrane signalling role (Royer and Reinherz, 1987) and is one of the most specific and useful markers of T-cell differentiation available. **Polyclonal CD3** used in paraffin sections is somewhat less sensitive or specific than the equivalent monoclonal antibodies used in cryostat sections.

CD4: *Antibodies:* T4 (Coulter), OKT4, Leu3 (Becton Dickinson)

The CD4 molecule acts a co-receptor with the TCR complex, and recognizes MHC class 2 molecules (Springer, 1990). It is a marker for T-helper cells and is the receptor for human immunodeficiency virus. The CD4+ T-cell subset is further divided into naive, helper-suppressor, and memory, helper-inducer subsets (Clement, 1992). Many phagocytic histiocytes and dendritic cells are also CD4+. This often renders interpretation of frozen sections difficult in the case of histiocyte-rich infiltrates. CD45RA antibody **OPD4** has been claimed to be specific for CD4+ T-cells, however this has not proven to be the case.

CD5: *Antibodies:* T1 (Coulter), OKT1, Leu1 (Becton Dickinson), RFT1

The CD5, a pan-T antigen, first appears on the surface of immature or stage 1 thymocytes. It is restricted to T-cells and small subpopulation of B-cells referred to as 'B-1 cells' (Kantor, 1991). In T-cells, it may function as an alternative activation receptor (Alberolaila et al., 1992). There is no equivalent antibody reactive in fixed, paraffin-embedded tissues.

CD7: *Antibodies:* 3A1 (Coulter), Leu9 (Becton Dickinson), RFT2, WT1

CD7 is the earliest antigen to be expressed in T-cell ontogeny, appearing in pre-thymic T-cell precursors and preceding CD2 expression. It is the most consistently expressed T-cell antigen in lymphoblastic leukaemias and lymphomas, and is specific for T-cell lineage. In mature, post-thymic T-cell tumours, it is the most common pan-T antigen to be aberrantly absent.

CD8: *Antibodies:* T8 (Coulter), OKT8, OKT5, Leu2 (Becton Dickinson)

The CD8 molecule functions as a TCR co-receptor on suppressor-cytotoxic T-cells, and recognizes MHC class 1 molecules (Springer, 1990). It is specific for T-cells, and is expressed in lymphoblastic lymphomas and a small percentage of post-thymic malignancies.

CD9: *Antibodies:* BA2, FMC8

CD9 is expressed on immature B-cells, monocytes and platelets. In tumour cell populations, CD9 is expressed in several B-cell malignancies including B lymphoblastic leukaemia and lymphoma, centrocytic lymphoma, follicle centre cell lymphoma and Burkitt's lymphoma (Lardelli et al., 1990). It is also found in mast cells (Horny et al., 1990b), and some DRCs (Carbone et al., 1987).

CD10: *Antibodies:* calla, J5 (Coulter), DakoCALLA, BA3

CD10 is normally expressed on pre B-cells, follicle centre cells and a small subpopulation of thymocytes, as well as mature neutrophils and a range of epithelia. It is now known to be a membrane associated enzyme, neutral endopeptidase (NEP) or enkephalinase (LeBien and McCormack, 1989). In tumours, it is expressed in common acute lymphoblastic leukaemia (cALL), follicle centre cell lymphomas, Burkitt's lymphoma, some forms of myeloma, and a percentage of T-lymphoblastic leukaemia and lymphoma (Durie and Grogan, 1985; Erber and Mason, 1988; Jaffe, 1990; LeBien and McCormack, 1989; Sheibani et al., 1987a).

CD11: CD11a *Antibodies:* MHM24 (Dako) CD11b *Antibodies:* MO1 (Coulter), Mac1, OKM1, CR3, Leu15 (Becton Dickinson), DakoC3biR

CD11c *Antibodies:* LeuM5 (Becton Dickinson), KiM1, KB23, BU15

Each of the three CD11 subtypes represents a different α chain, which when non-covalently linked to β2 (or CD18) glycoprotein, forms one of the β2 family of integrin adhesion receptors (see lymphocyte trafficking).

CD11a (or LFA-1) is expressed on B-cells, T-cells, NK cells, monocytes and granulocytes.

CD11b is the C3bi receptor, and is expressed on monocytes, granulocytes and some histiocytes.

CD11c is present on monocytes, tissue macrophages, granulocytes, some cytotoxic T-cells and a subset of B-cells. It is usually positive in histiocytic malignancies and in some B-cell lymphomas including hairy cell leukaemia and monocytoid B-cell lymphoma (Chadburn et al., 1990).

CD13: *Antibodies:* MY7 (Coulter), WM47 (Dako), LeuM7 (Becton Dickinson)

The CD13 antigen is thought to be an aminopeptidase which is expressed by myeloid and monocytic cells. It is present in myeloid leukaemia and in many of the histiocytic disorders.

CD14: *Antibodies:* MO2, MY4 (Coulter), LeuM3 (Becton Dickinson), FMC17

The CD14 antigen is expressed by monocytes and a percentage of histiocytes and dendritic cells. It is present in histiocytic malignancies and some cases of Langerhans cell histiocytosis. Antibody MY4 recognizes a different epitope to the other antibodies and shows a different pattern of reactivity. It is expressed in a small percentage of T-cell lymphomas, and approximately half of all B-cell lymphomas, including a majority of follicular lymphomas (Medeiros et al., 1991).

CD15: *Antibodies:* **DakoM1, LeuM1 (Becton Dickinson), Tü9**

The CD15 antigen corresponds to the Lewis X antigen or Lacto-N-fucopentaose III (LNF III), and is present in many cell types in a sialylated form, requiring prior digestion with neuraminidase to enable detection. Mature granulocytes and monocytes express the unsialylated molecule, and are CD15 positive without a requirement for prior digestion. It is found in myeloid and some monocytic malignancies as well as a minority of high grade T- and B-cell lymphomas. In Hodgkin's disease, it is expressed in over 85 per cent of non-lymphocyte predominance subtypes and takes the form of a paranuclear dot with variable membranous staining. In a sialylated form it is also present in lymphocyte predominance Hodgkin's disease and some dendritic cell malignancies. Many epithelial tumours are $CD15^{+}$, and **LeuM1** has been advocated as being useful in the differentiation of adenocarcinoma from mesothelioma.

CD16: *Antibodies:* Leu11b, FcγRIII

The CD16 antigen is the low affinity IgG Fc receptor and is found on NK cells, neutrophils and some histiocytic cells. It is characteristically present in Tγ lymphoproliferative disease, and in a small subgroup of T-lymphoblastic leukaemias and angiocentric lymphomas (Chan et al., 1992; Hollema and Poppema, 1989; Sheibani et al., 1987a).

CD19: *Antibodies:* B4 (Coulter), Leu12 (Becton Dickinson), DakoCD19

The CD19 antigen belongs to the Ig supergene family, and is a pan-B marker, appearing very early in B-cell development, before CD20, and at about the time of Ig gene rearrangement. It is present in most B-cell tumours and may be the only phenotypic evidence for B-cell lineage in immature lymphoblastic leukaemias.

CD20: *Antibodies:* B1 (Coulter), Leu16 (Becton Dickinson), **L26 (Dako)**

The CD20 antigen is also a pan-B marker, and appears in B-cell development after CD19. It is a transmembrane molecule and may be involved in ion transport. The monoclonal antibody L26 is strongly reactive in fixed tissues, exhibits excellent specificity and is currently one of the most useful antibodies available (Mason et al., 1990).

CD21: *Antibodies:* B2 (Coulter), CR2, **IF8 (Dako)**

The CD21 antigen is the receptor for C3D and EBV. It is expressed in mature resting B-cells and DRCs. Many B-cell lymphomas are variably positive for CD21 including, B-CLL, centrocytic and Burkitt's lymphoma. It may occasionally be detected in Langerhans cell histiocytosis. T-cell tumours do not express CD21. Antibody **IF8** is especially useful in paraffin sections, to identify the follicular networks of DRCs.

CD22: *Antibodies:* Dako panB, To15, Leu14 (Becton Dickinson)

The CD22 molecule appears in the cytoplasm of pre-B cells but is not expressed on the cell surface until later in development. Although showing a narrower range of expression in B-cell ontogeny than CD19 or CD20, it is present in the majority of B-cell lymphomas, and often stains more strongly in tissue sections. It is one of the most useful B-cell markers applicable in frozen section or cytospin preparations.

CD23: *Antibodies:* **BU38,** FcεRIIa, FcεRIIb

CD23 functions as the Fc receptor for IgE and lymphocyte growth factor. Following cross-linkage of antigen and Ig, CD23 is expressed and provides an autocrine stimulus driving B-cell proliferation (Raghoebier et al., 1991). It is therefore a marker of activated B-cells, but also stains some DRCs. FcεRIIa is largely B-cell restricted but FcεRIIb is found in a range of cell types including histiocytes, DRCs, some T-cells and NK cells, eosinophils and platelets. In tumour cell populations, CD23 is found in most low grade B-cell tumours and the within the Reed-Sternberg cells of Hodgkin's disease (Rowlands et al., 1990). Antibody **BU38**, effective in paraffin-sections, is useful as a marker for DRCs.

CD24: *Antibodies:* BA-1

The CD24 antigen is expressed by B-cells, granulocytes and some macrophages. It is present in a variable percentage of B-cell lymphomas and is also present in a subtytpe of T-ALL.

CD25: *Antibodies:* anti-TAC, Dako IL2R

CD25 is the interleukin receptor (Il-2R). It is therefore absent from resting cells, being expressed in activated T-cells, B-cells and macrophages. It is consistently found in hairy cell leukaemia and HTLV1-associated adult T-cell lymphoma/leukaemia as well as a variable percentage of other lymphomas and Hodgkin's disease (Erber and Mason, 1988).

CD29: *Antibodies:* β1 Integrin chain

CD29 is the VLA β1 chain (common to the β1 family of integrin receptors), which forms a heterodimer with one of at least 6 different a chains (see CDw49) (Zutter, 1991). The heterodimeric VLA molecules of the β1 family act as fibronectin, collagen and laminin receptors (Springer, 1990).

CD30: *Antibodies:* Ki-1, **BerH2**

The CD30 antigen is a transmembrane glycoprotein comprising a 90Kd precursor molecule, modified by addition of further 15kD or 30kD molecules. Ki-1 and BerH2 antibodies recognize different epitopes present on both the 90kD precursor molecule and the mature 105kD form (Moller et al., 1989b). The two antibodies therefore show different but related patterns of reactivity (Schwarting et al., 1989). Antibody Ki-1 is applicable only in frozen section material whereas **BerH2** is used in both paraffin and frozen section phenotyping. In general, **BerH2** stains frozen sections more intensely than Ki-1 and is itself, more effective in cryostat material than in paraffin sections.

Although initially thought to be specific for Reed-Sternberg cells and anaplastic large cell lymphoma, CD30 antigen expression has subsequently been identified in a number of cell types and is now generally regarded as an activation marker in lymphoid cells.

In non-neoplastic haemopoietic tissues, the CD30 antigen has been demonstrated in large transformed perifollicular cells (Stein et al., 1985), focally within the thymic medulla (Pallesen, 1990), and within a subset of plasma cells (Moller et al., 1989b) as well as in a number of reactive conditions such as toxoplasma lymphadenitis, infectious mononucleosis (Abbondanzo et al., 1990), Kikuchi's disease (Rivano et al., 1987) and virus-associated phagocytic syndrome (Pileri et al., 1990). Although the expression of CD30 on histiocytes has been reported to occur in certain circumstances (Andreeson et al., 1989), others ascribe this to cross-reactivity and claim that CD30 is never expressed in cells of histiocytic lineage.

In non-haemopoietic tissues, weak cytoplasmic staining for CD30 has been identified in melanoma, and some cases of carcinoma of the pancreas, salivary gland, breast, lung, stomach and endometrium (Schwarting et al., 1989). More significantly, strong staining has recently been reported to occur in a majority of cases of embryonal carcinoma

(Pallesen and Hamilton-Dutoit, 1988). Purkinje cells of the cerebellum and cortical neurons stain strongly for **Ber H2** in paraffin sections.

In haemopoietic malignancies, CD30 is expressed in almost all examples of anaplastic large cell (ALC) lymphoma, and in many cases of T-immunoblastic and T-pleomorphic lymphoma of medium and large cell type. It is also found within the large transformed cells of lymphomatoid papulosis (LYP) as well as in a minority of cases of B-immunoblastic, centroblastic and Burkitt's lymphoma (Pallesen, 1990; Piris et al., 1990). Although Langerhans cells, IRCs and DRCs are negative, some sarcomas of DRC origin have been reported to be positive for CD30 (Pallesen, 1990).

CDw32: *Antibodies:* 41H, KB61

The CDw32 antigen is present in a number of different isoforms and represents the FcγRII receptor (Miklem et al., 1990). It is expressed on granulocytes, monocytes, endothelium, platelets and most normal B-cells, with the exception of follicle centre cells (Pulford et al., 1986). It is present in all the diffuse low grade B-cell lymphomas including monocytoid B-cell, MALT and splenic marginal zone lymphoma, but is absent from follicle centre cell, Burkitt's, and lymphoblastic lymphoma.

CD33: *Antibodies:* MY9

The CD33 antigen is expressed in early myeloid progenitors and monocytes. It is a useful marker in frozen sections for myeloid tumours and mast cells, and is variably positive in a range of histiocytic disorders.

CD35: *Antibodies:* CR1, **Dako C3b receptor**

The C3b receptor CD35 is strongly expressed by DRCs, and more weakly expressed by mantle zone B-cells, granulocytes, some NK cells, red cells, and glomeruli. Preservation in fixed tissues makes the antigen a useful marker for DRCs.

CD37: *Antibodies*

The CD37 antigen is expressed strongly on B-cells, and weakly on T-cells and macrophages. It is often used as a B-cell marker in frozen sections.

CD38: Antibodies: T10, OKT10

The CD38 antigen is expressed in follicle centre B-cells, plasma cells, thymocytes and activated T-cells. It is found in corresponding B-cell lymphomas, T-lymphoblastic malignancies and in other high grade T-cell lymphomas.

CD43: *Antibodies:* **MT1, DFT1, (L60)Leu 22 (Becton Dickinson)**

The leucosialin or sialophorin (CD43) molecule is a large glycoprotein expressed on the surface of T-cells, monocytes, granulocytes and red cells. Its expression is defective in Wiskott–Aldrich syndrome and is thought to be important in lymphocyte adhesion. Although a sensitive and useful marker of T-cells in fixed tissues, it also stains a majority of diffuse low grade B-cell lymphomas as well as myeloid and some monocytic tumours (Segal et al., 1992). In the differentiation of high grade B-cell from T-cell lymphomas, the approximated test analysis parameters for CD43 (in paraffin section phenotyping) are as follows: sensitivity – 80 per cent, specificity – 88 per cent (Norton and Isaacson, 1989b).

CD44: *Antibodies:* Pgp-1, Hermes

The CD44 or extracellular matrix receptor (ECMRIII) antigen functions as a homing receptor, and is expressed by both white and red cells.

CD45

The CD45 or leucocyte common antigen is a leukocyte-restricted transmembrane glycoprotein expressed as one of several isoforms ranging in size from 180 to 220 kD (Trowbridge et al., 1991). It has a conserved cytoplasmic domain with tyrosine phosphatase activity, and a variable extracellular region; the product of three alternate exons (A, B and C), which undergoes post translational modification with alternate mRNA splicing to produce different isoforms related to lineage, state of differentiation and cell function. Evidence to date suggests that the different CD45 isoforms interact preferentially with other co-receptors in the plane of the cell membrane, to function as lineage and differentiation-related modulators of transmembrane signalling (Dianzani et al., 1992; Janeway, 1992). The CD45 antigen is both formalin resistant and leucocyte-restricted, making its isoforms particularly useful as markers of cell lineage and differentiation in paraffin sections.

Antibodies

CD45:	**2D1, 2B11**
CD45RO:	**UCHL1, A6, OPD4**
CD45RA:	**4KB5, MB1, MT2, Ki-B3,** 2H4
CD45RB:	**MT3, PD7/26**

CD45RA

The CD45RA group of antibodies recognize the 220 kD and 205 kD, high molecular weight variants of CD45 encoded by exon A. This isoform is normally expressed on the surface of most B-cells, as well as post-thymic, naive T-cells (Clement, 1992) and some medullary thymocytes. Antibodies **4KB5, MB1, KiB3,** 2H4 and **MT2** recognize different epitopes and exhibit different patterns of reactivity. Unlike **MB1, Ki-B3** and 2H4 which appear to bind to the peptide backbone of CD45RA, and are positive in mantle zone and follicle centre cells, antibody **MT2** is thought to recognize a carbohydrate moiety, and is negative in normal germinal centres (Lai et al., 1991). **Ki-B3**, differs from the other CD45RA antigens by being negative in splenic marginal zone cells. Weak positivity for histiocytic cells is often found with all the CD45RA antibodies.

The efficacy of different antibodies can be prepared by formal test analysis (see page 176). In the differentiation of low grade B-cell from T-cell lymphomas, the approximated test analysis figures for **4KB5, MB1** and **Ki-B3** are as follows: sensitivity – 90 per cent, specificity – 95 per cent, accuracy – 93 per cent. In high grade lymphomas, the equivalent parameters are: 70 per cent, 80 per cent, and 75 per cent respectively (Norton and Isaacson, 1989b). **MT2** differs from the other CD45RA antibodies in having a very low sensitivity for high grade B-cell tumours (40 per cent), and showing some discrimination between reactive and neoplastic follicles (Browne et al., 1991).

Anti-CD45RA antibodies are not lymphocyte specific and are frequently positive in myeloid leukaemia and mast cell infiltrates.

CD45RO

The CD45RO group of antibodies recognize the 180kD, low molecular weight variant of CD45, detectable only in the absence of expression of variable region exons A, B or C (Lai et al., 1991). This isoform is normally found in cortical thymocytes, post-thymic memory T-cells and monocytes. In peripheral blood, **UCHL1** stains over 70 per cent of $CD4^+$, and less than 40 per cent of $CD8^+$ T-cells (Norton et al., 1986).

In the differentiation of low grade B-cell from T-cell lymphomas, the approximated test analysis figures for **UCHL-1** are as follows: sensitivity – 95 per cent, specificity – 95 per cent, accuracy – 95 per cent. In high grade lymphomas, the equivalent parameters are: 80 per cent, 85 per cent and 83 per cent (Norton and Isaacson, 1989b).

Antibody **OPD4** is not, as originally claimed, a specific marker for $CD4^+$ T-cells and differs from **UCHL1** in having a low sensitivity (<50 per cent) for T-cell lymphoma (Cabecadas and Isaacson, 1991), and being unreactive with monocytic cells (Poppema et al., 1991). Antibody **A6** shows a similar range of reactivity to **UCHL1** and is claimed in a preliminary study to be a more sensitive T-cell marker (Berti et al., 1991).

CD45R0 is regularly expressed in most histiocytic and some myeloid malignancies.

CD45 and CD45RB

CD45RB antibodies **PD7/26** and **MT3** recognize the 190, 205 and 220 kD isoforms, and although useful as leucocyte common markers, do not have T-cell or B-cell specificity.

CD45

CD45 antibodies **2D1** and **2B11** recognize all four major variants of the leucocyte common antigen (220, 205, 190 and 220 kD), and are used as leucocyte specific markers.

Application of CD45 antibodies

Although CD45 isoforms are diagnostically useful in paraffin sections, their expression varies according to lymphocyte function and differentiation, and does not exhibit absolute lineage specificity. Most mature T-cells in adults are $CD45RO^+$, however it is important to remember that some normal T-cell subsets are constitutively $CD45RO^-$ and $CD45RA^+$. These include 'naive' $CD4^+$ T-cells (which predominate in neonates) and some $CD8^+$ or double negative ($CD4^-$ $CD8^-$) subsets, as found in intestinal intraepithelial T-cells, and enteropathy associated T-cell lymphoma. Furthermore, plasmacytic or secretory differentiation in B-cells is normally associated with a reciprocal 'switch' of isoform expression from CD45RA to CD45RO. This is seen in $CD45RO^+$ $CD45RA^-$ plasma cells, and is also evident in late differentiation stage B-cell tumours including immunoblastic and plasmacytic lymphomas. Some tumour cell populations in addition, show heterogeneity of CD45 isoform expression, with subpopulations showing reciprocal isoform inversions.

CDw49: *Antibodies:* VLRαb, VLRαd, VLRαf

The CDw49 antigen corresponds to the VLR alpha chain, which in one of three forms (b,d or f), complexes with CD29 (VLA β chain) to form integrin molecules.

CD54: *Antibodies:* ICAM-1

The adhesion molecule CD54 is the ligand for LFA-1 (CD11a) and is expressed by endothelial cells, activated lymphocytes and epithelia. It is the receptor for rhinovirus infection.

CD56: *Antibodies:* NKH1, Leu19 (Becton Dickinson)

The CD56 antigen is expressed by NK cells and is found in Tγ lymphoproliferative disease of NK lineage as well as some forms of sinonasal 'T-cell lymphoma'.

CD57: *Antibodies:* HNK1, **Leu7 (Becton Dickinson)**

The CD57 antigen is not leucocyte restricted, being expressed in prostatic epithelium, neural and neuroendocrine tissues. It is found in most cases of Tγ lymphoproliferative disease, as well as rare cases of T-lymphoblastic leukaemia.

CD58: *Antibodies:* LFA-3

The LFA-3 molecule is the ligand for CD2 and is present in many cell types.

CD68: *Antibodies:* **EBM11, KP1, Ki-M6, Ki-M7, Y-1/82A, PGM-1**

The above antibodies recognize different epitopes on this intracytoplasmic molecule which is is related to lysosomal granules, and is found diffusely within the cytoplasm of myeloid, histiocytic and mast cells. It is also expressed as a cytoplasmic dot-like reactivity in a majority of diffuse low grade B-cell lymphomas; a staining pattern which is distinctive and does not detract from the otherwise excellent specificity of these antibodies. CD68 is usually preserved in fixed tissues, and is a useful marker for myeloid and histiocytic tumours as well as plasmacytoid monocytes, in paraffin sections. Although Langerhans' cells do not express CD68, the antigen is none the less detectable in a percentage of the cells of Langerhans' cell histiocytosis (Ruco et al., 1989).

CD71: *Antibodies:* T9 (Coulter)

The CD71 antigen corresponds to the transferrin receptor and is present on activated, actively proliferating cells. The expression of CD71 correlates with tumour grade.

CD74: *Antibodies:* **LN2**

The CD74 antigen represents the HLA-Class II invariant chain, and is expressed on the cell membrane and within the cytoplasm of B-cells, histiocytes and epithelial cells. In formalin fixed tissues, antibody **LN2/** stains approximately 90 per cent and 20 per cent of low grade B and T-cell lymphomas respectively. In high grade malignancies, the corresponding figures are 85 per cent and 25 per cent respectively (Norton and Isaacson, 1989b) As a marker of B-cells therefore, the sensitivities are: 90 per cent for low grade, and 85 per cent for high grade lymphomas. The equivalent specificities are 80 per cent and 75 per cent respectively. The tumour cells of Hodgkin's disease also stain positively. The antigen lacks specificity for lymphoma subtyping.

CDw75: *Antibodies:* **LN1**

The CDw75 antigen is normally expressed in germinal centre B-cells and epithelial cells. The staining pattern is frequently membranous but may be cytoplasmic. It is a less sensitive but more specific marker than LN2, being expressed in approximately 80 per cent and 5 per cent of low grade B and T-cell malignancies, and 80 per cent and 8 per cent of high grade B and T-cell lymphomas respectively (Norton and Isaacson, 1989b). As a marker of B-cells therefore, the test sensitivity is: 80 per cent for low grade, and high grade lymphomas. The equivalent specificities are 95 per cent and 92 per cent for low and high grade lymphomas respectively.

Antibodies lacking a 'CD' designation

T-cell receptor antibodies-TCRαβ

Antibody βF1 recognizes a non-polymorphic, framework determinant of the TCR β chain, identifying the αβ TCR complex (Gaulard et al., 1990; Krajewski et al., 1989; Mori et al., 1990; Ng et al., 1988; Said et al., 1990; Weiss et al., 1988). With care, it can be used in fixed paraffin-embeded material, however it is most effective in frozen sections.

Antibody WT31 recognizes a different antigenic determinant on the TCR-$\alpha\beta$ and appears to be less sensitive than βF1 (Chan et al., 1988; Mori et al., 1990).

T-cell receptor antibodies-TCR$\gamma\delta$

Antibodies used to detect the gamma/delta TCR, include TCRδ-1, and δTCS1. The former recognises an invariant framework, or common variable determinant on the TCR δ chain, and the latter antibody reacts with a nondisulphide-linked subset of TCR$\gamma\delta$ cells. A further antibody, BB3 reacts with the complimentary disulphide-linked subset (Falini et al., 1989; Picker et al., 1988).

B-cell receptor antibodies

The recently described B-cell receptor is analogous to the TCR and consists of a heterodimeric transmembrane molecule. Recently available commercially, an antibody raised against one of the two BCR chains (mb-1) has been shown to be a specific, pan B-cell marker, expressed from early pre-B cells through to the plasma cell stage (Mason et al., 1991).

MB2

The antigen recognized by antibody **MB2** is not leucocyte restricted, being expressed on a range of epithelial tissues. Within the lymphomas, it is none the less a useful and sensitive marker for B-cells in paraffin sections. In the differentiation of high grade B-cell from T-cell lymphomas, the formal test analysis parameters for **MB2** are as follows: sensitivity – 80 per cent, specificity – 86 per cent (Hall and D'Ardenne, 1987; Norton and Isaacson, 1989b).

MAC387

Antibody **MAC387** recognizes calcium binding proteins (calgranulins), present on myeloid and histiocytic cells (Chilosi et al., 1990b). It is a relatively sensitive marker for myeloid and histiocytic cells in paraffin sections, but lacks specificity, being expressed by a wide range of malignancies, including epithelial tumours, soft tissue sarcomas and melanomas (Loftus et al., 1991). It should therefore be used only as part of a diagnostic panel of antibodies.

Ber-MAC3

This antibody recognizes a formol sensitive 140Kd antigen present on cells of histiocytic origin. It appears to be specifically expressed in histiocytic malignancies and leukaemias of M4 and M5 FAB subtype (Backe et al., 1991).

NP57 (anti-neutrophil elastase)

Antibody **NP57** is a useful marker of myeloid cells and is reactive against neutrophil elastase, a neutral protease which plays a role in microbial killing and has been localized to the primary (azurophil) granules of neutrophils (Horny et al., 1990a; Ralfkiaer et al., 1989). It is slightly more sensitive than a standard Leder's chloroacetate esterase stain, but appears later in myeloid development, and is less sensitive than myeloperoxidase (Pulford et al., 1988).

Anti-myeloperoxidase – MPO

The enzyme myeloperoxidase is regarded as the hallmark of the myeloid lineage, appearing early in myeloid cell development. Monoclonal antibody MPO has been developed against myeloperoxidase, and appears to be a highly sensitive and specific marker for myeloid cells (Buccheri et al., 1992).

AA1 (anti-mast cell tryptase)

Monoclonal antibody **AA1** raised against mast cells, is reactive with mast cell tryptase in paraffin sections, and appears to be a useful marker of mast cells, offering advantages over the use of toluidine blue (Backe et al., 1991).

HML-1, Ber-Act8

Monoclonal antibodies HML-1 and Ber-Act8 were initially thought to be specific for intraepithelial T-cells of the gut (Spencer et al., 1988). Subsequent studies have however shown that the antigen in fact represents a β7 integrin subunit (Krissansen et al., 1992; Micklem et al., 1991), and is expressed in a number of T-cell lymphomas as well as most cases of hairy cell leukaemia (Falini et al., 1991; Moller et al., 1990). It is characteristically found in enteropathy-associated T-cell lymphoma (EATCL).

bcl-2

The **bcl-2** gene is composed of two exons coding for closely related α and β proteins. It is expressed in many normal epithelial and lymphoid cells in which it appears to protect against apoptotic cell death (Hockenbery et al., 1991). In general, lymphomas characterized by t(14;18) stain strongly for the **bcl-2** gene product, consistent with the view that **bcl-2** is overexpressed in these conditions. Antibodies to the **bcl-2** gene product are therefore primarily of use in the differentiation of reactive from neoplastic follicles. The latter stain strongly for **bcl-2** gene product, whereas reactive follicles are negative, or weakly and focally positive, mainly within the light zone of the germinal centre (Gaulard et al., 1992; Pezzella et al., 1992; Zutter et al., 1991). Rare cases of **bcl-2** overexpression have also been detected in apparently reactive follicles, and the significance of marginally increased staining for **bcl-2** antibodies in such cases awaits elucidation. Although useful in the differentiation of follicular lesions, **bcl-2** gene expression is not limited to follicle centre cells, and the antibodies stain a number of other lymphomas including small lymphocytic lymphoma, hairy cell leukaemia and some high grade T-cell and anaplastic large cell lymphomas (Pezella et al., 1990).

UCL-3d3

Monoclonal antibody UCL-3d3 was raised against a follicular lymphoma but reacts with normal mantle zone cells, DRCs, and the tumour cells of centrocytic or intermediate lymphocytic lymphoma (Smith-Ravin et al., 1990; Spencer et al., 1988). It is negative in follicle centre cells and follicular lymphoma. UCL-3d3$^+$ cells usually coexpress IgM and IgD.

UCL-4d12

Monoclonal antibody UCL-4d12 was raised against a low grade lymphoma of MALT type and recognizes splenic marginal zone B-cells, small follicle centre cells, monocytoid B-cells and the perifollicular cells of Peyer's patches (Smith-Ravin et al., 1990; Spencer et al., 1988). In lymphomas, UCL-4d12 frequently stains the tumour cells of MALT lymphoma, follicular lymphomas, B-CLL and splenic marginal zone lymphoma (Schmid et al., 1992). Most B-cell populations show reciprocal positivity for UCL-3d3 or UCL-4d12, with less than 10 per cent showing a double positive or negative phenotype.

Leu 8

Monoclonal antibody Leu8 (and its equivalents MEL14 and LAM-1) recognize an adhesion molecule belonging to the LECAM-1 family of selectins, encoded on chromosome 1 (James et al., 1991; Springer, 1990). This molecule acts as a homing receptor and modulator of cell function for neutrophils and lymphocytes, and is expressed on T-cells, B-cells, monocytes and myeloid cells (Kansas et al., 1985). In normal T-cell populations, Leu8 is expressed by 80 per cent of CD4$^+$, and 60 per cent of CD8$^+$ T-cells (Rijlaarsdam et al., 1990; Slater, 1987). In B-cell populations, it is expressed on resting, mantle zone B-cells but is absent from follicle centre cells and plasma cells. In both B and T-cells, the molecule is downregulated during cell activation (James et al., 1991), and functionally, it is thought to act as a preferential homing receptor for lymph nodes rather than mucosal Peyer's patches (Butcher, 1990; Picker and Butcher, 1992). In tumour cell populations, Leu8 stains the cells of centrocytic, mantle zone, small lymphocytic and some MALT lymphomas and staining correlates with positivity for CD5 and IgD (Carbone et al., 1988a; Harris, 1991). In T-cell tumours, Leu8 negativity has been advocated as an indicator of neoplasia (Picker et al., 1987; Weiss et al., 1985), however this is an unreliable criterion as Leu8$^-$ T-cells are frequently found in reactive infiltrates due to cell activation (Rijlaarsdam et al., 1990), or predominance of Leu8$^-$ helper inducer cells (Ralfkiaer, 1991; Slater, 1990).

R4/23: *Antibody:* **Dako DRC**

This monoclonal antibody is unclustered and is a useful and specific marker for DRCs in cryostat sections.

Immunophenotypes of specific diseases

Given the poor reproducibility of current morphological classification systems, it must be anticipated that any attempt to correlate immunophenotypic features with morphological groups will be difficult from the outset. Consequently, phenotypic profiles reported for each lymphoma subtype often vary between different authors (Mason, 1987). Aside from determination of lineage, there are few instances in which a single antibody can accurately indicate the lymphoma subtype. In practice therefore, lymphoma diagnosis requires correlation of morphological features with an immunophenotypic 'profile' involving several antibodies.

B-cell lymphoma

Diffuse, low grade B-cell lymphoma

It is clear from Table 4.3, that there is significant disparity between the Kiel and Working Formulation subtypes. Thus, although most would equate lymphocytic lymphoma of intermediate differentiation (IDL) with centrocytic lymphoma (CC), there are some forms of B-CLL which, on the basis of nuclear irregularity , have been diagnosed as IDL. This emphasis on nuclear contour alone in the differentiation of B-CLL from centrocytic lymphoma is probably fallacious and as Weisenburger and colleagues have shown (Weisenburger et al., 1990; Weisenburger et al., 1991), lymphocytic lymphoma of intermediate differentiation (IDL) with proliferation centres is clinically similar to, and is better grouped with, B-CLL (B-SLL).

Similarly, a series of cases diagnosed as diffuse small cleaved cell lymphoma using the Working Formulation, is likely to include examples of follicle centre cell lymphoma (CB/CC) as well as centrocytic lymphoma (CC), and MALT lymphoma (Table 4.3).

Table 4.3. Low-grade B-cell lymphomas

Kiel	Working formulation
1. B-CLL	(B-SLL, IDL)
2. Lymphoplasmacytoid	(B-SLL – plasmacytic/ plasmacytoid)
3. Plasmacytic	(Plasmacytoma/Myeloma)
4. Prolymphocytic lymphoma	(Prolymphocytic)
5. Centrocytic	(IDL, DSCL, MZL)
6. Hairy cell leukaemia	(Hairy Cell Leukaemia)
7. MALT, monocytoid B-cell	(B-SLL, SL-plasmacytoid, IDL, DSCL)
8. Centroblastic/centrocytic – diffuse	(DSCL)

Notes: SLL = small lymphocytic lymphoma
IDL = lymphocytic lymphoma of intermediate differentiation
DSCL = diffuse small cleaved cell lymphoma
MZL = mantle zone lymphoma

Not only are the two major classifications incompatible, but within each system, there is a significant degree of overlap between the different entities. In a diagnostic setting, it is often difficult to allocate a given case to one morphological category and it is tempting to see the above lymphomas as a continuous spectrum of neoplastic disorders.

Against this impression, Zukerberg and colleagues (1991a) and Harris (1991), using the Kiel classification system, claim a diagnostically useful correlation between morphology and immunophenotype (Table 4.4).

Table 4.4. Low-grade B-cell lymphomas: phenotypic groups

1. B-CLL and variants	CD5$^+$	CD23$^+$	CD43$^+$	CD10$^-$	IgD$^+$
2. Centrocytic	CD5$^+$	CD23$^-$	CD43$^+$	CD10$^{-/+}$	IgD$^+$
3. MBCL/MALT	CD5$^-$	CD23$^-$	CD43$^{-/+}$	CD10$^-$	IgD$^-$
4. CB/CC / DSCL	CD5$^-$	CD23$^{+/-}$	CD43$^-$	CD10$^+$	IgD$^-$

Source: Zukerberg et al., 1991a
Notes: MBCL = Monocytoid β-cell lymphoma
MALT = Lymphoma of mucosa-associated lymphoid tissue
CB/CC = Centroblastic/centrocytic lymphoma
DSCL = Diffuse small cleaved cell lymphoma

A survey of the recent literature in this group of lymphomas reveals a number of apparent contradictions of immunophenotypic profile, however most of these can be traced to ambiguities in morphological nomenclature, and inherent incompatibilities between the Kiel and working formulation (WF) classifications.

B-CLL (small lymphocytic lymphoma/chronic lymphocytic leukaemia)

In Western countries, by far the majority of cases of CLL (>90%) are of B-cell origin. The tumour cells in most cases correspond phenotypically to a normal subset of immature, migratory, virgin B-cells, recently designated B-1 cells (see Normal B-cell Development, page 115). While B-CLL is analogous to migratory, CD5 positive immature B-cells, the lymphomatous counterpart (SLL) is analogous to a slightly more mature stage of development in which virgin B-cells settle in the secondary lymphoid organs in readiness for the primary immune response (Weisenburger, 1990).

In common with their normal counterpart, the proliferating cells of B-CLL are CD5 positive, and coexpress low density surface IgM and IgD, together with MHC class II, and the pan-B antigens CD19, 20, 22 and 24. CD20 may be absent or more weakly expressed than is usually seen in other forms of B-cell lymphoma (Kornstein et al., 1990; Salter et al., 1988; Weisenburger, 1990). Surface expression of CD21 (C3d receptor) is almost always present, (Salter et al., 1988) but may at times be weak, and more readily detected using flow cytofluorimetry. In contrast to follicle centre cell lymphomas, CD10 (calla) is almost always negative. Surface expression of CD43, CD23 and Leu8 is usually present. CD6 is variably positive, and CD9 (BA-2) is usually negative.

The T-cell associated antigens CD5 and CD43 are expressed on only a small subpopulation of normal B-cells in adults, and the presence of a large numbers of B-cells expressing these antigens is now accepted as useful immunophenotypic evidence for neoplasia (Picker et al., 1987). Proliferation centres differ from the remainder of the infiltrate by increased expression of the transferrin receptor (CD71) and proliferation antigens Ki-67 and DNA polymerase-α (PCNA) (Salter et al., 1988).

A minority of cases of B-CLL show a mature, or post follicular phenotype. As one would expect, these lymphomas show heavy chain class switching with expression of IgG, IgA and IgM, without CD5 or IgD.

In paraffin sections, the cells of B-CLL are positive for MB2 and CD20 (L26), although the latter may at times be expressed only weakly. The CD45 leucocyte common antigen is usually expressed as the high molecular weight form (CD45RA) commonly associated with B-cells (Salter et al., 1988), however rare cases of CD45RA negative, or even CD45RO positive B-CLL have been described (Norton and Isaacson, 1989b). BU-38, reactive against the CD23 antigen in paraffin sections, is positive (Murray et al., 1991).

CD43 (MT1, Leu22, DFT1) is demonstrable in paraffin sections of most cases of B-CLL, usually at an intensity less than that seen in adjacent T-cells. At present, there is no antibody available which is reactive against the CD5 antigen in fixed, paraffin-embedded sections. Although there is significant overlap between subsets staining for CD5 or CD43 in cryostat sections, antibodies to these antigens do not recognize identical subsets, and CD43 cannot be regarded as a substitute marker for CD5 in paraffin sections (Said et al., 1989; Stross et al., 1989).

CDw75 (LN1) is negative in the small neoplastic cells of B-CLL but it can be used to highlight proliferation centres (Norton and Isaacson, 1989b). The differentiation of proliferation centres from residual follicle centres can be further facilitated in paraffin sections by staining for follicular dendritic reticulum cells (DRCs) with antibodies to CD21 (IF8), CD23, CD35, laminin or Ki-FDC1P. Although DRCs are uniformly present within normal and neoplastic follicle centres, they are absent from proliferation centres (Carbone et al., 1987).

It is worth noting that antibodies to CD68 (e.g. KP1) used within immunophenotyping panels for the identification of macrophages, frequently stain the tumour cells of B-CLL. The staining pattern is distinctive however, and usually consists of a single dot-like focus of positivity (Warnke et al., 1989).

Variants of B-CLL

The 'paraimmunoblastic' or 'tumour forming' variant of B-CLL/small lymphocytic lymphoma has striking morphological features, often leading to a misdiagnosis of small non-cleaved or large cell lymphoma. Its close relationship to B-CLL proper, however, is supported by a similar immunophenotypic profile and positivity for CD5 (Pugh et al., 1988).

Prolymphocytoid transformation occurs in approximately 15 per cent of cases of B-CLL. Changes in the peripheral blood, in which there is a marked increase in circulating prolymphocytoid tumour cells in addition to the B-CLL cells, are well described, however accompanying changes within lymphoid organs are not well documented, and may take the form of large cell transformation or a dominant pseudofollicular pattern (Pugh et al., 1988).

In prolymphocytoid and large cell transformation (Richters syndrome), the transforming tumour cells as one would predict, usually retain the pattern of light chain restriction of the parent clone, however this is not a universal finding and there are many reported examples of Richter's syndrome in which a phenotypically distinct B-cell tumour supervenes, either as an incidental, unrelated malignancy, or presumably from a common stem cell progenitor or pro-B-cell (Nakamine et al., 1992; Suster and Rywlin, 1987).

Rarely, transformation of B-CLL may produce a lymphoma which is both morphologically and immunophenotypically indistinguishable from Hodgkin's disease. In a series of eight such cases, Brecher and Banks (1990) demonstrated a phenotype typical for Hodgkin's disease, with positivity for CD15 and absence of staining for CD45 or B-cell or T-cell antigens within the Hodgkin's cells.

Common clonality has not been demonstrated in any such cases to date, and it is possible that this form of phenotypically disparate transformation is also a chance collision of what are, after all, two common types of lymphoma.

Lymphoplasmacytoid lymphoma (SLL with plasmacytic/plasmacytoid differentiation)

This category consists of all cases of B-CLL or small lymphocytic lymphoma which show plasmacytic differentiation.

Although not subcategorized in the working foundation (WF) system, lymphoplasmacytoid lymphoma (LPL) is traditionally divided into three subtypes within the Kiel system: (1) Lymphoplasmacytic; (2) Lymphoplasmacytoid; (3) Polymorphic subtype. The lymphoplasmacytic type contains the typical cells of B-CLL together with mature plasma cells with the same light chain restriction. When plasma cells are abundant, this is also referred to as 'immunocytoma'. The plasmacytoid form is similar but contains a broader range of cell types, including plasmacytoid cells and occasional plasma cell precursors and immunoblasts.

The polymorphic variant is much more variable, containing many admixed centroblasts, immunoblasts and other cell types including histiocytes (Patsouris et al., 1990). This third, polymorphic category is controversial. Some cases, in addition to the presence of centroblasts, also contain DRCs, and many now reclassify such tumours as pleomorphic or polymorphic variants of centroblastic lymphoma (Hall et al., 1987).

In common with B-CLL, most cases correspond to pre-follicular, virgin B-cells of the primary immune response and express IgM, sometimes with coexpression of IgD (though less frequently than with B-CLL). A variable percentage, particularly those in extranodal sites, express IgG or IgA. As with most B-cell lymphomas, kappa light chains are more frequently expressed than lambda. In B-CLL, immunoglobulin is expressed weakly on the cell surface and occasionally, focally within the perinuclear space. In LPL, however, the pattern of Ig staining parallels that of normal plasma cell differentiation, with diffuse cytoplasmic Ig staining and a reduction in surface Ig expression. If the tumour is mainly plasmacytic (immunocytoma), the reduction in surface immunoglobulin intensity may prevent detection of light chain restriction by flow cytofluorimetry. Secretion of immunoglobulin commonly occurs, with detectable levels of paraprotein. As this is usually of IgM class, the clinical syndrome of Waldenstrom's macroglobulinaemia often results. The frequent presence of an associated haemolytic anaemia is not surprising given the known propensity for B-1 lineage cells to produce autoreactive antibodies (Kantor, 1991; Kipps et al., 1990) (see p. 115).

Surface staining for B-cell restricted antigens including CD19, 20, 22 and 24 is usually found in cryostat sections, however in common with normal plasma cell differentiation, this expression may be lost in a percentage of cases. In contrast to B-CLL without plasmacytoid differentiation, CD5 is usually reported to be absent (Sundeen et al., 1992; Weisenburger, 1990), or present in a minority of cases, where its presence may correlate with the propensity for peripheral blood lymphocytosis (Hall et al., 1987). CD10(calla) is consistently negative, while CD21 and KB61 are variably present. The degree of terminal differentiation in the plasmacytic and plasmacytoid cells is paralleled by the expression in some cases, of plasma cell antigens PCA-1 and PC-1 as well as CD38(T10).

In fixed, paraffin-embedded sections, the expression of CD20(L26) parallels that seen in frozen sections. MB2 is usually positive. As with all tumours showing plasmacytic differentiation, CD45 and variants are unreliable as indicators of lineage. CD45RA may be lost entirely or may revert to a low molecular weight form (CD45RO). CD45 itself may be negative and the plasmacytic cells may become positive for epithelial membrane antigen (EMA). Staining for CD30 (BerH2) may also occur (Moller et al., 1989b). CD43 (MT1, Leu22) stains most cases of LPL as it does B-CLL. This seems to be particularly so with the lymphoplasmacytoid form (Norton and Isaacson, 1989b).

Plasmacytic (plasmacytoma/myeloma)

Lymphoproliferative diseases showing exclusively plasmacytic differentiation usually express IgG (60 per cent), IgA (25 per cent), or rarely IgD or IgE (<1 per cent), and in 10 per cent of cases, light chains only (Bartl et al., 1987). The tumour cells are analogous to normal secretory, post-follicular B-cells of the secondary immune response, and not surprisingly, show a similar predeliction for the bone marrow (Weisenburger, 1990).

Predictably, in cryostat sections, the tumour cells exhibit cytoplasmic staining for immunoglobulin with light chain restriction. Surface immunoglobulin expression is very weak, often preventing detection of light chain restriction when using untreated cells with flow cytofluorimetry. In line with normal B-cell secretory differentiation, the tumour cells often show loss of pan B-cell antigens CD19, 20, and 22, while retaining expression of MHC class II antigen (HLA-DR). CD21 is usually negative. The acquisition of CD38 and antigens recognized by the plasma cell antibodies PCA-1 and PC-1 is also in accord with the level of secretory differentiation (Anderson et al., 1984; Salter et al., 1988).

Unfortunately, this view of myeloma as a neoplasm of terminally differentiated plasma cells, although accounting for most of the observed features, is oversimplistic. The occurrence of 'primitive' phenotypes, and the finding of circulating B-lymphocytes with the same idiotype in some cases of myeloma, both point towards an underlyng abnormality of pre-B or stem cells (Epstein, 1992; Grogan, 1989). The expression of CD10 (calla), terminal deoxynucleotidyl transferase (TdT), and transferrin receptors (CD71) in some cases of myeloma is well described, and appears to be associated with a significantly reduced prognosis (Durie and Grogan, 1985). Further evidence for a stem cell abnormality is found in the 'aberrant' myelomonocytic phenotypes which may precede the development of leukaemia in myeloma patients.

In fixed, paraffin-embedded sections, CD20 (L26) is usually negative. Leucocyte common antigen is also negative and often switches to a T-cell pattern, with expression of the low molecular weight form (CD45RO/UCHL1) with loss of the high molecular weight (CD45RA/4KB5) variety. Ki-B3, may be an exception to this rule. In addition to being negative for leucocyte common antigen, most cases are positive for EMA and CD30 (BerH2). Rare reports have claimed positivity with anti-keratins, underscoring the importance of morphological assessment of such cases (Norton and Isaacson, 1989b). CD43 (MT1, Leu22) and CDw75 (LN1) may, on occasion, be positive.

MB2 has been reported to be negative by some authors, (Norton and Isaacson, 1989b) however Dehou and colleagues (1990) have recently demonstrated positivity for MB2 in over 90 per cent of a series of 59 myeloma cases.The same authors have indicated that MB2 may discriminate between myeloma and monoclonal gammopathy of uncertain significance (MGUS) and that MB2 negative cases of myeloma may have a worse prognosis than those which are MB2 positive.

Prolymphocytic leukaemia

Approximately 80 per cent of cases of prolymphocytic leukaemia are of B-cell origin and phenotypically correspond to an activated or slightly more mature form of B-CLL. Seen predominantly in elderly males, it is characterized by prominent splenomegaly with a high lymphocyte count of which more than 55 per cent are prolymphocytes (Peterson, 1991). A close association with B-CLL is emphasized by the fact that B-CLL may undergo prolymphocytoid transformation; transitional forms exist; and *in vitro* activation of B-CLL can produce a prolymphocytic appearance and phenotype (Peterson, 1991; Weisenburger, 1990).

In common with B-CLL, IgM and IgD are usually coexpressed with some examples expressing IgG. The surface immunoglobulin expression is intermediate in intensity between B-CLL and centrocytic lymphoma. Pan B-cell antigens CD19 and CD20 are positive while CD21 and CD25 (Tac) expression is variable. In contrast to B-CLL, the majority of cases are CD5 and CD23 negative and FMC7 positive. CD10 (calla) and CD38 are negative (Deegan, 1989; Kamat et al., 1990).

Mantle cell lymphoma – centrocytic lymphoma (lymphocytic lymphoma of intermediate differentiation)

Centrocytic lymphoma (CC) in the Kiel system and intermediate lymphocytic lymphoma (IL) represent two closely overlapping but historically non-identical sets. 'Lymphocytic lymphoma of intermediate differentiation' was originally defined by Berard and colleagues as an alkaline phosphatase positive variant of lymphocytic lymphoma showing nuclear profiles and sIg expression intermediate between small lymphocytic and small cleaved cell lymphoma. The presence of alkaline phosphatase was suggested as evidence for origin from the mantle zone or primary follicles (Namba et al., 1977). Subsequently, others have used terms such as 'intermediate lymphocytic lymphoma' but have included examples of B-CLL or prolymphocytic leukaemia showing nuclear irregularity as well as cases of centrocytic/centroblastic lymphoma containing sparse centroblasts. The Kiel group produced a tight definition for the entity but unfortunately coined the term 'centrocytic', mistakenly assuming homology with small cleaved follicle centre cells.

Following a meeting in London in 1991, it was agreed that all these categories (centrocytic, intermediate lymphocytic lymphoma, and lymphocytic lymphoma of intermediate differentiation) should be unified under the single title of 'mantle cell lymphoma' (MCL) (Banks et al., 1992).

In current usage, the criteria originally proposed by Berard and co-workers are retained, but refined by the exclusion of cases showing proliferation centres, paraimmunoblasts, prolymphocytic differentiation or centroblastic cells (Gaulard et al., 1990; Lardelli et al., 1990; Weisenburger et al., 1990; Weisenburger et al.,

1991). Although the typical case consists of a monotonous population of small to intermediate sized lymphocytes with irregular or indented nuclear borders, admixed histiocytes may be prominent, and blastic or pleomorphic forms are well described and may constitute up to 20 per cent of cases (Lardelli et al., 1990; Lennert and Mohri, 1978). Thus defined, CC or MCL has characteristic clinical and immunophenotypic features, and its validity is further supported by frequent association with t(11;14)(q13;q32), related to the *bcl-1* breakpoint on chromosome11, and possibly linked to the proto-oncogene Prad-1 (Frizzera et al., 1991; Rosenberg et al., 1991).

The disease often presents as stage III or IV disease, usually in older men with generalized lymphadenopathy and splenomegaly, and occasionally, extranodal disease (Lardelli et al., 1990; Weisenburger, 1990). Gastrointestinal disease, with multiple lymphomatous polyposis is an uncommon but distinctive form of presentation (O'Briain et al., 1989). CC/MCL responds poorly to therapy but is generally regarded as a low grade lymphoma. Blastic or pleomorphic variants with a high proliferative index behave more aggressively (Lardelli et al., 1990).

Morphologically and immunophenotypically, the tumour cells closely resemble normal immature B-cells of the primary follicle or mantle zone and as such are intermediate in differentiation between the cells of B-CLL and centrocytic / centroblastic lymphoma. Surface immunoglobulin is correspondingly of intermediate intensity, while cytoplasmic immunoglobulin is usually not detected. In keeping with the analogy of immature B-cells, over 90 per cent of cases express IgM, two thirds IgD, and approximately half coexpress IgM and IgD (Lardelli et al., 1990; Mori et al., 1988; Strickler et al., 1988; Swerdlow et al., 1983; Van den Oord et al., 1986b; Weisenburger, 1990; Weisenburger et al., 1991). Interestingly, most studies have demonstrated a reversal of the usual kappa:lambda ratio, and a predominance of lambda light chains is a feature of centrocytic and intermediate lymphocytic lymphoma.

In the vast majority of cases, CD5 is strongly expressed and CD10 (calla) is negative, however a minority may coexpress CD5 and CD10 . Leu8 is positive but in contrast to B-CLL, CD23 is usually negative (Manconi et al., 1987; Salter et al., 1988; Zukerberg et al., 1991a). CD9 (BA-2) has been reported to be positive in approximately 50 per cent of cases (Jaffe et al., 1987; Lardelli et al., 1990; Strickler et al., 1988; Swerdlow et al., 1983). CD9 and CD10 are not in themselves specific, however their presence is good evidence against B-CLL, while their coexpression with CD5 argues strongly against follicular lymphoma (Lardelli et al., 1990).

Pan B-cell antigens CD19, 20, 22, and 24 and MHC class II antigens are positive in by far the majority of cases while the C3d receptor, CD21 is reported to be positive in most series (Close and Lauder, 1990; Harris and Bhan, 1985; Hollema and Poppema, 1988; Salter et al., 1988; Strickler et al., 1988) but negative in others (Weisenburger et al., 1987). CD38 is consistently negative, while Il-2 receptors (CD25) are variably and weakly expressed (Salter et al., 1988). FMC7 is usually positive (Pombo de Oliveira et al., 1989). Antibody UCL-3D3 which is reported to stain normal mantle zone cells, is also claimed to be positive in centrocytic lymphoma (Spencer et al., 1988). CDw32 (KB61) is positive, as it is in most low grade B-cell lymphomas of non-follicle centre cell origin.

In fixed, paraffin-embedded sections, the tumour cells are positive for CD20 (L26), and CD74 (LN2), but negative for CDw75 (LN1) (Mori et al., 1988; Weisenburger et al., 1991). LN5, which stains normal mantle zone cells, is surprisingly negative (Weisenburger et al., 1991). CD43 (MT1, Leu22) in common with the findings in B-CLL, is positive in most cases, whereas antibody BU-38, reactive against CD23 is negative (Murray et al., 1991).

The pattern of staining for DRCs (IF8, BU38) is distinctive and may be of diagnostic use (Manconi et al., 1987). DRCs are present within the normal follicle mantle zone where the cell processes form an ill-defined meshwork. Furthermore, normal mantle zone DRCs are reported to have a distinctive phenotype which distinguishes them from those of the follicle centre, being CD9(BA-2) and CD14 (LeuM3) negative (Carbone et al., 1988b). This intriguing zonal variation of DRC phenotype persists in the neoplastic state, and DRCs in follicular lymphomas are CD9 and CD14 positive whereas those in centrocytic lymphoma are negative for both antigens (Carbone et al., 1987). Thus, B-CLL is negative for DRCs, except for occasional residual follicle centres; follicular centroblastic/centrocytic lymphoma contains tightly clustered DRCs as an integral component of the follicular architecture; and centrocytic lymphoma exhibits an intermediate pattern having ill-defined loose DRC networks with blurred outlines (Manconi et al., 1987).

This DRC pattern accords with the observation of a vaguely nodular pattern within many cases of centrocytic lymphoma, and fits with the concept of a primary follicle cell phenotype. At the same time, a nodular pattern in centrocytic lymphoma can create difficulties in differentiation from follicular small cleaved cell lymphoma, best resolved by staining for CD5. In fact, rare reports of rearrangement of bcl-1 in follicular lymphomas suggest that a small subset may occur independently of the usual bcl-2 rearrangement, and may in fact be more closely related to centrocytic or mantle cell lymphoma (Frizzera et al., 1991; Weisenburger, 1990).

Although now proposed as a unifying term for all forms of centrocytic and intermediate lymphocytic lymphoma, the term 'mantle cell lymphoma' was first introduced by Weisenburger and colleagues (Weisenburger et al., 1981; Weisenburger and Rappaport, 1982) to indicate a distinctive pattern of growth around reactive follicles in a subset of intermediate lymphocytic lymphomas. Subsequently, it was shown that such 'mantle zone lymphomas' may progress to diffuse intermediate lymphoma, and that this pattern merely represented the earliest stage of nodal involvement (Lardelli et al., 1990; Weisenburger, 1991; Weisenburger et al., 1991).

Conceptually, if centrocytic/mantle cell lymphoma were to express the homing characteristics of its normal cellular counterpart, then early involvement of a secondary lymphoid organ would result in a mantle zone pattern. Progressive replacement would lead to sheets of diffuse centrocytic/intermediate lymphocytic lymphoma containing only occasional naked reactive follicles. Recapitulation of primary follicle differentiation with attendant DRCs could provide a follicular or nodular pattern. Thus, all three observed architectural patterns of MCL are accounted for.

A number of lymphoproliferative conditions may mimic mantle cell lymphoma, and in a diagnostic setting, it is important to be able to make a clear distinction between them (Close and Lauder, 1990; Harris and Bhan, 1985).

Follicular lymphomas may on occasion produce a mantle zone pattern (Harris and Bhan, 1985) and are distinguished by the presence of monotypic immunoglobulin within the follicle centre. Monocytoid or MALT lymphomas, in common with mantle cell lymphoma, have reactive follicles however in the former, there is progressive neoplastic infiltration of the follicles, gradually leading to monotypia and positivity for MT2 (Isaacson et al., 1991). Furthermore, they may be identified by the presence of lymphoepithelial lesions, plasmacytic differentiation and lack of CD5 or CD10.

Occasionally, B-CLL or prolymphocytic lymphoma may produce a mantle zone pattern (Carbone et al., 1992) but this can be identified by the presence of prolymphocytes, paraimmunoblasts, and proliferation centres, lack of CD10 or CD9, and presence of CD23.

Castleman's disease should be distinguished by morphological criteria, and rare cases of mantle zone hyperplasia can be excluded by the demonstration of monotypic immunoglobulin or other immunophenotypic criteria for malignancy such as the coexpression of CD43 (MT1, Leu22), or CD5 with pan B-cell antigens such as CD20 (L26).

Hairy cell leukaemia

Controversy surrounding the cell of origin of hairy cell leukaemia has been largely due to the expression by the neoplastic cells of both B-cell and monocytic features. The latter include cell adherence, phagocytosis, the presence of cytoplasmic enzymes such as non-specific esterases (fluoride sensitive), tartrate resistant acid phosphatase, and the presence of surface antigens such as CD11c and CD68 (Chang et al., 1992; Naeim, 1988). None the less, hairy cell leukaemia (HCL) is now widely accepted to be a B-cell tumour corresponding in differentiation to normal pre-plasma cells (Weisenburger, 1990). This view is supported by the membranous expression of monotypic immunoglobulin and pan B-cell antigens, as well as immunoglobulin gene rearrangement studies (Naeim, 1988). Moreover, the concept of HCL as a B-cell tumour, intermediate in level of differentiation between IgG^+/IgA^+ B-CLL and myeloma is supported by the fact that B-CLL cells can be induced to express features of HCL following exposure to phorbol ester, and some cases of HCL have been associated with production of a paraprotein (Anderson et al., 1985; Naeim, 1988).

The majority of cases of HCL bear surface IgG or IgA, and are negative for IgM and IgD. They therefore correspond to late-maturation cells of the secondary immune response, although sIgM and sIgD positive cases are also described. CD5 is consistently negative. CD10 is weak or negative in Western countries, but it has been suggested that HCL in Japan is phenotypically different and is often CD10 positive. MHC class II, FMC7 and pan-B antigens, CD19, 20, 22 ,24 and 37 are consistently positive, and in addition PCA-1, a plasma cell antigen is also expressed. CD38, also a feature of plasmacytic differentiation, is however, negative (Salter et al., 1988). CD21 is negative (Jaffe, 1990).

A striking feature of diagnostic value, is the strong and consistent expression of CD25 (Tac, IL-2 receptors). Soluble IL-2 receptors are also detectable within the peripheral blood, and may be partly responsible for the associated NK cell dysfunction (Chilosi et al., 1989; Naeim, 1988). Antibody SHCL-3 (Leu-M5) was originally raised against cells from a patient with hairy cell leukaemia (Schwarting et al., 1985) and it strongly stains the all neoplastic cells in this disease, however the antigen it recognizes (CD11c) is present on a number of cell types including monocytes and activated CD8+ T-cells (Chadburn et al., 1990). Coexpression of CD11c with pan-B antigens provides some specificity for HCL and has been widely used for this purpose however, monocytoid B-cell lymphoma and the recently described B-cell lymphoma with villous lymphocytes may also be positive and requires differentiation (see below) (Carbone et al., 1989; Schwarting et al., 1985; Traweek et al., 1989; Vardiman et al., 1988). Other myeloid or monocytic antigens which may be positive include CD68 (KP1, EBM11) and CD11b (OKM1) (Pulford et al., 1989; Schwarting et al., 1985; Warnke et al., 1989).

T-cell restricted antigens are negative but interestingly, antibodies HML-1 and BerAct8 which recognize mucosal T-cells, are positive in most cases of HCL. This finding is of interest as most other forms of B-cell lymphoma are negative, however specificity and sensitivity studies have not been reported to date and its diagnostic usefulness is uncertain (Kruschwitz et al., 1991; Moller et al., 1990). Positive stainings with the recently reported antibody LF-61 is also of unproven significance (Flenghi et al., 1990).

Two new antibodies (GHI/75 and VMP55) have been described, raised against glycoprotein enriched lysate of hairy cell leukaemia (Pulford et al., 1991). The antibodies show strong reactivity with hairy cells and plasma cells, but have not yet been subjected to extensive analysis, and their diagnostic value also remains unproven.

Fixed paraffin-embedded sections, are usually of bone marrow and decalcified. Consequently, the phenotypic profile obtained will depend to a significant extent upon the fixation and decalcification regimen used. Leucocyte common antigen (CD45) is consistently positive and may be a valuable aid for the identification of low levels of residual disease. There may be an enhanced appreciation of cell surface positivity due to the configuration of the cell membrane in this disease, however claims for a specific membrane staining pattern in HCL (Martin et al., 1988) have not been substantiated by other authors (Strickler et al., 1990). Leucocyte common antigen is expressed in the high molecular weight form usually associated with B-cells however there may be some variability between different CD45R antibodies. Thus while Ki-B3 and MB1 are usually present, 4KB5 and MT2 may be more variably expressed (Davey et al., 1990). CD45RO (UCHL1, A6) is consistently negative (Davey et al., 1990; Hall et al., 1988a; Norton and Isaacson, 1989b; Strickler et al., 1990).

L26 (CD20) is expressed in almost all cases of HCL (Davey et al., 1990; Norton and Isaacson, 1989b) however ocasional cases may be negative in decalcified bone marrow sections (Strickler et al., 1990). MB2 and CD74(LN2), although not as specific as CD20, appear to be the most sensitive B-cell markers in this disease. Antibody KB61 (CDw32) which recognizes low grade B-cell lymphomas other than those of follicle centre cell origin, was raised against HCL cells, and is consistently positive. A related CD32 antibody (41H) is also positive. CDw75(LN1), usually a marker of follicle centre B-cells, is also frequently present but may be obscured by the numerous erythrocytes often present in HCL which are also positive (Davey et al., 1990; Hall et al., 1988a; Norton and Isaacson, 1989b).

Unlike many other low grade B-cell lymphomas, hairy cell leukaemia is consistently negative for CD43 (MT1), (Davey et al., 1990; Hall et al., 1988a; Strickler et al., 1990) a feature which may be of diagnostic use. A number of antibodies showing variable specificity for monocytic cells are consistently negative in HCL. These include anti-lysosyme, anti-cathepsin B, α1-antitrypsin, α1-antichymotrypsin, and MAC 387. CD68 (KP1) is present in most cases of HCL as it is in other low-grade B-cell malignancies. Characteristically, this takes the form of small cytoplasmic dots of reactivity rather than the diffuse pattern seen in monocytic cells (Pulford et al., 1989; Warnke et al., 1989). S100 protein has been reported to be positive in some cases of HCL (Naeim et al., 1987; Norton and Isaacson, 1989b) however other studies have failed to confirm this finding (Strickler et al., 1990). Recently, a new antibody DBA.44 has been described which is reactive against HCL in paraffin sections (Hounieu et al., 1992). Although not entirely specific, it is useful in fixed paraffin sections to differentiate small lymphocytic lymphoma from HCL.

Tartrate resistant acid phosphatase (TRAP) can be detected in fixed tissue and may be a useful corroborative test if positive (Therkildsen, 1986). None the less, the technique has a low sensitivity in paraffin sections and depends upon prior enzyme digestion. It is rendered completely ineffective following decalcification (Strickler et al., 1990; Therkildsen, 1986).

Several closely related lymphoproliferative diseases require consideration in the differential diagnosis of hairy cell leukaemia. A number of B-cell lymphoproliferative disorders have been described which also coexpress CD11c and pan-B antigens. These include the rare splenic lymphoma with villous lymphocytes (SLVL), a related familial CD11c+ B-lymphocytosis and an uncommon CD11c+ variant of B-CLL. SLVL may present with similar clinical features but preferentially involves the splenic white pulp rather than the red pulp, is consistently negative for CD25, and may express CD10 (Bassan et al., 1991; Vardiman et al., 1988). B-CLL should be morphologically distinctive, and, unlike HCL is positive for CD5 and usually CD43, but is negative for FMC7 and usually CD25.

Rare T-cell and bi-phenotypic hairy cell lymphomas have been reported, some associated with HTLV-II, however they have little in common phenotypically with HCL as described above, and are probably unrelated (Naeim, 1988).

The differentiation of mast cell disease may present problems, particularly as both may be positive for CD45, CD45RA and CD68, however mast cells, unlike hairy cells, are positive for anti-lysosyme and are negative for B-cell specific antigens such as CD20 (Strickler et al., 1990).

Finally, monocytoid B-cell lymphoma (MBCL) is phenotypically and morphologically similar to HCL, being positive for pan-B antigens and CD11c, and similarly negative for CD5,10,38 and 43 in most cases. Acid phosphatase is also present in MBCL but is not tartrate resistant. Phenotypically, the most significant difference is the lack of CD25 expression in MBCL, while clinically, the two diseases have little similarity, either in clinical presentation or tissue distribution (Carbone et al., 1989; Traweek et al., 1989).

Monocytoid B-cell lymphoma and MALT lymphoma

In the early 1980s, observations on cases of immunoproliferative small intestinal disease (IPSID) and low-grade primary B-cell lymphoma of the stomach, prompted Isaacson and Wright (1983) to describe a distinctive type of lymphoma which they designated low grade malignant lymphoma of mucosa associated lymphoid tissue (MALT). These so-called MALT lymphomas exhibited an unusual histological pattern and range of cell types which have been well summarized elsewhere (Harris, 1991; Isaacson and Spencer, 1987; Isaacson et al., 1985; Wright and Isaacson, 1989). Briefly, the entity entails reactive follicles, surrounded by neoplastic B-cells with a distinctive appearance ranging from small 'centrocyte-like' cells, to larger monocytoid cells. Characteristically, these infiltrate mucosal epithelium, giving rise to so-called 'lymphoepithelial lesions', and in roughly one third of cases, there are zones of monotypic plasma cell maturation within the tumour cell population. The authors propose that as the lesion develops, there is a progressive influx of tumour cells into the reactive follicles, mimicking follicular lymphoma; a process referred to as 'follicular colonization' (Isaacson et al., 1991). Subsequently, the concept of low-grade MALT lymphoma has been extended to include many other sites including the lung, salivary gland, thyroid, thymus, orbit, Waldeyer's ring, bladder, female genital tract and breast. Some of these sites are not strictly mucosal, however most occur in association with some form of glandular epithelium, and significantly, they are all extranodal (Addis et al., 1988; Anscombe and Wright, 1985; Hyjek and Isaacson, 1988; Hyjek et al., 1988; Isaacson, 1990; Isaacson et al., 1990; Isaacson and Spencer, 1987; Li et al., 1990; Medeiros and Harris, 1989; Pelstring et al., 1991).

The group of lymphomas so defined has no direct equivalent within the Working Formulation classification, and one may be excused for asking where this new lymphoma came from. Many such cases had previously been diagnosed as reactive or 'pseudolymphoma' and their neoplastic or clonal nature became apparent only when immunotechniques became sensitive enough to demonstrate low density immunoglobulin within the paranuclear space of tumour cells. It is therefore not surprising that most MALT lymphomas present with stage I disease and follow an indolent course. Other cases of MALT lymphoma are equivalent to the Working Formulation categories of small lymphocytic lymphoma (particularly the lymphoplasmacytic variety), lymphocytic lymphoma of intermediate differentiation, or diffuse small cleaved cell lymphoma. Furthermore, those cases showing well-developed follicular colonization may have been diagnosed as follicular lymphoma (Harris, 1991; Isaacson et al., 1991).

In addition to the morphological features described above, an integral part of the MALT concept is the idea that this group of lymphomas is derived from mucosa associated lymphoid tissue, and thus exhibits homing characteristics appropriate for this compartment of the immune system. Some support for this notion is found in the tendency of MALT lymphomas to remain localized, or relapse at other mucosal sites. Although the tumour cells were initially thought to be derived from follicle centre cells, later studies have demonstrated phenotypic homology with marginal zone B-cells. (see below) (Isaacson, 1990; Isaacson and Spencer, 1987; Myhre and Isaacson, 1987) The MALT concept has not been fully or universally accepted, and some authors have questioned its validity and clinical relevance, particularly when applied to high grade mucosal B-cell lymphomas (Chan et al., 1990; van Krieken et al., 1989a; Villuendas et al., 1991). Notwithstanding this controversy, the distinctive morphological and immunophenotypic features, described by Isaacson and Wright in mucosal sites, are closely paralleled in the American literature by subsequent reports of an unusual parafollicular lymphoma arising in lymph nodes and referred to as monocytoid B-cell lymphoma (MBCL) (Agnarsson and Kadin, 1987; Cousar et al., 1987; Ngan et al., 1989; Sheibani et al., 1988).

Monocytoid B-cell lymphoma primarily involves lymph nodes, but in other respects is remarkably similar histologically and immunophenotypically to low grade MALT lymphoma. In fact, when low grade MALT lymphoma involves a regional lymph node, the appearances may be indistinguishable from those of MBCL (Harris, 1991; Isaacson, 1990; Nizze et al., 1991). The tumour shows a perifollicular or sinusoidal distribution consisting of either small or medium-sized lymphoid cells with well defined cell borders. The former type consists of small or intermediate-sized cells, phenotypically and morphologically similar to marginal zone B-cells and 'centrocyte-like' cells of MALT lymphoma. The latter type contains larger, medium-sized cells resembling the monocytoid B-cells originally described as 'immature sinus histiocytes' in toxoplasma lymphadenitis and subsequently identified in a range of reactive and neoplastic disorders including AIDS-related lymphadenopathy. Both MBCL and MALT lymphomas have in common, a tendency towards a marginal zone pattern, in which abundant reactive follicles with a cuff of small mantle zone lymphocytes, are surrounded by a third zone of pale-staining 'centrocyte-like' or 'monocytoid cells'. When the infiltrate surrounds naked or primary follicles, an 'inside-out' follicular pattern may result. This marginal zone pattern is also seen in primary splenic marginal zone lymphomas which appear to be closely related. MBCL also shares with MALT lymphoma, the presence of plasmacytic differentiation in approximately one third of cases and progressive infiltration of reactive follicles by neoplastic cells (follicular colonization).

Phenotypically, MBCL and low grade MALT lymphoma are remarkably similar.

In frozen sections, low-grade MALT lymphoma and MBCL share the following phenotype: CD19$^+$, 20$^+$, 22$^+$, 32 (KB61, 41H)$^+$, and CD5$^-$, 9$^-$, 10$^-$, 23$^-$, 25$^-$, 38$^-$, PCA-1$^-$. Both have a low proliferative index, and on average, only 10 per cent of cells are positive for Ki-67. CD11c and 24 are reported to be positive in most cases of MBCL but the findings in MALT lymphomas have not been widely reported. CD21 is frequently recorded as being negative in MBCL but is variably positive in MALT lymphomas. Leu8 is variably positive in both lymphomas. T-cell antigens CD2, 3, 4, 5, 7 and 8 are consistently negative. In MBCL, IgM is the most frequently expressed heavy chain, while in low-grade lymphomas of MALT type, IgM or IgA and occasionally IgG are expressed. In contrast to centrocytic lymphoma, both MBCL and lymphomas of MALT are IgD negative (Banerjee et al., 1991; Isaacson, 1990; Isaacson et al., 1990; Isaacson and Spencer, 1987; Ngan et al., 1991; Nizze et al., 1991; Sheibani et al., 1988; Shin et al., 1991; Traweek et al., 1989; Wotherspoon et al., 1990).

In paraffin sections, both low grade lymphoma of MALT and MBCL have the following phenotype: L26 (CD20)$^+$, MB2$^+$, CD45RA (4KB5, MB1)$^+$ and CD45RO (UCHL1)$^-$ (Banerjee et al., 1991). In contrast to many other low-grade B-cell lymphomas, CD43 (MT1, Leu22) is usually negative, but rare positive cases ($<$10 per cent) have been reported for both MALT lymphoma and MBCL (Li et al., 1990; Medeiros and Harris, 1990; Ngan et al., 1991). Staining for antibody Ki-B3, thought to represent an epitope on the CD45RA antigen, is variable. Although preferentially staining mantle zone B-cells, and sometimes stated to be negative in MALT lymphomas, it has been reported to be present in a significant percentage of cases (Li et al., 1990; Myhre and Isaacson, 1987; Van Krieken et al., 1989b). In MBCL, Ki-B3 has been detected in the larger, or medium-sized monocytoid variants, but appears to be negative in the smaller, or centrocyte-like variants of MBCL. LN1 (CDw75) and LN2 (CD74) are both expressed in MBCL (Carbone et al., 1989; Nizze et al., 1991). In MALT lymphomas, LN1 is variably expressed and tends to stain the larger, or blastic variants of centrocyte-like cells most intensely (Myhre and Isaacson, 1987). The recently reported antibody KiM1p, which reacts with macrophages in fixed, paraffin-embedded tissues, is also found to be postive in MBCL (Nizze et al., 1991). Surface immunoglobulin is difficult to identify in paraffin sections, however with the use of sensitive techniques, cytoplasmic immunoglobulin may be detectable within the paranuclear space.

What then, is the relationship between MBCL and MALT lymphomas? As discussed, the two may be virtually indistinguishable phenotypically and morphologically. The major difference historically has been the site of tumour presentation; the former characteristically presenting itself in American lymph nodes, and the latter appearing in English mucosae. Even this distinction has become blurred as MALT lymphomas are described in non-mucosal sites, and MBCL is reported in extranodal sites including mucosae and soft tissues. A single lymphoma of the salivary gland for example could legitimately be diagnosed as MBCL or a low-grade MALT lymphoma depending on ones point of view. A significant percentage of MBCL presenting in lymph nodes may been shown to have an associated low-grade lymphoma of MALT type in a mucosal site, while up to 25 per cent of cases of MALT lymphoma will have the changes of MBCL in a draining lymph node (Cogliatti et al., 1990; Nizze et al., 1991). Both lymphomas appear to lack t(14;18) or bcl-2 overexpression typical of follicular lymphomas; both are CD5, CD10, CD23 and largely CD43 negative, and both have have been likened phenotypically to splenic marginal zone cells. Leaving questions of nomenclature aside, Sundeen and colleagues (Sundeen et al., 1992) have recently demonstrated a significant correlation between CD5 negativity and extranodal presentation in low-grade B-cell lymphomas; providing indirect support for the idea of a distinctive group of low-grade, extranodal, B-cell lymphomas, not catered for in the working formulation or standard Kiel classifications.

The differential diagnosis of MBCL or low-grade MALT lymphoma includes reactive hyperplasia, centrocytic lymphoma, follicular lymphoma, CLL with plasmacytic differentiation and hairy cell leukaemia.

Reactive hyperplasia may be distinguished by a lack of monotypic immunoglobulin in the paranuclear space of centrocyte-like or monocytoid cells. MT2 may also offer a 'soft' indicator, as it is more likely to be positive in neoplastic, than reactive follicle centres (Norton et al., 1989). Centrocytic lymphoma unlike MBCL and MALT lymphoma, consistently lacks expression of immunoglobulin in the paranuclear space, and expresses surface IgD. The frequent expression of CD5, CD10 and CD43 in centrocytic lymphoma is also diagnostically useful.

Follicular lymphoma usually lacks the presence of parafollicular centrocyte-like or monocytoid cells with zones of plasmacytic differentiation. Phenotypically, it is usually CD10 and often CD23 positive. Antibodies to bcl-2 gene product are usually positive in follicular lymphomas, but negative in MALT/MBCL lymphomas (Ngan et al., 1988a).

CLL is characteristically CD5 and CD23 positive, and often expresses CD43 and/or IgD. Hairy cell leukaemia is phenotypically similar to MALT or MBCL lymphomas except that the tumour cells express CD25 and plasma cell related antigens PCA-1 and CD38. Moreover, while both groups of lymphoma may express acid phosphatase, only the isoform present in HCL is tartrate resistant.

Follicle centre cell lymphoma

This group includes both follicular and diffuse forms of the following entities; all of which show a follicle centre cell phenotype:

1. ML predominantly small cleaved cell type (centroblastic/centrocyticCB/CC);
2. ML mixed small and large cell type (centroblastic/centrocyticCB/CC);
3. ML predominantly large cell (centroblastic).

A distinction should be made between follicular lymphoma and follicle centre cell lymphoma. As discussed in a preceding section, a nodular pattern is often encountered in centrocytic lymphoma. The nodules contain DRC meshworks and express a mantle zone phenotype, closely resembling primary lymphoid follicles. Thus, although centrocytic lymphomas are in the strictest sense follicular, they are morphologically and phenotypically quite dissimilar to follicle centre cell lymphomas which recapitulate secondary lymphoid follicles, and are considered separately.

Recently, the cytogenetic abnormality t(14;18) (q32;q21) and associated overexpression of bcl-2 protein has offered a unifying concept for follicle centre cell lymphomas. It has been demonstrated in up to 80 per cent of follicular lymphomas in Western societies, and is thought to protect transforming follicle centre B-cells from apoptotic cell death (Ngan et al., 1988b; Ott et al., 1991; Pan et al., 1989; Shibata et al., 1990). In normal follicles, transforming B-cells are selected for bcl-2 expression and consequent rescue from apoptosis, by cross-linking of surface Ig, or stimulation by CD40 or the 25kDa subunit of CD23 (Liu et al., 1991). The translocation t(14;18) leads to unregulated or abnormal bcl-2 expression with consequent lymphoproliferative disease in the form of follicular lymphoma. Support for this concept is found in the observation that neoplastic follicles exhibit reduced apoptotic figures and a lower mitotic count than reactive equivalents (Hollowood and Macartney, 1991). The overexpression of bcl-2 is diagnostically useful, as anti-bcl-2 antibodies are found to stain neoplastic follicles in almost all follicular lymphomas, whereas they are very rarely or only focally positive in reactive follicles (Ott et al., 1991). Recently, the finding of the bcl-1 translocation, t(11;14)(q13;q32) in a small subgroup of follicular lymphomas suggests that there may be some genotypic heterogeneity within this group (Frizzera et al., 1991).

In frozen sections, follicle centre cell lymphomas, whether follicular or diffuse, mixed or large cell type, generally express the following phenotype: CD 5$^-$, CD9$^+$, CD10$^+$, CD19$^+$, CD20$^+$, CD22$^+$, HLA-DR$^+$. CD10 is generally expressed more intensely than in reactive follicles. CD21 (C3d receptors) are strongly expressed on DRCs in a dendritic pattern which often obscures cellular staining of tumour cells. None the less, approximately one third of follicular lymphomas of mixed cell type are reported to be CD21 positive (Garcia et al., 1986a; Hollema and Poppema, 1988; Jaffe, 1990). Large cell lymphomas, whether follicular or diffuse, are rarely positive (Williamson et al., 1986). CD23 is present in a majority of low-grade follicular (CC/CB) lymphomas, but is usually negative in higher grade CB lymphoma, follicular or diffuse (Murray et al., 1991). CD24 (BA-1), is found to be negative in most series. CD25 (Tac) is weakly expressed in roughly 50 per cent of cases, or negative (Garcia et al., 1986a). CD32 (KB61, 41H) is variably reported. Antibody KB61 is said not to stain follicle centre cell lymphomas (Pulford et al., 1986), yet antibody 41H has been reportedly positive in most cases of follicular lymphoma (CC/CB). CD38, which is present on the surface of activated B-cells and plasmacytic cells, has been variably reported to be present in a minority of follicular lymphomas, but is more likely to be detected by flow cytofluorimetric analysis.

Immunoglobulins may be detected in the perinuclear space or rarely, on the cell surface. Approximately one third of follicle centre cell lymphomas are immunoglobulin negative. This is in keeping with the observation that a significant percentage of normal follicle centre cells are also Ig negative (Strauchen and Mandeli, 1991). Most cases express IgM with or without IgD. A significant number of cases will show isotype switch with expression of IgG or rarely, IgA.

In general, the findings in large cell or centroblastic lymphoma are similar to those in mixed small and large cell type (CC/CB) except that the centroblastic phenotypes are more likely to be aberrant, with loss of both pan-B antigens and immunoglobulin expression. Antigens such as CD21 and CD23 are likely to be negative and occasional or rare cases may express CD30 or CD43.

In fixed, paraffin-embedded sections, most follicle centre cell lymphomas stain positively for MB2, L26 (CD20) (Figs 4.3 and 4.4), LN1 (CDw75), and LN2 (CD74). Antibodies 4KB5 and MB1 are positive in over 2/3 of cases but other CD45RA variants including KiB3 and MT2 are less sensitive and show some variability (Davey et al., 1990; Hall et al., 1988a; Norton and Isaacson, 1987; West et al., 1986). Antibody BU38, which recognizes CD23 in fixed tissues, is positive in over 80 per cent of low-grade follicular lymphomas, but is negative in centroblastic lymphoma (Murray et al., 1991). With rare exceptions, antibody MT1, reactive against CD43, is negative in almost all follicle centre cell lymphomas (Hall et al., 1988a). Detection of immunoglobulin in paraffin sections of follicle centre cell lymphoma is often difficult. It is claimed that by using sensitive techniques, up to 80 per cent of cases can be shown to express monotypic immunoglobulin in the paranuclear space. In practice however, this is rarely achievable.

In cases with ill-defined nodularity, the follicular nature of an infiltrate may be confirmed by the identification well-formed DRC meshworks using formalin-resistant antibodies to any of the following antigens: CD21 (1F8), CD23 (BU38), or CD35 (C3bR).

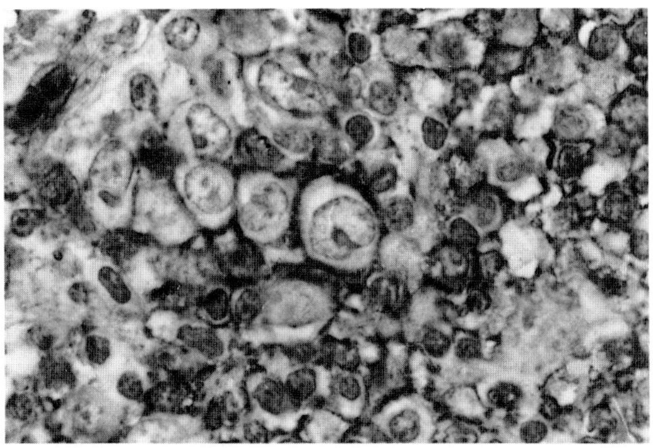

Fig. 4.3. Follicle centre cell lymphoma of mixed small and large cell type (centroblastic/centrocytic), showing strong membranous staining for CD20 (anti-L26, X1000).

The differential diagnosis of follicular lymphoma includes reactive follicular hyperplasia, monocytoid/low-grade MALT lymphoma, progressive transformation of follicle centres (PTGC) and centrocytic lymphoma. Positivity for CD5, negativity for CD10, and the monomorphous character of the cellular infiltrate in centrocytic lymphoma distinguishes it from follicular lymphomas. Monocytoid and MALT lymphomas are CD10 and CD23 negative, and exhibit a range of cellular differentiation not encountered in follicular lymphomas. Progressive transformation of germinal centres is distinguished by lack of monotypic immunoglobulin, the coexistence of normal reactive follicles (not usually present in follicular lymphomas), and follicular disruption caused by an influx of mantle zone cells, characteristic for PTGC (see page 174).

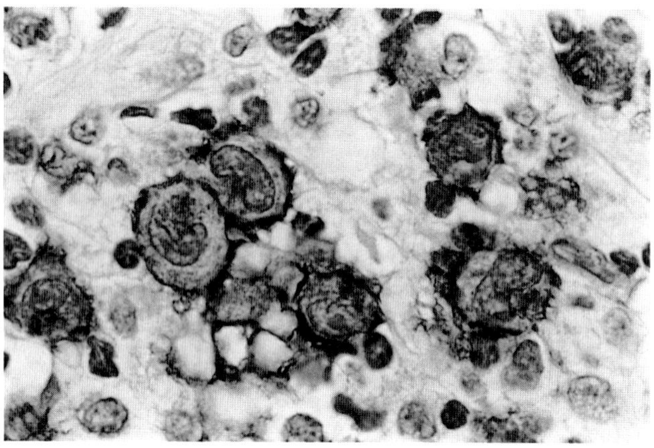

Fig. 4.4 Pleomorphic large cell lymphoma of follicle centre cell type (centroblastic lymphoma), showing strong membranous staining for CD20. Most of the smaller cells are CD20 negative T-cells (anti-L26, ×1000).

Finally, reactive hyperplasia is best distinguished by lack of monotypic immunoglobulin. In practice, this is often difficult in paraffin sections, and it is sometimes necessary to rely on morphological assessment. Other evidence in favour of neoplasia includes (in decreasing order of significance) demonstration of clonal immunoglobulin gene rearrangement, the immunohistochemical detection of bcl-2 protein, using anti-bcl-2 antibodies, and positivity for antibody MT2. This latter antibody is reported to be negative in almost all cases of reactive follicular hyperplasia yet positive in the majority of follicular lymphomas (Browne et al., 1991; Norton et al., 1989). It is therefore of potential but as yet unproven value in the distinction of follicular lymphoma from reactive hyperplasia. Antibody MY4 which recognizes an epitope on the CD14 molecule is also reported to be positive in follicular lymphoma but negative in reactive follicles (Medeiros et al., 1991). Formal test analysis has not yet been conducted however, and the diagnostic usefulness of this finding is so far undetermined.

A cuff of reactive, small mantle zone B-cells is almost always present in follicular lymphoma and a polytypic mantle cannot therefore be used as evidence against a diagnosis of follicular neoplasia.

Multilobated B-cell lymphoma

Multilobated lymphomas are usually of B-cell phenotype (Fig. 4.5) (Von Baarlen et al., 1988), and are generally considered to be variants of centroblastic or large, follicle centre cell lymphoma (Chan et al., 1986; O'Hara et al., 1986; Pettit et al., 1990). Typically, the nuclear irregularity is unlike the rounded, embryo-like lobulation seen in anaplastic large cell lymphoma, or Hodgkin's disease, and consists of small knobbly, or sharp projections from the nuclear surface. Isolated multilobated cells may be noted in many follicle centre cell lymphomas. However those given this designation usually comprise 30 per cent or more multilobated cells (Von Baarlen et al., 1988; Westermann et al., 1990). The phenotype and prognosis appears to be similar to that of centroblastic lymphoma.

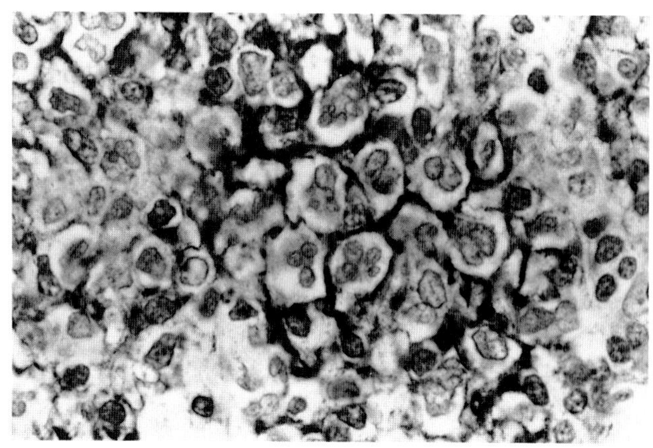

Fig. 4.5. Multilobated B-cell lymphoma showing typical tightly formed nuclear lobations. This is a variant of centroblastic lymphoma which in this case was partly follicular (anti-L26, X1000).

B-immunoblastic lymphoma

This high grade B-cell lymphoma is, in most cases, analogous with B-immunoblasts of the primary or secondary plasma cell reaction. It usually presents de novo but may also occur as a result of transformation of many other B-cell lymphomas. This concept of a 'final common pathway' implies a degree of heterogeneity which is further accentuated by current criteria for morphological diagnosis.

Although a classical example of plasmacytoid IBL with amphophilic cytoplasm and large central nucleoli is readily recognizable, there are many lymphomas in which it is difficult to differentiate morphologically between immunoblastic and centroblastic lymphoma. The finding of t(14;18) translocations in a small but significant percentage of IBL cases may partly be a reflection of this diagnostic difficulty (Weisenburger, 1990). Fortunately, with current treatments, there seems to be little difference in the prognosis of the two groups (Kwak et al., 1991). The number of different morphological subtypes of immunoblastic lymphoma included in the working formulation is, itself indicative of the groups heterogeneity. In fact, using current criteria, any large B-cell lymphoma which is neither anaplastic nor of follicle centre cell type is obligatorily either immunoblastic or unclassifiable.

In general, B-immunoblastic lymphoma is phenotypically similar to centroblastic lymphoma but is more likely to show phenotypic aberrancy and a pattern of antigen expression reflecting the degree of plasmacytic differentiation.

In frozen sections, B-immunoblastic lymphoma usually expresses the following phenotype: $CD5^-$, $CD19^+$, $CD20^+$, $CD21^-$, $CD22^+$, $CD23^-$, $CD24^-$, however any of the pan-B antigens CD19, 20 and 22 may be absent (Jaffe, 1990). Antibody B1 in particular, which recognizes CD20 in cryostat sections often stains weakly. CD10, a feature of follicle centre cell differentiation, is present in a minority of cases (Dobson et al., 1987; Jaffe, 1990). CD5 is almost always negative, but rare examples of CD5 positive immunoblastic lymphoma have been described, and may reflect inclusion of paraimmunoblastic variants of B-CLL in this group. CD25 may be weakly positive in some cases. As with centroblastic lymphoma, CD30 may be positive in a small percentage (<20 per cent) of cases (Hall et al., 1988a; Norton and Isaacson, 1989b; Salter et al., 1988). CD38 is usually negative (Jaffe, 1990) unless the tumour shows pronounced plasmacytic differentiation. Transferrin receptor (CD71) is more frequently expressed than in lower grade B-cell lymphoma (Salter et al., 1988). IgM is the most commonly expressed heavy chain subclass, however IBL may be immunoglobulin negative in up to 40 per cent of cases (Strauchen and Mandeli, 1991).

In fixed, paraffin-embedded sections, at least three-quarters of B-IBL cases are positive for L26(CD20) (Figs 4.6 and 4.7), LN2(CD75) and MB2 (Davey et al., 1990; Hall et al., 1988a; Ngan et al., 1989a; Norton and Isaacson, 1989b). In common with normal immunoblastic cells, expression of the high molecular weight form of leucocyte common antigen (CD45RA) may be lost, or even revert to the 180 kD CD45RO form. Consequently, antibodies 4KB5, MB1 and KiB3, reactive against CD45RA variants, are negative in up to 50 per cent of B-IBL cases, and antibody UCHL1 (principally used as a T-cell marker and reactive against CD45RO) is positive in over 10 per cent of cases (Davey et al., 1990; Norton and Isaacson, 1989b). Antibody MT2, although recognizing the CD45RA antigen, is less sensitive than MB1, 4KB5 and KiB3, being negative in most cases of B-IBL (Hall et al., 1988a). As it is positive in most low-grade B-cell lymphomas, its presence correlates inversely with tumour grade (Hall et al., 1989b).

Antibodies IF8 (CD21) and BU38 (CD23) do not show DRC meshworks except for residual follicles; and tumour

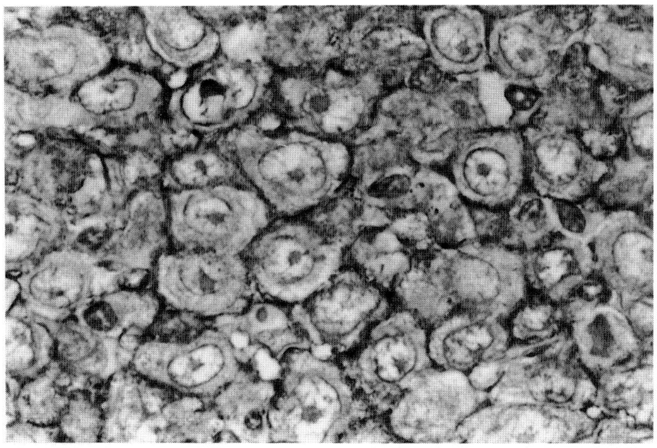

Fig. 4.6. B-immunoblastic lymphoma with central, prominent nucleoli. Membranous staining for CD20 (anti-L26, X1000).

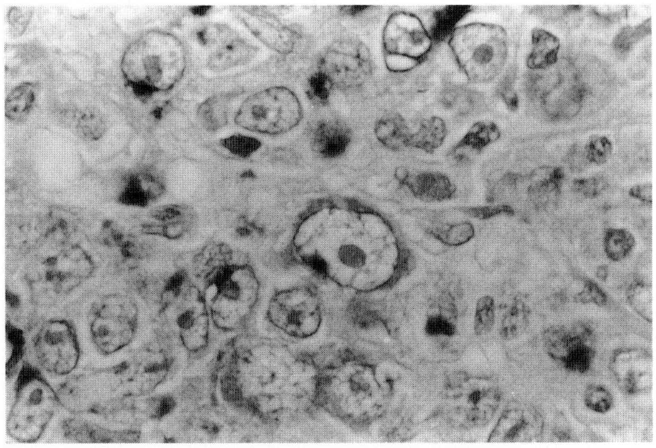

Fig. 4.7. B-immunoblastic lymphoma showing strong light chain expression within the perinuclear space (anti-lambda light chain, X1000).

cells are negative for both antibodies in the vast majority of cases (Jaffe, 1990; Murray et al., 1991; Salter et al., 1988). LeuM1 (CD15) and BerH2 (CD30) are positive in approximately 5 per cent to 10 per cent of cases (Hall et al., 1988a; Norton and Isaacson, 1989b). Antibody LN1 (CDw75) is expressed in roughly three-quarters of cases (Davey et al., 1990; Hall et al., 1988a; Norton and Isaacson, 1987). Finally, antibody MT1 (CD43), which is generally used as a T-cell marker, is positive in slightly more than 10 per cent of cases of B-immunoblastic lymphoma (Davey et al., 1990; Dobson et al., 1987; Norton and Isaacson, 1987; Norton and Isaacson, 1989b).

Miscellaneous B-cell lymphomas

T-cell – rich B-cell Lymphoma

This term was first used by Ramsay and colleagues in 1988 (Ramsay et al., 1988) to describe a distinctive group of B-cell neoplasms which frequently simulate peripheral T-cell lymphoma or Hodgkin's disease, and were referred to in earlier reports as 'pseudo T-cell lymphoma' (Jaffe et al., 1984; Mirchandani et al., 1985).

Both the clinical and pathological features are quite variable, suggesting heterogeneity, and the term 'T-cell-rich B-cell lymphoma' (TCRBCL) is probably best viewed as a pathological descriptor, rather than indicating a single disease entity (Macon et al., 1992b).

As the name implies, most cases have an overwhelming admixture of reactive T-cells, usually amounting to 90 per cent or more of the total cell population. Often, these reactive T-cells are 'activated' and slightly larger than small resting T-cells, adding to the confusion with T-cell lymphoma (Ng et al., 1989). The infiltrate is typically polymorphous, with abundant admixed histiocytes, plasma cells and eosinophils. On occasion, the degree of histiocytic infiltration may cause initial confusion with lymphoepithelioid, or Lennert's lymphoma (Ramsay et al., 1988). Recently, a series of 6 such cases with abundant histiocytes has been described as 'histiocyte-rich B-cell lymphoma'. The clinical features in this small series were distinctive, with male predominance, splenomegaly and a tendency for progression to higher grade lymphoma, and it has been suggested that this group may be a singular entity, more closely related to nodular lymphocyte predominant Hodgkin's disease (Delabie et al., 1992).

The sparsely distributed tumour cells may represent less than 5 per cent of the total population, and usually show centroblastic morphology, often with multilobation, but may on occasion resemble Reed–Sternberg cells or variants. The pattern of nodal infiltration may be diffuse, but is not uncommonly interfollicular with reactive lymphoid follicles, and prominent high endothelial venules (HEVs).

Using flow cytofluorimetry alone, the neoplastic nature of the infiltrate is usually missed, because the neoplastic cells are present in numbers below the threshold for detection. In cryostat tissue sections, interpretation is compromised by the problems usually encountered with polymorphous lymphomas, using this modality (see pages 174 & 175). These include inability to recognize the individual tumour cells due to poor morphology, and a high level of background staining due to large numbers of histiocytes bearing Fc receptors.

It is in fixed, paraffin-embedded sections that the nature of the disease is best revealed. L26 (CD20), and to a lesser extent LN1 (CDw75), stain the tumour cells strongly and outline them clearly against the background of reactive cells. Immunoglobulin stains are especially useful, and cytoplasmic staining, with light chain restriction can be demonstrated in the majority of cases of TCRBCL (Macon et al., 1992; Osborne et al., 1990a; Ramsay et al., 1988). LeuM1 (CD15), UCHL1 (CD45RO), MT1 (CD43) and EMA are negative.

The pathogenesis of TCRMCL remains unclear, however it is generally assumed that in common with most other lymphomas of polymorphous pattern, cytokine production by tumour cells leads to recruitment of a varied and dominant, reactive cell population (Ng et al., 1989; Macon et al., 1992a). In experimental models at least, there is some evidence to support this concept (Willoughby et al., 1988). More recently, it has been suggested that the reactive cells could be a host response to EBV-infected, neoplastic cells (Loke et al., 1992).

T-cell-rich B-cell lymphoma should be considered in the differential diagnosis of any polymorphous infiltrate, as well as some of the more monomorphous lymphomas. TCRBCLs have, in the past been included with ML: diffuse, mixed small and large cell type (Katzin et al., 1989), ML: lymphoplasmacytoid (polymorphic subtype), some follicular lymphomas, Hodgkin's disease, and a wide range of T-cell lymphomas, including Lymphoepithelioid T-cell (Lennert's) lymphoma, T-zone lymphoma, and angioimmunoblastic (AILD-like) T-cell lymphoma. Paraffin section immunophenotyping is extremely effective in

TCRBCL and readily excludes all the T-cell lymphomas and non-lymphocyte predominance forms of Hodgkin's disease. TCRBCL and classical HD show reciprocal staining patterns for CD15, CD20, CD30, and usually, CD45. Although L26 staining of HD cells has been reported (Schmid et al., 1991a), the reaction is weak compared with the intense membranous staining encountered in TCRBCL.

The most difficult problem immunophenotypically, may be the differentiation of TCRBCL from nodular lymphocyte predominance Hodgkin's disease (NLPHD). EMA may be of some help (present in NLPHD, absent from TCRBCL), and the typical immunophenotypic features of progressively transformed germinal centres may also favour NLPHD. Light chain restriction, if found, favours TCRBCL. Although reported one recent series of NLPHD (Schmid et al., 1991b), all other studies have been unable to demonstrate clonality for light chains in the hyperlobate cells of NLPHD. When in doubt, the two diseases should be separable using morphological criteria.

Finally, diffuse lymphocyte predominance Hodgkin's disease (DLPHD) is a heterogenous group (see page 167) which is thought to include a diffuse form of NLPHD (so-called 'diffuse paragranuloma'). Like NLPHD, diffuse paragranuloma is a B-cell disease. It differs however, by the absence of associated progressive transformation of germinal centres, and in having a predominantly T-cell environment. The diffuse form of NLPHD (or diffuse paragranuloma) is therefore in effect, a form of TCRBCL.

T-cell-rich B-cell lymphoma is not included in any of the major classification schemes, and its categorisation is controversial (Jaffe et al., 1991). Using the Working Formulation system TCRBCL is classified as ML: Mixed Small and Large cell type. A more recent view is that these tumours should be categorized as large cell lymphoma, since the neoplastic component consists exclusively of large cells (Osborne et al., 1990a). With this approach, immunophenotyping would then be a mandatory requirement for the classification of all lymphomas of diffuse, mixed, small and large cell type. Given the extreme biologic heterogeneity of this group, it could be argued that all such lymphomas should be phenotyped anyway.

Mediastinal B-cell lymphoma of sclerosing, or clear cell type

After Hodgkin's disease and T lymphoblastic malignancy, large B-cell lymphoma is the commonest lymphoid neoplasm of the mediastinum (Moller et al., 1989a). The disease predominates in young females (median age 32), but is also seen in older men (median age 50 years; sex ratio at least 3:2, F:M) (Lamarre et al., 1989).

Clinically, the patients often present with cough, chest pain, dyspnea, and signs of venous obstruction (Moller et al., 1987). Origin from the thymus is often not demonstrable, as the tumours are locally aggressive with invasion of surrounding structures . The disease rarely disseminates widely but is difficult to cure with conventional chemotherapy, and it has been suggested, but not proven, that local resection may be of some value (Lavabrebertrand et al., 1992).

Histologically, all cases are of diffuse, large cell type. The cell nuclei are ovoid but may be multilobated, and often contain one or two nucleoli. Abundant clear cytoplasm is typically present, and the sclerotic bands often impart an alveolar or compartmentalized appearance (Davis et al., 1990; Menestrina et al., 1986). The tumours are difficult to categorize using conventional classification schemes, however, most have been designated ML: Diffuse, large non-cleaved cell; or ML: Diffuse, large cell, immunoblastic (Lamarre et al., 1989).

Immunophenotypically, the tumours resemble normal medullary thymic B-cells and express the following phenotype: HLA-DR$^{+/-}$, CD1$^-$, CD2$^-$, CD3$^-$, CD5$^-$, CD9$^-$, CD10$^-$, CD11c$^{+/-}$, CD19$^+$, CD20$^+$, CD21$^-$, CD22$^+$, CD23$^{+/-}$, CD25$^-$, CD30$^-$, CDw32$^-$, CD35$^-$, CD37$^+$ (Davis et al., 1990; Lamarre et al., 1989; Lavabrebertrand et al., 1992; Menestrina et al., 1986; Moller et al., 1989a). In some cases, there is expression of CD38 and PC-1, a marker of plasmacytic differentiation, and it has been suggested that mediastinal B-cell lymphoma is a tumour of pre-plasmacytic differentiation (Moller et al., 1987). Light chain restriction is demonstrable in as few as 17 per cent of paraffin section cases, and 32 per cent of cases examined by cryostat section (Davis et al., 1990). Most cases are immunoglobulin negative, and it is claimed that the immunoglobulin expression is a feature of the disease in older men, all the females being Ig-negative (Lamarre et al., 1989).

In fixed paraffin-embedded tissues, the cells strongly express L26 (CD20). Rare cases have been reported to be MT1 or Leu22 (CD43)$^+$ (Davis et al., 1990), however UCHL1 (CD45RO) is consistently negative.

With the use of simple paraffin section immunophenotyping, the diagnosis is usually straightforward. It is worth noting however, that epithelial thymomas may have an associated proliferation of L26$^+$ asteroid B-cells; a source of potential confusion, particularly when interpreting the results of flow cytofluorimetry (Taubenberger et al., 1991).

Recently, low grade thymic lymphomas with features of so-called MALT lymphoma have been described (Isaacson et al., 1990; Takagi et al., 1992). These are slightly different phenotypically from thymic large B-cell lymphoma, and express CDw32. None the less the possibility of a relationship between the two is worthy of investigation.

Burkitt's lymphoma

It is now generally agreed that small non-cleaved cell (SNC), or Burkitt's lymphoma (BL) corresponds phenotypically to an early stage of follicle centre cell differentiation (van der Valk and Meijer, 1988; Weisenburger, 1990). Not only is there evidence of germinal centre involvement in some cases (Pavlova et al., 1987), but examples of transformation from FCC lymphoma to Burkitt's or SNC lymphoma are well-described (Mintzer et al., 1984). Moreover, Gregory and colleagues (1987) have identified a subset of normal follicle centre cells which match the cells of BL morphologically and phenotypically.

Endemic Burkitt's lymphoma is strongly associated with Epstein–Barr virus (EBV), however sporadic cases are not. Recently, both post-transplantation and AIDS patients have been shown to have a high incidence of immunoblastic and BL (or Burkitt's-like) lymphoma (Hamilton-Dutoit et al., 1991; Pedersen et al., 1991). Post-transplantation, or immunosuppressed patients tend to have oligoclonal or polyclonal immunoblastic proliferations with a very high EBV association, and express EBV latent membrane protein and Epstein–Barr nuclear antigen (EBNA) (Pallesen et al., 1991). AIDS patients show the same propensity, but in addition, have a higher incidence of EBV-unrelated Burkitt's lymphoma, which resembles sporadic rather than endemic disease and is apparently not related to immunosuppression (Hamilton-Dutoit et al., 1991; Pedersen et al., 1991).

In frozen sections, Burkitt's lymphoma is generally found to have the following phenotype: CD5$^-$, CD9$^+$, CD10$^+$, CD19$^+$, CD20$^+$, CD22$^+$, CD23$^-$, CD24$^+$, CD25$^-$, and CD32(41H)$^+$,TdT$^-$ (Erber and Mason, 1988; Garcia et al., 1986b; Gregory et al., 1987; Jaffe, 1990). CD21 is positive in a significant percentage of cases, and its presence seems to correlate with EBV integration. CD38 positivity is variably reported. As would be expected in such a proliferative tumour, Ki-67 is usually expressed in approximately 80 per cent of the tumour cells. In contrast with centroblastic and immunoblastic lymphoma, immunoglobulin heavy chain expression is largely limited to surface and cytoplasmic IgM with occasional coexpression of surface IgD. Heavy chain class switching, with expression of IgG or IgA is uncommon, in keeping with the concept that BL corresponds to an early follicle centre cell level of differentiation (Garcia et al., 1986b; Jaffe, 1990; Pavlova et al., 1987; Strauchen and Mandeli, 1991). EBV transformed B-cells are known to express CD30 (Abbondanzo et al., 1990; Schwarting et al., 1989), and not surprisingly therefore, positivity is found in cases of endemic BL, as well as approximately 20 per cent of sporadic cases (Pallesen, 1990; Schwarting et al., 1989). In BL, the CD30 staining may be due to cytoplasmic production of an antigenically similar, but independently synthesized, and smaller (57kD) molecule than that encountered on the cell surface in anaplastic large cell lymphoma, or Hodgkin's disease (Diehl et al., 1990).

In fixed, paraffin-embedded tissue sections, the cells of Burkitt's lymphoma usually express the following phenotype: L26 (CD20)$^+$, MB2$^+$, LN2 (CD74)$^+$, LN1 (CDw75)$^+$, and MAC 387$^-$ (Hall et al., 1988a; Norton and Isaacson, 1987). CD45 is generally expressed as the high MW isoform (CD45RA) and antibodies 4KB5, MB1 and KiB3 are usually positive, while antibody UCHL1 (reactive against CD45RO) is negative. None the less, CD45 isoform inversion may occur in Burkitt's lymphoma, particularly in HIV related disease (Hamilton-Dutoit et al., 1991). Anti-CD43 antibodies produce variable results; MT1 is reported to be negative in most cases, but Leu22 is said to be positive (Hall et al., 1988a; Norton and Isaacson, 1987; Said et al., 1989). Cytoplasmic IgM may be detectable in many cases. BerH2 (CD30) is often expressed in endemic Burkitt's, but is variably expressed in sporadic cases. Antibody KB61 which is thought to react with CD32, and is positive in most B-cell lymphomas except those of follicular origin, is reported to be negative in BL (Pulford et al., 1986).

B-lymphoblastic lymphoma/leukaemia

Approximately 80 per cent of acute lymphoblastic leukaemias (ALL), and 20 per cent of lymphoblastic lymphomas, are of B-cell lineage (Foon and Todd, 1986;

Jaffe, 1990; Sheibani et al., 1987a; Weiss et al., 1986), the remainder being of T-cell type. Lymphoblastic lymphoma (LBL) of B-lineage is clinically quite unlike its T-cell equivalent, lacking a mediastinal mass, often presenting in bone or cutaneous sites, and possibly having a less aggressive course. This distinctive pattern of tissue involvement is such that despite the relative rarity of B-lymphoblastic lymphoma, those cases presenting primarily in the skin or bone marrow, are usually of B-cell lineage (Sander et al., 1991).

Virtually all cases have rearranged heavy chain genes, but light chain genes are in germline configuration or at varying stages of rearrangement. This is in keeping with the concept that non-T ALL and pre-B lymphoblastic lymphoma (LBL) correspond to the earliest stages of B-cell development: that of marrow-based pre-B cells which are undergoing immunoglobulin gene rearrangement (Weisenburger, 1990). The immunophenotypic findings add further support to this view.

Non-T ALL can been divided into 6 immunophenotypic groups (Anderson et al., 1984; Foon and Todd, 1986), all of which contain the enzyme terminal deoxynucleotidyl transferase (TdT). The most immature type expresses HLA-DR without B-cell antigens, and is heterogenous, including tumours other than those of B-cell lineage. The 5 remaining types are exclusively of B-cell lineage and are defined by the successive expression of CD19, CD10 (calla), CD20, Cμ, and finally SIgM. CD10 expression may be lost in the most mature of these immunophenotypic groups. As a general rule, tumours with a lymphomatous, rather than leukaemic presentation will belong to one of the more mature phenotypic groups.

In cryostat sections therefore, although virtually all cases of non-T ALL and LBL contain TdT, and over 95 per cent express CD19, the expression of other pan-B antigens, CD10 and immunoglobulin depends upon the level of tumour cell differentiation. Approximately 10 per cent express CD19 only; 30 per cent express CD19 and CD10; 30 to 40 per cent express CD19, CD10 & CD20; while approximately 20 to 30 per cent of cases contain cytoplasmic μ heavy chains as well as CD19 and CD20 (Anderson et al., 1984; Weisenburger, 1990). Examples of lymphoblastic lymphoma expressing a B-cell (sIg$^+$), rather than pre-B phenotype (cμ^+) are rare (Sheibani et al., 1987a). CD1,2,3,4,5,7,8,21 and 38 are virtually always negative, and CD25(Tac) is expressed in $<$10 per cent of cases. B-cell antigen CD22 is acquired in B-cell ontogeny later than CD19 and CD20, and is therefore present in the more mature phenotypic subgroups of non-T ALL. CD9(BA-2) and CD24(BA-1) are expressed in most cases of ALL and LBL of B-cell lineage.

In fixed, paraffin-embedded tissues, L26 (CD20) is a specific marker for B-cell lineage, however as discussed above, it is expressed in only 50 per cent of cases of B-lineage ALL or LBL and is therefore a specific but relatively insensitive marker (Norton and Isaacson, 1989b). μ heavy chain may be detected within the perinuclear cytoplasm if sensitive immunostaining techniques are used. The CD45 leucocyte common antigen is usually expressed as the high molecular weight isoform. Consequently, UCHL1 and OPD4 (CD45RO) are negative while 4KB5, MB1, (CD45RA) are usually positive (Dobson et al., 1987; Hall et al., 1988a; Norton and Isaacson, 1989b). None the less, CD45RA antibodies are not invariably positive; positive staining for MT2 is found infrequently, and antibody KiB3 may react with LBL of T-cell lineage. Antibody MB2 (unclustered) also lacks specificity in lymphoblastic lymphoma as it may be positive in some T-lineage tumours (Norton and Isaacson, 1989b). Anti-CD43 antibodies MT1, Leu 22 and DFT1 may be positive in lymphoblastic tumours of B- as well as T-cell lineage and therefore lack specificity (Picker et al., 1987; Said et al., 1989). LN2 (CD74) is usually positive, but also lacks specificity. LN1(CDw75) is expressed in only a small percentage of cases while LeuM1 (CD15), BerH2 (CD30) and EMA are negative (Hall et al., 1988a; Norton and Isaacson, 1987). Antibody KB61 (CDw32) is negative in pre-B ALL (Pulford et al., 1986).

The differential diagnosis of lymphoblastic malignancies is discussed in the next section.

T-cell lymphoma

T-lymphoblastic lymphoma/leukaemia

Approximately 80 per cent of lymphoblastic lymphomas (LBL), and only 20 per cent of lymphoblastic leukaemias (ALL) are of T-cell origin, the remainder being of B-cell lineage. The T lymphoblastic malignancies, perhaps better than most other forms of lymphoma, epitomize the concept that lymphomas are morphologically and immunophenotypically analogous to normal lymphoid cells 'frozen' at a given stage of development. T-ALL and T-LBL correspond to T-cells at the earliest stages of development; that of intra-thymic T-cells, and therefore generally exhibit genotypic and phenotypic expression resembling pro-thymocytes, immature (stage I) thymocytes, common (stage II) thymocytes, or medullary (stage III) thymocytes. (See normal T-cell development, page 115).

As a general rule, T-ALL cases have a less mature phenotype than T-LBL (Weiss et al., 1986). Roughly two thirds of T-ALL cases express a pro-thymocyte or immature thymocyte phenotype, while the remaining one third resemble common thymocytes. Medullary or stage II phenotypes are rare in T-ALL. In contrast, two thirds of T-LBL cases express a common thymocyte phenotype, while the remaining one third resemble medullary thymocytes (Jaffe, 1988; Knowles, 1989). Although normal thymocyte development provides a framework for the understanding of T-lymphoblastic malignancies, it is important to note that there is significant intra- and inter-case variability, and that some cases express an apparently aberrant phenotype for which there is no known normal counterpart (Sheibani et al., 1987a).

In frozen sections therefore, while CD2, CD7, TdT and CD71 are usually present, the expression of HLA-DR, CD1, CD3, CD4, CD5, CD8, CD10 and CD38 depends upon the stage of development emulated (Drexler et al., 1989; Jaffe, 1990; Sheibani et al., 1987a; Weiss et al., 1986). As most cases of T-LBL express a common thymocyte phenotype, they are usually positive for CD1 and CD5. In contrast, T-ALL is usually CD1 negative, and is less likely to express CD5. CD10 is found in slightly more than half of all T-ALL cases, and approximately one fifth of all cases of T-LBL. Its presence is reported to be associated with a better prognosis, and an increased likelihood of HLA-DR and CD9 expression (Dowell et al., 1987; Hollema and Poppema, 1989; Sheibani et al., 1987a; Weiss et al., 1986). CD3 is identifiable in slightly less than one half of T-ALL and two thirds of T-LBL cases. Although it appears in the cytoplasm of stage II corticothymocytes, it is not detectable on the cell surface until the later medullary thymocyte stage. As a result, many lymphoblastic lymphomas may be reported to be CD3 positive in cryostat sections but CD3 negative using flow cytofluorimetry. Antibody βF1, reactive against an invariant region of the T-cell receptor β chain, stains positively in slightly less than one half of cases of T-LBL or T-ALL (Mori et al., 1990; Ng et al., 1988; Said et al., 1990).

CD9 and HLA-DR are present in a small minority of cases (<20 per cent) of T-ALL (Dowell et al., 1987; Pittaluga et al., 1986). CD14, CD15, CD25 and CD30 are virtually always negative (Weiss et al., 1986). Natural killer cell antigens CD16 (Leu11) and Leu7 are present in a minority of cases and may identify a distinctive clinicopathological group within T lymphoblastic malignancies, apparently being associated with non-white females and an aggressive clinical course (Hollema and Poppema, 1989; Sheibani et al., 1987a). CD38 is expressed by a narrow majority of T-ALLs and T-LBLs. Interestingly, antibody HML-1, reactive against intraepithelial T-cells of the gastrointestinal tract, and apparently recognizing a novel integrin, is also positive in rare cases of T-lymphoblastic malignancy (Falini et al., 1991; Krissansen et al., 1992; Spencer et al., 1988)). With rare exceptions, B-restricted antigens (CD19, CD20) are virtually always negative in T-ALL.

In fixed, paraffin-embedded tissue sections, most of the antigens characteristic of T lymphoblastic malignancy are not detectable. Although some reports have claimed success in staining for TdT in paraffin sections (Said et al., 1988), other useful antigens including CD1, CD2, CD5, CD10 and CD38 are masked or lost following fixation. Consequently, apart from the detection of TdT, paraffin section immunophenotyping is largely restricted to determination of tumour lineage. The vast majority of cases are positive for CD45 (Hall et al., 1988a; Norton and Isaacson, 1986), which is usually expressed as the low molecular weight form (CD45RO), recognised by antibodies UCHL1 and OPD4. These two antibodies are generally positive in T-LBL, but may be negative in a significant number of cases, particularly in the more immature or leukaemic malignancies (Cabecadas and Isaacson, 1991; Clark et al., 1990; Davey et al., 1990; Hall et al., 1988a; Krajewski et al., 1988; Norton and Isaacson, 1986) In normal T-cell development, the CD45 antigen is initially expressed as a high molecular weight isoform (CD45RA) and the switch to a low MW form (CD45RO) which we normally associate with mature T-cells, occurs following the conversion of T-cells from 'naive' to 'memory' status (Clement, 1992). Consequently, a large percentage of normal thymocytes are CD45RA positive (West et al., 1986). Despite this finding, MB1, 4KB5, KiB3 and MT2 are usually negative in T-LBL (Clark et al., 1990; Dobson et al., 1987; Hall et al., 1988a; Krajewski et al., 1988; Norton and Isaacson, 1986; Norton and Isaacson, 1989b). Polyclonal CD3 antibody, in theory, is a valuable T-cell specific marker which should stain the majority of T lymphoblastic lymphomas (Anderson et al., 1991; Cabecadas and Isaacson, 1991; Davey et al., 1990). In practice, although many laboratories have reported success, the antibody may present technical difficulties and CD3 is more readily detected in cryostat sections using monoclonal antibodies. Antibody βF1 is reported to stain fixed tissues in a percentage of cases, but with less efficacy than in cryostat sections (Cabecadas and Isaacson, 1991; Krajewski et al., 1989).

CD43 is expressed by a majority of T-lymphoblastic malignancies (Fig. 4.8) and is more likely to be positive in those with a more mature phenotype (Said et al., 1989). In the lymphoblastic tumours, however, it is not T-cell restricted and can be identified in a percentage of cases of B-lineage lymphoblastic malignancies (Dobson et al., 1987; Hollema and Poppema, 1989; Krajewski et al., 1988; Norton and Isaacson, 1989b; West et al., 1986). B-cell related antigen MB2 is usually negative but its expression has been reported in rare cases. Antibodies L26 (CD20), LN1 (CDw75), LN2 (CD74), LeuM1 (CD15), BerH2 (CD30), MAC387 and EMA are negative (Hall et al., 1988a; Hollema and Poppema, 1989; Norton and Isaacson, 1986; Strickler et al., 1987).

Lymphoblastic lymphoma and leukaemia can be distinguished from non-haemopoietic malignancies by the high frequency of CD45 expression and absence of other antigens often seen in other small cell malignancies including keratins, neurofilaments, desmin, specific actins, desmoplakins, EMA, etc. Acute myeloid leukaemia (AML) is identifiable by the expression of CD13, CD33 and other myeloid antigens, and the absence of TdT expression. This enzyme is virtually restricted to the lymphoid leukaemias, except for a rare subgroup of AML.

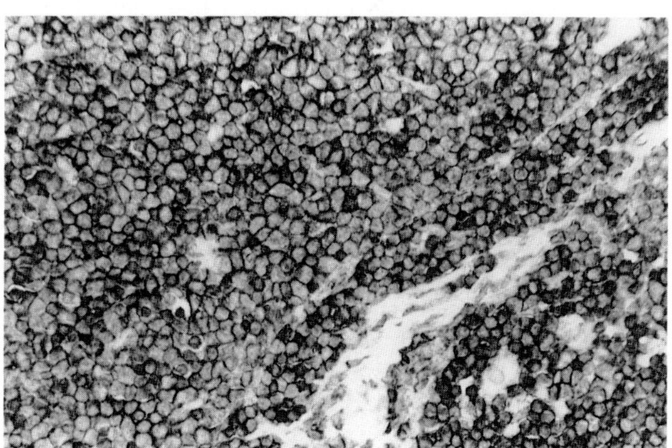

Fig. 4.8 T-lymphoblastic lymphoma showing staining for CD43. Note the slightly stronger staining of scattered resident thymocytes. Although CD43 is more consistently and strongly expressed in T- rather than B-lymphoblastic lymphoma, it may be positive in the latter in some cases. This case also expressed CD3 and CD2 (anti-MT1, ×400)

In the differentiation of T-cell from B-cell disease, some indication of lineage may be gained from the clinical features. Primary mediastinal lymphoblastic lymphoma is virtually always of T-lineage, while primary cutaneous disease is usually of B-lineage (Sander et al., 1992; Sander et al., 1991). T-cell antigens βF1, CD2, 3, 5, and B-cell antigens CD19 and 20, exhibit excellent specificity. Furthermore, CD19 and CD20 are present in over 90 per cent, and 50 per cent of B lineage lymphoblastic malignancies repectively, while CD7 is present on virtually all cases of T-ALL and T-LBL.

Phenotyptic ambiguity (so-called 'lineage infidelity') is a well-known phenomenon in some of the more immature types of leukaemias. AML may uncommonly express CD7, or B-cell antigens, however this is rarely a problem with the lymphomas.

Finally, it is worth noting for the unwary, that the reactive lymphoid infiltrate in a thymoma expresses a thymic phenotype which could be confused with T-ALL or LBL, particularly if the epithelial component is obscured. In such cases, a stain for keratins may be illuminating.

Mature, post-thymic T-cell malignancies

As the name implies, this group consists of T-cell lymphomas which express a mature or post-thymic phenotype. Many examples, however, express an 'aberrant' phenotype quite unlike that of most normal, mature T-cells, and in practice, the term is usually applied to any T-cell lymphoma which is not of immature, or lymphoblastic type.

Due to the prevalence of HTLV1 infection, this group is the commonest form of lymphoid malignancy in some parts of Japan and the Carribean, but represents less than 20 per cent of lymphomas diagnosed in Western countries. In the working formulation (WF) scheme, most T-cell lymphomas with a mature, post-thymic phenotype are classified as either ML: diffuse, mixed, small and large cell, or ML:immunoblastic, (often clear cell or polymorphous subtype). This division of mature T-cell lymphomas into two types appears to be of some prognostic value but it is clearly simplistic, and in addition, contributes to the marked biologic heterogeneity of these two WF groups which also include follicle centre cell lymphomas and B-immunoblastic lymphomas respectively. The morphological subclassification of T-cell lymphomas has long been frustrated by a remarkable histological diversity, which may also be expressed in successive biopsies from

Table 4.5. T-cell lymphomas: classifications

	USA*	Updated Kiel†
1.	T-cell chronic lymphocytic leukaemia T-cell prolymphocytic leukaemia	Lymphocytic – T-CLL Prolymphocytic leukaemia
2.	Cutaneous T-cell lymphoma: mycosis fungoides, Sezary's syndrome	Small cerebriform cell: mycosis fungoides, Sezary's syndrome
3.	Peripheral T-cell lymphoma (PTCL)	Lymphoepithelioid (Lennert's lymphoma) Angioimmunoblastic (AILD, LgX) T-zone lymphoma Pleomorphic, small cell (+/− HTLV1) Pleomorphic, medium and large cell (+/− HTLV1) Immunoblastic (+/− HTLV1)
4.	Adult T-cell leukaemia/lymphoma (ATLL)	
5.	Angiocentric immunoproliferative lesions: Lymphomatoid granulomatosis, Angiocentric lymphoma	
6.	Anaplastic large cell (Ki-1 +)	Anaplastic large cell (Ki-1 +)

Sources: * Jaffe, 1990; Knowles, 1989
† Stansfield et al., 1988

a given case. Based upon a wide range of experience of HTLV1-related lymphomas in Japan, Suchi and colleagues (Suchi et al., 1987) proposed a largely morphological system of classification for T-cell lymphomas which was subsequently included in the updated Kiel classification (Stansfield et al., 1988; Wright, 1989). On the other side of the Atlantic, a related but slightly different classification developed (Jaffe, 1990; Knowles, 1989). The major categories of each classification are given in the attached table (Table 4.5).

It is clear that although most groups are directly comparable, the Kiel system differs in two major respects. First, the angiocentric immunoproliferative lesions are not recognized, and secondly, Adult T-cell Lymphoma/Leukaemia (ATLL) is denoted by the postcript (+/− HTLV1) rather than being separately categorized.

In general, each of the 6 major groups indicated above has distinctive clinical, histopathological and immunophenotypic features warranting separate discussion. Cutaneous T-cell lymphoma and anaplastic large cell lymphoma will be discussed in a later section.

T-cell chronic lymphocytic leukaemia; small lymphocytic T-CLL

In Western countries, a small percentage of cases of CLL, or small lymphocytic lymphoma (<15 per cent) are of T-cell origin. Early reports of T-CLL showed a wide variability in clinical behaviour, histology and immunophenotype, however it subsequently became clear that this group, as originally described, was heterogenous and that most cases thought to be T-CLL were in fact examples of Tγ lymphoproliferative disease or T-prolymphocytic leukaemia (Knowles, 1989). Lennert and colleagues, recognizing this heterogeneity in 1982 (Lennert et al., 1982), subdivided the T-cell, small lymphocytic malignancies into 4 main groups: 'knobby', azurophilic, pleomorphic, and T prolymphocytic leukaemia (Table 4.6).

Table 4.6. T-CLL and variants

1. 'Knobby' type	T-CLL
2. Azurophilic type 3. Pleomorphic type	Tγ lymphoproliferative disease
4. T-prolymphocytic leukaemia	T-prolymphocytic lymphoma

Sources: Column 1, Lennert et al., 1982; column 2, Knowles, 1989

It appears likely that the 'knobby' type is equivalent to T-CLL proper, while the azurophilic and pleomorphic subtypes correspond to Tγ lymphoproliferative disease (see Table 4.6).

'True' T-CLL, T-cell small lymphocytic lymphoma Tumours of this type represent the minority of T-cell small lymphocytic malignancies and are presumed to be equivalent to resting naive or memory T-cells of post thymic phenotype. In contrast to T-prolymphocytic leukaemia and Tγ lymphoproliferative disease, lymphadenopathy is a common feature, and therefore in surgical pathology laboratories, it is more commonly seen than T-PLL or Tγ LPD. Histologically, the tumour differs from its B-cell counterpart by the absence of proliferation centres, and a more irregular ('knobby') nuclear profile.

In frozen section material, the tumour cells are CD1 and TdT negative and usually express a 'helper/inducer' phenotype: $CD2^+$, $CD3^+$, $CD4^+$, $CD5^+$, $CD7^+$, $CD8^-$ (Knowles, 1989; Krajewski et al., 1988; Suchi et al., 1987). Occasional cases may show anomalous subset expression or loss of one or more pan T-cell antigens, however phenotypic 'aberrancy' is less common than in other peripheral T-cell, and anaplastic large cell lymphomas. Expression of CD38 has been rarely recorded, however other activation antigens such as CD25 are usually negative.

In fixed paraffin-embedded material, the tumour cells are usually positive for LCA (CD45), UCHL1 (CD45RO), MT1, Leu22 (CD43) and polyclonal CD3. Use of antibody βF1 has not been widely reported in this context. B-cell associated markers L26 (CD20), LN1 (CDw75), and MB2 (unclustered) are usually negative (Clark et al., 1990; Dobson et al., 1987; Krajewski et al., 1988; Macon et al., 1991; Said et al., 1989). CD45RA antibodies MT2, KiB3 and MB1 are usually negative although occasional examples of MB1 positivity have been recorded (Hall et al., 1988a). HLA-DR, LeuM1 (CD15), BerH2 (CD30) and EMA are negative.

T-prolymphocytic leukaemia Approximately 20 per cent of cases of prolymphocytic leukaemia (PLL) are of T-cell lineage. Clinically, the patients present with a high lymphocyte count and splenomegaly but minimal or absent lymphadenopathy. The disease follows a more aggressive course than that of T-CLL. Morphologically, the tumour cells usually exhibit the typical features of a prolymphocyte, i.e. cytoplasmic basophilia, a single prominent nucleolus, and a cell size slightly larger than that of T-CLL (Suchi et al., 1987). Recently however, Matutes and colleagues (Matutes et al., 1991), have described small cell and other variants of T-PLL which may be misinterpreted morphologically as T-CLL, emphasizing both the heterogeneity of T-PLL and the importance of immunophenotyping and cytogenetic analysis (Brunning, 1991). In common with the B-cell equivalents, transitional forms exist between T-CLL and T-PLL, and T prolymphocytic leukaemia may supervene in T-CLL as a transformational event.

In frozen sections, the tumour cells exhibit a mature post thymic phenotype, being negative for CD1 and TdT. The pan-T antigens CD2, CD3, CD5, and CD7 are usually expressed. Positive staining for CD7 in particular, appears to be a feature of T-PLL and contrasts with the frequently negative staining seen in ATLL. Subset expression is variable. Approximately two thirds of T-PLL cases express a helper phenotype ($CD4^+$ $CD8^-$). Roughly one fifth show a suppressor phenotype ($CD4^-$ $CD8^+$), and the remainder are double positive ($CD4^+$ $CD8^+$). T-cell activation antigens T9 (CD71), T10 (CD38), Il-2R (CD25) and HLA-DR are usually negative, but may be found in a minority of cases. Markers of natural killer cells or large granular lymphocytes (CD11b, CD57, CD16) are almost always negative (Brunning, 1991; Erber and Mason, 1988; Knowles, 1989; Matutes et al., 1991).

At the time of writing, there is little published information available concerning the immunophenotype of T-PLL in paraffin sections, however it is worth noting that slightly more than half are reported to coexpress CD45RA and CD45R0, and therefore antibodies to CD45 variants may give misleading results in determining the lineage of prolymphocytic leukaemia (Matutes et al., 1991).

Tγ lymphoproliferative disease (TγLPD)-Lymphoproliferative disease of large granular lymphocytes (LDLGL) This term encompasses a group of low grade, chronic lymphoproliferative disorders, named in the days before monoclonal antibodies became available, for the ability of the tumour cells to form E rosettes (CD2), and express receptors for the Fc portion of IgG (CD16). Morphologically, the component cells contain azurophilic cytoplasmic granules and are referred to as large granular lymphocytes (LGL). Functional assays in most cases show that the tumour cells are capable of MHC independent cytotoxicity, i.e. they have natural killer (NK) function. Clinically, most patients present with a chronic lymphocytosis, anaemia and neutropenia with recurrent infections and autoimmune manifestations. Hepatosplenomegaly and marrow involvement are usually present without lymphadenopathy (McKenna, 1992).

Despite the common clinical features, recent immunophenotypic and genotypic studies have demonstrated that lymphoproliferative disorders of LGL are heterogenous with regard to immunophenotype, lineage and clonality (Knowles, 1989). The disease is now broadly divided into two morphologically indistinguishable categories: CD3+ tumours of T-cell lineage, and CD3− tumours of NK lineage (Chan et al., 1992).

The T-cell form of TγLPD represents approximately 80 per cent of cases. These exhibit clonal rearrangement of the T-cell receptor, and express a mature, post thymic, T-suppressor phenotype: CD1−, TdT−, CD2+, CD3+, CD4−, CD8+, CD5+. The NK related antigen CD57 (Leu7, HNK-1) is present in most cases while CD56 (NKH-1) is usually negative. Recently, McDaniel and colleagues have drawn attention to an uncommon CD16− variant which also apparently lacks clonal rearrangement of the TCR (Mcdaniel et al., 1992). This has reawakened earlier controversy, in which the neoplastic status of some forms of LDLGL is questioned. In paraffin sections, the tumour cells are usually positive for antibodies reactive against CD43, CD45RO, and in some cases S-100β (Hanson et al., 1991).

In Tγ LGL disease of NK lineage, (20 per cent of cases), the TCRβ and TCRγ chains are in the germline configuration, and the tumour cells express the phenotype: CD2+, CD3−, CD4−, CD5−, CD16+ and CD56+, often with positivity for CD11b. Some cases also express CD57 (Leu7), a finding which may be of prognostic significance (Mcdaniel et al., 1992).

Peripheral T-cell lymphoma (PTCL)

This term was originally coined by Waldron and colleagues (Waldron et al., 1977), to indicate lymphomas of T-cell lineage other than those of thymic or 'central' origin. In the strict sense of the definition therefore, it also includes T-CLL, T-PLL, ATLL, angiocentric lymphomas, and T-anaplastic large cell lymphoma, however in common usage these are often considered as separate entities. The peripheral T-cell lymphomas (PTCL) are a diverse group of malignancies which remain poorly understood (Jaffe, 1990; Knowles, 1989). In the updated Kiel classification, the equivalent tumours are divided into low grade: lymphoepithelioid (Lennert's), angioimmunoblastic, T-zone; and high grade categories: pleomorphic small cell, pleomorphic medium and large cell, and immunoblastic (Stansfield et al., 1988; Wright, 1989). This nomenclature remains the most recent and detailed attempt to subtype post-thymic T-cell malignancies, however in practice, it is often difficult to apply. Suchi and colleagues have themselves commented that 'One may be almost be driven to conclude that in classifying the T-cell lymphomas, we require as many categories as the number of cases we see' (Suchi et al., 1987). Recently, the reproducibility of the T-cell categories within the updated Kiel system has been questioned (Hastrup et al., 1991), and it has been further suggested that the division into high and low grades may not be statistically significant (Chott et al., 1990a; Noorduyn et al., 1990), and that stage at presentation, not morphology, is the more significant pathological variable in these diseases (Noorduyn et al., 1990).

Unfortunately, within the PTCL, there appears to be little correlation between morphological subtype and immunophenotype (Knowles, 1989; Krajewski et al., 1988; Weiss et al., 1985). The immunophenotypic findings of this group will therefore be discussed as a whole.

In frozen section material, the tumour cells, being of post thymic phenotype are, with rare exceptions (Hastrup et al., 1989), CD1 and TdT negative. Expression of the mature, pan T-cell antigens CD2, CD3, CD5 and CD7 is variable, and 'aberrant' phenotypes lacking one or more pan-T antigens (see below) are found in the majority of cases (Armitage et al., 1989; Chott et al., 1990a; Hastrup et al., 1989; Hollema and Poppema, 1989; Knowles, 1989; Krajewski et al., 1988; Picker et al., 1987; Weis et al., 1986; Weiss et al., 1985). In decreasing order of frequency, the deletions involve CD7, CD5, CD3, and CD2. Approximately one third, one quarter and one fifth are negative for one, two or three pan-T antigens respectively (Picker et al., 1987). The presence of such 'aberrant' phenotypes is uncommon in normal or reactive populations, and is therefore a useful indicator of malignancy. The use of CD7 in this context however should be treated with caution, as it is not strictly speaking, a pan T-cell antigen, being expressed on approximately 85 per cent of normal mature T lymphocytes. CD7− T-cells may in fact predominate in some reactive infiltrates, particularly in cutaneous sites (Kernohan and Smart, 1990; Ralfkiaer, 1991; Slater, 1990).

The majority (approximately two thirds) of PTCL express the CD4+ CD8− helper subset. The remaining one third of cases are roughly divided equally between the CD4− CD8+ suppressor/cytotoxic subset, and CD4− CD8− double negatives. The double positive CD4+ CD8+ subset, although frequently seen in lymphoblastic lymphomas, is uncommon in PTCL (Hastrup et al., 1989; Picker et al.,

1987; Weiss et al., 1985). The relative frequencies reported for these subsets depends upon the cases selected for study, as T-anaplastic large cell lymphomas have a relatively high prevalence of double negative subsets (Chott et al., 1990a).

T-cell activation antigens such as CD38, CD71 and HLA-DR are expressed in most cases of PTCL, while CD25 is found in a minority of cases (Krajewski et al., 1988; Raziuddin et al., 1991; Sheibani et al., 1987b; Su and Kadin, 1989). CD30, also considered by many to be an activation antigen, is identified in a small minority of non-anaplastic PTCL, including T-pleomorphic medium and large cell lymphoma, and T-immunoblastic lymphoma. In contrast with anaplastic large cell lymphoma, CD30 positive PTCL usually show only focal positivity (Chott et al., 1990a; Pallesen, 1990; Piris et al., 1990).

T-cell receptor antibodies A number of antibodies are now available, which react with antigenic determinants on the αβ, and γδ subtypes of the T-cell receptor (TCR).

TCR αβ Greater than 95 per cent of normal mature T-cells show rearrangement and expression of the TCRαβ. In PTCL however, approximately one third fail to show detectable TCR expression.

Antibody βF1 is one of the most frequently used antibodies of this type, and recognizes a non-polymorphic, framework determinant of the TCR β chain, identifying the αβ TCR complex (Gaulard et al., 1990; Krajewski et al., 1989; Mori et al., 1990; Ng et al., 1988; Said et al., 1990; Weiss et al., 1988).

In frozen section material, the antibody is highly specific, but lacks sensitivity as a marker for T-cells. In most series, βF1 expression is found in approximately 70 per cent of cases (Gaulard et al., 1990; Krajewski et al., 1989; Mori et al., 1990). The frequency of βF1 positivity appears to be significantly reduced in extranodal PTCL, particularly those of sinonasal origin (Ng et al., 1988).

Antibody WT31 recognizes a different antigenic determinant on the TCR-αβ and appears to be less sensitive than βF1 (Chan et al., 1988; Mori et al., 1990). Moreover, WT31 may react with framework determinants on the TCRγδ, indicating that although specific for T-cells, it may not be specific for those bearing the TCRαβ (Falini et al., 1989; Inghirami et al., 1990).

In T-cell ontogeny, transcription of the CD3 genes precedes that of the TCR β chain, which itself precedes α chain transcription (Royer and Reinherz, 1987). Normal mature T-cells then, obligatorily express the TCR on the cell membrane in conjunction with CD3. Numerous studies have however, demonstrated discordant expression of the TCR and CD3 in T-cell neoplasia (Krajewski et al., 1989; Ng et al., 1988; Picker et al., 1988; Picker et al., 1987; Raziuddin et al., 1991). All four possible combinations of TCR and CD3 expression are found in PTCL as follows:

1. $CD3^{+}\beta F1^{+}$
2. $CD3^{+}bF1^{-}$
3. $CD3^{-}\beta F1^{+}$
4. $CD3^{-}\beta F1^{-}$

The first group constitutes slightly more than half of PTCL cases. Groups 2 and 3 account for approximately one third of cases, and the remainder express neither CD3 nor βF1 (Picker et al., 1987). It was initially suggested that $CD3^{+}\beta F1^{-}$ cases of T-cell lymphoma may represent tumours in which productive rearrangements of the TCRγδ rather than TCRαβ were involved, however it has been subsequently shown that tumours of γδ T-cells are uncommon, and constitute less than 5 per cent of T-cell tumours (Picker et al., 1988). The fourth group shows a high incidence of NK antigen expression, and is probably heterogenous, including the following (Ng et al., 1988):

1. tumours of NK rather than T-cell lineage;
2. immature (early thymic) types;
3. T lymphomas with marked aberrancy.

TCRγδ Most studies suggest that in normal adults, less than 5 per cent of peripheral blood T-cells have productive rearrangement of the TCRγδ, although this percentage may be significantly higher in some organs such as the spleen (Inghirami et al., 1990).

Antibodies used to detect the gamma/delta TCR, are usually those reactive against the δ chain. These include antibodies TCRδ-1, and δTCS1. The former recognizes an invariant framework, or common variable determinant on the TCR δ chain, and therefore reacts with all cells bearing the TCRγδ (Picker et al., 1988). The latter antibody reacts with a nondisulphide-linked subset of TCRγδ cells and a further antibody, BB3 reacts with the complimentary disulphide-linked subset (Falini et al., 1989).

In studies of PTCL, positive staining for TCRδ-1 is uncommon, and has been found in only 2/14 (Picker et al., 1988), 0/30 (Falini et al., 1989), and 6/67 cases tested (Gaulard et al., 1990).

TCR variable region antibodies Genes coding for the TCR β chain include variable (V), constant (C), diversity—

(D) and joining (J) regions (Royer and Reinherz, 1987). The gene cluster for the variable region of the TCR β chain (Vβ) contains approximately 60 different Vβ genes, which are grouped into approximately 20 families according to the level of DNA sequence homology (Kimura et al., 1986). In reactive lymphoid populations therefore, an antibody to any one of the Vβ families should only react with approximately 5 per cent of T-cells.

A number of antibodies reactive against the products of these Vβ gene families are now commercially available and it has been suggested that dominant expression of one Vβ family may provide an indicator of clonality (Clark and Boylston, 1989; O'Grady et al., 1990; Poppema and Hepperle, 1991). The list of antibodies includes: 1C1 (Vb5.2 and 5.3), W112 (Vb5.3), 16G8 (Vb8), S511 (Vb12), OT145 (Vb6.7), LC4 (Vb5.1) and 5REX9H5 (Vb8). In a recent series utilizing a limited panel of antibodies, 29 per cent of TCR-positive lymphomas were found to have restricted Vβ gene usage (Poppema and Hepperle, 1991), suggesting that employment of a more complete panel may be useful for the diagnosis of both malignancy and lineage (O'Grady et al., 1990). It is also feasible however, that certain foreign antigens may induce dominant expression of one Vβ gene family even in reactive lymphoid populations, and at present therefore, the use of TCR Vβ antibodies is largely restricted to research. The recent demonstration of Vβ gene overexpression, even in the absence of detectible clonal TCR rearrangements, awaits elucidation (Smith et al., 1992a).

Phenotypic 'aberrancy' The pathogenetic significance of 'aberrant' or 'abnormal' phenotypes is unresolved. In some cases, phenotypes which were initially thought to be aberrant such as double negative ($CD4^-CD8^-$) T-cells, were subsequently found to represent clonal expansion of otherwise small subpopulations of T-cells (Lanier et al., 1986). Other cases of 'aberrancy' may be attributable to disorders of the genome, or gene transcription associated with the neoplastic state (Su et al., 1988); however a third possible mechanism involves changes of antigen expression which normally occur upon lymphocyte activation. Surface expression of antigens such as the CD3/T-cell receptor complex for example, is markedly reduced following activation in normal T-cells (Royer and Reinherz, 1987; Su et al., 1988). Evidence supporting antigen modulation as a possible mechanism for aberrancy, is the observation that such phenotypes are more frequently seen, and are more extreme in high grade T-cell lymphomas bearing activation antigens such as CD25 (Hollema and Poppema, 1989; Su and Kadin, 1989). This is best exemplified by T-anaplastic large cell lymphomas (Chott et al., 1990a).

Subtypes of peripheral T-cell lymphoma

The above comments apply to all PTCL, however in some cases, there are additional immunophenotypic findings which may be diagnostically useful.

Angioimmunoblastic or AILD-like Lymphoma Angioimmunoblastic lymphadenopathy, originally thought to be an abnormal immune reaction or preneoplastic condition, has subsequently been shown to have frequent non-random cytogenetic abnormalities and clonal rearrangement of the TCR (Feller et al., 1988; Lipford et al., 1987; Weiss et al., 1986). The typical case, showing angioproliferation, polyclonal B-cell proliferation, absent or 'burnt out' follicles, deposition of periodic acid Schiff (PAS) +ve eosinophilic material, and clinical features such as hypergammaglobulinaemia and immune dysfunction; is now generally categorized as angioimmunoblastic, or AILD-like lymphoma; the commonest form of PTCL (Chott et al., 1990a; Suchi et al., 1987). The proliferating T-cells in most cases, are of $CD4^+CD8^-$ helper phenotype, however in a small percentage of cases, a $CD4^-CD8^+$ suppressor phenotype is found. Most cases also show an activated phenotype with expression of HLA-DR and often, CD25 (Chott et al., 1990a; Jaffe, 1990).

A distinctive feature of this form of PTCL is the presence of large numbers of Ki67-positive follicular dendritic reticulum cells (DRCs), which often proliferate diffusely in a sheet-like fashion. These are identifiable using anti-DRC antibodies or immunostains specific for CD21, CD23 or CD35, and contrast with the tightly formed follicular dendritic patterns seen in the reactive follicles of hyperimmune reactions which constitute the main differential diagnosis in this disease (Suchi et al., 1987).

Lymphoepithelioid (Lennert's) lymphoma Double immunostaining techniques have demonstrated that the proliferating element in this lymphoma consists largely of $CD4^+$ T helper cells, and it is currently regarded as a $CD4^+$ PTCL (Chott et al., 1990a; Feller et al., 1986; Patsouris et al., 1988; Suchi et al., 1987). In comparison with other PTCL there are numerous epithelioid histiocytes present which stain positively with a number of histiocyte related antibodies including Ki-M1, Ki-M6, and

Ki-M8 (Feller et al., 1986). It is distinguished from the variants of angioimmunoblastic lymphoma which have a high content of epithelioid histiocytes, by the absence of clinical and morphological features of AILD, and the lack of proliferating DRCs (Patsouris et al., 1989a). It may also resemble lymphoplasmacytoid B-cell lymphoma with a high content of epithelioid histiocytes, from which it may be distinguished by a lack of plasmacytic cells showing light chain restriction (Patsouris et al., 1990). The most challenging differential diagnosis is that of Hodgkin's disease, particularly as LeuM1 (CD15)$^+$, Reed–Sternberg like cells may be found in lymphoepithelioid lymphoma (Patsouris et al., 1988; Patsouris et al., 1989b). The distinction must often be made on clinical and morphological grounds, however the detection of immunophenotypic aberrancy in the background T-cell population, when found, is diagnostic of T-cell lymphoma.

T-zone lymphoma The proliferating element in this subtype also consists of CD4$^+$ T helper cells (Suchi et al., 1987). It is distinguished from the other PTCL, at least in the early phase of tumour infiltration, by the presence of prominent reactive B-cell follicles which are readily detected by antibodies reactive against DRCs. The major differential diagnosis in this subtype is that of reactive hyperplasia or even follicular lymphoma. Apart from the detection of cytological atypia in the T-lymphocytes of the interfollicular zone, the T-cell infiltrate may be examined for evidence of immunophenotypic aberrancy, and the follicles, for evidence of light chain restriction, indicative of follicular lymphoma. In the early stages, genotypic analysis may be vitally important to establish the diagnosis.

Plasmacytoid T-cell lymphoma This tumour, once thought to be of T-cell lineage on the basis of CD4 positivity, is now known to be a tumour of plasmacytoid monocytes (Koo et al., 1990).

Angiocentric immunoproliferative disorders The term angiocentric immunoproliferative lesion (AIL) has been used to indicate a spectrum of lymphoproliferative disease which is usually of T-cell type and exhibits a striking angiocentric lymphoid infiltration with necrotizing lesions (Jaffe, 1985). This group includes polymorphic reticulosis, lymphomatoid granulomatosis of Liebow, and angiocentric lymphoma. It frequently presents in the paranasal sinuses, lung, and less commonly, other extranodal sites (Lipford et al., 1988). On the basis of morphological criteria, the spectrum of AIL has been subdivided into grades 1, 2 and 3, which appear to have prognostic significance (Jaffe, 1990).

The AILs are not recognized in the updated Kiel classification, in which they are included with the pleomorphic T-cell lymphomas of medium and large cell type (Suchi et al., 1987). Notwithstanding this, there appear to be both clinical and pathological features which justify consideration of the AILs as a separate entity.

Clinically, patients present with a slow, unremitting course, often commencing with nasal stuffiness, hoarse voice or cough, progressing to ulcerating, necrotizing and destructive lesions of the respiratory tract and paranasal sinuses. The AILs therefore represent one of the causes of the 'lethal midline granuloma' syndrome. In a small percentage of cases, the AILs may terminate in a fulminant, reactive haemophagocytic syndrome (Boyd et al., 1988; Jaffe et al., 1983; Kueck et al., 1989; Ng et al., 1986).

Histologically, the low grade lesions are characterized by a polymorphous leucocytic infiltrate which shows slight cytological atypia and infiltration and occlusion of vessels with extensive tissue necrosis. Many cases are mistaken initially for inflammatory processes.

In Asian populations, such lesions are almost always of T-cell phenotype and constitute the most common lymphoma of the nasal sinuses; the second most common site of extranodal lymphoma after the gastrointestinal tract (Chan et al., 1987a; Ho et al., 1990; Ng et al., 1988). In Western communities, the situation is less clear. The majority of studies have, in the past, indicated that angiocentric T-cell lymphomas are uncommon in the nasal sinuses in Western communities, and that most lymphomas at this site are of B-cell phenotype (Fellbaum et al., 1989; Frierson et al., 1989). More recently however, a number of authors have shown that with careful case selection, T-cell tumours predominate at this site in Western as well as in Asian communities (Chott et al., 1988; Ferry et al., 1991; Gaulard et al., 1988; Knowles, 1989; Lipford et al., 1988; Ratech et al., 1989).

Apart from rare examples of some B-cell lymphomas showing an angiocentric pattern, B-cell antigens are negative, and the AILs express a mature T-cell, or T-cell-like phenotype which is TdT and CD1 negative. Most cases express a CD4$^+$CD8$^-$ T-helper phenotype however CD4$^-$CD8$^+$ phenotypes may occur, and double negative CD4$^-$CD8$^-$ cases are relatively common in some series (Chott et al., 1988; Ho et al., 1990). Pan-T antigens CD2,

CD3, CD5 and CD7 are commonly expressed, however phenotypic aberrancy is unusually frequent in sinonasal T-cell lymphomas, and in some cases, CD2 expression is the only indication of T-cell lineage (Chan et al., 1987a; Lippman et al., 1987). Antibody βF1, in contrast with the findings in nodal PTCL, is usually negative, and NK antigens including CD16 and CD56 may be expressed (Ng et al., 1988). T-cell activation antigens such a CD25 and HLA-DR are usually present. In contrast with nodal PTCL, most genotypic studies have shown clonal TCR-β rearrangement in only a relatively small percentage of cases (Medeiros et al., 1991).

A number of hypotheses have been advanced to explain these unusual pathological findings. Firstly, the relatively frequent finding of TCRδ expression suggests that some cases may be tumours of gamma/delta T-cells (Gaulard et al., 1990; Ng et al., 1988). Secondly, the relatively frequent double negative $CD4^-CD8^-$ phenotype with expression of NK antigens and absence of CD3, suggests that some cases may be of NK lineage (Medeiros et al., 1991; Wong et al., 1992). Natural Killer function has been demonstrated in at least one such case (Boyd et al., 1988). Finally, Epstein Barr virus is frequently found in association with the AILs (Weiss et al., 1992), and it has been suggested that the frequent absence of clonal TCRβ rearrangement, may indicate that some AILs are a polyclonal, EBV driven proliferation analagous to the post-transplantation lymphoproliferative disorders (Medeiros et al., 1991).

Adult T-cell lymphoma/leukaemia (ATLL) Despite a remarkable morphological diversity, this condition is a clinicopathological entity, and is characterized by distinctive clinical features and the presence of HTLV1 infection.

Commonest in areas of endemic HTLV1 infection, such as southwest Japan and the Caribbean, the tumour is usually manifest as a leukaemia of markedly pleomorphic lymphoid cells. Sites of organ involvement include skin, liver, lungs, gastrointestinal tract and the central nervous system. Infiltration of lymphoid organs usually occurs in a leukaemic distribution.

Given the known tropism of HTLV1 for $CD4^+$ T-cells, it is not surprising that ATLL expresses a $CD4^+$, mature T-cell phenotype. Curiously however, the tumour cells exhibit suppressor function (Knowles, 1989). HTLV1 infection, possibly due to gene products encoded in the *tat* region of the HTLV1 genome, induces the expression of Il-2 receptors as well as the production of Il-2, establishing an autocrine feedback loop. It is not surprising therefore, that positivity for CD25 is a constant feature of ATLL, as well as the expression of other activation antigens such as HLA-DR, CD71 and/or CD38. Loss of CD7, commonly seen in many PTCL is thought to be particularly characteristic.

Enteropathy-associated T-cell lymphoma (EATCL)

This disease was originally designated 'malignant histiocytosis of the intestine', on the basis of positivity for α1-antitrypsin and morphological features of histiocytes, including erythrophagocytosis, sinusoidal involvement of regional lymph nodes, and the presence of cytoplasmic lysosomal granules. Subsequent phenotypic and genotypic studies however, have clearly demonstrated the T-cell nature of this disorder (Isaacson et al., 1985; Stein et al., 1988). It has no place within the working formulation, or revised Kiel classification schemes, yet the distinctive clinical, morphological and immunophenotypic features suggest a unique entity worthy of inclusion.

The disease typically presents with malabsorption and abdominal pain. Macroscopically, ulcerating masses, often multiple, are found anywhere within the small intestine. On occasions, the lesions may be essentially ulcerative, without obvious tumour formation. Such appearances may be indistinguishable from ulcerative jejunitis, often necessitating many biopsies to achieve a diagnosis. Involvement of mesenteric nodes is common and occurs early in the course of the disease. Microscopically, the infiltrate is extremely variable, often including pleomorphic and multinucleate tumour cells with admixed plasma cells, lymphocytes and eosinophils. Erythrophagocytosis by both histiocytes and tumour cells may be present, and the tumour cells often exhibit an angiocentric distribution (Wright and Isaacson, 1989). Intra-epithelial tumour cells are frequently seen, and the adjacent uninvolved mucosa often shows crypt hyperplastic villous atrophy.

The tumour cell immunophenotype resembles that of intra-epithelial lamina propria T-cells. This specialized arm of the T-cell immune system differs from normal peripheral T-cells in the following ways:

1. >90 per cent express a $CD4^-$ $CD8^+$ phenotype;
2. >5 per cent are subset double-negative ($CD4^-$ $CD8^-$);
3. many are $CD5^-$;
4. all are $HML\text{-}1^+$;
5. increased utilization of the γδ TCR.

Although some report a $CD4^+$ phenotype in EATCL (Salter et al., 1986), the commonest phenotype is subset double-negative, as follows: $CD2^+$, $CD3^{+/-}$, $CD4^-$, $CD5^-$,

CD7+, CD8−, HML-1+ . In paraffin sections, the tumour cells usually express polyclonal CD3, while L26 (CD20) is negative. CD45 isoforms usually follow the pattern expected for a T-cell tumour, however inversions are not uncommon, and neither CD45RA (4KB5, KiB3, MB1, KiB3) nor CD45RO (UCHL1, A6, OPD4) should be used as sole discriminants of lineage in this context. Antibody HML-1 and subsequently Ber-Act8 were originally thought to be specific for intra-epithelial T-cells of the gut, and EATCL (Spencer et al., 1988). They have since been shown to be expressed on hairy cell leukaemia, some B-cell lymphomas, and T-lymphoblastic lymphoma (Falini et al., 1991; Moller et al., 1990; Pallesen and Hamilton-Dutoit, 1990). Recent studies have shown that this antibody in fact recognizes a β7 integrin molecule, possibly induced in intraepithelial T-cells as a homing receptor (Micklem et al., 1991; Parker et al., 1992).

Cutaneous T-cell lymphoma The immunophenotypic findings in cutaneous lymphoproliferative disease are discussed in a separate chapter.

Immunophenotyping in paraffin sections The choice of antibodies reactive against T-cells in fixed paraffin-embedded sections includes CD43 (MT1, Leu22/L60, T2/48, DF-T1); CD45RO (UCHL1, OPD4, A6); polyclonal CD3 and βF1.

In most recent studies, CD43 antibodies Leu22 and MT1 are found to be marginally more sensitive, but less specific markers for T-cells in paraffin sections than the CD45RO antibody UCHL1 (Macon et al., 1991; Wieczorek et al., 1988). Polyclonal CD3 antibody is a specific but less sensitive marker, while βF1 is highly specific, but insensitive, technically difficult to use and produces variable results depending on fixation and digestion schedules (Cabecadas and Isaacson, 1991).

CD43 is expressed in approximately 85 per cent to 90 per cent of PTCLs overall, however this is dependent on the cases selected for study, and the fixation procedure adopted (Chott et al., 1990a; Hall et al., 1988a; Krajewski et al., 1988; Poppema et al., 1987; Said et al., 1989; Strickler et al., 1987; Stross et al., 1989). In low grade lesions the frequency of staining approaches 95 per cent or better, while in high grade lesions, the frequency of staining is probably closer to 80 per cent (Norton and Isaacson, 1989b).

The specificity of CD43 is unfortunately quite low, as it is normally expressed in myeloid, megakaryocytic, and erythroid precursors, as well as mature myeloid and monocytic cells (Poppema et al., 1987; Said et al., 1989; Stross et al., 1989; van der Valk et al., 1989). In tumour cell populations, a majority (approximately two thirds) of low grade B-cell lymphocytic lymphomas are strongly positive for CD43, while in high grade B-cell lymphomas, approximately 10 per cent of cases are CD43 positive (Norton and Isaacson, 1989b). Anti-CD43 antibodies therefore, should not be used to assess the lineage of low grade lymphomas. In high grade lymphomas however, the dramatic improvement in specificity for T lineage is gained at the expense of a only a small reduction in sensitivity, and CD43 is therefore very useful in distinguishing between high grade B and T-cell lymphomas. In the diagnosis of undifferentiated malignancies, CD43 is of little diagnostic value, as it is expressed in a wide range of myeloid and monocytic malignancies, as well as a number of non-haemopoietic tumours including some carcinomas, melanomas and mesotheliomas (Andrade et al., 1988; Ng et al., 1988; Said et al., 1989; Segal et al., 1992). In well fixed tissues, specific staining with anti-CD43 antibodies occurs in a crisp, membranous pattern which is readily recognizable. Cytoplasmic staining is usually seen in non-lymphoid cells and is best disregarded.

Anti-CD45RO antibody UCHL1 is expressed in approximately 95 per cent of low grade, and greater than 70 per cent of high grade T-cell lymphomas (Fig. 4.9) (Cabecadas and Isaacson, 1991; Chott et al., 1990a; Clark et al., 1990; Hall et al., 1988a; Macon et al., 1991; Norton and Isaacson, 1989b), although some series report a slightly lower sensitivity (Wieczorek et al., 1988).

The complex biology of CD45 isoform expression has important implications for the immunodiagnosis of T-cell lymphomas in paraffin sections (see CD45 antibodies page 125).

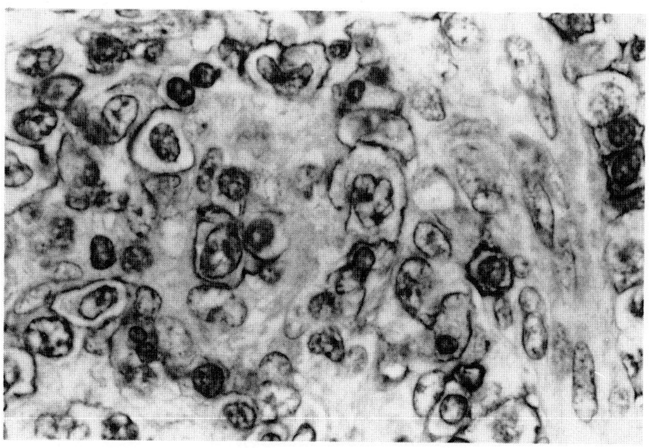

Fig. 4.9. T-pleomorphic lymphoma, medium and large cell type. Clear membranous staining for CD45RO. This case also expressed CD3 and CD43 (anti-UCHL1, X1000).

First, anti-CD45RO antibodies are not 'pan-T markers'. The switch from CD45RA to CD45RO expression is an integral part of the conversion from 'naive' to 'memory' T-cells (Clement, 1992), causing a modulation TCR function (Janeway, 1992). Therefore, although most mature T-cells in adults are reactive with UCHL1, the reverse is true in immunologically 'naive' neonates.

Secondly, many tumour populations show heterogeneity of CD45 isoform expression. This usually involves small subpopulations, but may on occasion involve a significant percentage of tumour cells, potentially causing diagnostic confusion.

Thirdly, in normal T-cell populations, CD45RO is preferentially expressed on normal $CD4^+$ rather than $CD8^+$ cells (72 per cent versus 36 per cent respectively) (Norton et al., 1986). In T-cell tumours therefore it is not surprising that anti-CD45RO antibodies are less frequently positive in $CD4^-CD8^+$ suppressor cell, and double-negative $CD4^-CD8^-$ tumours (Norton and Isaacson, 1989a).

Finally, as the lack of CD45RO expression in many T-cell tumours may be a functional rather than 'aberrant' phenomenon, it is frequently associated with reciprocal positivity for CD45RA. This switch of CD45 isoform expression is potentially misleading as it delivers a doubly 'false' signal to the unwary pathologist.

The specificity of CD45RO antibodies in the differentiation of T-cell from B-cell lymphoma is greater than 95 per cent for low grade, but closer to 85 per cent for high grade lymphomas (Norton and Isaacson, 1989b). This reduced specificity in high grade lesions is largely due to the expression of CD45RO in B-immunoblastic lymphoma, a consequence of CD45 isoform switch which occurs normally during B-cell plasmacytic differentiation.

CD45RO is leucocyte restricted, and is therefore of value in the diagnosis of undifferentiated malignancies, however, it is also expressed on myeloid and monocytic cells (Cabecadas and Isaacson, 1991). It is identifiable on the surface of normal immature myeloid cells and is strongly expressed in the myelocyte stage, staining both the cell membrane and cytoplasmic granules. In tumour populations it is present on the surface of most cases of CML and a variable percentage of AML cases (Caldwell et al., 1991; Kurec et al., 1990).

Antibody OPD4 was originally proposed as a specific marker for $CD4^+$ cells (Yoshino et al., 1989), however this has not been substantiated. More recent studies have indicated that it is unreactive with monocytic cells but otherwise exhibits a similar range of reactivity to UCHL1 (O'Grady et al., 1991; Poppema et al., 1991). Moreover, it is relatively insensitive, and stains less than 50 per cent of T-cell lymphomas in some series (Cabecadas and Isaacson, 1991).

Antibody A6 also reacts with CD45RO and shows a range of tissue reactivities similar to UCHL1. An initial paraffin section study claims a higher sensitivity for T-cells than UCHL1, however this requires confirmation (Berti et al., 1991).

Polyclonal anti-CD3 antibody, raised against a synthetic amino acid sequence derived from the epsilon chain of the CD3 molecule (Mason et al., 1988), is a specific but slightly insensitive marker of T-cells in paraffin sections (Cabecadas and Isaacson, 1991). In most published studies, approximately two thirds of T-cell lymphomas are found to be positive, however it is significantly less sensitive than an equivalent monoclonal anti-CD3 antibody used in frozen sections and the efficacy of this staining depends upon the fixation and digestion methods used (Anderson et al., 1991; Mason et al., 1989).

Antibody βF1 is highly specific for T-cells, but shows variable sensitivity when used in fixed, paraffin-embedded tissue sections. Although some reports have claimed positive staining in up to two thirds or even three quarters of T-cell lymphomas tested (Krajewski et al., 1989; Said et al., 1990), others have found staining in less than 50 per cent of cases (Cabecadas and Isaacson, 1991). It is important to remember that polyclonal CD3 and βF1 should be used cautiously in the differentiation of T-cell lymphoma from Hodgkin's disease, as either may be expressed in up to one third of cases of Hodgkin's disease (see page 163).

The B-cell antibody L26 (CD20) is virtually always negative in low grade T-cell lymphomas, while in high grade malignancies, it is positive in less than 4 per cent of cases (Elghetany et al., 1991; Mason et al., 1990). MB2 (unclustered) is positive in less than 4 per cent of low grade and 12 per cent of high grade T-cell lymphomas (Norton and Isaacson, 1989b). Anti-CD45RA antibodies MB1, MT2, KiB3 and 4KB5 are subject to reciprocal inversions with UCHL1, and are best avoided in high grade malignancies.

Anaplastic large cell lymphoma

In the early 1980s, a distinctive group of large cell lymphomas was identified by the coexpression of Ki-1

(CD30) and leucocyte common (CD45) antibodies and acquired the title: 'Ki-1 Lymphoma' (Stein et al., 1985). The histological features included a striking sinusoidal distribution, a cohesive growth pattern and pleomorphic cytology with lobated nuclei, prominent nucleoli, and basophilic cytoplasm. Many had been previously misdiagnosed as malignant histiocytosis, carcinoma, melanoma or sarcoma.

Subsequently, it became apparent that CD30 is not specific for this entity and is expressed on a number of cell types including a significant percentage of high grade T and B-cell lymphomas. As a result, this group of lymphomas has been redefined morphologically and as such has been incorporated into the revised Kiel classification system (Stansfield et al., 1988; Suchi et al., 1987). At the same time the term 'Ki-1 Lymphoma' has been replaced by anaplastic large cell (ALC) lymphoma. Recently, a distinction has been made between primary and secondary ALC, the latter ocurring as a complication in a CD30 negative lymphoma such as mycosis fungoides or follicular lymphoma. The distinction may be of prognostic importance (Kaudewitz et al., 1989).

Anaplastic large cell (ALC) lymphoma has been accepted as a clinicopathological entity and appears to be one of the more reproducible groups within the Kiel system (Hastrup et al., 1991) yet a number of morphological variants have recently been described (Chan et al., 1989; Chott et al., 1990b), some of which may difficult to distinguish from pleomorphic forms of immunoblastic and centroblastic lymphoma. Moreover, even the more typical examples may be difficult to distinguish from the syncytial variant, or lymphocyte depleted forms of Hodgkin's disease.

Immunophenotyping in this group is therefore concerned with the following:

1. What antigens are expressed in ALC?
2. How is it distinguished from non-lymphoid malignancy?
3. How is it distinguished from CD30+ve lymphomas other than ALC?
4. How is it distinguished from Hodgkin's disease?

Immunophenotypic profile of ALC

Approximately 60 per cent are of activated T-cell phenotype (Agnarsson and Kadin, 1988; Chan et al., 1989; Chott et al., 1990b; Kinney et al., 1990; Stein et al., 1985), and in cryostat sections show variable positivity for βF1, CD4 and pan T-cell antigens: CD2, CD3, CD5 and CD7 (Chott et al., 1990b). Activation associated antigens CD25, HLA-DR and transferrin receptors are expressed in almost all cases (Agnarsson and Kadin, 1988). Probably because of the level of cellular activation, ALC has a very high frequency of phenotypic 'aberrancy' with loss of one or more pan-T antigens in the great majority of cases. Paraffin sections reveal expression of CD45RO (UCHL1) and/or CD43 (MT1, DFT1, Leu22) in a small majority of cases (Chott et al., 1990b; Norton and Isaacson, 1989b).

Of the remaining cases of ALC, approximately 15 per cent are of B-cell and 25 per cent are of 'null' phenotype. The former express CD19, CD20 and CD22 in frozen sections and L26 (CD20), MB2, MB1 and/or MT2 (CD45RA) in paraffin sections. Immunoglobulin with light chain restriction may be weakly expressed (Chott et al., 1990b).

'Null cell' forms of ALC are of indeterminate lineage. Some may represent T-cell or B-cell neoplasia with extreme aberrancy, however rare cases may be of true histiocytic origin (Banks et al., 1990), particularly as CD30 expression appears to be inducible in histiocytes (Andreesen et al., 1989). In this context, expression of CD45RO or CD43 alone is not diagnostic of T-cell lineage, as either may be expressed on histiocytic cells.

CD30 (BerH2, Ki-1) is not specific for ALC, nor is it an absolute prerequisite for the diagnosis. In a recent series of 500 lymphomas (Piris et al., 1990), 11 per cent were found to be CD30+ve. Of these CD30+ve tumours, only 32 per cent (or 3.4 per cent of the total) were considered to be anaplastic large cell lymphomas. In general, ALC shows more diffuse and intense staining for CD30, usually involving more than 80 per cent of the tumour cells (Fig. 4.10). Most series report CD30 positivity in all cases of ALC however rare CD30 negative cases are described.

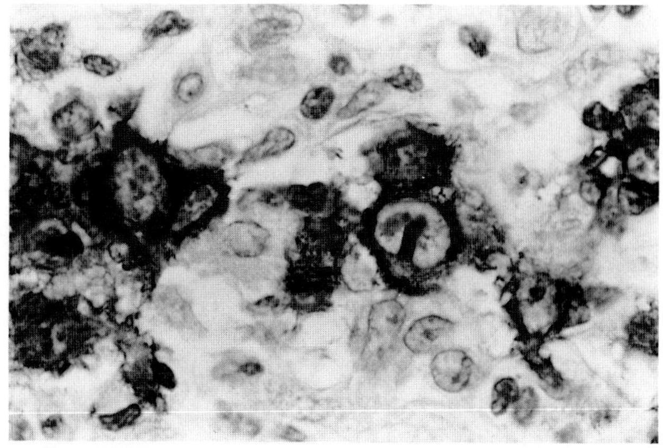

Fig. 4.10. Anaplastic large cell lymphoma showing perinuclear and membranous expression of CD30 (anti-BerH2, X1000).

EMA expression is reported in most examples of ALC, varying from 58 per cent (Chott et al., 1990b) to 91 per cent (Leoncini et al., 1990) of cases (Fig. 4.11). Some series have suggested a correlation with T-cell phenotype (Kinney et al., 1990) however EMA+ve examples of B-ALC and Null-ALC are not infrequent. The expression of EMA probably correlates with the level of activation.

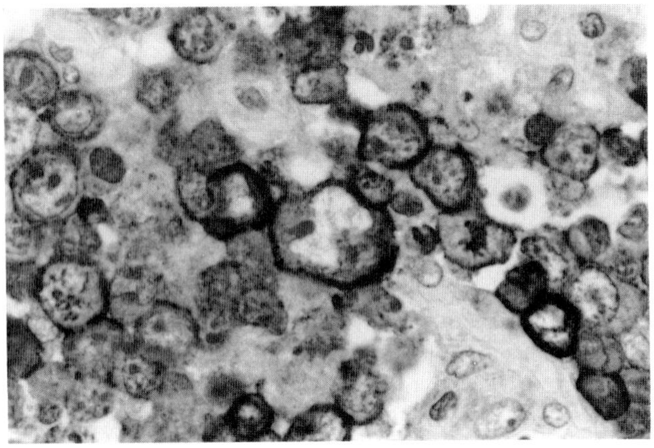

Fig. 4.11. Anaplastic large cell lymphoma within a lymph node subcapsular sinus and showing membranous expression of EMA (anti-EMA, X1000).

CD45, or LCA was initially described as being positive in almost all cases of ALC. More recent series however, have clearly indicated positivity in only two thirds of cases, (range 50 per cent to 87 per cent) (Burns and Dardick, 1990; Chan et al., 1989; Chott et al., 1990b; Falini et al., 1990; Hall et al., 1988b; Kinney et al., 1990; Leoncini et al., 1990; Piris et al., 1990). The number of positive cases increases in frozen section material, and the low rate of CD45 expression in paraffin sections may be a threshold effect, due to relatively weak CD45 expression in activated ALC cells.

CD15 (LeuM1,Tu9) is negative in the majority of ALC lymphomas, however most series have demonstrated CD15 positivity in a range from 20 per cent to 50 per cent of cases (Chan et al., 1989; Kinney et al., 1990; Leoncini et al., 1990; Lukes and Tindle, 1975; Norton and Isaacson, 1989b). The number of positive cases is increased if sections are first predigested with trypsin (Hall et al., 1988b).

Differentiation of ALC from non-lymphoid malignancy

In the presence of CD45 (LCA) antigen, localized to the cell membrane, the diagnosis of lymphoma is straightforward, as membranous staining is almost never seen in non-lymphoid cells. In the absence of such staining, the distinction may be difficult. Neither EMA nor Leu-M1 are of any diagnostic value in this context. Positive staining for keratins will in general, indicate an epithelial tumour however some caution should be exercised, as rare keratin-positive, vimentin-negative examples of ALC have been described, and some of these are CD45 negative (Gustmann et al., 1991; Norton and Isaacson, 1989b). The differentiation of ALC from amelanotic melanoma should also be approached with caution. Although S100 is generally negative in ALC, and a positive reaction would argue in favour of melanoma, rare cases have been described in which there is expression of S100 or neuron specific enolase (NSE).

In difficult cases, resort to acetone-fixed cryostat sections may demonstrate low levels of CD45 antigen or a coherent pattern of expression of B- or T-cell restricted antigens. Expression of desmoplakins may also favour a non-lymphoid tumour however this has not been fully investigated in the context of ALC lymphomas. Some cases may require demonstration of clonally rearranged T-cell receptor or immunoglobulin genes.

Differentiation of ALC from other CD30+ve lymphomas

ALC is now a morphologically defined entity (Pallesen, 1990; Suchi et al., 1987), and this distinction is therefore not made immunophenotypically. None the less, the range of morphological appearances encountered in ALC is diverse (Chan et al., 1989; Chott et al., 1990b) and some forms of CD30+ve, pleomorphic T-cell, immunoblastic, or centroblastic lymphomas may be difficult to distinguish from ALC. In this context, the presence of LeuM1 (CD15), BerH2 (CD30), LCA (CD45) or B- or T-cell antigens has no discriminatory value. In general, ALC lymphomas show strong staining for CD30 in more than 80 per cent of tumour cells, whereas other CD30+ve lymphomas express the antigen in a minority of cells. Unfortunately, this is not an absolute criterion as some ALC mimics may exhibit widespread staining. EMA may be helpful, as it is present in approximately two thirds of ALC cases but is negative in other CD30+ve, non-Hodgkin's lymphomas (Piris et al., 1990). More recently, antibody BNH9 (reactive against blood group related antigens) has been shown to be positive in 51 per cent of cases of ALC while staining less than 6 per cent of other lymphomas and Hodgkin's disease (Delsol et al., 1991).

Differentiation of ALC from Hodgkin's disease.

The syncytial variant of nodular sclerosing Hodgkin's disease and lymphocyte depleted forms may be difficult to distinguish from ALC morphologically. The lymphocyte predominant and mixed cellularity subtypes generally do not resemble ALC morphologically and will not be discussed here.

BerH2 (CD30) has no discriminatory value in this context, being present in over 90 per cent of cases of Hodgkin's disease and almost all cases of ALC.

In a typical example, a case of Hodgkin's disease will be positive for LeuM1 (CD15) but negative for LCA (CD45) and EMA. A typical example of ALC would give the reverse pattern. If such a phenotypic profile is found, then the diagnosis is straightforward. Unfortunately however, indeterminate phenotypes such as the coexpression of CD15 with CD45 or EMA are found in a significant number of cases and present a difficult diagnostic problem (Carbone et al., 1992). By the application of formal test analysis (Hall and D'Ardenne, 1987) (see page 176) the diagnostic discriminatory value of each antibody in this context can be assessed, enabling the interpretation of antibody stains in a weighted fashion. To this end, the operating characteristics (sensitivity, specificity, test accuracy) of each antibody 'test' will be approximated for each of the following relevant antigens.

LeuM1 (CD15) is positive in approximately 90 per cent of cases of Hodgkin's disease excluding lymphocyte predominant forms (Hall and D'Ardenne, 1987; Leoncini et al., 1990; Norton and Isaacson, 1989b). In contrast, anaplastic large cell lymphomas express CD15 in at least 20 per cent, and in some series, up to 50 per cent of cases (see above). The significance of these figures is best appreciated by formal test analysis (Hall and D'Ardenne, 1987). Assuming an equal prevalence for the two diseases and a best case of only 20 per cent CD15 'false positives' in ALC, the sensitivity of CD15 in distinguishing ALC from Hodgkin's disease is at best, 90 per cent while the specificity is at most, 80 per cent. (A 50 per cent result would indicate that the test had contributed no information). The predictive value of a positive result would be 81 per cent while the predictive value of a negative result would be 89 per cent. Translated in terms of betting odds, these figures indicate that a negative result for CD15 would favour ALC with odds of at best, 8:1, while a positive result would favour Hodgkin's disease with odds of, at best, 4.5:1. In practice therefore, a negative stain has some diagnostic value however a positive result offers a poor discriminatory ratio compared with most other antibodies. The overall efficiency or accuracy of this 'test' is 85 per cent. In practice, the actual probability of a given disease is also affected by the relative prevalence of the two diseases.

LCA (CD45) is positive in approximately 65 per cent of ALC lymphomas. In non-lymphocyte predominant forms of Hodgkins disease, it is reported to be positive in 8–12 per cent of cases (Leoncini et al., 1990; Lukes and Tindle, 1975; Norton and Isaacson, 1989b). The operating characteristics for CD45 in this context therefore are as follows: sensitivity – 65 per cent; specificity – 90 per cent; predictive value of a positive result – 87 per cent; predictive value of a negative result – 72 per cent; accuracy – 78 per cent. The low accuracy and sensitivity are due to the high frequency of negative staining for CD45 in ALC. None the less, assuming equal disease prevalence, a positive result would favour ALC with odds approaching 7:1. A negative result would favour Hodgkin's disease with odds of as little as 2.5:1. In this context therefore, a negative CD45 is of little diagnostic use.

EMA is negative in most examples of non-lymphocyte predominant Hodgkin's disease. Most series report positive staining for EMA in a range from 11 to 24 per cent of such cases (Chittal et al., 1988; Hall et al., 1988b; Norton and Isaacson, 1989b). In contrast, anaplastic large cell lymphomas are positive for EMA in somewhere between 58 per cent and 91 per cent of cases (see above). Using cumulative figures up to 1989 (Norton and Isaacson, 1989b), the operational characteristics would be as follows: sensitivity – 90 per cent; specificity – 80 per cent; predictive value of a positive result – 83 per cent (or 4.9:1); predictive value of a negative result – 89 per cent, (or 8:1); accuracy – 96 per cent.

The use of T-cell and B-cell restricted antibodies is of limited use in this context, as a significant percentage of cases of non-lymphocyte predominant Hodgkin's disease are positive for T- and B-cell markers including CD3, L26 (CD20), and MB2. None the less, CD43 and some of the CD45 variants exhibit quite good operating characteristics. MT1 (CD43) is positive in T-ALC in at least 64 per cent of cases (Agnarsson and Kadin, 1988; Chott et al., 1990b; Leoncini et al., 1990; Norton and Isaacson, 1989b). In contrast, membrane positivity for CD43 has been infrequently reported in Hodgkin's disease (Chittal et al., 1988; Lukes and Tindle, 1975; Said et al., 1989; Wieczorek et al., 1988). If one assumes a level of CD43 positivity in Hodgkin's disease of 5 per cent (which is more than most series report), the operating characteristics would be as follows: sensitivity – 64 per cent; specificity – 95 per cent; predictive value of a positive result – 93 per cent (or 13:1); predictive value of a negative result – 73 per cent (or 2.7:1); accuracy – 80 per cent. The overall accuracy for CD43 is low, and the sensitivity is poor, (a negative CD43 being of little diagnostic value), however the specificity is higher than for most other antibodies, and membrane positivity for CD43 therefore makes a diagnosis of Hodgkin's disease most unlikely.

UCHL1 is reported to be positive in approximately 5 per cent of cases of non-lymphocyte predominant Hodgkin's disease (Norton and Isaacson, 1989b). Positivity for UCHL1 is reported in 76 per cent of cases of T-cell ALC. In the context of this differential diagnosis, the operating characteristics for UCHL1 therefore are: sensitivity – 76 per cent; specificity – 95 per cent; predictive value of a positive result – 94 per cent (or 19:1); predictive value of a negative result – 79 per cent (or 4:1); accuracy – 86 per cent.

In summary, in the presence of indeterminate morphology, the distinction of ALC from Hodgkin's disease may be possible by the use a number of immunostains, having regard for their varying specificities and sensitivities. In descending order, the most useful discriminants are as follows: +ve MT1, or +ve UCHL1 (each approximately 95 per cent predictive value for ALC); −ve EMA or −ve LeuM1 (89 per cent predictive value for Hodgkin's disease or ALC respectively); +ve LCA (87 per cent predictive value for ALC); +ve EMA (83 per cent predictive value for ALC), +ve LeuM1 (81 per cent predictive value for Hodgkin's disease), −ve UCHL1 (80 per cent predictive value for Hodgkin's disease), −ve MT1 (73 per cent predictive value for Hodgkin's disease) and −ve LCA (72 per cent predictive value for Hodgkin's disease).

Hodgkin's disease

In his publication of the macroscopic findings in six cases of splenomegaly and lymphadenopathy in 1832, Thomas Hodgkin gave the first description of lymphoma reported in the English language. Since that time, the taxonomy of lymphoproliferative disease has largely progressed by the gradual recognition and separation of discrete clinicopathological entities, starting last century with the group of monomorphous lymphomas, referred to at that time as 'lymphadenoma' or 'lymphosarcoma'; later to become known as 'Non-Hodgkin's Lymphoma'. It is ironic that this latter group, which is now so well characterized in terms of lineage and immunophenotype is still defined collectively, by a negative qualification of the disease whose lineage and phenotype we know least about – Hodgkin's disease.

Hodgkin's disease largely remains an enigma; a malignancy of uncertain lineage, widely thought to be heterogenous, and showing a polymorphous cellular infiltrate including reactive lymphocytes, polymorphs, histiocytes and fibroblastic elements, in which the tumour cells may represent less than 1 per cent of the cellular complement, yet having distinctive clinical features, empirically curable in two thirds of cases, with characteristic sites of tumour involvement and patterns of dissemination.

The immunophenotyping of Hodgkin's disease, and polymorphous lymphomas in general, is one of the more interesting and challenging fields of diagnostic haematopathology. The paucity of tumour cells within involved tissues often renders flow cytofluorimetry ineffective. Fibroblastic cells, tissue necrosis, Fc receptors expressed by the numerous histiocytes, and the rosettes of T-cells surrounding Reed–Sternberg cells often obscure membrane staining of sparse tumour cells in cryostat sections. Consequently, the diagnosis of Hodgkin's disease is usually made by a combination of morphological assessment and paraffin section, or cytospin immunochemistry.

Histogenesis

Many theories regarding the 'cell of origin' in Hodgkin's disease have been proposed. Despite compelling immunophenotypic, and molecular genetic evidence favouring a lymphoid origin, (Diehl et al., 1990; Jaffe, 1989; Naumovski et al., 1990) a monocytic or interdigitating cell origin has not been entirely refuted (Hsu, 1990). This uncertainty is due partly to the paucity of tumour cells in involved tissues, (often at the limits of sensitivity of molecular assays) but probably also reflects heterogeneity within Hodgkin's disease itself. Moreover, it is a reflection of the uncertainty surrounding the significance of phenotypic 'aberrancy' in which myeloid or monocytic cell lines and malignancies are known to express lymphoid antigens, and vice versa (Diehl et al., 1990; Falk et al., 1987; Hsu and Hsu, 1989).

Aside from these misgivings, the prevailing view is that Hodgkin's disease is a malignancy of B-cells, and in some cases probably of T-cells, characterized by transformation of immature lymphocytes, at about the time of immunoglobulin or T-cell receptor rearrangement. The neoplastic cells then express an activated phenotype, prematurely superimposed upon an immature genotype (Falk et al., 1987; Herbst et al., 1989). Concomitant with the level of cellular activation, the tumour cells then express a wide range of cytokines which may account for the complex tumour-host interactions and polymorphous patterns of cellular infiltration (Hsu and Hsu, 1990; Hsu et al., 1990; Kadin et al., 1990; Newcom et al., 1990).

Support for this view is found in the activated phenotype of Hodgkin cells, the frequent presence of immunoglobulin gene rearrangements, and occasionally T-cell receptor rearrangements in Hodgkin's disease, the weak expression of lymphoid antigens by Hodgkin's tumour cells, and the observation that EBV transformation of immature lymphoid cells may give rise to a similar dissociation of phenotype and genotype.

Immunophenotyping of Hodgkin's disease

Just as 'lymphadenoma' or 'lymphosarcoma', the forerunner of non-Hodgkin's lymphomas was cleaved from Hodgkin's disease in the last century, so the process continues.

Recent immunophenotypic findings (Pinkus and Said, 1985; Pinkus and Said, 1988; Regula et al., 1987; Stein et al., 1986; Timens et al., 1986) have confirmed earlier morphological studies (Lennert and Mohri, 1978) showing that the nodular lymphocyte predominance type (paragranuloma) is dissimilar from other forms of Hodgkin's disease. Not only is it clinically and morphologically a distinct entity (Banks, 1990; Tefferi et al., 1990) but it is the only form of Hodgkin's disease for which a B-cell lineage has been established beyond any doubt.

In the following discussion therefore, the findings in nodular lymphocyte predominance Hodgkin's disease (NLPHD or nodular paragranuloma) will be considered separately from those of the mixed cellularity, lymphocyte depleted and nodular sclerosing forms of 'classical' Hodgkin's disease (MCHD, LDHD and NSHD).

Although most studies have emphasized the phenotype of the atypical (H-RS) cells, the lymphocyte predominance form also differs significantly from other forms of Hodgkin's disease in the composition its reactive cellular milieu. As will be discussed, this may be of diagnostic value.

'Classical' Hodgkin's disease: (mixed cellularity, nodular sclerosing and lymphocyte depleted forms)

Early studies showed a distinctive immunophenotypic profile for H-RS cells which, it was hoped, would prove diagnostic for Hodgkin's disease. Unlike most other forms of lymphoma, the neoplastic cells of Hodgkin's disease were found to be negative for CD45, B-cell and T-cell specific antigens, while showing positivity for LeuM1 (CD15) and Ki-1 (CD30) (Hsu and Jaffe, 1984c; Hsu et al., 1985). Many subsequent reports however, have questioned the diagnostic usefulness of each of these antigens, particularly when used independently of each other.

CD15 CD15 or Leu M1, although initially thought to be specific for Hodgkin's disease, has subsequently been identified in a significant number of high grade T-cell, and to a lesser extent, high grade B-cell lymphomas. The percentage of high grade T-cell lymphomas staining positively for CD15 varies widely in published reports, reflecting different selection criteria and enzymatic digestion methods (Hall P.A. et al., 1988b) and ranges from 20 per cent to 67 per cent (Pinkus et al., 1985; Sheibani et al., 1986; Swerdlow and Wright, 1986; Wieczorek et al., 1985). Cumulative series, however, indicate an overall positivity for CD15 in approximately 20 per cent of peripheral T-cell lymphomas and approximately 5 per cent of high grade B-cell lymphomas when tested in paraffin sections (Norton and Isaacson, 1989b). The specificity of CD15 depends in part, upon the pattern of staining encountered. H-RS cells show a distinctive paranuclear and membranous distribution which is usually lacking in myeloid and other cell types (Pinkus et al., 1985; Sheibani et al., 1986). None the less, a small percentage of T-cell lymphomas contain Hodgkin's-like cells with a staining pattern for CD15 which is indistinguishable from that of Reed–Sternberg cells (Wieczorek et al., 1985). This is particularly evident in the R-S like cells of lymphomatoid papulosis (Kadin et al., 1985).

The sensitivity of CD15 for HD is reported in most series to be between 80 per cent and 94 per cent (Fig. 4.12), however if the lymphocyte predominance forms are excluded, the sensitivity approaches the latter figure (Frierson and Innes, 1985; Norton and Isaacson, 1989b; Pinkus et al., 1985). Formal test analysis of immunostaining for CD15 in the differentiation of Hodgkin's disease from NHL has indicated an overall sensitivity of 80 per cent, specificity: 80 per cent, test accuracy: 80

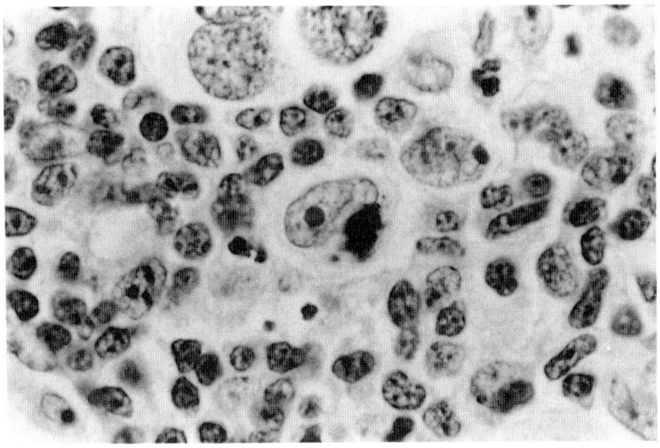

Fig. 4.12. Nodular sclerosing Hodgkin's disease. Strong perinuclear expression of CD15 within an atypical H-RS variant (anti-LeuM1, X1000).

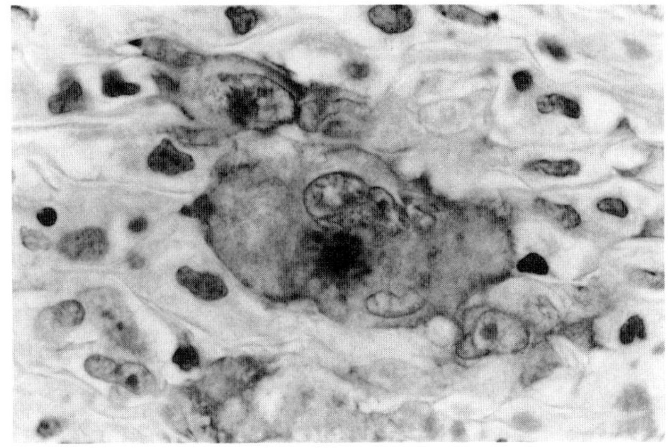

Fig. 4.13. Nodular sclerosing Hodgkin's disease. Perinuclear globular and weak membranous expression of CD30 by an H-RS variant (anti-BerH2, X1000).

per cent, predictive value of a positive result: 86 per cent, and predictive value of a negative result: 73 per cent (Hall and D'Ardenne, 1987). In practical terms, these figures indicate that, given an equal prevalence of HD and T-cell lymphoma, the use of CD15 immunostains alone, will give misleading results in approximately one of every five cases tested.

CD15 can be induced in normal mitogen-activated T4 cells and is more likely to be expressed in T-cell lymphomas bearing an activated phenotype and containing large atypical, pleomorphic tumour cells (Wieczorek et al., 1985). As CD15 immunostaining is more likely to be used in situations where atypical and Hodgkin's-like cells are present, it is likely that the use of the test will select for T-cell tumours with a high probability for CD15 positivity. In practical terms therefore, a positive CD15 is likely to be of less predictive or diagnostic value than even the quoted specificity figures would suggest.

CD30 CD30 (BerH2, Ki-1), was initially thought to be specific for Hodgkin's disease (Fig. 4.13) and anaplastic large cell lymphoma, (Stein et al., 1985) but is now regarded as a marker of cellular activation, and has been identified in many high grade T- and B-cell lymphomas as well as non-lymphoid tumours including embryonal carcinoma. In the differentiation of classical Hodgkin's disease from anaplastic large cell lymphoma, CD30 has no discriminatory value, being positive in 90–95 per cent of HD and nearly 100 per cent of ALC. Similarly, it is of limited usefulness in the differentiation of HD from non-anaplastic high grade T-cell lymphomas, as it can be identified in paraffin sections in up to 60 per cent of such cases (Norton and Isaacson, 1989b). CD30 is therefore, a sensitive but relatively non-specific marker for Hodgkin's disease. Consequently, a negative result has a greater predictive value than a positive result (85–90 per cent vs 60-80 per cent respectively).

Although many series have reported absence of staining for CD45 (LCA) in classical HD, (Bishop et al., 1991; Schmid et al., 1991a) cumulative and other large series indicate that CD45 may be found in approximately 8 to 12 per cent of cases (Diehl et al., 1990; Hall et al., 1988b; Leoncini et al., 1990). Many of these exhibit cytoplasmic, rather than membranous staining, and the 'false positive' rate in paraffin sections is actually lower than 8 per cent if only membranous staining is considered (Chittal et al., 1988; Schmid et al., 1991a). If more sensitive techniques are used, such as PLP-fixation and frozen sections or plastic-embedding, a much higher percentage of cases of Hodgkin's disease can be shown to express CD45 (Agnarsson and Kadin, 1989; Casey et al., 1989). In the differentiation of Hodgkin's disease from other lymphomas therefore, the diagnostic usefulness of CD45 stains is restricted to the interpretation of membranous staining in paraffin-embedded sections. The predictive value of a negative stain for CD45 is also influenced by 'false negative' results in a percentage of non-Hodgkin's lymphomas. Although well over 90 per cent of all NHL are positive for CD45 overall, between 20 and 30 per cent of high grade T-cell and anaplastic large cell lymphomas are negative for CD45, at least in paraffin sections (Falini et al., 1990; Norton and Isaacson, 1989b). In the differentiation of high grade T-cell or anaplastic large cell lymphoma from Hodgkin's disease in paraffin sections therefore, a negative CD45 stain has a relatively poor predictive value of approximately 75 per cent (3:1), assuming an equal incidence for the two diseases. Membrane positivity for CD45 in this context, however, has a diagnostically useful predictive value, approaching 95 per cent (Fig. 4.14).

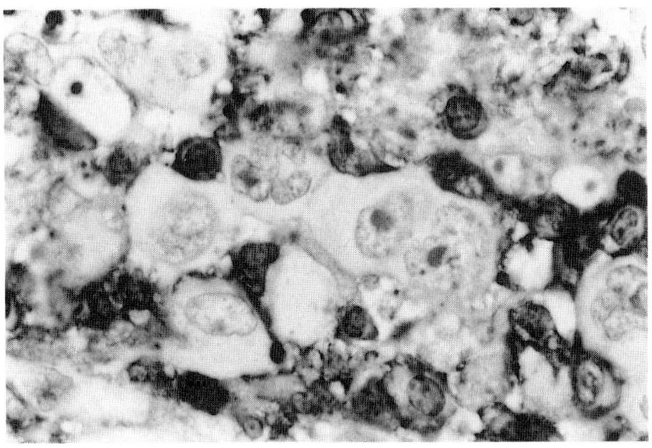

Fig. 4.14. Nodular sclerosing Hodgkin's disease. Stains for CD45 are often difficult to interpret due to staining of the surrounding lymphocytes. A search for two or more H-RS cells in apposition is often necessary to appreciate the CD45 negative phenotype of H-RS cells (anti LCA, X1000).

T-cell antigens The atypical cells of Hodgkin's disease were initially thought to be negative for T- and B-cell antigens, however subsequent reports, often using more sensitive techniques, have clearly shown that H-RS cells can express lineage-specific lymphoid markers (Angel et al., 1987; Diehl et al., 1990). In formalin-fixed, paraffin-embedded tissue sections, up to one third of cases may stain positively with polyclonal anti-CD3 antibodies (Cibull et al., 1989). The staining pattern is usually cytoplasmic, and paranuclear with weak or absent membrane staining (a distribution which may reflect the level of cellular activation present in H-RS cells (Su et al., 1988). Although such staining could be due to cross-reactivity, particularly as the antibody is polyclonal, similar results have been found using monoclonal anti-CD3 antibodies in cytospin preparations, PLP-fixed frozen sections, and plastic embedded sections (Agnarsson and Kadin, 1989; Casey et al., 1989; Falini et al., 1987; Kadin et al., 1988). Furthermore, monoclonal antibody βF1, which recognizes a framework determinant on the T-cell receptor β chain has been shown to stain the membrane of H-RS cells of non-predominance, or 'classical' Hodgkin's disease in 21 to 41 per cent of cases (paraffin-embedded and cryostat sections respectively (Dallenbach and Stein, 1989)). Other T-cell associated or restricted antigens, including CD2, CD4, CD5, CD7 and CD8 have been demonstrated in a high percentage of H-RS cells, using PLP-fixed cryostat sections, but are not generally found using routine techniques (Agnarsson and Kadin, 1989; Falini et al., 1987; Kadin et al., 1988).

Anti-CD43, Anti-CD45RO and anti-CD45RA antibodies including MT1, Leu22, DFT1, UCHL1, 4KB5, MB1, MT2, and KiB3 are almost invariably negative in formalin-fixed paraffin-embedded sections of classical Hodgkin's disease, being expressed in less than 5 per cent of cases (Norton and Isaacson, 1989b). In the rarely reported cases of positivity, the staining is usually cytoplasmic rather than membranous, and it is a useful guide that if tumour cells exhibit membrane positivity for any of these antibodies, a diagnosis of Hodgkin's disease is unlikely (Chittal et al., 1988).

B-cell antigens B-cell specific antigens including CD19, CD20, CD22, and CD24, have been variably demonstrated in mixed cellularity and nodular sclerosing Hodgkin's disease. The percentage of positive cases varies widely from one series to another (15 to 87 per cent) and is greater if cryostat sections rather than paraffin sections are used (Agnarsson and Kadin, 1989; Angel et al., 1987; Casey et al., 1989; Diehl et al., 1990; Falini et al., 1987; Norton and Isaacson, 1989b; Schmid et al., 1991a; Zukerberg et al., 1991b). In paraffin sections, CD20 (L26) is generally reported to be positive on H-RS cells in approximately 15 per cent of cases, however a recent study has claimed a much higher incidence of 58 per cent (Schmid et al., 1991a) (Fig. 4.15). L26 may be coexpressed with LeuM1 (CD15), and in a minority of cases, may be coexpressed with T-cell markers such as polyclonal CD3 or βF1 (Schmid et al., 1991a; Zukerberg et al., 1991b). The significance of T- and B-cell antigen expression in HD remains unclear, and there is no clear cut correlation between the subtype of 'classical' Hodgkin's disease (MC, NS or LD), and the expression of lymphoid markers, although, several authors have noted that they are more commonly expressed in syncytial or monomorphous variants containing large numbers of H-RS cells (Agnarsson and Kadin, 1989; Zukerberg et al., 1991b). Furthermore, there is still disagreement as to whether H-RS cells more commonly express T-cell (Diehl et al., 1990) or B-cell (Schmid et al., 1991a) antigens.

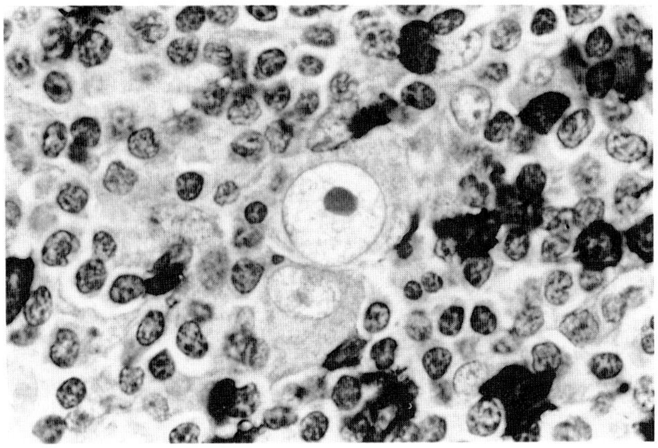

Fig. 4.15. Nodular sclerosing Hodgkin's disease, negative for CD20. Although CD20 is reportedly expressed in a significant number of cases of classical Hodgkin's disease, most cases show negative or very weak staining of H-RS cells in routine preparations. Strong staining for CD20 should prompt a consideration of other diagnoses such as nodular lymphocyte predominance Hodgkin's disease or T-cell-rich B-cell lymphoma (anti-L26, X1000).

Other B-cell related antigens such as MB2 and CDw75 (LN1) may also be detected in paraffin sections of 'classical' Hodgin's disease in a minority of cases. Cumulative series suggest a rate of positivity approaching 20 per cent (Norton and Isaacson, 1989b), although some studies claim a rate of greater than 33 per cent (Schmid et al., 1991a).

Other antigens Epithelial Membrane Antigen (EMA) is commonly expressed in most cases of anaplastic large cell lymphoma and lymphocyte predominance Hodgkin's disease, but it is found in only 8 to 24 per cent of the mixed cellularity, nodular sclerosing, or lymphocyte depleted forms (Chittal et al., 1988; Hall et al., 1988b; Leoncini et al., 1990; Norton and Isaacson, 1989b).

In keeping with the view of H-RS cells as activated lymphoid cells, activation markers CD25 (Tac or Il-2 receptors) and CD71 (transferrin receptors) as well as MHC class II antigens (HLA-DR) are almost invariably expressed (Diehl et al., 1990; Hsu et al., 1990).

CD23 antigen which functions as an IgE receptor and B-cell growth factor, can be identified in paraffin sections using antibody BU38. Its presence has been reported in H-RS cells in over 85 per cent of cases of Hodgkin's disease (Rowlands et al., 1990), however other studies have indicated a much lower rate of positivity, closer to 15 per cent.

Other assorted antigens regularly expressed on H-RS cells include: CD54 (ICAM-1), CD58 (CD2 ligand), peanut agglutinin (PNA), alpha napthyl acetate esterase (ANAE) and alpha 1 anti-trypsin (A1AT) (Diehl et al., 1990).

A wide range of cytokines may be produced by H-RS cells, including Il-1, Il-2, Il-5, Il-6, TNF-α, TNF-β, IFN-γ, GM-CSF, G-CSF, M-CSF, and TGF-β, and many of these can be identified in tissue sections using the appropriate antibodies (Diehl et al., 1990; Kadin et al., 1990; Newcom et al., 1990; Tabibzadeh et al., 1989).

Proliferation antigens Studies of proliferation antigens such as Ki-67 in cryostat sections and cyclin (PCNA), in paraffin sections have demonstrated similar proliferation rates in Reed-Sternberg cells and the mononuclear variants. The growth fraction is reportedly as high as 80 per cent and is therefore similar to that of high grade NHL (Wu et al., 1990), however mitotic rate and S-phase analysis has shown a significantly higher level of proliferation in peripheral T-cell lymphoma than in Hodgkin's disease (Osborne et al., 1990b). Interestingly, anti-cyclin antibody PCNA, which reacts with DNA polymerase-α, shows an 'aberrant' cytoplasmic distribution in H-RS cells (Benjamin and Gown, 1991), the significance of which is unclear.

The status of lymphocyte depleted Hodgkin's disease

With the advent of new, specific monoclonal antibodies, particularly those applicable in paraffin sections, it became possible to reassess retrospectively, large series of cases of Hodgkin's disease which had been diagnosed on morphological criteria alone. In one such study of 198 cases of lymphocyte depletion Hodgkin's disease, Kant and colleagues (Kant et al., 1986) demonstrated that many cases previously diagnosed as lymphocyte depletion Hodgkin's disease were in fact T-cell lymphomas, and that primary lymphocyte depletion Hodgkin's disease is a very uncommon disease. More importantly, following the removal of these T-cell lymphomas from the survival statistics, the cases of true lymphocyte depletion Hodgkin's disease behaved little differently from the other subtypes.

Reactive cells The reactive cellular milieu in 'classical' Hodgkin's disease is well described and includes lymphocytes, histiocytes, plasma cells, eosinophils and fibroblasts. The lymphocytes throughout the infiltrate are predominantly $CD4^+$ T-cells and a characteristic rosette of $CD4^+$ T-cells surrounds each H-RS cell. These are mainly $CD45RO^+$, $CD45RA^-$, and $CD38^+$, i.e. activated, helper-inducer T-cells (Poppema, 1989). The rosetting is often well demonstrated in paraffin sections with the use of anti-CD43 or CD45RO antibodies. In contrast to most T-cell lymphomas, the background T-cells in Hodgkin's disease, being reactive, do not exhibit aberrant phenotypes. Furthermore, the lack of a continuous morphological spectrum between the background T-cells and H-RS cells in Hodgkin's disease, (sometimes referred to as a 'neoplastic cellular hiatus'; (Banks, 1990) is characteristic.

Nodular lymphocyte predominance Hodgkin's disease (paragranuloma)

Nodular lymphocyte predominance Hodgkin's disease is separable from other subtypes using clinical, morphological and immunophenotypic features.

The clinical presentation in a young male with stage 1, axillary, or cervical disease is characteristic (Tefferi et al., 1990). Long-term remission following simple local excision is frequently encountered, and recurrences are as the lymphocyte predominance form, without transformation into mixed cellularity or other subtypes (Banks, 1990). The propensity for transformation, however, into a high grade, large cell, often pleomorphic B-cell lymphoma is now well documented in a small percentage of cases (<5 per cent) (Hansmann et al., 1989; Sundeen et al., 1986).

Morphologically, the nodularity, association with progressively transformed germinal centres, 'garlands' of histiocytes, and the typical morphology of 'L and H' or 'popcorn' variants of Reed–Sternberg cells, are characteristic. The classical description of rare or infrequent Reed–Sternberg cells in this disease is now challenged by a number of authors who deny their existence in this form of Hodgkin's disease (Nicholas et al., 1990).

Immunophenotypically, the 'L and H' or 'popcorn' cells of NLPHD regularly express a B-cell phenotype, usually with coexpression of LCA (CD45) and EMA, and absence of LeuM1 (CD15) and BerH2 (CD30). This pattern is the reverse of that generally seen in the classical, non-lymphocyte predominance subtypes (see above) (Bishop et al., 1991; Chittal et al., 1988; Hall et al., 1988b; Nicholas et al., 1990; Norton and Isaacson, 1989b; Pinkus and Said, 1985; Timens et al., 1986).

B-cell and T-cell antigens B-cell specific antigens including CD19, CD20 (L26) (Fig. 4.16), CD22, CDw75 (LN1) and MB2, are strongly expressed in most cases of NLPHD, although the frequency of expression varies significantly in different series. A number of reports have demonstrated B-cell antigens in 100 per cent of cases studied (Hall et al., 1988b; Norton and Isaacson, 1989b; Pinkus and Said, 1985; Pinkus and Said, 1988), however the most recent cumulative survey indicates positivity for B-cell antigens in approximately 70 per cent of cases (Bishop et al., 1991). As the non-lymphocyte predominance subtypes of Hodgkin's disease may also express B-cell antigens (range 20 to 76 per cent; (Norton and Isaacson, 1989b; Schmid et al., 1991a), it is apparent that B-cell antigen expression alone, is unlikely to differentiate NLPHD from the other Hodgkin's disease subtypes.

CDw75 (LN1) is expressed in 20 to 55 per cent of cases of non-lymphocyte predominance forms of Hodgkin's disease (Norton and Isaacson, 1989b; Schmid et al., 1991a), but it is regularly found in NLPHD and suggests follicle centre cell differentiation. CD45RA (4KB5, MB1, MT2 and KiB3) is rarely expressed in this or any other form of Hodgkin's disease, and its absence in the 'L and H variant' B-cells of NLPHD is further evidence for a follicle centre cell derivation (Hall et al., 1988b; Norton and Isaacson, 1989b). Leu8, reportedly expressed on H-RS cells of most forms of HD, is usually negative in NLPHD, also suggesting follicle centre cell differentiation (Timens et al., 1986).

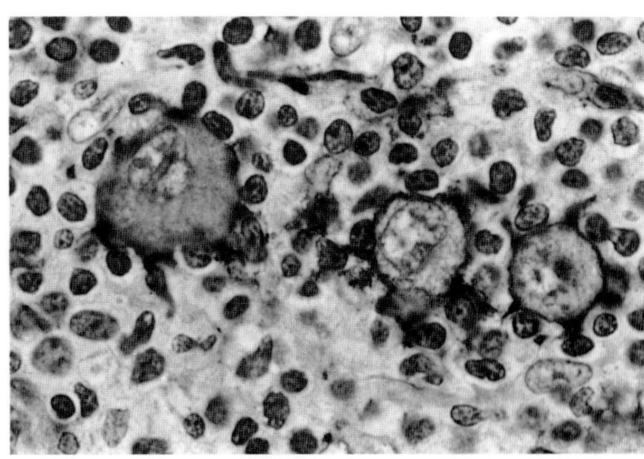

Fig. 4.16. Nodular lymphocyte predominance Hodgkin's disease. The H-RS variants typically show strong membranous staining for B-cell antigens such as CD20, CDw75 and MB2 (anti-L26, X1000).

T-cell associated or specific antigens (CD43, CD45RO, CD3, βF1) are consistently negative, or very rarely positive (Bishop et al., 1991; Cibull et al., 1989; Dallenbach and Stein, 1989; Kadin et al., 1988; Norton and Isaacson, 1989b). Cytoplasmic J chain expression has been demonstrated (Stein et al., 1986), and is a clear indication of B-cell lineage. Cytoplasmic lambda and kappa light chains have been identified in L and H cells (Timens et al., 1986), possibly reflecting uptake of exogenous immunoglobulin. Numerous studies have failed to demonstrate light chain restriction, and molecular studies have failed to demonstrate clonal rearrangement of immunoglobulin genes or expression of bcl-2 gene products (Algara et al., 1991; Knowles et al., 1986; Linden et al., 1988; Said et al., 1991). In a recent paraffin section study, Schmid and colleagues claim to have demonstrated light chain restriction in a majority of cases of nodular lymphocyte predominance Hodgkin's disease (Schmid et al., 1991b). Curiously, all cases expressed kappa light chain. This finding has not been reproduced elsewhere, and the status of NLPHD as a neoplasm therefore, remains unresolved (Nicholas et al., 1990; Said et al., 1991). In fact, the earlier Jackson and Parker term 'paragranuloma,' adopted by European authors and implying a 'granuloma-like process', may yet prove to be particularly apt.

CD45 Membrane expression of leucocyte common antigen (CD45) by 'L and H' cells has been reported in approximately 75 per cent of cases of nodular lymphocyte predominance Hodgkin's disease in paraffin sections (range: 55 to 100 per cent). By comparison, less than 10 per cent of Hodgkin's -RS cells in the non-lymphocyte predominant forms of HD show membrane positivity in paraffin sections (Norton and Isaacson, 1989b; Poppema et al., 1991).

CD15 CD15 (LeuM1) expression is seen in approximately 25 per cent of cases of NLPHD (Bishop et al., 1991; Norton and Isaacson, 1989b) compared with expression by H-RS cells in approximately 90 per cent of other forms of Hodgkin's disease. CD15 antigen is in fact present in NLPHD but it is masked by sialylation. Pretreatment with neuraminidase unmasks the antigen and 'L and H' cells then stain positively for CD15 (Hsu et al., 1986). The expression of unsialylated CD15 in the non-predominance forms of 'classical' HD may in fact, reflect altered metabolism of the neoplastic state.

CD30 BerH2 (CD30) is expressed on the surface membrane of 'L and H' cells in 14 to 45 per cent of cases (Bishop et al., 1991; Norton and Isaacson, 1989b). This contrasts with 90 to 95 per cent for the other subtypes of Hodgkin's disease.

EMA EMA is expressed in approximately 15 per cent of cases of non-lymphocyte predominance Hodgkin's disease (range 8 to 24 per cent), however cumulative series indicate positivity in 55 to 60 per cent of NLPHD (Bishop et al., 1991; Norton and Isaacson, 1989b) (Fig. 4.17).

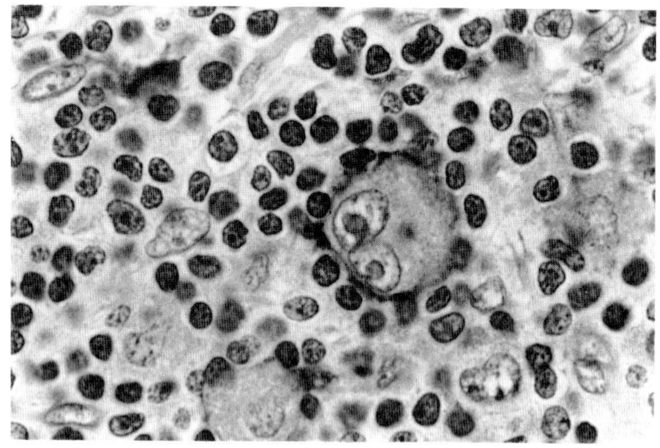

Fig. 4.17. Nodular lymphocyte predominance Hodgkin's disease. Expression by H-RS variants of EMA (anti-EMA, X1000).

Reactive cells The reactive cellular milieu in nodular lymphocyte predominance Hodgkin's disease is characteristic, and may be of diagnostic value. In most forms of Hodgkin's disease, CD4+ve T-cells constitute the major reactive lymphoid component, however nodular lymphocyte predominance Hodgkin's disease, develops in the context of progressively transformed germinal centres (PTGC) and has a predominantly B-cell milieu (see Progressive Transformation of Germinal Centres). Despite the B-cell predominance, $CD4^+$ T-cells form a rosette around single 'L and H' variants, much as they do in the other forms of Hodgkin's disease (Figs 4.18a and 4.18b).

A large proportion of the $CD4^+$ T-cells within the nodules are also $Leu7^+$ and $Leu8^-$. This unique T-cell subset is normally confined to follicle centres, is present in PTGC, NLPHD, and follicular lymphomas, and is thought to be important in supporting B-cell differentiation. In cases of Hodgkin's disease where the nodular architecture is indistinct, the identification of $CD4^+$, $Leu7^+$ T-cells may therefore provide useful evidence in support of nodular paragranuloma.

Epithelioid cell clusters, often forming 'garlands' around the follicle mantle zones, are present in roughly one quarter of cases of PTGC, but are usually present in NLPHD and may be an early sign of Hodgkin's disease (Hansmann et al., 1990; Poppema, 1989; Timens et al., 1986).

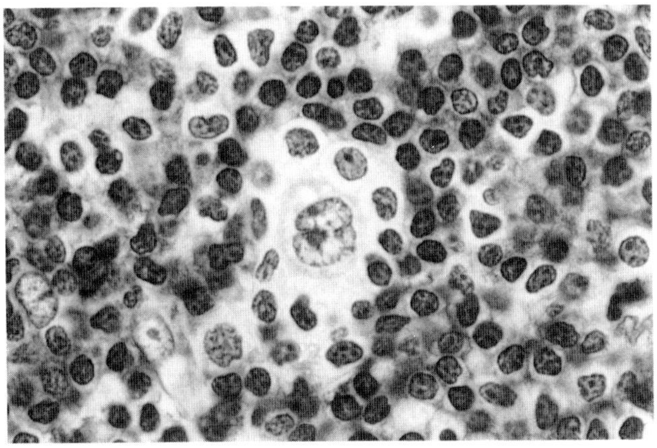

Fig. 4.18a. Nodular lymphocyte predominance Hodgkin's disease. Unlike classical HD, the nodular lymphocyte predominance form has a predominantly B-cell reactive milieu. Note the CD45RA negative zone surrounding the central H-RS variant (anti-4KB5, X1000).

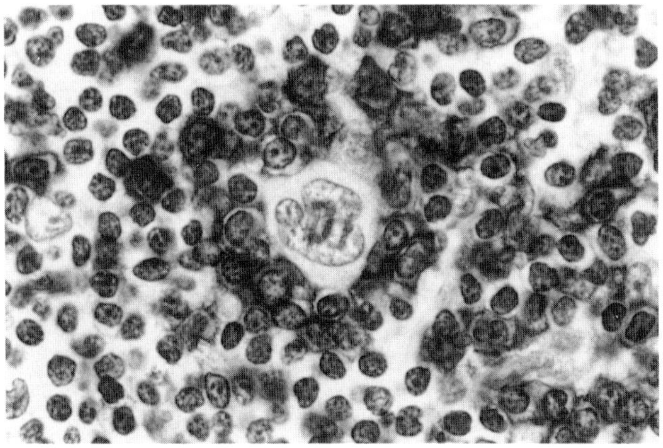

Fig. 4.18b Nodular lymphocyte predominance Hodgkin's disease. The same case stained for CD45RO shows that despite having a predominantly B-cell reactive environment, the H-RS cells of NLPHD have a T-cell rosette typical of all forms of HD (anti-UCHL1, ×1000).

Diffuse lymphocyte predominance Hodgkin's disease (HD)

Although NLPHD or nodular paragranuloma is now a clinicopathological entity, distinct from other forms of Hodgkin's disease, and probably related to follicle centre B-cells, the status of the diffuse form (diffuse paragranuloma) remains unproven.

A number of studies have examined the clinical, morphological and immunophenotypic features of diffuse lymphocyte predominance Hodgkin's disease, but have yielded conflicting results (Bishop et al., 1991; Nicholas et al., 1990; Regula et al., 1987; Regula et al., 1988; Tefferi et al., 1990).

These discrepancies are not surprising if, as suggested by Poppema and colleagues (1979), DLPHD is seen as a heterogenous group, of which 'diffuse paragranuloma' is only one form.

In Hodgkin's disease, a diffuse pattern with lymphocyte predominance may develop in at least three ways:

1. a diffuse counterpart to NLPHD ie. 'diffuse paragranuloma';
2. a lymphocyte-rich form of mixed cellularity HD, (referred to by some European authors as 'diffuse non-paragranuloma');
3. early, or interfollicular involvement by mixed cellularity HD.

Most authors have suggested that diffuse paragranuloma is closely related to the nodular form, sharing the same cytological features, immunophenotypic profile for B-cell antigens, CD15, CD30, CD45 and EMA, and a similar protracted clinical course. Moreover, cases have been described in which both nodular and diffuse areas coexist. (Nicholas et al., 1990; Regula et al., 1987). The latter two forms of diffuse lymphocyte predominance HD on the other hand, belong with 'classical' HD, sharing the typical immunophenotypic profile of MCHD and propensity for clinical and histological progression.

Distinguishing between these three forms of DLPHD, is one of the most difficult diagnostic tasks within haematopathology. Morphology alone, is an unreliable guide (Bishop et al., 1991), however Nicholas and colleagues (1990) have demonstrated that by using a combination of cytological features and immunophenotype, a diagnostic distinction is possible, and that diffuse paragranuloma, so-defined, is an uncommon disease (Nicholas et al., 1990).

Although the reactive cells in nodular paragranuloma are predominantly B-cells, the diffuse form has consistently been shown to be associated with a T-cell environment. All three forms of diffuse lymphocyte predominance Hodgkin's disease therefore, exist within a predominantly T-cell milieu (Bishop et al., 1991; Nicholas et al., 1990). Diffuse paragranuloma therefore is, in effect, a form of T-cell-rich B-cell lymphoma (Chittal et al., 1991).

Histiocytic disorders

There are probably no terms in haematopathology that have suffered greater abuse than 'histiocytic' and 'histiocytosis'. Before the advent of immunophenotyping, it was assumed that any lymphoma of large cell size, exhibiting phagocytic properties or showing a sinusoidal distribution in secondary lymphoid organs, was of histiocytic origin. Thus, all large cell lymphomas were once designated as 'histiocytic', and the term 'malignant histiocytosis' encompassed a wide range of conditions including tumours of lymphoid origin such as Anaplastic Large Cell lymphoma. Histiocytic Medullary Reticulosis is a clinicopathological identity exhibiting all three of these characteristics, in combination with the clinical features of a haemophagocytic syndrome. It is now seen as a heterogenous disorder, most commonly a reactive, lymphokine induced, phagocytic syndrome secondary to infection or an underlying T-cell lymphoma (Boyd et al., 1988; Craig et al., 1992; Daum et al., 1987; Jaffe et al., 1983; Komp and Perry, 1991; Kueck et al., 1989; Miyashita et al., 1991; Smith et al., 1992b).

With the development in the late 1970s, of polyclonal antibodies to a limited range of enzymes, the diagnostic emphasis became over dependent upon antibodies such as α-1-antitrypsin, α-1-antichymotrypsin and lysozyme. Consequently, a number of lymphoid conditions such as Enteropathy Associated T-cell Lymphoma (EATCL), and childhood malignancies, were mistakenly assumed to be of histiocytic origin (Ornvold et al., 1992).

Since that time, improvements in our understanding of lymphocyte biology have identified a number of lymphoid conditions erroneously included within the 'histiocytic' disorders. Unfortunately, our knowledge of monocyte ontogeny and function has not kept pace with these advances, and what remains of the histiocytic disorders is a collection of uncommon diseases, poorly defined, and including both neoplastic conditions and proliferations of undetermined clonality and cause.

Currently, the most widely accepted classification of the histiocytic disorders is that advocated by the Writing Group of the Histiocyte Society (the Writing Group of the Histiocyte Society, 1987, Komp and Perry, 1991) (Table 4.7).

Class 1 histiocytoses – Langerhans' cell histiocytosis

Of the Class 1 and 2 histiocytoses, Langerhans' cell histiocytosis (LCH) is the most important in terms of prevalence, morbidity and mortality. There is no evidence that the disorder is a clonal neoplasm and DNA studies have not detected evidence of aneuploidy (Favara, 1991). Most authors view the disease as being the result of immune disregulation, with localised or occasionally diffuse activation and proliferation of histiocytic cells showing a LC phenotype.

According to the Writing Group of the Histiocyte Society (1987), a 'presumptive diagnosis' of LCH is made when conventional stains reveal a typical histological pattern. A 'designated' diagnosis is made when at least two of the following are present: ATPase +ve, S100 +ve, α-d-mannisodase +ve, or peanut lectin +ve. A 'definitive diagnosis' requires the presence of Birbeck granules or expression of CD1.

Despite the close phenotypic and ultrastructural similarities between LC and the pathological Langerhans' cells of LCH, there is no evidence that LCH derives directly from Langerhans' cells. It may equally arise from the induction of LC characteristics in proliferating monocytes, histiocytes or dendritic cells. The phenotype of LCH cells in fact differs slightly from that of normal epidermal LCs and more closely resembles that of node-based LCs in dermatopathic lymphadenopathy (Ruco et al., 1989).

In frozen section material, LCH cells regularly stain for Class 1 and Class 2 MHC antigens, CD1, vimentin, S-100, peanut lectin, ATPase, and α-d-mannosidase. More variable positivity is found with antibodies to CD4, CD14, CD15, CD16, CD25, CD30, CD45, CD21, CD35, CD74, and EMA (Favara, 1991; Ornvold et al., 1990; Ruco et al., 1989). CD15 is normally present in a sialylated form and its demonstration requires prior digestion with neuraminidase (Santamaria et al., 1988). Antibody Ki-M1 may also stain some cases of LCH. CD57 (transferrin receptor), CD68 and γ interferon, are frequently present and discriminate between LCH cells and normal LCs.

CD1 is a sensitive marker for LCH, being expressed in all cases. It is not entirely specific however, and can be found in some marrow derived cells and IRCs.

Birbeck granules, the gold standard LCH diagnosis, are identified in a variable percentage of LCH cells and appear to arise from the endocytosis of cell membrane antigens following their cross-linkage. Their formation may be dependent upon prior exposure to epithelium (Shamoto et al., 1992).

In fixed paraffin-embedded sections, antibodies to S100 are a sensitive marker for LCH, and have some specificity in $CD45^{+}$ tumours. Caution should be exercised in the

Table 4.7. The histiocytic disorders

Class	1 Histiocytoses	
	Langerhans cell histiocytosis (histiocytosis X)	
	includes:	Eosinophilic Granuloma
		Hand-Schuller Christian disease
		Letterer-Siwe disease
Class	2. Histiocytoses	
	Haemophagocytic syndromes	
	includes:	Infection associated haemophagocytic syndrome
		Familial haemophagocytic lymphohistiocytosis
		Sinus histiocytosis with massive lymphadenopathy
Class	3. Histiocytoses	
	Malignant histiocytic conditions	
	Leukaemias	
	Acute Myelomonocytic Leukaemia (M4)	
	Acute Monocytic Leukaemia (M5)	
	Chronic Myelomonocytic Leukaemia (CMML)	
	Malignant Histiocytosis	
	Ordinary histiocytic type	
	Dendritic cell types	
	Langerhans' cells	
	Interdigitating cell type	
	Non-specific dendritic cell type	
	True Histiocytic Lymphoma	
	Ordinary histiocytic type	
	Dendritic cell types	
	Langerhans' cells	
	Interdigitating cell type	
	Non-specific dendritic cell type	

Source: Modified from: The Writing Group of the Histiocyte Society, 1987, and Favara, 1991

interpretation of S100 positivity alone however, as polyclonal S100 antibodies may stain some T-cell lymphomas (Hanson et al., 1991; Ruco et al., 1984; Takahashi et al., 1985), myeloid leukaemias (Elliott et al., 1989; Horny et al., 1990a), neoplasms of dendritic cells (Delabie et al., 1991; Monda et al., 1986), and some examples of Sinus Histiocytosis with Massive Lymphadenopathy (Miettinen et al., 1987). Furthermore, positive staining for S100 is not universally present in LCH (Ruco et al., 1989). Anti-CD68 antibodies such as KP1, are positive in most cases, but in less than one third of the LCH cells (Ruco et al., 1989). This finding parallels the identification in frozen sections, of histiocytic markers such as CD14 in a minority of cells. Antibodies to enzymes such as lysozyme and α1-antichymotyrypsin stain less than 20 per cent of cells in most cases and are of little diagnostic value.

Class 2 histiocytoses – reactive haemophagocytic syndromes (RHS)

Although haemophagocytic syndromes may rarely be due to direct phagocytosis by tumour cells as described in malignant histiocytosis, the majority of cases are due to activation and proliferation of reactive histiocytes, either secondary to infection or an underlying lymphoma (Chan et al., 1987b). The resulting syndrome accounts for many of the cases previously designated as histiocytic medullary reticulosis, and is characterized by fevers, pancytopaenia, hepatosplenomegaly, coagulopathy and frequently, death (Jaffe et al., 1983).

Infection associated haemophagocytic syndrome, originally described by Risdall in relation to viral infection (Risdall et al., 1979), is now known to occur following a range of viral, bacterial and fungal infections including

Epstein-Barr virus, Influenza A virus, Dengue fever, salmonellosis, tuberculosis and leishmaniasis (Chan et al., 1987b; Daum et al., 1987; Miyashita et al., 1991; Ohshima et al., 1991; Potter et al., 1991; Wong et al., 1991). An underlying immunological deficiency is usually thought to be the cause. Familial Haemophagocytic Lymphohistiocytosis appears to be a closely related disorder occurring in infants and young children, possibly as a result of an autosomally inherited immune defect (Loy et al., 1991). The terminal phase of Chediak–Higashi syndrome also exhibits similar features.

T-cell lymphomas, particularly those of angiocentric type, may occasionally present, or terminate with a secondary reactive haemophagocytic syndrome (RHS) (Boyd et al., 1988; Craig et al., 1992; Jaffe et al., 1983; Kueck et al., 1989; Ng et al., 1986; Smith et al., 1992b).

In all the above, it is hypothesized that dysregulated lymphokine production by T-cells directly leads to the haemophagocytic manifestations. In a significant percentage of cases however, no underlying cause is found.

Sinus histiocytosis with massive lymphadenopathy (SHML, or Rosai–Dorfman disease) is characterized by nodal and extranodal infiltrates of histiocytes, often showing prominent emperipolesis, and frequently associated with an underlying immune defect. Localized extranodal masses involving skin, respiratory tract, bone, genitourinary system and soft tissues often dominate the clinical picture (Foucar et al., 1990; Montgomery et al., 1992).

Phenotypically, the proliferating cells in all the above conditions show the phenotype expected for phagocytic histiocytes. In frozen sections there is positivity for CD4, CD11c, CD25, CD45 and CD68. Variable positivity is found with antibodies to CD11b, CD13, CD14 and CD33. In paraffin sections, anti-CD68 antibodies (KP1, EBM11) and MAC387 are positive within the phagocytic cells while lymphoid markers are negative (Smith et al., 1992b). Anti-CD45RO and CD43 antibodies (UCHL1 and MT1) may however show weak staining. SHML differs slightly from the other class 2 histiocytoses in that the phagocytic cells are usually positive for S100 protein (Miettinen et al., 1987; Montgomery et al., 1992; Paulli et al., 1992).

Apart from confirming the histiocytic nature of the phagocytic cells in these conditions, phenotyping currently has little value, and in conditions other than SHML, the diagnostic process is strongly focused upon the search for an infective agent. In idiopathic cases, an underlying lymphoma should be sought as this is often occult or remote from the site of phagocytic activity (Boyd et al., 1988; Jaffe et al., 1983). In either event, the prognosis in a full-blown haemophagocytic syndrome is grave.

Class 3 histiocytoses – malignant histiocytic conditions

Histiocytic malignancies other than the leukaemias are extremely rare and, it is generally agreed, constitute less than 1 per cent of all 'lymphomas' (Levine et al., 1991; Ralfkiaer et al., 1990). Historically, the term 'malignant histiocytosis' (MH), coined by Rappaport in 1966, refers to an aggressive malignancy, often haemophagocytic, and systemic from the outset, whilst 'true histiocytic lymphoma' (THL) has been used to indicate a localised nodal or extranodal 'lymphoma' bearing morphological and immunophenotypic hallmarks of histiocytic, rather than lymphoid lineage. In current usage, the differences between the two have become blurred, and some authors make no distinction. The earlier term of 'histiocytic medullary reticulosis' (HMR) (Scott and Robb-Smith, 1939) is analogous to MH but probably included a majority of cases which we would now designate as reactive haemophagocytic syndromes.

Since the development of hybridoma technology, and later genotypic analysis, it has become possible in most cases to distinguish between lymphoid and histiocytic tumours with accuracy.

Most would now require for a diagnosis of histiocytic malignancy, the absence of specific T-cell or B-cell antigens, coupled with the expression of histiocyte-related antigens and enzymes (Levine et al., 1991). Ralfkiaer and colleagues (1990), extended this definition to include the requirement that the TCR and imunoglobulin genes should be in the germline state, and in a series of 925 malignant lymphomas, found only 4 cases which satisfied these criteria (0.4 per cent). All 4 cases in this tightly defined subset presented with cutaneous involvement and showed an aggressive course with rapid dissemination and early death.

In the extended classification of the histiocytic disorders given (see Table 4.7), both MH and THL are further subdivided according to whether the tumour cells show phagocytic or accessory cell differentiation. The latter group includes cases of putative IRC (Chan and Zaatari, 1986; Nakamura et al., 1988; Weiss et al., 1990; Yamakawa et al., 1992), DRC (Monda et al., 1986), and LC sarcoma (Benezra et al., 1991; Delabie et al., 1991).

Phenotypic differences between MH and THL have not been clearly defined, however it has been suggested that THL is less likely to express CD11b or CD14 than MH, analogous to tissue histiocytes, whereas the cells of MH more closely resemble peripheral blood monocytes (Hsu et al., 1991).

In frozen sections, histiocytic malignancies other than those of dendritic cell type, show the following phenotype: HLA-DR$^+$, CD1$^-$, CD2$^-$, CD3$^-$, CD4$^+$, CD5$^-$, CD7$^-$, CD8$^-$, CD11b$^{+/-}$, CD11c$^+$, CD13$^{+/-}$, CD14$^{+/-}$, *CD15*$^{+/-}$, CD19$^-$, CD20$^-$, CD22$^-$, CD25$^+$, *CD30*$^{+/-}$, CDw32$^{+/-}$, CD33$^{+/-}$, CD45$^+$, CD45RO$^+$, CD68$^+$, β*F1*$^-$, TCRδ-1$^-$, DakoDRC(R4/23)$^-$, NSE$^+$, S100$^-$, Lysozyme$^{+/-}$, α1-antichymotrypsin$^{+/-}$, (Cattoretti et al., 1990; Hanson et al., 1989; Hsu et al., 1991; Ralfkiaer et al., 1990; Roholl et al., 1988). Italicized CD groups are those in which the findings depend upon the case selection criteria. CD30 in particular is found to be positive in a majority of some series of so-called MH, in which EMA$^+$, TCR$^+$ cases of anaplastic large cell (ALC) lymphoma are included. In this context, ALC lymphomas are a controversial area. Although many cases of T or B lineage ALC have been erroneously designated as MH in the past, there is evidence that a small number of ALC lymphomas may in fact be of histiocytic lineage (Banks et al., 1990; Carbone et al., 1990; Gogusev et al., 1991). This is further supported by the finding that macrophages are capable of CD30 expression (Andreesen et al., 1989).

Evidence for IRC differentiation would include the expression of S100 and ATPase. DRC differentiation would be favoured by weak or negative S100 expression with positivity for antibody Dako DRC (R4/23) or Ki-M4. CD1 expression would favour LC differentiation, however it is not entirely specific for LCs or LCH cells and may occasionally be detected in interdigitating reticulum and other cells (Andersen et al., 1992).

In fixed, paraffin-embedded sections, the histiocytic malignancies (other than those of dendritic cell type) show the following phenotype: CD45$^+$, CD45RO$^+$, CD68 (EBM11, KP1, Ki-M6)$^+$, Mac387$^+$, LN4$^+$, LN5$^+$, Ber MAC3$^+$, S100$^-$, NSE$^{+/-}$, EMA$^{+/-}$ (Backe et al., 1991; Bhoopat et al., 1988; Hanson et al., 1989; Kelly et al., 1988b; Micklem et al., 1989; Warnke et al., 1989).

If one excludes the characteristic dot-like cytoplasmic positivity seen with anti-CD68 antibodies (KP1 and EBM11) in low grade B-cell lymphomas, the antigen has demonstated a high level of specificity and sensitivity for histiocytic tumours in a number of series (Gloghini et al., 1990; Horny et al., 1990b; Kelly et al., 1988a; Kelly et al., 1988b; Micklem et al., 1989; Pulford et al., 1989; Warnke et al., 1989). MAC387 is more sensitive in some series, but lacks specificity and is not leucocyte restricted (Loftus et al., 1991).

When only paraffin sections are available, the presence of S100 positivity in a CD45$^+$ malignancy may be perplexing. The differential diagnosis then includes malignancies of IRC, LC, T-cell, and myeloid or myelomonocytic origin. If leukaemia can be excluded, and T-cell antigens are absent, the lesion is usually assumed to be a tumour of dendritic origin and a search for Birbeck granules is the best recourse.

Extramedullary myeloid and myelomonocytic tumours – (chloroma)

Extramedullary myeloid or myelomonocytic malignancy enters into the differential diagnosis of all diffuse lymphomas of large cell or Burkitt's type and should be seriously considered whenever a lymphoma exhibits atypical morphological or phenotypic features.

In frozen section material, the tumour cells express myeloid or monocytic antigens including CD11, CD13, CD15, CD33, CD45 and CD68. Variable results are found with antibodies to CD4, CD14 and CD25. T-cell specific (CD2, CD3, CD5, CD7, CD8, βF1, TCRδ-1) and B-cell specific (CD19, CD20, CD22, CD37), and other antibodies (CD10, TdT, CD30) are negative, although examples of so-called lineage infidelity, with expression of CD2, CD19 or CD20, are well described, and TdT may be found in rare cases of acute myeloid leukaemia. The enzymes myeloperoxidase and chloroacetate esterase are positive.

In fixed, paraffin-embedded material, antibody MAC387, anti-lysozyme, and anti-CD68 antibodies stain the majority of cases of acute myeloid leukaemia (AML) FAB subtypes M2, M3, M4 and M5, while monoclonal antibodies to glycophorin C label FAB subtype M6 (Kurec et al., 1990). Antibody NP57, raised against neutrophil elastase, an enzyme located within the primary azurophilic granules of neutrophils, is positive in approximately three quarters of AML FAB subtypes M1-5 (Pulford et al., 1988; Ralfkiaer et al., 1989). The enzyme myeloperoxidase appears earlier in myeloid development than neutrophil elastase, and anti-myeloperoxidase antibody MPO has been shown to be a highly sensitive and specific reagent, complimentary to NP57 and effective in decalcifed bone marrow sections

(Buccheri et al., 1992; Pinkus and Pinkus, 1991; Pulford et al., 1988). Megakaryoblastic cells may be identified in fixed tissues with the use of monclonal antibody Y2/51, reactive against platelet glycoprotein IIIA. Anti-CD43 antibodies MT1, DFT1 and Leu 22 stain a majority of cases of AML (Andrade et al., 1988; Horny et al., 1990a; Said et al., 1989). Anti-CD15 antibody LeuM1 is expressed, often focally within a small majority of cases (Davey et al., 1988). Antibodies to lysozyme stain positively in approximately half of AML cases (Kurec et al., 1990).

Antibodies to CD45 are weakly positive in most cases. Isoforms of CD45 are variably expressed according to the degree of monocytic differentiation. Normal myeloid cells are all CD45RO positive, while CD45RA is expressed by 3–15 per cent of cells (Caldwell et al., 1991). In myeloid leukaemias however, anti-CD45RA antibodies Ki-B3, 4KB5 and MB1 are frequently positive (Elghetany et al., 1991; Horny et al., 1990a). Other antibodies which may stain myeloid proliferations include Ber MAC3, MB2, LN2 and S100 (Andrade et al., 1988; Backe et al., 1991; Elliott et al., 1989; Horny et al., 1990a; Ng et al., 1988; Ng et al., 1987b).

A traditional Leder's chloroacetate esterase preparation remains one of the most useful stains in this context, surpassed in sensitivity only by antibodies MPO and NP57 (Ralfkiaer et al., 1989).

Mast cell disease

Mast cell disease may be considered in the differential diagnosis of a number of conditions including Hairy cell leukaemia and some cutaneous infiltrates. Normal and neoplastic mast cells express HLA-DR, CD45, CD9, CD33, lysozyme, α1-antitrypsin, α1-antichymotrypsin, and chloroacetate esterase (Horny et al., 1990b; Horny et al., 1988). CD25, CD45RA (4KB5) and CD43 (MT1, Leu22) may be expressed in some cases (Anstey et al., 1991; Said et al., 1989). Anti-CD68 antibodies such as KP1 stain the granules of normal and neoplastic mast cells and are a reliable marker (Warnke et al., 1989). MAC387 is negative in all cases, and it has been suggested that a combination of MAC387 and chloroacetate esterase stain may be useful to differentiate between neutrophils, monocytic cells and mast cells (Chilosi et al., 1990b; Horny et al., 1990b). Recently, monoclonal antibody AA1 specific for human mast cell tryptase has been produced and may prove to be of diagnostic use (Walls et al., 1990).

Kikuchi – Fujimoto disease (histiocytic necrotizing lymphadenitis)

Originally described in Japan, Kikuchi–Fujimoto disease has subsequently been reported from many parts of the world. Widely thought to be a response to a viral infection (resembling an autologous mixed lymphocyte reaction), the histological appearances are closely mimicked by systemic lupus erythematosus (Medeiros et al., 1989), and are significant for being easily confused with large cell lymphoma (Chamulak et al., 1990; Facchetti et al., 1988). The diagnosis can usually be made with some confidence with good routine H & E sections and an appropriate clinical history, however the unique immunophenotypic findings provide valuable confirmation of the diagnosis.

The disease typically presents in young women with posterior cervical lymphadenopathy, often preceded by a mild systemic illness with fever and myalgia. Histologically, the sheets of large cells with angulated nuclei, admixed blasts and areas of necrosis, may be mistaken for large cell lymphoma. Clues to the correct diagnosis include: (i) preserved architecture with partial involvement; (ii) reactive hyperplasia within the remaining node; (iii) absence of neutrophils or true necrosis and the presence of apoptotic debris; (iv) characteristic cytology of the histiocytic cells and (v) the presence of plasmacytoid monocytes surrounding the affected zone. Appearances vary according to the timing of biopsy in this short-lived disease. In early involvement, there may be little or no necrosis (or apoptosis), and the risk of misdiagnosis is high.

The infiltrate consists, in varying proportions, of necrotic or apoptotic cells, macrophages, plasmacytoid monocytes, immunoblasts and lymphocytes. In most cases, macrophages predominate and are stained with CD68, MAC387, and lysozyme. In frozen sections they are positive for CD4 and HLA-DR with variable positivity for CD11b, CD11c, CD14 and CD38.

Plasmacytoid monocytes (PM) are usually a major component, and stain strongly for MT1, Leu22 (CD43), KP1 (CD68), LN2 (CD74) and Ki-M1P in paraffin sections (Hansmann et al., 1992). Variable expression is found for LN1 (CDw75), but MAC387 is negative. In frozen sections, PM express CD4, CD36, CD38, CD71 and HLA-DR.

The accompanying lymphoid infitrate is reported in some instances to consist predominantly of B-cells (Chamulak et al., 1990). In the experience of this laboratory however, and in most other studies, T-cells constitute by far the majority of the accompanying lymphocytes and immunoblasts. These are found to be positive for CD2, 3, 4, 5, 8, 38 and 71 in frozen sections, and MT1 or Leu22 (CD43) in paraffin sections. CD8$^+$ cells usually predominate over CD4$^+$ T-cells, in keeping with the concept of a cytotoxic reactive process (Facchetti et al., 1989).

The infitrate in Kikuchi's disease therefore consists of CD68$^+$, CD43$^+$, MAC387$^-$, Ki-M1P $^+$ plasmacytoid monocytes, CD68$^+$, MAC387$^+$ macrophages, with scattered T-cells, B-cells, T-immunoblasts and infrequent B-immunoblasts. This contrasts with large cell lymphoma, which consists largely of CD20$^+$ B-cells, or rarely of CD45R0$^+$, CD3$^+$ T-cells, which practically never express CD68.

Angiofollicular lymph node hyperplasia (AFLNH) – Castleman's disease

The eponymous title 'Castleman's disease' suggests a degree of singularity which, unfortunately, is entirely lacking in this disease, and conceals marked clinical and pathological heterogeneity.

Histologically, both hyaline vascular and plasma cell variants feature 'regressively transformed follicles', in which hypocellular germinal centres are surrounded by expanded mantle zones, often showing a distinctive 'onion ring' lamination. The former variant is characterized by follicle vascular proliferation with hyalinization, while the latter shows interfollicular plasmacytic proliferation. Either form may be solitary or multicentric, however multicentric types are more commonly of the plasma cell variety.

Clinically, the plasma cell type in particular, is associated with systemic autoimmune manifestations including fevers, night sweats, anaemia, thrombocytopaenia, skin rashes, peripheral neuropathy and renal dysfunction. Changes of AFLNH have been described in lymph nodes of patients with autoimmune disorders including rheumatoid arthtitis and POEMS syndrome and have been described in association with Kaposi's sarcoma, AIDS and malignant lymphoma (West, 1989).

Although cases with solitary nodal involvement frequently undergo spectacular remission of symptoms following simple surgical excision, multicentric variants not uncommonly follow a rapid downhill course with a high mortality.

Genotypic and immunophenotypic studies have shown that while the hyaline vascular form is polyclonal with germline immunoglobulin genes, the plasma cell variant not infrequently shows clonal immunoglobulin gene rearrangement and immunoglobulin light chain restriction, sometimes with clonal TCR rearrangement (Hanson et al., 1988).

Immunophenotypically, the concentric rings of mantle zone cells express CD19, 20, 22, w32, 45 and HLA-DR with coexpression of surface IgM and IgD. Hall and colleagues (Hall et al., 1989a) have suggested that these cells are also CD5$^+$. Although not yet corroborated, this finding fits with the concept that CD5$^+$ B-cells (so-called 'B-1' cells), which are frequently involved in the production of auto-antibodies and autoimmune phenomena, may be fundamental to the pathogenesis of Castleman's disease (Bhat et al., 1992; Inghirami et al., 1991; Isaacson, 1989; Kantor, 1991). Monotypia has not been demonstrated within the small, IgM$^+$ IgD$^+$ mantle zone B-cells.

The regressively transformed germinal centres of both forms of AFLNH contain CD21$^+$, CD23$^+$, CD35$^+$, laminin$^+$ and R4/23$^+$ DRCs. A recent study of the hyaline vascular variant of AFLNH has demonstrated abnormal morphology, and hyperplasia of DRCs, with anomalous expression of adhesion molecules CD54, VCAM-1, and ELAM-1 (Ruco et al., 1991). In addition to these changes of DRC structure and function, the significance of which is not clear, there is a significant reduction in numbers of CD4$^+$ T-cells within the follicle centre; and CD57$^+$ (Leu7$^+$) T-cells, normally a feature of follicle centres, are absent.

In the plasma cell form of the disease, the interfollicular zone is infiltrated by IgG$^+$ or IgA$^+$ plasma cells which may, or may not show light chain restriction (Radaszkiewicz et al., 1988). Intriguingly, most of the monoclonal cases reported, show lambda light chain restriction; a reversal of the usual findings in B-cell neoplasms, and commonly found in autoimmune disorders associated with B-1 cells (Knight et al., 1986). Interfollicular T-cells are predominantly of $CD4^+$ helper subset, often admixed with $CD68^+$ histiocytes.

Progressive transformation of germinal centres

Progressive transformation of germinal centres (PTGC), originally described by Lennert and Muller-Hermelink (Lennert and Muller-Hermelink, 1975), is most commonly seen as an incidental finding in reactive lymph nodes removed from the cervical, inguinal or axillary regions of otherwise asymptomatic young men (Hansmann et al., 1990). In approximately 15 to 25 per cent of cases, PTGC is associated with Hodgkin's disease (HD), usually of nodular lymphocyte predominance subtype (Poppema et al., 1979). This finding initially led to concerns about the risk of development of HD in cases of PTGC, however subsequent studies have consistently shown that while PTGC may recur in up to 50 per cent of cases, it rarely progresses, and that those cases which are associated with HD have usually declared themselves at the outset (Ferry et al., 1992; Osborne et al., 1992).

Histologically, progressively transformed germinal centres are considerably larger than the surrounding germinal centres and are characterized by disruption of the follicle centre by a proliferation and progressive influx of small lymphocytes. Follicle centre cells become separated into isolated clusters, and in some cases, particularly children, groups of epithelioid histiocytes appear around the periphery of the affected follicle.

Immunophenotypically, PTGC is characterized by a progressive influx of B-cells into the follicle centres with disruption of the DRC network. These polyclonal B-cells, which gradually expand and replace the follicle, express CD45RA (4KB5, MB1, Ki-B3) and coexpress surface IgM and IgD similar to normal mantle zone B-cells, but are probably activated, being Leu8 negative and expressing CD38 and transferrin receptor CD71. The DRC meshwork, readily identifiable in paraffin sections with anti CD21, CD23 or CD35 antibodies, is both expanded and fenestrated, the defects or 'holes' being filled with mantle zone T- and B-cells rather than follicle centre cells. The polyclonal immunoglobulin which adorns the DRC meshwork of reactive follicles is curiously missing from the involved follicles in PTGC, as it is in follicular lymphomas and nodular lymphocyte predominance Hodgkin's disease (nodular paragranuloma).

Diagnostic application

Investigational modalities and division of tissue

Investigation of lymphoproliferative disorders may involve any of the following techniques:

1. frozen section;
2. paraffin section;
3. flow cytofluorimetry;
4. cytological preparations:
   - imprints
   - cytospins
   - fine needle aspiration;

5 genotyping.

Each method has advantages and disadvantages. In many cases, accurate phenotyping may require the use of two or more complimentary modalities.

Frozen sections have the advantage that specimen fixation is controlled and a full range of well characterized and specific antibodies can be used, often enabling the use of immunophenotypic criteria for neoplasia. All cell types are labelled and can be examined in an architectural context. The major disadvantage of cryostat sections is the poor preservation of cytological detail which in some cases prevents morphological identification of neoplastic cells. Moreover it is often difficult to determine if staining is interstitial or membranous, and in the latter case, which cell it belongs to. This is often a problem with polymorphous lymphomas which contain an intimate admixture of cell types. These and other histiocyte-rich tumours are also often difficult to visualize clearly due to non-specific staining of histiocytes expressing surface Fc receptors.

Paraffin sections are now the most frequently employed modality in lymphoma immunophenotyping. The recent development of relatively specific antibodies which recognise formalin-resistant epitopes has meant that even in small laboratories, determination of cell lineage can be performed with a reasonable level of accuracy. The preservation of cell detail often results in a crisp membranous staining pattern, which can usually be ascribed to a particular cell. For this reason, paraffin sections are particularly useful in the immunophenotyping of

Hodgkin's disease and other polymorphous lymphomas where correlation of individual cell morphology and immunophenotype is important. The major disadvantage of paraffin sections is that many of the antibodies exhibit relative, rather than absolute specificity and the diagnostic context has to be carefully controlled to achieve accuracy. Weak sensitivity may also be a problem with some antibodies, particularly immunoglobulins. With regard to sensitivity, it is important to remember that the generic term 'paraffin sections' conceals great heterogeneity, including cases which have undergone carefully standardized fixation, processing and enzymatic digestion, as well as others which have been left in fixative or paraffin blocks for unknown periods ranging from days to years. Consequently, quoted sensitivities for many of the paraffin section markers may not be achieved in all cases.

Flow cytofluorimetry is now routinely used in haematology laboratories, and can provide extremely useful quantitative information cost-effectively with a wide range of antibodies. This modality achieves the same antibody specificity as cryostat sections with similar or better sensitivity (Witzig et al., 1990), and avoids the problem of interstitial staining. Double or triple staining techniques are easily applied, enabling the application of immunophenotypic criteria for malignancy. Disadvantages of flow cytofluorimetry include the lack of an architectural or cytological context, sampling problems, and the fact that fragile or adhesive tumour cells may be preferentially lost in preparation. Furthermore, tumours in which the neoplastic cells are sparse, such as Hodgkin's disease and some polymorphous lymphomas, may be missed. It is important to remember that cytoplasmic antigens are not detected in routine flow cytofluorimetry and light chain restriction in immunoblastic or plasmacytic tumours may be overlooked.

Cytological preparations are unique in allowing preservation of both morphology and antigenicity. Imprints and fine needle aspiration specimens both suffer some background staining due to adherent serum. Cytospin preparations largely obviate this problem and are an excellent adjunct to paraffin section phenotyping; enabling the use of more specific antibodies under conditions of maximum sensitivity. This method is especially useful for the determination of surface immunoglobulin light chain restriction. In common with flow cytofluorimetry however, there may be some preferential loss of tumour cells during preparation, due to cell fragility or adhesiveness.

Genotyping now has an important role to play in the diagnosis of a percentage of lymphomas (Cossman et al., 1991; Papadopoulos et al., 1989; Sklar, 1990; Wu et al., 1990). Consequently, preservation of fresh tissue for DNA harvest is an important consideration at the time of specimen accession. Some success has been achieved in the extraction of relatively short segment DNA from paraffin blocks however the yield is usually reduced and subject to the length of fixation and storage time. Moreover, some fixatives such as Carnoy's fluid and mercuric fixatives such as B5 render tissue almost useless for genotyping.

Division of tissue is therefore according to the following priorities:

1. transverse sections (3 mm) for histology:
   formalin
   mercuric if preferred;
2. transverse sections for cryostat section immunophenotyping;
3. imprints;
4. fresh tissue for:
   flow cytofluorimetry
   genotyping
   cytospin preparation
   cytogenetics (if available)
   culture (as indicated).

Diagnostic interpretation

The process of diagnostic interpretation involves first determining the immunophenotype of any given lymphoid population, and secondly evaluating the diagnostic significance of these findings.

In the determination of immunophenotype, the importance of adequate positive and negative controls is self evident. In many tissues, residual normal lymphoid tissue provides a good internal positive and negative control for most antibodies.

It is important to have an understanding of the normal cellular pattern of staining for any given antibody . Specific staining with CD45 variants for example is membranous. Diffuse cytoplasmic staining for these and a number of other antibodies is usually an indicator of non-specific reactivity. Similarly, when using anti-CD68 antibodies, a dot-like, rather than diffuse/granular cytoplasmic staining should be a clue that the lesion in question is a low grade B-cell lymphoma rather than a histiocytic lesion.

Formal test analysis

In the evaluation of the significance of phenotypic findings, it is a common practice among pathologists to ignore, or not report negative staining results, and make a diagnosis only on the basis of positive reactions. However, if biopsy sections have a valid, internal positive control population, and the tumour cells are negative, then this finding is significant. In fact formal test analysis shows that for some antibodies, a negative test result has a greater predictive value than a positive result (Hall and D'Ardenne, 1987; Sox, 1987). Furthermore, when the results of several antibody stains suggest conflicting diagnoses, formal test analysis may show that certain antibodies are more powerful discriminants than others. By utilizing cumulative figures derived from multiple series, it is possible to estimate the diagnostic significance, or operating characteristics for any given antibody and diagnostic context (Table 4.8).

This quantitative approach enables more rigorous assessment, and highlights the limitations underlying all immunohistochemical testing, i.e. the operating characteristics for any given antibody depend upon the definition adopted for the reference test (in this context, histological diagnosis), as well as the criteria for selection of test cases (frequently not defined). These two factors are principally responsible for the wide variation of staining pattern sometimes reported for the same antibody in different case series.

Wherever possible in the accompanying descriptions of lymphoproliferative disease, the operating characteristics of each antibody have been estimated according to the diagnostic context, and data given in the cited references. The actual predictive value of a result, depends upon the local disease prevalence. Where the predictive values have been quoted in the text, it has been assumed for illustrative value, that the diseases have equal prevalence. The operating characteristics are important not only in the interpretation of immunophenotypic findings, but also for the rational choice of an appropriate diagnostic panel of antibodies for use in a given histological context (see Pattern Immunodiagnosis).

Immunophenotypic criteria for neoplasia

Reactive and neoplastic lymphoproliferative diseases are usually differentiated morphologically, however in difficult cases, immunophenotyping may provide confirmatory evidence of neoplasia. Genotypic and cytogenetic

Table 4.8. Formal test analysis

		Reference Test	
	New test	**Positive**	**Negative**
Positive	**a** (True positive)	**b** (False positive)	**a+b**
Negative	**c** (False negative)	**d** (True negative)	**c+d**
	a+c	**b+d**	**N = a+b+c+d**

Operating characteristics:
Sensitivity = a/(a+c)
Specificity = d/(b+d)
Predictive value of a positive result = a/(a+b)
Predictive value of a negative result = d/(c+d)
Accuracy = (a+d)/N
(The actual predictive value of a positive or negative result in any given case is also dependent upon the disease prevalence in the community or population being tested.)

Source: Reproduced from Hall and D'Ardenne, 1987

studies are particularly useful, but are beyond the scope of this chapter. Immunophenotypic criteria operate as indicators of clonal expansion, phenotypic 'aberrancy', or a combination of the two.

Indicators of clonality

Lineage predominance

Most lymphoid infiltrates comprise 40 to 80 per cent T-cells and 20 to 60 per cent B-cells. Overwhelming B-cell or T-cell predominance may on occasion, be taken as evidence in favour of neoplasia. The marked variability encountered in T-cell and B-cell response to different antigens, however, makes this an unreliable criterion, which is better used only to ascribe lineage to a morphologically obvious lymphoma.

Light chain restriction

This remains the gold standard in the immunodiagnosis of B-cell neoplasia but is often difficult to demonstrate. Surface immunoglobulin (sIg) is best demonstrated using cryostat sections, cytospin preparations or flow cytofluorimetry. In paraffin section material, sIg is rarely identifiable and evidence of cytoplasmic light chain restriction must be sought. In B-cell tumours showing plasmacytic or immunoblastic differentiation this is usually not a problem. In all other B-cell lymphomas except Burkitt's and centrocytic lymphoma, light chain restriction can often be detected by careful scrutiny of the tumour cell perinuclear space (Norton and Isaacson, 1987).

Light chain negative B-cells

A percentage of normal follicle centre B-cells and lymphomas derived thereof, are immunoglobulin light chain negative (Hsu and Jaffe, 1984b; Ngan et al., 1989b). In diffuse lymphoid infiltrates therefore, the presence of light chain negative B-cells has been advocated as immunophenotypic evidence for neoplasia. In practice however, the interpretation of light chain staining can be very difficult, especially in the presence of background or interstitial staining, and this is rarely useful diagnostically (Picker et al., 1987).

CD5 positive B-cells

$CD5^+$ B-cells represent a small subpopulation, currently designated 'B-1' cells (Bhat et al., 1992). In normal adults, they represent a small fraction of B-cells within peripheral blood and lymphoid organs. A significant increase in the number of cells coexpressing CD5 and pan-B antigens such as CD20, is strong evidence for neoplasia, usually a diffuse low grade B-cell lymphoma or B-CLL. It is important to remember that 'B-1' cells constitute the major pool of circulating B-cells following bone marrow transplantation and in normal neonates. In either of these contexts therefore, the presence of $CD5^+$ B-cells has little diagnostic significance.

Leu8 positive B-cells

In normal B-cell populations, Leu8 expression is limited to the mantle zone. A large population of $Leu8^+$ B-cells may therefore suggest clonal expansion, as is seen in B-cell small lymphocytic, centrocytic, or mantle zone lymphoma.

Restricted use of TCR variable region genes

A number of studies have demonstrated the usefulness of antibodies to products of the TCR variable region genes (Bahler et al., 1992; Hunt et al., 1992; Jack et al., 1990; Poppema and Hepperle, 1991; Ralfkiaer et al., 1991; Smith et al., 1992a). There are 18 Vβ and 19 Vα gene families. Therefore in reactive populations, unless there is preferential usage related to specific antigens (Clark and Boylston, 1989), any one Vβ or Vα family should represent between 1 and 5 per cent of the total T-cell population (O'Grady et al., 1990). T-cell neoplasms can be identified by the clonal expression of only one Vβ and one Vα gene. Although potentially of great use as clonotypic markers in T-cell neoplasia, their use is currently limited by the relatively small repertoire of antibodies available (Ralfkiaer et al., 1991), and uncertainty surrounding some reported cases in which there is preferential V region usage, apparently in the absence of clonal T-cell expansion (Smith et al., 1992a). Moreover, the antibodies are unlikely to be of use in the 20 per cent or so, of T-cell lymphomas which do not express TCR gene products (O'Grady et al., 1990).

T-cell subset anomalies

In most lymphoid infiltrates, $CD4^+$ cells predominate over $CD8^+$ cells in a ratio of 2 or 3:1. A major imbalance of the normal $CD4^+$:$CD8^+$ ratio may suggest neoplasia but is also seen in some reactive conditions including HIV-related disease, and is not diagnostic per se (Knowles, 1989).

Double negative ($CD4^-CD8^-$) T-cells comprise less than 5 per cent of normal peripheral T-cell populations (Lanier et al., 1986); mainly contained within the γδ subset. The finding of a high percentage of double negative T-cells is therefore strongly indicative of neoplasia. In rare individuals, certain anti-CD4 antibodies may be non-reactive with normal $CD4^+$ T-cells, due to genetic polymorphism. This artefactual cause of double negative T-cells can be distinguished by the apparent lack any normal $CD4^+$ cells in the affected patients, and is corrected by the use of a different anti-CD4 antibody clone.

Double positive ($CD4^+CD8^+$) T-cells are normally encountered only during intra-thymic development, and the finding of a significant percentage of double positive T-cells, particularly in peripheral lymphoid organs, is very strong evidence in favour of neoplasia.

Immature phenotype

The detection of a dominant intrathymic T-cell phenotype (including expression of CD1or TdT) is usually strong evidence for lymphoblastic lymphoma or leukaemia, especially when sampled from a mass lesion in an adult. In general, however, immature phenotypes detected in young children should be interpreted cautiously (Kamat et al., 1990). Furthermore, it should be remembered that normal thymic T-cells, and the background lymphocytes in thymoma, also exhibit immature phenotypes; a potential source of diagnostic confusion.

Phenotypic 'aberrancy'

Aberrant or abnormal phenotypes are those for which there is no known normal counterpart, best exemplified by deletion of pan-B or pan-T antigens (see PTCL-phenotypic aberrancy). In mature B-cell populations therefore, absence of HLA-DR, CD11a, CD19, CD20 or CD22 is virtually diagnostic of malignancy. Similarly, expression of CD43 in any B-cells, or CDw32(41H) in proliferating B-cell populations (>10 per cent $Ki\text{-}67^+$) is also strongly indicative of neoplasia (Picker et al., 1987). In mature T-cell populations, absence of one or more pan-T antigens CD2, CD3, CD5, or of both TCRαβ and TCRγδ indicates aberrancy and is also virtually diagnostic of malignancy.

In the past, $CD7^-$ and $Leu8^-$ T-cell phenotypes have also been labelled as aberrant. CD7 is present in 70 to 90 per cent of normal T-cell populations and is not strictly speaking a pan-T antigen. Its absence from T-cells in peripheral lymphoid tissues is therefore suggestive but not diagnostic of neoplasia. In cutaneous sites, where reactive T-cell infiltrates are not uncommonly $CD7^-$, it is of little diagnostic value.

Leu8 is expressed by most T-cells, and the presence of $Leu8^-$ T-cell populations has therefore been advocated as evidence for neoplasia. In fact however, Leu8 expression by normal T-cells is lost during activation, and normal helper-inducer $CD4^+$ T-cells are constitutively $Leu8^-$ (Rijlaarsdam et al., 1990). Leu8 negativity is therefore not an indicator of T-cell aberrancy, and is of limited use in the diagnosis of T-cell malignancy (Ralfkiaer, 1991).

CD45 isoform anomalies, specifically CD45RA (MB1) positivity in T-cells have also been shown to be a useful criterion for malignancy (Picker et al., 1987).

Follicular lesions

In the special case of follicular lesions, additional immunophenotypic criteria apply.

Antibodies to the bcl-2 gene product have recently become available and provide a useful indicator of bcl-2 gene expression. Normal follicle centre B-cells are bcl-2 antibody-negative, expressing the gene product only after specific cross-linking of surface immunoglobulin, or certain other activation pathways (Liu et al., 1991). Antibodies to the bcl-2 gene product are therefore only focally and weakly positive in reactive follicles. The (14;18) translocation characteristic of follicular lymphoma, however, causes constitutive overexpression of the bcl-2 gene and widespread positivity for the antibody (Gaulard et al., 1992; Ngan et al., 1988b).

Other findings which favour follicular neoplasia rather than hyperplasia, include positivity for antibodies MT2 (Browne et al., 1991; Norton et al., 1989) and MY4 (Medeiros et al., 1991), as well as absence of immunoglobulin staining of the DRC meshwork normally seen in reactive follicles (Timens et al., 1986). Chilosi and colleagues (Chilosi et al., 1990a), in a detailed study of over 30 reactive, and neoplastic lymph nodes, demonstrated strong MT2 staining in 1908 of 2288 neoplastic follicles, but negative or weak, focal staining in all 2329 reactive follicles examined. Such findings are potentially useful but are unfortunately subject to the vagaries of specimen fixation and digestion protocols, which may create artificial staining thresholds. The validity of MT2 staining in this context should therefore be tested, and the sensitivity and specificity of the test defined for any given laboratory.

Immuno-architectural anomalies

Assessment of lymphoid architecture, often the cornerstone of morphological diagnosis, is significantly enhanced with the use of immunostains.

In florid paracortical immunoblastic reactions, normal lymphoid architecture may be grossly distorted by preferential expansion of some immunological compartments at the expense of others, often giving the impression in H & E stains, of diffuse architectural effacement. Use of a simple panel of antibodies such as CD45RO, CD20, CD21 and CD68 in these cases, often reassuringly outlines the normal immunological elements, enabling critical reassessment of the cellular cytology of each compartment.

Conversely, in cases with apparently normal architecture, immunophenotyping may demonstrate anomalous immunoarchitecture. Appreciation of clonality or aberrancy as detailed above, may be enhanced by close histological examination of individual immunological compartments. Furthermore, even in the absence of demonstrable clonality or aberrancy, neoplasia may be suggested by either *loss of normal immunological compartmentalization* or the finding of *a phenotype or lineage inappropriate for a given compartment*. An example of the latter is the replacement of the paracortical or T-cell zone of lymph nodes by B-cells in B-CLL.

Pattern diagnosis of lymphoproliferative disease

The purpose of this section is to provide a morphological framework in which to choose and interpret diagnostic antibody panels. In contrast to the detail of the preceding sections, and at the risk of offending those with a detailed knowledge of haematopathology, this section has been designed in tabulated form as a guide to the diagnosis of immunoproliferative disease. To this end, immunoproliferative diseases can been divided into six morphological groups, defined by asking three questions (Fig. 4.19). For each category, a checklist of differential diagnoses is suggested, together with a table of useful antibody panels. Figures 4.20 through to 4.32 illustrate a diagnostic approach through the pattern of involvement and the cellular composition. In each case, antibodies reactive in fixed tissues are emphasized in **bold** typeface. The six groups have been chosen because they represent to a large extent, the morphological contexts in which lymphoma immunodiagnosis is usually made.

Morphological classifications such as the Rappaport scheme have in the past, defined lymphomas according to:

1. The low power, or architectural pattern of infiltration;
2. The nature or size of the infiltrating cells (e.g. Follicular, large cell type).

The approach outlined here is similar, however whereas such schemes recognized only follicular and diffuse infiltrates, there is now a need to include several others, including mantle zone, marginal zone, and interfollicular

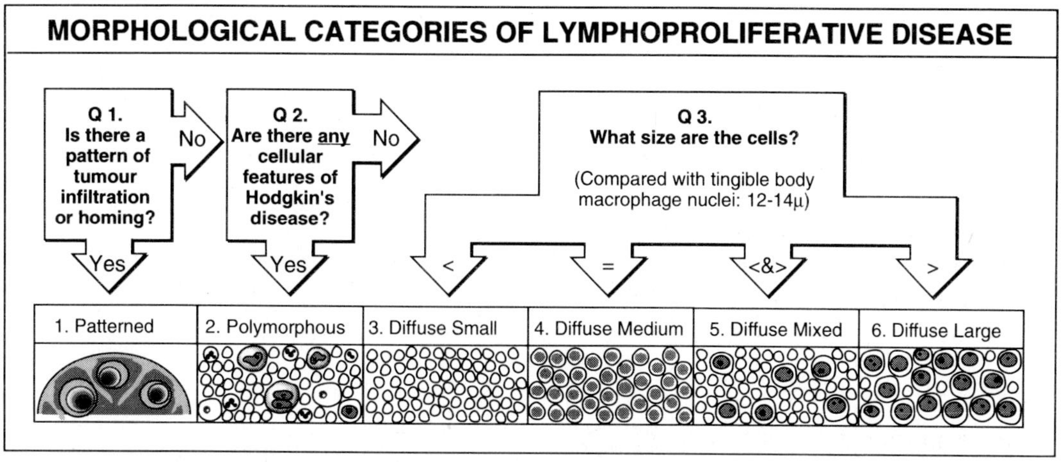

Fig. 4.19. By posing three questions, it is possible to divide lymphoproliferative diseases into 6 major morphological categories. The individual category can then be examined and a checklist of differential diagnoses can be explored using the appropriate antibodies.

1. PATTERNED INFILTRATE

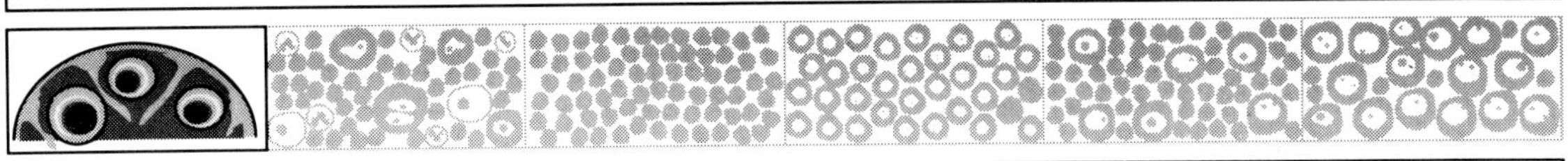

Architectural Pattern | **Disease Checklist** | Immunophenotype

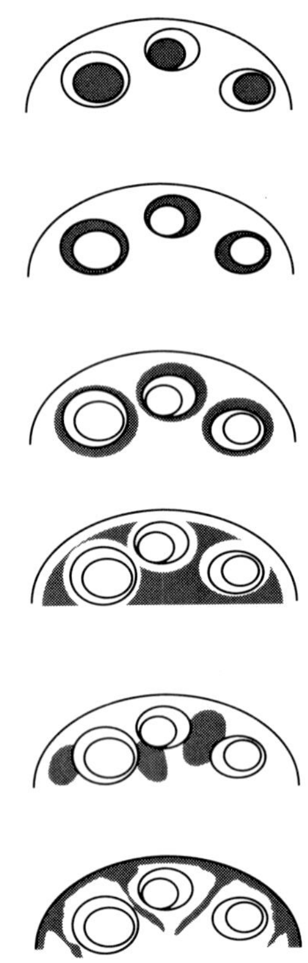

Disease Checklist	CD20	CD45RO	DRC+ ¶	Clonal Ig	CD43	CD68	bcl-2	CD23	SIgM+D+	UCL3d3	UCL4d12
Follicular Pattern											
Reactive Follicular Hyperplasia	+	-	+	-	-	-	-	+	-		
Progressive Transformation of GC	+	-	+	-	-	-	-	-	+	+	
Nodular Lymphocyte Predom. HD	+	-	+	See: Polymorphous Patterns							
Follicular Lymphoma	+	-	+	+	-	-	+	+/-	-	-	+
Pseudofollicular (B-CLL/SL)	+	-	-	+	+	§	+/-	+	+	-	+/-
Mantle Zone Pattern											
Mantle Zone Hyperplasia	+	-	-	-	-	-		-	+	+	-
Mantle Zone Lymphoma (Centrocytic)	+	-	-	+	+	§		-	+	+	-
CLL/Small Lymphocytic Lymphoma	+	-	-	+	+	§		+	+	-	+/-
Castleman's Disease											
Hyaline Vascular	+	-	-	-	-	-			+		
Plasma Cell Type	+	-	-	+/-	-	-			+		
Marginal Zone Pattern											
Marginal Zone Hyperplasia	+	-	-	-	-	-		-	-	-	+
Marginal Zone Lymphoma (Spleen)	+	-	-	+	-	-		-	-	-	+
Monocytoid B-cell Lymphoma	+	-	-	+	-	-		-	-	-	+
MALT Lymphoma	+	-	-	+	-	-		-	-	-	+
Interfollicular Pattern											
Paracortical Hyperplasia	-	+	-	-	+	-		-	-	-	-
Castleman's Disease (Plasma Cell Type)	+	-	-	+/-	-	-			-		
T-cell Lymphoma (espec. T-zone)	-	+	-	-	+	-		-	-	-	-
Some cases of CLL/SL	+	-	-	+	+	§		+	+	+/-	
Some T-cell-rich B-cell Lymphomas	+	-	-	+	-	-		+/-	-		
Hodgkin's Disease	Refer to Polymorphous Patterns										
Paracortical Nodular Pattern											
Reactive: Monocytoid B-cell Clusters	+	-	-	-	-	-		-	-	-	+
Plasmacytoid Monocytes	-	-/+	-	-	+	+		-	-		
Kikuchi-Fujimoto Disease	-	-/+	-	-	+	+		-	-		
Dermatopathic	-	+	-	-	+	-		-	-		
Early Interfollicular Pattern	See Interfollicular Pattern above										
Metastatic Disease (Melanoma etc.)	-	-	-	-	-	-		-	-		
Sinusoidal Pattern											
Reactive: Sinus Histiocytosis	-	-	-	-	-	+		-	-		
Histiocytoses	-	-	-	-	-/+	+		-	-		
Anaplastic Large Cell Lymphoma	-/+	+/-	-	-	+/-	-		-	-		
Metastatic Disease (Melanoma etc.)	-	-	-	-	-	-		-	-		

Fig. 4.20. In this first group, recognizable immuno-architectural patterns of infiltration or homing, provide clues to the diagnosis. Antibodies reactive in fixed tissues are emphasized with bold typeface.

Note: § Low grade B-cell lymphomas may express dot-like cytoplasmic $CD68^+$. ¶ DRC^+ indicates that $CD21^+$ or $CD23^+$, Follicular Dendritic Reticulum Cells proliferate in follicular aggregates as part of the infiltrate, rather than within uninvolved follicles. Diffuse or ill-defined DRC proliferation is found in centrocytic lymphoma and some T-cell lymphomas.

1. Castleman's disease may be viewed as a predominantly mantle zone, or interfollicular pattern. Coexpression of SIgM and SIgD is seen in the mantle zones of both variants. Plasma cells in the interfollicular zone of the plasma cell variant express IgG or IgA, often with light chain restriction. 2. In the determination of lineage, CD20 could be replaced by MB2, or in frozen sections, CD19 or 22. Similarly, CD45RO could be replaced by polyclonal CD3 or in frozen sections, βF1,CD2, 3, or 7. 3. Small lymphocytic lymphoma (SLL) or CLL may on occasions, show a mantle or interfollicular pattern depending upon the degree of involvement. Pseudofollicular growth centres of B-cell SLL / CLL are distinguished from genuinely follicular patterns by the absence of DRC^+ staining patterns, detected in paraffin sections by CD21, CD23 or CD35. 4. Anti-bcl-2 antibodies stain a wide range of tumours including some high grade T-cell lymphomas, and are mainly useful in the differentiation of reactive from neoplastic follicles. Antibodies MT2 and MY4 may be used similarly, but their specificity and sensitivity has not been established.

patterns. Moreover, with the recognition that Hodgkin's disease is probably a neoplasm of activated lymphocytes, with B-cell and T-cell simulants, as well as intermediate, or indeterminate forms, there is a need to integrate the diagnosis of HD and NHL into one schematic overview. The essence of both Hodgkin's disease and simulants is the presence of a polymorphous infiltrate,which includes atypical, hyperlobate mononuclear cells with prominent nucleoli, but is dominated by reactive cells, in a symbiotic exchange of cytokines. The term 'polymorphous' is

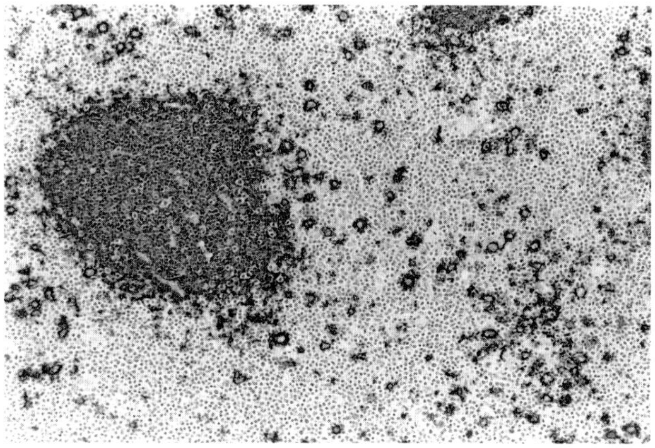

Fig. 4.21a. Interfollicular involvement by T-cell-rich B-cell lymphoma. A stain for CD20 shows a reactive follicle and a number of large CD20 positive cells within the interfollicular zone (anti-L26, X1000).

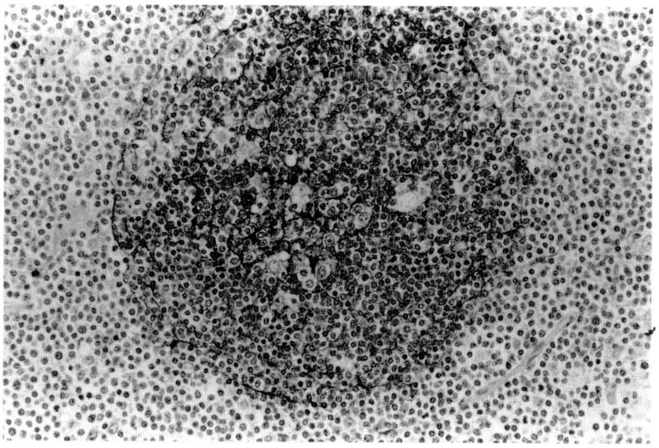

Fig. 4.21b. Interfollicular involvement by T-cell-rich B-cell lymphoma. The follicular nature of the CD20+ area is confirmed by CD21 expression (anti-IF8, X200).

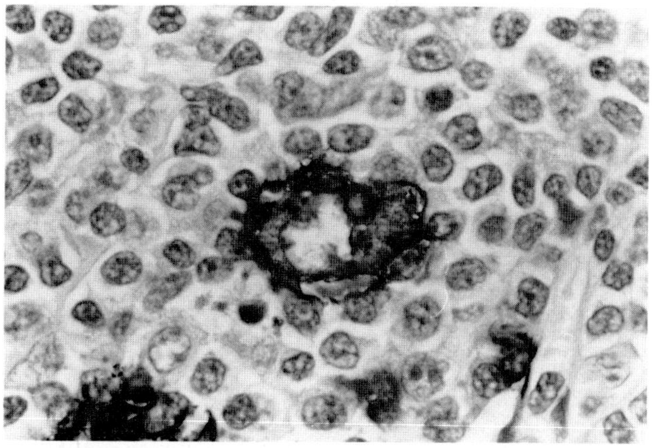

Fig. 4.21c. T-cell-rich B-cell lymphoma. The isolated B-cell blasts (surrounded by reactive T-cells) show strong expression of CD20 (anti-L26, X1000).

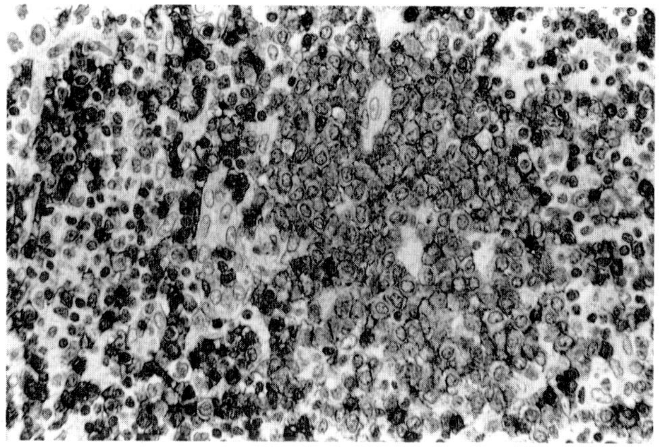

Fig. 4.22a. Paracortical nodule of plasmacytoid monocytes within a reactive lymph node. The cells stain positively for CD43 and CD45RA (anti-MT1, X400).

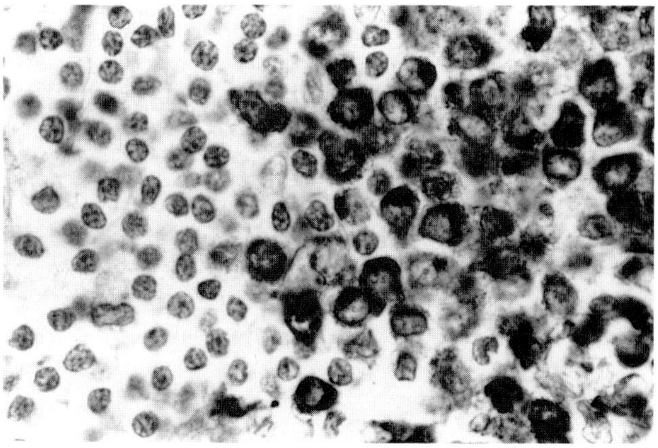

Fig. 4.22b. Paracortical nodule of plasmacytoid monocytes within a reactive lymph node. The same cells show strong expression of CD68 (anti-KP1, X1000).

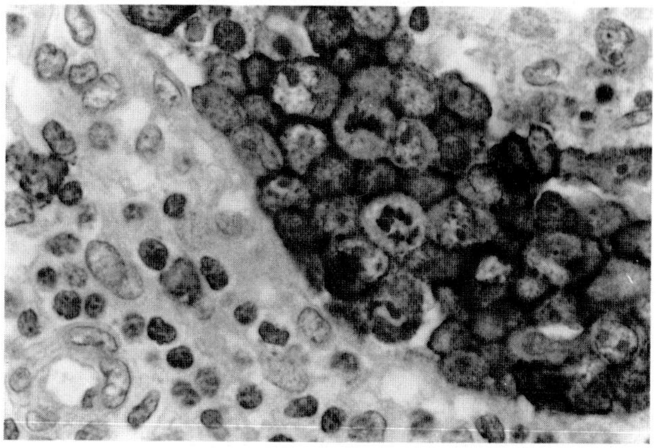

Fig. 4.23. Sinusoidal pattern of nodal infiltration by anaplastic large cell lymphoma (anti-EMA, X1000).

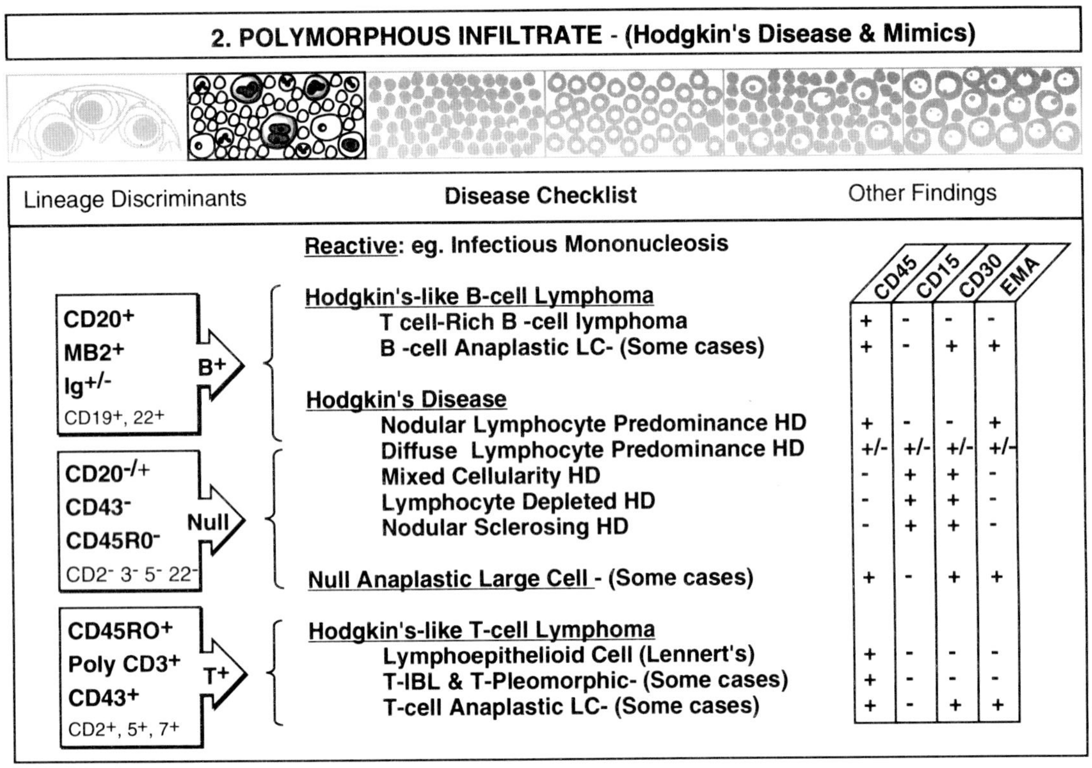

Disease	CD45	CD15	CD30	EMA
T cell-Rich B -cell lymphoma	+	-	-	-
B -cell Anaplastic LC- (Some cases)	+	-	+	+
Nodular Lymphocyte Predominance HD	+	-	-	+
Diffuse Lymphocyte Predominance HD	+/-	+/-	+/-	+/-
Mixed Cellularity HD	-	+	+	-
Lymphocyte Depleted HD	-	+	+	-
Nodular Sclerosing HD	-	+	+	-
Null Anaplastic Large Cell - (Some cases)	+	-	+	+
Lymphoepithelioid Cell (Lennert's)	+	-	-	-
T-IBL & T-Pleomorphic- (Some cases)	+	-	-	-
T-cell Anaplastic LC- (Some cases)	+	-	+	+

Fig. 4.24 Polymorphous infiltrates include Hodgkin's disease, related malignant lymphomas and a number of reactive conditions, particularly EBV-related. The above findings represent the most common phenotype for each disease. Exceptions are detailed in the accompanying text. Diffuse Lymphocyte Predominance Hodgkin's Disease is immunophenotypically heterogenous, incorporating several different biological entities (See page 167). Antibodies reactive in fixed tissues are emphasized with bold typeface.

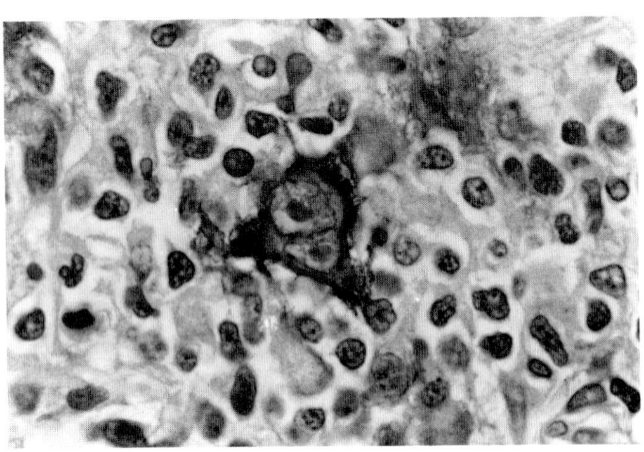

Fig. 4.25 Polymorphous infiltrate with CD30 positive R-S cell. This is a case of infectious mononucleosis. The hyperlobate cells are frequently CD30+, but are often CD20+ and almost always CD15 negative (anti-BerH2, X1000).

used here to link HD and simulants together under a unifying pattern descriptor, while the reciprocal term 'monomorphous' serves to describe all other lymphomas without resort to the negative terminology of 'non-Hodgkin's lymphoma'.

Finally, in judging the character of infiltrating cells, it is important not to confuse the terms 'pleomorphic' and 'polymorphous'. Nuclear pleomorphism may be a feature of almost any lymphoma, and does not necessarily imply the type of mixed, reactive infiltrate characteristic of polymorphous lymphomas.

For the minimalist: constructing a minimum useful antibody panel

It should be apparent from the foregoing discussions that there is almost no limit to the number of antibodies that can be applied in the investigation of lymphoproliferative disease. Not all of these are of relevance to diagnostic laboratories, which usually conduct immunophenotyping for the following reasons:

3. DIFFUSE - SMALL / INTERMEDIATE-SIZED INFILTRATE

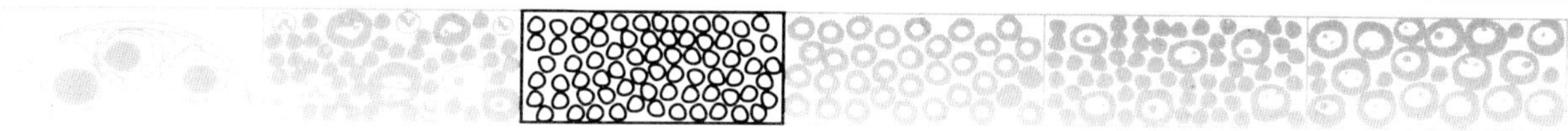

Lineage Discriminants | **Disease Checklist** | Other Findings

B⁺ lineage discriminants: **CD20⁺**, **MB2⁺**, **Ig(Cytoplasmic)⁺**, Ig (Surface)⁺, CD19, 22⁺

Disease Checklist	CD5, **43**	SIgM+D-	**CD23**	CD10	CDw32	TRAP	CD11c	FMC7	UCL3d3	UCL4d12	CD1	TdT
B-Small Lymphocytic / CLL	+	+	+	-	+	-	-	-	-	+/-	-	-
Lymphoplasmacytic	-/+	+	+	-	+	-	-	-	-	+/-	-	-
Lymphoplasmacytoid	-/+	+	+	-	+	-	-	-	-	+/-	-	-
Mantle Zone Lymphoma (Centrocytic)	+	+	-	-	+	-	-	+	+	-	-	-
Centroblastic/Centrocytic (CB/CC)	-	-	+/-	+	-	-	-		-	+	-	-
B-Prolymphocytic	-	+	-	-	+	-	-	+			-	-
Hairy Cell Leukaemia	-	-		-/+	+	+	+	+			-	-
MALT/ Monocytoid B-Cell Lymphoma	-	-	-	-	+	-	-		-	+	-	-
Plasmacytic (Myeloma/ Plasmacytoma)	-	-	-	-/+	-	-	-				-	-
B-Lymphoblastic	-*	-	-	+	-	-	-				-	+

T⁺ lineage discriminants: **CD45R0⁺**, **poly CD3⁺**, **βF1⁺**, CD2, 3, 7⁺

Disease Checklist	CD5, **43**	SIgM+D-	**CD23**	CD10	CDw32	TRAP	CD11c	FMC7	UCL3d3	UCL4d12	CD1	TdT
T-Small Lymphocytic / CLL	+	-	-	-	-	-	-	-			-	-
Tγ Lymphoproliferative Disease (CD3⁺)	+	-	-	-	-	-	-	-			-	-
T-Prolymphocytic	+	-	-	-	-	-	-	-			-	-
Lymphoepithelioid Cell (Lennert's)	+	-	-	-	-		-	-			-	-
T-Pleomorphic Small Cell	+	-	-	-	-	-	-	-			-	-
T-Lymphoblastic	+	-	-	-/+	-	-	-	-			+	+

Fig. 4.26. Diffuse infiltrates of small or intermediate size. The frequent expression of CD5⁺ and 43⁺ in low grade B-cell lymphomas precludes their use as markers of lineage in this category.
Note: 1. Hairy Cell Leukaemia is consistently and strongly CD25⁺. *2 Some B-Lymphoblastic lymphomas are CD43⁺. Antibodies reactive in fixed tissues are emphasized with bold typeface.

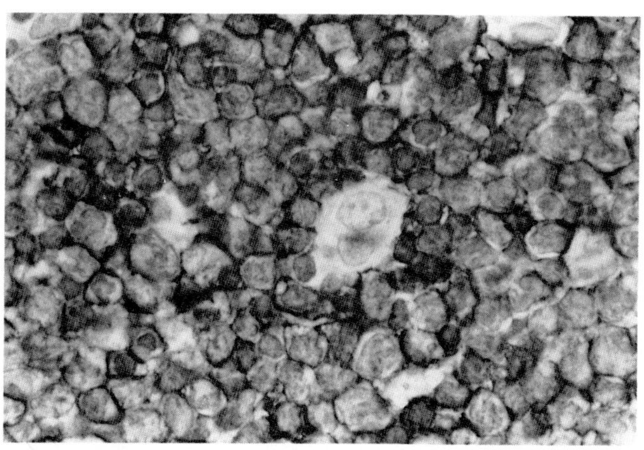

Fig. 4.27. Diffuse small / intermediate-sized infiltrate: T-lymphoblastic lymphoma. Note the small size of the tumour cells compared with the Tingible body macrophage nucleus (anti-MT1, X1000).

1. differentiation of lymphoid from non-lymphoid lesions;
2. determination of leucocyte lineage (T-cell, B-cell, monocytic and myeloid) and differentiation of Hodgkin's disease (HD) from other lymphomas;
3. differentiation of reactive from neoplastic infiltrates;
4. precise lymphoma subclassification.

It is generally true that the cost/benefit ratio increases disproportionately in a stepwise fashion from 1 to 4, and in choosing an antibody panel, it is important to clearly define the purpose of the exercise. Most non-specialized laboratories, utilizing a minimal panel of antibodies, should be able to achieve items1 and 2 with reasonable accuracy.

Undifferentiated tumours

Virtually all laboratories now routinely differentiate lymphoid from non-lymphoid tumours with the use of antibodies to leucocyte common antigen and keratins. It is ironic that this, the simplest and cheapest of all antibody panels, has had by far the greatest impact upon tumour diagnosis and patient management (Gatter et al., 1985).

Minimum panel: CD45, Broad spectrum anti-keratin antibody

4. DIFFUSE - MEDIUM SIZED INFILTRATE

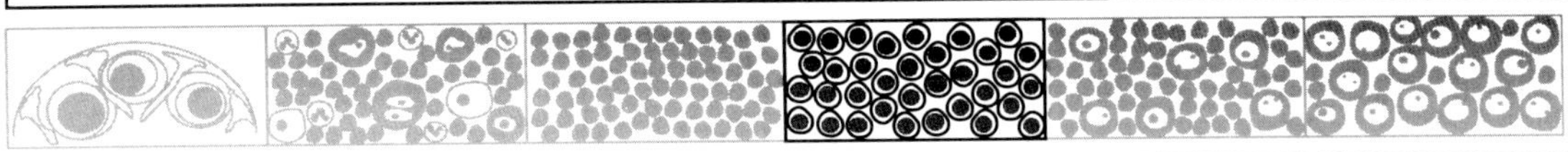

Lineage Discriminants		Disease Checklist	CD45RA	CD45RO	CD43	MAC387	CD68	CD15	NP57	MPO	AA1	CD13	CD33
CD20+, CIgM+ CD19+ 22+	**B+**	**Burkitt's Lymphoma**	+	-	-	-	-	-	-	-	-	-	-
polyCD3+ CD2+ 3+ 5+ 7+	**T+**	**T-Pleomorphic Medium- size**	-	+	+	-	-	-/+	-	-	-	-	-
CD3- 5- 7- 19- **20**- 22- **Leder's+**	**Null**	**Myeloid/monocyticLeukaemia**	+/-	+/-	+/-	+/-	+/-	+/-	+	+	-	+	+
		Mast Cell Disease	+/-	+/-	+/-	-	+	+/-	-	-	+		+

(Other Findings)

Fig. 4.28 Diffuse infiltrates of medium size. Note: CD43, CD45RA , CD45RO , MB2, CD74 (LN2) and S-100 are frequently positive in myeloid/monocytic proliferations, and may give misleading results if used in isolation. Antibodies reactive in fixed tissues are emphasized with bold typeface.

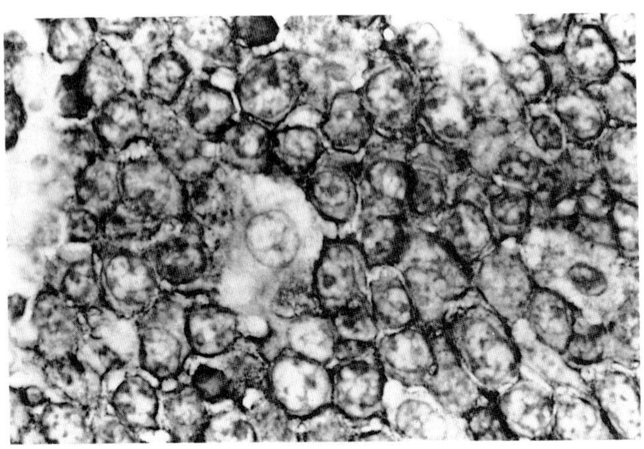

Fig. 4.29. Diffuse infiltrate of medium size: Small-non-cleaved cell, or Burkitt's lymphoma, CD20 positive. Note the approximation of tumour cells to the macrophage nucleus (anti-L26, X1000).

Leucocyte lineage

In the further determination of lineage, the most intensely staining, and reliable B-cell antigens are CD22 or CD37 in frozen sections (FS) and L26 or MB2 in paraffin sections (PS). Because MB2 stains non-lymphoid, and some myeloid tumours, L26 is probably preferable. Immunoglobulin (Ig) heavy and light chain antibodies have the advantage of demonstrating clonality as well as indicating lineage. For the demonstration of T-cells in FS, the most useful antibodies are CD3 and CD2. In PS, polyclonal CD3, is the most specific, but least sensitive marker, and CD45RO or CD43, offer the best compromise between specificity and sensitivity. As the latter two antigens, particularly CD43, may be expressed on myeloid and monocytic tumours, the panel should include either histochemical stains or antibodies reactive with myeloid and monocytic cells. These could include neutrophil elastase (NP57), myeloperoxidase (MPO), CD13, CD33, MAC387 or anti-CD68 antibodies. Antigens most useful in the differentiation of HD from other lymphomas include many of the above, as well as CD15, CD30, and EMA.

In non-specialized and private laboratories, PS are often used in in preference to FS, both for convenience, and because of difficulty in controlling the way in which tissue is presented to the laboratory. In general, for the determination of lineage, the above antibodies used in PS are now approaching the specificity and sensitivity of FS antibodies, and are adequate for a minimum panel. None the less, FS offer advantages in immunoglobulin detection, and the ability to test for highly specific antigens.

5. DIFFUSE - MIXED SMALL & LARGE CELL INFILTRATE

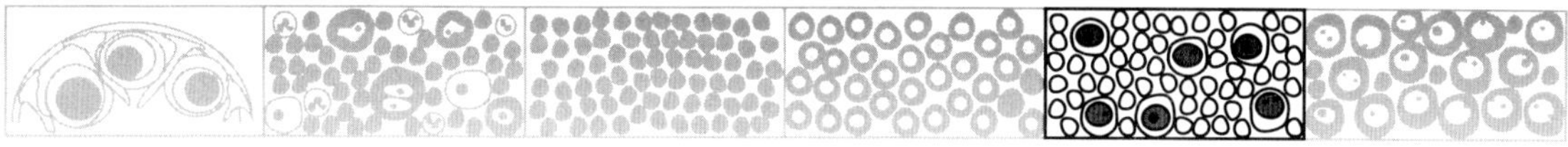

Lineage Discriminants	Disease Checklist	CD45RA	CD43	CDw75	CD5	CD10	CD23-DRC
CD20+ MB2+ CD19+ 22+ **CIg+** SIg+ → B+	**CB/CC (Mixed small & Large)**	+	-	+	-	+	-/+
	Small Lymphocytic (Paraimmunoblastic variant)	+	+/-	-*	+	-	-
	T cell- rich B-cell Lymphoma	+	-	+	-	-	-
CD45RO+ **polyCD3+** CD2+ 3+ 5+ 7+ → T+	**T-Pleomorphic Medium and Large Cell**	-	+	-	+	-	-
	T-Zone Lymphoma	-	+	-	+	-	-
	Angioimmunoblastic (AILD- like) T-cell Lymphoma	-	+	-	+	-	+

(Other Findings)

Fig. 4.30 Diffuse infiltrates of mixed small and large cell type. Note: 1. Reactive infiltrates may on occasion, have a monomorphous, mixed infiltrate which appears diffuse. In almost all such cases, stains for DRCs, T-cells, B-cells, plasma cells and monocytes will reveal an underlying architectural pattern. 2. In diffuse CB/CC lymphoma, some residual DRCs meshworks may persist. In AILD-like lymphoma, there is a diffuse proliferation of DRCs recognized with antibodies to CD21, 23 or 35. 3. CDw75 * (LN1) is negative in the small cells, but highlights the paraimmunoblasts of small lymphocytic lymphoma. Antibodies reactive in fixed tissues are emphasized with bold typeface.

6. DIFFUSE - LARGE CELL INFILTRATE

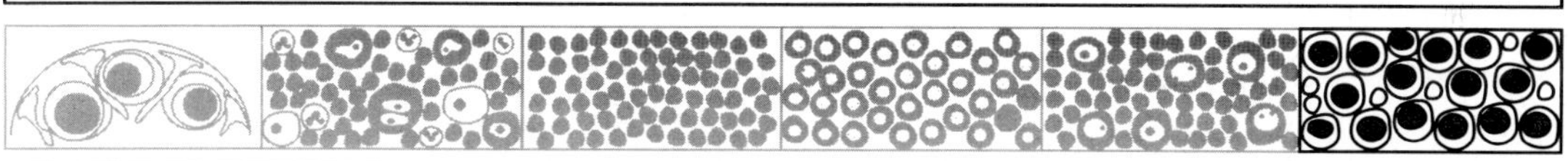

Lineage Discriminants	Disease Checklist	CD43	CD45RA	CDw75	CD30	CD68	MAC387	S-100	CD1	NP57	MPO
CD20+ MB2+ CD19+ 22+ **CIg+** SIg+ → B+	**Centroblastic (Large non-cleaved)**	-	+	+	-	-	-	-	-	-	-
	B-Immunoblastic	-	+/-	+	-	-	-	-	-	-	-
	B-Anaplastic Large Cell	-	+/-	+	+	-	-	-	-	-	-
	Reactive: B-Immunoblastic Proliferations	-	+	+	-/+	-	-	-	-	-	-
CD45RO+ **polyCD3+** CD2+ 3+ 5+ 7+ → T+	**T-Pleomorphic Large Cell**	+	-	-	-/+	-	-	-	-	-	-
	T-Immunoblastic	+	-	-	-/+	-	-	-	-	-	-
	T-Anaplastic Large Cell	+	-	-	+	-	-	-	-	-	-
	Reactive: T-Immunoblastic Proliferations	+	-	-	-/+	-	-	-	-	-	-
CD20- MB2- CD19- 22- **CIg-** SIg- **CD45RO+/-** **polyCD3-** CD2- 3- 5- 7- → Null	**Null-Anaplastic Large Cell**	-	-	-	+	-	-/+	-	-	-	-
	Myeloid/Myelomonocytic Leukaemia	+	+/-	-	-	+	+	+/-	-	+	+
	Histiocytoses:										
	Langerhans Cell Histiocytosis	-	-	-	-	+	-	+	+	-	-
	Haemophagocytic Syndromes	-/+	-	-	-	+	+	+/-	-	-	-
	Histiocytic Malignancy										
	True Histiocytic Lymphoma:	-/+	-	-	-	+	+	-	-	-	-
	Dendritic Cell Sarcoma (IRC/DRC/LC)	-/+	-	-	-	-/+	-	+	-/+	-	-
	Reactive: Kikuchi - Fujimoto Disease	+	-	+/-	-	+	-/+	-	-	-	-

(Other Findings)

Fig. 4.31. Diffuse infiltrates of large cell type. Note:1. The above findings represent the most common phenotype for each disease. Exceptions are detailed in the accompanying text. Antibodies reactive in fixed tissues are emphasized with bold typeface.

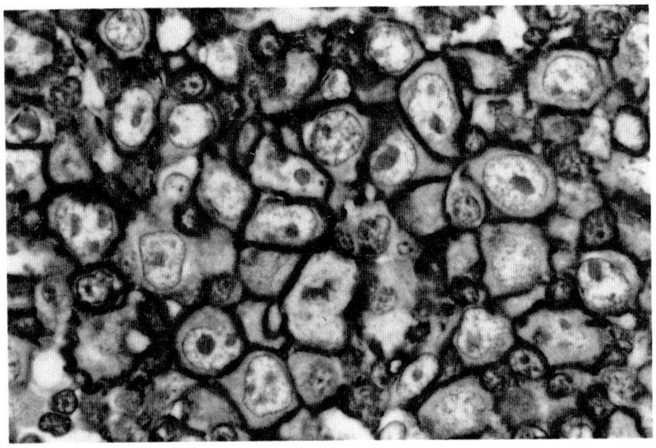

Fig. 4.32. Diffuse infiltrate of large cell type: Reactive B-immunoblastic proliferation of tonsillar infectious mononucleosis (anti-L26, X1000).

Minimum panel: L26(CD20), (+/− MB2)
Immunoglobulins
CD45RO
CD43
CD68 or MAC387
CD15
CD30, (+/− EMA)
Chloroacetate esterase stain, antibody NP57 or MPO

Reactive vs neoplastic

Both CD43 and Immunoglobulins are included in the above antibody list, and in some cases, may indicate neoplasia without recourse to a more expensive panel (see immunophenotypic criteria for neoplasia). Beyond this, other antibodies which could be useful as indicators of malignancy, are (in order of diminishing return): bcl-2, MT2, MY4, CD5, CD2, CD3, CD4, CD8, Leu8, and TCR variable region antibodies.

Further subtyping

In determining the precise subtype of lymphoproliferative disease, a prohibitively large repertoire of antibodies is available (see Immunophenotypes of specific immunoproliferative diseases). None the less, certain antibodies are particularly useful. The ability to detect follicle centres, with the use of stains for DRCs such as CD21, CD23, CD35 or laminin, is extremely useful in assessing the overall architecture of lymphoid organs; and antibodies to one of the above should be included in a minimum panel. All are effective, however CD23 is also useful in the differentiation of low grade B-cell lymphomas, and in Hodgkin's disease. Some consideration should be given to immature lymphoid tumours, and a minimum panel should be able to confirm a lymphoblastic phenotype. This could be achieved with the use of TdT antibodies, or a combination of CD10, CD1, and T-cell antigens 2, 3, 4, 5, 7, and 8. Clearly an antibody to TdT offers the simplest solution, however CD1, CD5, and CD10 are also valuable in the differentiation of Langerhans cell histiocytosis, low grade B-cell lymphomas, and follicular lymphomas respectively, and may be a better alternative. Finally, the immunophenotypic identification of hairy cell leukaemia may require the use of either tartrate resistant acid phosphatase (TRAP) or an anti-CD11c antibody.

Minimum panel: CD23 (or CD21, CD35)
+/− CD1, CD5 and CD10
TRAP or CD11c

References

Abbondanzo, S.L., Sato, N., Straus, S. and Jaffe, E.S. (1990). Acute infectious mononucleosis. CD30 (Ki-1) antigen expression and histologic correlations. *American Journal of Clinical Pathology* **93**, 698–702.

Acuto, O., Fabbi, M., Bensussan, A., Milanese, C., Campen, T.J., Royer, H.D. and Reinherz, E.L. (1985). The human T-cell receptor. *Journal of Clinical Immunology* **5**, 141–57.

Addis, B.J., Hyjek, E. and Isaacson, P.G. (1988). Primary pulmonary lymphoma. A re-appraisal of its histogenesis and its relationship to pseudolymphoma and interstitial pneumonia. *Histopathology* **13**, 1–17.

Agnarsson, B.A. and Kadin, M.E. (1987). An unusual B-cell lymphoma simulating hairy cell leukaemia. *American Journal of Clinical Pathology* **88**, 752–9.

Agnarsson, B.A. and Kadin, M.E. (1988). Ki-1 positive large cell lymphoma: A morphologic and immunologic study of 19 cases. *American Journal of Surgical Pathology* **12**, 264–74.

Agnarsson, B.A. and Kadin, M.E. (1989). The immunophenotype of Reed-Sternberg cells. A study of 50 cases of Hodgkin's disease using fixed frozen tissues. *Cancer* **63**, 2083–7.

Alberolaila, J., Places, L., Cantrell, D.A., Vives, J. and Lozano, F. (1992). Intracellular events involved in CD5-induced human T cell activation and proliferation. *Journal of Immunology* **148**, 1287–93.

Alexandre, D. and Lefranc, M.P. (1992). The Human gamma/delta+ and alpha/beta+ T-cells – A branched pathway of differentiation. *Molecular Immunology* **29**, 447–51.

Algara, P., Martinez, P., Sanchez, L., Villuendas, R., Orradre, J.L. and Oliva, H. (1991). Lymphocyte predominance Hodgkin's disease (nodular paragranuloma) – A bcl-2 negative germinal centre lymphoma. *Histopathology* **19**, 69–75.

Andersen, W.K., Knowles, D.M. and Silvers, D.N. (1992). CD1 (OKT6)-positive juvenile xanthogranuloma – OKT6 is not specific for Langerhans cell histiocytosis (histiocytosis-X). *Journal of the American Academy of Dermatology* **26**, 850–4.

Anderson, C., Rezuke, W.N., Kosciol, C.M., Pastuszak, W.T. and Cartun, R.W. (1991). Identification of T-cell lymphomas in paraffin-embedded tissues using polyclonal anti-CD3 antibody: Comparison with frozen section immunophenotyping and genotypic analysis. *Modern Pathology* **4**, 358–62.

Anderson, K.C., Bates, M.P., Slaughenhoupt, B.L., Pinkus, G.S., Schlossman, S.F. and Nadler, L.M. (1984). Expression of human B cell-associated antigens on leukaemias and lymphomas. A model of B cell differentiation. *Blood* **63**, 1424–33.

Anderson, K.C., Boyd, A.W., Fischer, D.C., Leslie, D., Schlossman, S.F. and Nadler, L. (1985). Hairy cell leukemia: A tumour of pre-plasma cells. *Blood* **65**, 620.

Andrade, R.E., Wick, M.R., Frizzera, G. and Gajl-Peczalska, K.L. (1988). Immunophenotyping of hematopoietic malignancies in paraffin sections. *Human Pathology* **19**, 394–402.

Andreesen, R., Brugger, W., Lohr, G.W. and Bross, K.J. (1989). Human macrophages can express the Hodgkin's cell-associated antigen Ki-1 (CD30). *American Journal of Pathology* **134**, 187–92.

Angel, C.A., Warford, A., Campbell, A.C., Pringle, J.H. and Lauder, I. (1987). The immunohistology of Hodgkin's disease. Reed-Sternberg cells and their variants. *Journal of Pathology* **153**, 21–30.

Anscombe, A.M. and Wright, D.H. (1985). Primary malignant lymphoma of the thyroid-a tumour of mucosa associated lymphoid tissue: review of seventy-six cases. *Histopathology* **9**, 81–97.

Anstey, A., Lowe, D.G., Kirby, J.D. and Horton, M.A. (1991). Familial mastocytosis – A clinical, immunophenotypic, light and electron microscopic study. *British Journal of Dermatology* **125**, 583–7.

Armitage, J.O., Greer, J.P. and Levine, A.M. (1989). Peripheral T-cell lymphoma. *Cancer* **63**, 158–63.

Ashman, L.K. and Aylett, G.W. (1991). Expression of CD31-epitopes on human lymphocytes – CD31-monoclonal antibodies differentiate between naive (CD45RA+) and memory (CD45RA-) CD4–positive T-cells. *Tissue Antigens* **38**, 208–212.

Backe, E., Schwarting, R., Gerdes, J., Ernst, M. and Stein, H. (1991). Ber-MAC3 – new monoclonal antibody that defines human monocyte macrophage differentiation antigen. *Journal of Clinical Pathology* **44**, 936–45.

Bahler, D.W., Berry, G., Oksenberg, J., Warnke, R.A. and Levy, R. (1992). Diversity of T-cell antigen receptor variable genes used by mycosis fungoides cells. *American Journal of Pathology* **140**, 1–8.

Banerjee, S.S., Harris, M., Eyden, B.P., Radford, J.A., Harrison, C.J. and Mainwaring, A.R. (1991). Monocytoid B cell lymphoma. *Journal of Clinical Pathology* **44**, 39–44.

Banks, P.M. (1990). The pathology of Hodgkin's disease. *Seminars in Oncology* **17**, 683–95.

Banks, P.M., Chan, J., Cleary, M.L., Delsol, G., Dewolfpeeters, C., Gatter, K., Grogan, T.M., Harris, N.L., Isaacson, P.G., Jaffe, E.S., Mason, D., Pileri, S., Ralfkiaer, E., Stein, H. and Warnke, R.A. (1992). Mantle cell lymphoma – A proposal for unification of morphologic, immunologic, and molecular data. *American Journal of Surgical Pathology* **16**, 637–40.

Banks, P.M., Metter, J. and Allred, D.C. (1990). Anaplastic large cell (Ki-1) lymphoma with histiocytic phenotype simulating carcinoma. *American Journal of Clinical Pathology* **94**, 445–52.

Bartl, R., Frisch, B., Fateh-Moghadam, A., Kettner, G., Jaeger, K. and Sommerfeld, W. (1987). Histologic classification and staging of multiple myeloma: a retrospective and prospective study of 674 cases. *American Journal of Clinical Pathology* **87**, 342–55.

Bassan, R., Neonato, M.G., Abbate, M., Motta, T., Barbui, T. and Rambaldi, A. (1991). Monoclonal lymphocytosis with villous lymphocytes – A chronic lymphoproliferative disease of CD11c+ B-cells. *Leukemia* **5**, 799–806.

Benezra, J., Bailey, A., Azumi, N., Delsol, G., Stroup, R., Sheibani, K. and Rappaport, H. (1991). Malignant histiocytosis-X – A distinct clinicopathologic entity. *Cancer* **68**, 1050–60.

Benjamin, D.R. and Gown, A.M. (1991). Aberrant cytoplasmic expression of proliferating cell nuclear antigen in Hodgkin's disease. *American Journal of Surgical Pathology* **15**, 764–8.

Berti, E., Aversa, G.G., Soligo, D., Cattoretti, G., Delia, D., Aiello, A., Parravincini, C., Hall, B. and Caputo, R. (1991). A6 – A new monoclonal antibody for immunostaining of paraffin-embedded tissues. *American Journal of Clinical Pathology* **95**, 188–93.

Bhat, N.M., Kantor, A.B., Bieber, M.M., Stall, A.M., Herzenberg,

L.A. and Teng, N.N.H. (1992). The ontogeny and functional characteristics of human B-1 ($CD5^{+}B$) cells. *International Immunology* **4**, 243–52.

Bhoopat, L., Turner, R.R., Stathopoulos, E., Meyer, P.R., Taylor, C.R., Marder, R.J. and Epstein, A.L. (1988). Immunohistochemical characterization of two new monoclonal antibodies (LN-4, LN-5) reactive with human macrophage subsets and derived malignancies in B5-fixed, paraffin-embedded tissues. *Blood* **71**, 1079–85.

Bishop, P.W., Harris, M., Smith, A.P. and Elsam, K.J. (1991). Immunophenotypic study of lymphocyte predominance Hodgkin's disease. *Histopathology* **18**, 19–24.

Bordessoule, D., Gaulard, P. and Mason, D.Y. (1990). Human lymphocytes bearing g/d T cell receptor localise preferentially to the red pulp of the spleen. *Journal of Clinical Pathology* **43**, 461–4.

Boyd, A.W., Ellis, D.W., Kannourakis, G., Begley, C.G., Mackay, I.R. and Burns, G.F. (1988). Activated killer cell lymphoma: An erythrophagocytic syndrome simulating histiocytic medullary reticulosis. *Pathology* **20**, 265–270.

Brecher, M. and Banks, P.M. (1990). Hodgkin's disease variant of Richter's syndrome. Report of eight cases. *American Journal of Clinical Pathology* **93**, 333–9.

Browne, G., Tobin, B., Carney, D.N. and Dervan, P.A. (1991). Aberrant MT2 positivity distinguishes follicular lymphoma from reactive follicular hyperplasia in B5- and formalin-fixed paraffin sections. *American Journal of Clinical Pathology* **96**, 90–4.

Brunning, R.D. (1991). T-Prolymphocytic Leukemia. *Blood* **78**, 3111–13.

Buccheri, V., Shetty, V., Yoshida, N., Morilla, R., Matutes, E. and Catovsky, D. (1992). The role of an anti-myeloperoxidase antibody in the diagnosis and classification of acute leukaemia – A comparison with light and electron microscopy cytochemistry. *British Journal of Haematology* **80**, 62–8.

Burns, B.F. and Dardick, I. (1990). Ki-1-positive non-Hodgkin's lymphomas: An immunophenotypic, ultrastructural, and morphometric study. *American Journal of Clinical Pathology* **93**, 327–32.

Butcher, E.C. (1990). Cellular and molecular mechanisms that direct leukocyte traffic. *American Journal of Pathology* **136**, 3–11.

Cabecadas, J.M. and Isaacson, P.G. (1991). Phenotyping of T-cell lymphomas in paraffin sections – Which antibodies? *Histopathology* **19**, 419–24.

Caldwell, C.W., Patterson, W.P., Toalson, B.D. and Yesus, Y. (1991). Surface and cytoplasmic expression of CD45 antigen isoforms in normal and malignant myeloid cell differentiation. *American Journal of Clinical Pathology* **95**, 180–7.

Carbone, A., Gloghini, A., De Re, V., P., T., Boiocchi, M. and Volpe, R. (1990). Histopathologic, immunophenotypic and genotypic analysis of Ki-1 anaplastic large cell lymphomas that express histiocyte-associated antigens. *Cancer* **66**, 2547–56.

Carbone, A., Gloghini, A., Pinto, A., Attadia, V., Zagonel, V. and Volpe, R. (1989). Monocytoid B-cell lymphoma with bone marrow and peripheral blood involvement at presentation. *American Journal of Clinical Pathology* **92**, 228–36.

Carbone, A., Gloghini, A. and Volpe, R. (1992). Paraffin section immunohistochemistry in the diagnosis of Hodgkin's disease and anaplastic large cell ($CD30^{+}$) lymphomas. *Virchows Archives A – Pathological Anatomy and Histopathology* **420**, 527–32.

Carbone, A., Manconi, R., Poletti, A., Gloghini, A., De Paoli, P. and Volpe, R. (1988a). Expression of Leu 8 surface antigen in B-cell lymphomas: Correlation with other B-cell markers. *Journal of Pathology* **154**, 133–40.

Carbone, A., Manconi, R., Poletti, A. and Volpe, R. (1988b). Heterogenous immunostaining patterns of follicular dendritic reticulum cells in human lymphoid tissue with selected antibodies reactive with different cell lineages. *Human Pathology* **19**, 51–6.

Carbone, A., Pinto, A., Gloghini, A., Volpe, R. and Zagonel, V. (1992). B-zone small lymphocytic lymphoma – a morphologic, immunophenotypic, and clinical study with comparison to well-differentiated lymphocytic disorders. *Human Pathology* **23**, 438–48.

Carbone, A., Poletti, A., Manconi, R., Gloghini, A. and Volpe, R. (1987). Heterogenous in situ immunophenotyping of follicular dendritic reticulum cells in malignant lymphomas of B-cell origin. *Cancer* **60**, 2919–26.

Casey, T.T., Olson, S.J., Cousar, J.B. and Collins, R.D. (1989). Immunophenotypes of Reed–Sternberg cells: A study of 19 cases of Hodgkin's disease in plastic-embedded sections. *Blood* **74**, 2624–8.

Cattoretti, G., Villa, A., Vezzoni, P., Giardini, R., Lombardi, L. and Rilke, F. (1990). Malignant histiocytosis. A phenotypic and genotypic investigation. *American Journal of Pathology* **136**, 1009–19.

Chadburn, A., Inghirami, G. and Knowles, D.M. (1990). Hairy cell leukemia-associated antigen LeuM5 (CD11c) is preferentially expressed by benign activated and neoplastic CD8 cells. *American Journal of Pathology* **136**, 29–37.

Chamulak, G.A., Brynes, R.K. and Nathwani, B.N. (1990). Kikuchi-Fujimoto disease mimicking malignant lymphoma. *American Journal of Surgical Pathology* **14**, 514–23.

Chan, J.K.C., Ng, C.S., Hui, P.K., Leung, T.W., Lo, E.S.F., Lau, W.H. and McGuire, L.J. (1989). Anaplastic large cell Ki-1 lymphoma: Delineation of two morphological types. *Histopathology* **15**, 11–34.

Chan, J.K.C., Ng, C.S. and Isaacson, P.G. (1990). Relationship between high grade lymphoma and low grade B-cell mucosa associated lymphoid tissue lymphoma (MALToma) of the stomach. *American Journal of Pathology* **136**, 1153–64.

Chan, J.K.C., Ng, C.S., Lau, W.H. and Lo, S.T.H. (1987a).

Most nasal/nasopharyngeal lymphomas are peripheral T-cell neoplasms. *American Journal of Surgical Pathology* **11**, 418–29.

Chan, J.K.C., Ng, C.S., Law, C.K., Ng, W.F. and Wong, K.F. (1987b). Reactive hemophagocytic syndrome: A study of 7 fatal cases. *Pathology* **19**, 43–50.

Chan, J.K.C., Ng, C.S. and Tung, S. (1986). Multilobated B-cell lymphoma, a variant of centroblastic lymphoma. Report of four cases. *Histopathology* **10**, 601–12.

Chan, W.C., Borowitz, M.J., Hammami, A., Wu, Y.J. and Ip, S.J. (1988). T cell receptor antibodies in the immunohistochemical studies of normal and malignant lymphoid cells. *Cancer* **62**, 2118–24.

Chan, W.C., Gu, L.B., Masih, A., Nicholson, J., Vogler, W.R., Yu, G. and Nasr, S. (1992). Large granular lymphocyte proliferation with the natural killer-cell phenotype. *American Journal of Clinical Pathology* **97**, 353–8.

Chan, W.C. and Zaatari, G. (1986). Lymph node interdigitating reticulum cell sarcoma. *American Journal of Clinical Pathology* **85**, 739–44.

Chang, K.L., Stroup, R. and Weiss, L.M. (1992). Hairy cell leukemia – current status. *American Journal of Clinical Pathology* **97**, 719–38.

Chilosi, M., Mombelli, A., Menestrina, F., Gilioli, E., Manfrin, E., Pizzolo, G. and Fiore-Donati, L. (1990a). Immunohistochemical differentiation of follicular lymphomas from florid reactive follicular hyperplasia with monoclonal antibodies reactive on paraffin sections. *Cancer* **65**, 1562–9.

Chilosi, M., Mombello, A., Montagna, L., Benedetti, A., Lestani, M., Semenzato, G. and Menestrina, F. (1990b). Multimarker immunohistochemical staining of calgranulins, chloroacetate esterase, and S-100 for simultaneous demonstration of inflammatory cells on paraffin sections. *Journal of Histochemistry and Cytochemistry* **38**, 1669–75.

Chilosi, M., Semenzato, G., Vinante, F., Menestrina, F., Piazzola, E., Focchiatti, V., Sabbioni, R., Zanotti, R. and Pizzolo, G. (1989). Increased levels of soluble interleukin-2 receptor in non-Hodgkin's lymphomas. Relationship with clinical, histologic and phenotypic features. *American Journal of Clinical Pathology* **92**, 186–91.

Chittal, S.M., Brousset, P., Voigt, J.J. and Delsol, G. (1991). Large B-cell lymphoma rich in T-cells and simulating Hodgkin's disease. *Histopathology* **19**, 211–20.

Chittal, S.M., Caveriviere, P., Schwarting, R., Gerdes, J., Al Saati, T., Rigal–Huguet, F., Stein, H. and Delsol, G. (1988). Monoclonal antibodies in the diagnosis of Hodgkin's disease. The search for a rational panel. *American Journal of Surgical Pathology* **12**, 9–21.

Chott, A., Augustin, I., Wrba, F., Hanak, H., Ohlinger, W. and Radaskiewicz, T. (1990a). Peripheral T-cell lymphomas: A clinicopathological study of 75 cases. *Human Pathology* **21**, 1117–25.

Chott, A., Kaserer, K., Augustin, I., Vesely, M., Heinz, R., Oehlinger, W., Hanak, H. and Radaszkiewicz, T. (1990b). Ki-1 positive large cell lymphoma. A clinicopathologic study of 41 cases. *American Journal of Surgical Pathology* **14**, 439–48.

Chott, A., Rappersberger, K., Schlossarek, W. and Radaszkiewicz, T. (1988). Peripheral T cell lymphoma presenting primarily as lethal midline granuloma. *Human Pathology* **19**, 1093–101.

Cibull, M.L., Stein, H., Gatter, K.C. and Mason, D.Y. (1989). The expression of CD3 antigen in Hodgkin's disease. *Histopathology* **15**, 597–605.

Clark, D.M. and Boylston, A.W. (1989). T-cell antigen receptor beta-chain variable region families: A study of their distribution in normal and reactive tissues. *Journal of Pathology* **158**, 9–12.

Clark, J.R., Williams, M.E. and Swerdlow, S.H. (1990). Detection of B- and T-cells in paraffin-embedded tissue sections. Diagnostic utility of commercially obtained 4KB5 and UCHL-1. *American Journal of Clinical Pathology* **93**, 58–69.

Clement, L.T. (1992). Isoforms of the CD45 common leukocyte antigen family – Markers for human T-cell differentiation. *Journal of Clinical Immunology* **12**, 1–10.

Close, P. and Lauder, I. (1990). Editorial. Mantle zone lymphoma – Is it an entity? *Journal of Pathology* **160**, 279–81.

Cogliatti, S.B., Lennert, K., Hansmann, M.L. and Zwingers, T.L. (1990). Monocytoid B cell lymphoma: clinical and prognostic features of 21 patients. *Journal of Clinical Pathology* **43**, 619–25.

Cooper, M.D. (1987). B Lymphocytes. Normal development and function. *New England Journal of Medicine* **317**, 1452–6.

Cossman, J., Zehnbauer, B., Garrett, C.T., Smith, L.J., Williams, M., Jaffe, E.S., Hanson, L.O. and Love, J. (1991). Gene rearrangements in the diagnosis of lymphoma/leukemia. Guidelines for use based on a multiinstitutional study. *American Journal of Clinical Pathology* **95**, 347–54.

Cousar, J.B., McGinn, D.L., Glick, A.D., List, A.F. and Collins, R.D. (1987). Report of an unusual lymphoma arising from parafollicular B-lymphocytes (PBLs) or so-called 'monocytoid' lymphocytes. *American Journal of Clinical Pathology* **87**, 121–8.

Craig, F.E., Clare, C.N., Sklar, J.L. and Banks, P.M. (1992). T-cell lymphoma and the virus-associated hemophagocytic syndrome. *American Journal of Clinical Pathology* **97**, 189–94.

Dallenbach, F.E. and Stein, H. (1989). Expression of T-cell receptor beta chain in Reed-Sternberg cells. *Lancet* **ii**, 828–30.

Daum, G.S., Sullivan, J.L., Ansell, J., Mulder, C. and Woda, B.A. (1987). Virus-associated hemophagocytic syndrome: Identification of an immunoproliferative precursor lesion. *Human Pathology* **18**, 1071–4.

Davey, F.R., Elghetany, M.T. and Kurec, A.S. (1990). Immunophenotyping of hematologic neoplasms in paraffin-embedded tissue sections. *American Journal of Clinical Pathology* **93** (Suppl. 1), S17–S26.

Davey, F.R., Olsen, S., Kurec, A.S., Eastman-Abaya, R., Gottlieb, A.J. and Mason, D.Y. (1988). The immunophenotyping of extramedullary myeloid cell tumours in paraffin-embedded tissue sections. *American Journal of Surgical Pathology* **12**, 699–707.

Davis, R.E., Dorfman, R.F. and Warnke, R.A. (1990). Primary large-cell lymphoma of the thymus: A diffuse B-cell neoplasm presenting as primary mediastinal lymphoma. *Human Pathology* **21**, 1262–8.

Deegan, M.J. (1989). Membrane antigen analysis in the diagnosis of lymphoid leukemias and lymphomas: Differential diagnosis, prognosis as related to immunophenotype, and recommendations for testing. *Archives of Pathology and Laboratory Medicine* **113**, 606.

Dehou, M.-F., Schots, R., Lacor, P., Arras, N., Verhavert, P., Kloppel, G. and van Camp, B. (1990). Diagnostic and prognostic value of the MB2 monoclonal antibody in paraffin-embedded bone marrow sections of patients with multiple myeloma and monoclonal gammopathy of undetermined significance. *American Journal of Clinical Pathology* **94**, 287–91.

Delabie, J., Vandenberghe, E., Kennes, C., Verhoef, G., Foschini, M.P., Stul, M., Cassiman, J.J. and de Wolf-Peeters, C. (1992). Histiocyte-rich B-cell lymphoma – a distinct clinicopathologic entity possibly related to lymphocyte predominant Hodgkin's disease, paragranuloma subtype. *American Journal of Surgical Pathology* **16**, 37–48.

Delabie, J., de Wolf-Peeters, C., de Vos, R., Vandenberghe, E., Kennes, K., de Jonge, I. and Desmet, V. (1991). True histiocytic neoplasm of Langerhans' cell type. *Journal of Pathology* **163**, 217–23.

Delsol, G., Blancher, A., Alsaati, T., Ralfkiaer, E., Lauritzen, A., Bruigeres, L., Brousset, P., Rigalhuguet, F., Mazerolles, C., Robert, A. and Chittal, S.M. (1991). Antibody BNH9 detects red blood cell-related antigens on anaplastic large cell ($CD30^+$) lymphomas. *British Journal of Cancer* **64**, 321–6.

Dembic, Z. (1991). Specificity and function of gammadelta T-Cells. *Periodicum Biologorum* **93**, 591–9.

Dianzani, U., Redoglia, V., Malavasi, F., Bragardo, M., Pileri, A., Janeway, C.A. and Bottomly, K. (1992). Isoform-specific associations of CD45 with accessory molecules in human lymphocytes-T. *European Journal of Immunology* **22**, 365–71.

Diehl, V., von Kalle, C., Fonatsch, C., Tesch, H., Juecker, M. and Schaadt, M. (1990). The cell of origin in Hodgkin's disease. *Seminars in Oncology* **17**, 660–72.

Dinarello, C.A. and Mier, J.W. (1987). Lymphokines. Current concepts. *New England Journal of Medicine* **317**, 940–5.

Dobson, C.M., Myskow, M.W., Krajewski, A.S., Carpenter, F.H. and Horne, C.H.W. (1987). Immunohistochemical staining of non-Hodgkin's lymphoma in paraffin sections using the MB1 and MT1 monoclonal antibodies. *Journal of Pathology* **153**, 203–12.

Dowell, B.L., Borowitz, M.J., Boyett, J.M., Pullen, D.J., Crist, W.M., Quddus, F.F., Russell, E.C., Falletta, J.M. and Metzgar, R.S. (1987). Immunologic and clinicopathologic features of common acute lymphoblastic leukemia antigen positive childhood T-cell leukemia: A pediatric oncology group study. *Cancer* **59**, 2020–6.

Drexler, H.G., Jones, D.B., Diehl, V. and Minowada, J. (1989). Is the Hodgkin cell a T- or B-lymphocyte? Recent evidence from geno- and immunophenotypic analysis and in vitro cell lines. *Haematology and Oncology* **7**, 95.

Duijvestijn, A.M., Horst, E. and Pals, S.T. (1988). High endothelial differentiation in human lymphoid and inflammatory tissues defined by monoclonal antibody HECA-452. *American Journal of Pathology* **130**, 147–55.

Durie, B.G.M. and Grogan, T.M. (1985). Calla-positive myeloma: An aggressive subtype with poor survival. *Blood* **66**, 229–32.

Editorial (1991). Gamma/delta T-cell receptors. *Lancet* **337**, 207–8.

Elghetany, M.T., Kurec, A.S., Schuehler, K., Forbes, B.A., Duggan, D.B. and Davey, F.R. (1991). Immunophenotyping of non-Hodgkin's lymphomas in paraffin-embedded tissue sections. A comparison with genotypic analysis. *American Journal of Clinical Pathology* **95**, 517–25.

Elliott, C.J., McCarthy, K.P., Carter, R.L. and Davies, P. (1989). Granulocytic sarcoma: Misleading immunohistological staining with MT1 and S-100 protein antibodies. *Journal of Clinical Pathology* **42**, 188–90.

Epstein, J. (1992). Myeloma Phenotype – Clues to disease origin and manifestation. *Hematology – Oncology Clinics of North America* **6**, 249–56.

Erber, W. and Mason, D.Y. (1988). Expression of the interleukin-2 (Tac antigen / CD25) in hematologic neoplasms. *American Journal of Clinical Pathology* **89**, 645–8.

Facchetti, F., de Wolf-Peeters, C., Mason, D.Y., Pulford, K., van den Oord, J.J. and Desmet, V.J. (1988). Plasmacytoid T cells: immunohistochemical evidence for their monocyte-macrophage origin. *American Journal of Pathology* **133**, 15–21.

Facchetti, F., De Wolf-Peeters, C. and Van Den Oord, J.J. (1989). Plasmacytoid monocytes (so-called plasmacytoid T-cells) in Kikuchi's lymphadenitis. An immunohistologic study. *American Journal of Clinical Pathology* **92**, 42–50.

Falini, B., Flenghi, L., Fagioli, M., Pelicci, P.G., Stein, H., Bignerna, B., Pileri, S. and Martelli, M.F. (1991). Expression of the intestinal T-lymphocyte associated molecule HML-1: analysis of 75 non-Hodgkin's lymphomas and description of the first HML-1 positive T-lymphoblastic tumour. *Histopathology* **18**, 421–6.

Falini, B., Flenghi, L., Pileri, S., Pelicci, P., Fagioli, M., Martelli, M.F., Moretta, L. and Ciccone, E. (1989). Distribution of T cells bearing different forms of the T cell receptor g/d in normal and pathological tissues. *Journal of Immunology* **143**, 2480–8.

Falini, B., Pileri, S., Stein, H., Dieneman, D., Dallenbach, F., Delsol, G., Minelli, O., Poggi, S., Martelli, M.F., Pallesen, G. and Palestro, G. (1990). Variable expression of leucocyte-common (CD45) antigen in CD30 (Ki-1)- positive anaplastic large cell lymphoma: Implications for the differential diagnosis between lymphoid and nonlymphoid malignancies. *Human Pathology* **21**, 624–9.

Falini, B., Stein, H., Pileri, S., Canino, S., Farabbi, R., Martelli, M.F., Grignani, F., Fagioli, M., Minelli, O., Ciani, C. and Flenghi, L. (1987). Expression of lymphoid-associated antigens on Hodgkin's and Sternberg-Reed cells of Hodgkin's disease. An immunocytochemical study on lymph node cytospins using monoclonal antibodies. *Histopathology* **11**, 1229–42.

Falk, M.H., Tesch, H., Stein, H., Diehl, V., Jones, D.B., Fonatsch, C. and Bornkamm, G.W. (1987). Phenotype versus immunoglobulin and T-cell receptor genotype of Hodgkin's-derived cell lines: Activation of immature lymphoid cells in Hodgkin's disease. *International Journal of Cancer* **40**, 262–9.

Favara, B.E. (1991). Langerhans' cell histiocytosis pathobiology and pathogenesis. *Seminars in Oncology* **18**, 3–7.

Fellbaum, C., Hansmann, M.-L. and Lennert, K. (1989). Malignant lymphomas of the nasal cavity and paranasal sinuses. *Virchows Archives (Anatomy, Pathology)* **414**, 399–405.

Feller, A.C., Griesser, G.H., Mak, T.W. and Lennert, K. (1986). Lymphoepithelioid lymphoma (Lennert's lymphoma) is a monoclonal proliferation of helper/inducer T cells. *Blood* **68**, 663–7.

Feller, A.C., Griesser, G.H., Von Schilling, C., Wacker, H.H., Dallenbach, F., Bartels, H., Kuse, R., Mak, T. and Lennert, K. (1988). Clonal gene rearrangement patterns correlate with immunophenotype and a different clinical course in patients with angioimmunoblastic lymphadenopathy. *American Journal of Pathology* **133**, 549–56.

Ferry, J.A., Sklar, J., Zuckerberg, L.R. and Harris, N.L. (1991). Nasal lymphoma: A clinicopathologic study with immunophenotypic and genotypic analysis. *American Journal of Surgical Pathology* **15**, 268–79.

Ferry, J.A., Zukerberg, L.R. and Harris, N.L. (1992). Florid progressive transformation of germinal centers – a syndrome affecting young men, without early progression to nodular lymphocyte predominance Hodgkin's disease. *American Journal of Surgical Pathology* **16**, 252–8.

Flenghi, L., Spinozzi, F., Stein, H., Krushwitz, M., Pileri, S. and Falini, B. (1990). LF61: A new monoclonal antibody directed against a trimeric molecule (150, 125, 105kD) associated with hairy cell leukaemia. *British Journal of Haematology* **76**, 451–9.

Foon, K.A. and Todd, R.F. (1986). Immunologic classification of leukaemia and lymphoma. *Blood* **68**, 1–31.

Foucar, E., Rosai, J. and Dorfman, R. (1990). Sinus histiocytosis with massive lymphadenopathy (Rosai-Dorfman disease): Review of the entity. *Seminars in Diagnostic Pathology* **7**, 19–73.

Foucar, K. and Foucar, E. (1991). The mononuclear phagocytic and immunoregulatory effector (M-PIRE) system: evolving concepts. *Seminars in Diagnostic Pathology* **7**, 4–18.

Frierson, H.F. and Innes, D.J. (1985). Sensitivity of anti-Leu-M1 as a marker in Hodgkin's disease. *Archives of Pathology and Laboratory Medicine* **109**, 1024–8.

Frierson, H.F., Innes, D.J., Mills, S.E. and Wick, M.R. (1989). Immunophenotypic analysis of sinonasal non-Hodgkin's lymphomas. *Human Pathology* **20**, 636–42.

Frizzera, G., Sakurai, M., Notohara, K. and Konishi, H. (1991). t(11;14)(q13;q32) in B-cell lymphomas (intermediately differentiated lymphocytic and follicular). A report of four cases. *American Journal of Clinical Pathology* **95**, 684–91.

Garcia, C.F., Warnke, R.A. and Weiss, L.M. (1986a). Follicular large cell lymphoma: An immunophenotypic study. *American Journal of Pathology* **123**, 425–31.

Garcia, C.F., Weiss, L.M. and Warnke, R.A. (1986b). Small non-cleaved cell lymphoma: An immunophenotypic study of 18 cases and comparison to large cell lymphoma. *Human Pathology* **17**, 454.

Gatter, K.C., Alcock, C., Heryet, A. and Mason, D.Y. (1985). Clinical importance of analysing tumours of uncertain origin with immunohistological techniques. *Lancet* **1**, 1302.

Gaulard, P., Bourquelot, P., Kanavaros, P., Haioun, C., Le Couedic, J.P., Divine, M., Goosens, M., Zafrani, E.S., Farcet, J.P. and Reyes, F. (1990). Expression of the alpha/beta and gamma/delta T-cell receptors in 57 cases of peripheral T-cell lymphomas. Identification of a subset of g/d T-cell lymphomas. *American Journal of Pathology* **137**, 617–28.

Gaulard, P., Dagay, M.F., Peuchmaur, M., Brousse, N., Gisselbrecht, C., Solalceligny, P., Diebold, J. and Mason, D.Y. (1992). Expression of the bcl-2 gene product in follicular lymphoma. *American Journal of Pathology* **140**, 1089–95.

Gaulard, P., Henni, T., Marolleau, J.P., Haioun, C., Henni, Z., Voisin, M.-C., Divine, M., Goosens, M., Farcet, J.P. and Reyes, F. (1988). Lethal midline granuloma (polymorphic reticulosis) and lymphomatoid granulomatosis. Evidence for a monoclonal T-cell lymphoproliferative disorder. *Cancer* **62**, 705–10.

Gloghini, A., Volpe, R. and Carbone, A. (1990). Ki-M6 immunostaining in routinely processed sections of reactive and neoplastic human lymphoid tissue. *American Journal of Clinical Pathology* **94**, 734–41.

Gogusev, J., Barbey, S. and Nezelof, C. (1991). Human malignant histiocytosis CD30+ DEL cell line differentiates into macrophage-like cells when treated with a Phorbol Diester. *Cancer Research* **51**, 5712–15.

Gregory, C.D., Tursz, T., Edwards, C.T., Tetaud, C., Talbot, M., Caillou, B., Rickinson, A.B. and Lipinski, M. (1987). Identification of a subset of normal B-cells with a Burkitt's lymphoma. (BL)-like phenotype. *Journal of Immunology*, **139**, 313–18.

Grogan, T.M. (1989). Immunophenotypic properties of myeloma cells. *American Journal of Surgical Pathology* **13**, 164–5.

Gustmann, C., M., A., Osborn, M., Griesser, H. and Feller, A.C. (1991). Cytokeratin expression and vimentin content in large cell anaplastic lymphomas and other non-Hodgkin's lymphomas. *American Journal of Pathology* **138**, 1413–22.

Hall, P.A. and D'Ardenne, A.J. (1987). Value of CD15 immunostaining in diagnosing Hodgkin's disease: A review of published literature. *Journal of Clinical Pathology* **40**, 1298–304.

Hall, P.A., D'Ardenne, A.J., Richards, M.A. and Stansfeld, A.G. (1987). Lymphoplasmacytoid lymphoma: An immunohistological study. *Journal of Pathology* **153**, 213–23.

Hall, P.A., d'Ardenne, A.J. and Stansfeld, A.G. (1988a). Paraffin section immunohistochemistry. 1. Non-Hodgkin's lymphoma. *Histopathology* **13**, 149–60.

Hall, P.A., D'Ardenne, A.J. and Stansfield, A.G. (1988b). Paraffin section immunohistochemistry. II. Hodgkin's disease and large cell anaplastic (Ki-1) lymphoma. *Histopathology* **13**, 161–9.

Hall, P.A., Donaghy, M., Cotter, F.E., Stansfield, A.G. and Levison, D.A. (1989a). An immunohistological and genotypic study of the plasma cell form of Castleman's disease. *Histopathology* **14**, 333–46.

Hall, P.A., Gregory, W.M. and Stansfield, A.G. (1989b). MT2 immunoreactivity, cellular proliferation and prognosis in B-cell non-Hodgkin's lymphoma. Histopathology **14**, 523–36.

Hamilton-Dutoit, S.J., Pallesen, G., Franzmann, M.B., Karkov, J., Black, F., Skinhoj, P. and Pedersen, C. (1991). AIDS-related lymphoma: Histopathology, immunophenotype, and association with Epstein-Barr virus as demonstrated by in situ nucleic acid hybridization. *American Journal of Pathology* **138**, 149–63.

Hansmann, M.-L., Stein, H., Fellbaum, C., Hui, P.K., Pawaresch, M.R. and Lennert, K. (1989). Nodular paragranuloma can transform into high-grade malignant lymphoma of B type. *Human Pathology* **20**, 1169–75.

Hansmann, M.L., Fellbaum, C., Hui, P.K. and Moubayed, P. (1990). Progressive transformation of germinal centers with and without association to Hodgkin's disease. *American Journal of Clinical Pathology* **93**, 219–26.

Hansmann, M.L., Kikuchi, M., Wacker, H.H., Radzun, H.J., Nathwani, B.N., Hesse, K. and Parwaresch, M.R. (1992). Immunohistochemical monitoring of plasmacytoid cells in lymph node sections of Kikuchi-Fujimoto disease by a new pan-macrophage antibody Ki-M1P. *Human Pathology* **23**, 676–80.

Hanson, C.A., Bockenstedt, P.L., Schnitzer, B., Fox, D.A., Kueck, B. and Braun, D.K. (1991). S100-positive, T-cell chronic lymphoproliferative disease – an aggressive disorder of an uncommon T-cell subset. *Blood* **78**, 1803–13.

Hanson, C.A., Frizzera, G., Patton, D.F., Peterson, B.A., McLain, K.L., Gajl-Peczalska, K.J. and Kersey, J.H. (1988). Clonal rearrangement for immunoglobulin and T-cell receptor genes in systemic Castleman's disease. Association with Epstein-Barr virus. *American Journal of Pathology* **131**, 84–91.

Hanson, C.A., Jascz, W., Kersey, J.H., Astorga, M.G., Peterson, B.A., Gajl-Peczalska, K.J. and Frizzera, G. (1989). True histiocytic lymphoma: Histopathologic, immunophenotypic and genotypic analysis. *British Journal of Haematology* **73**, 187–98.

Harris, N.L. (1991). Extranodal lymphoid infiltrates and mucosa-associated lymphoid tissue (MALT) – A unifying concept. *American Journal of Surgical Pathology* **15**, 879–84.

Harris, N.L. and Bhan, A.K. (1985). Mantle zone lymphoma. A pattern produced by lymphomas of more than one cell type. *American Journal of Surgical Pathology* **9**, 872–82.

Hastrup, N., Hamilton-Dutoit, S., Ralfkiaer, E. and Pallesen, G. (1991). Peripheral T-cell lymphomas: An evaluation of reproducibility of the updated Kiel classification. *Histopathology* **18**, 99–105.

Hastrup, N., Ralfkiaer, E. and Pallesen, G. (1989). Aberrant phenotypes in peripheral T cell lymphomas. *Journal of Clinical Pathology* **42**, 398–402.

Herbst, H., Tippelmann, G., Anagnostopoulos, I., Gerdes, J., Schwarting, R., Boehm, T., Pileri, S., Jones, D.B. and Stein, H. (1989). Immunoglobulin and T-cell receptor gene rearrangements in Hodgkin's disease and Ki-1-positive anaplastic large cell lymphoma: dissociation between phenotype and genotype. *Leukemia Research* **13**, 103–16.

Ho, F.C.S., Choy, D., Loke, S.L., Kung, I.T., Fu, K.H., Liang, R., Todd, D. and Khoo, R.K.K. (1990). Polymorphic reticulosis and conventional lymphomas of the nose and upper aerodigestive tract: A clinicopathologic study of 70 cases and immunophenotypic study of 16 cases. *Human Pathology* **21**, 1041–50.

Hockenbery, D.M., Zutter, M., Hickey, W., Nahm, M. and Korsmeyer, S.J. (1991). BCL2 protein is topographically restricted in tissues characterized by apoptotic cell death. *Proceedings of the National Academy of Sciences of the United States of America* **88**, 6961–5.

Hofmann, W.J., Momburg, F. and Moller, P. (1988). Thymic medullary cells expressing B lymphocyte antigens. *Human Pathology* **19**, 1280–7.

Hollema, H. and Poppema, S. (1988). Immunophenotypes of malignant lymphoma centroblastic-centrocytic and malignant lymphoma centrocytic: An immunohistologic study indicating a derivation from different stages of B-cell differentiation. *Human Pathology* **19**, 1053–9.

Hollema, H. and Poppema, S. (1989). T-lymphoblastic and

peripheral T-cell lymphomas in the northern part of the Netherlands. An immunological study of 29 cases. *Cancer* **64**, 1620–8.

Hollowood, K. and Macartney, J.C. (1991). Reduced apoptotic cell death in follicular lymphoma. *Journal of Pathology* **163**, 337–42.

Horny, H.-P., Campbell, M., Steinke, B. and Kaiserling, E. (1990a). Acute myeloid leukaemia: Immunohistologic findings in paraffin-embedded bone marrow biopsy specimens. *Human Pathology* **21**, 648–55.

Horny, H.-P., Schaumburg-Lever, G., Bolz, S., Geerts, M.L. and Kaiserling, E. (1990b). Use of monoclonal antibody KP1 for identifying normal and neoplastic human mast cells. *Journal of Clinical Pathology* **43**, 719–22.

Horny, H.P., Reimann, O. and Kaiserling, E. (1988). Immunoreactivity of normal and neoplastic human tissue mast cells. *American Journal of Clinical Pathology* **89**, 335–40.

Hounieu, H., Chittal, S.M., Alsaati, T., Demascarel, A., Sabattini, E., Pileri, S., Falini, B., Ralfkiaer, E., Letourneau, A., Selves, J., Voigt, J.J., Laurent, G., Diebold, J. and Delsol, G. (1992). Hairy cell leukemia – diagnosis of bone marrow involvement in paraffin-embedded sections with monoclonal antibody DBA.44. *American Journal of Clinical Pathology* **98**, 26–33.

Hsu, S.-M. (1990). The never-ending controversies in Hodgkin's disease. *Blood* **75**, 1742–50.

Hsu, S.-M., Ho, Y.-S. and Hsu, P.-L. (1991). Lymphomas of true histiocytic origin: expression of different phenotypes in so-called true histiocytic lymphoma and malignant histiocytosis. *American Journal of Pathology* **138**, 1389–404.

Hsu, S.-M., Ho, Y.-S., Li, P.-J., Monheit, J., Ree, H.J., Sheibani, K. and Winberg, C.D. (1986). L & H variants of Reed-Sternberg cells express sialylated Leu M1 antigen. *American Journal of Pathology* **122**, 199–203.

Hsu, S.-M. and Hsu, P.-L. (1989). Aberrant expression of T cell and B cell markers in myelocyte/monocyte/histiocyte-derived lymphoma and leukaemic cells: Is the infrequent expression of T/B cell markers sufficient to establish a lymphoid origin for Hodgkin's Reed–Sternberg cells? *American Journal of Pathology* **134**, 203–12.

Hsu, S.-M. and Hsu, P.-L. (1990). Lack of effect of colony-stimulating factors, interleukins, interferons, and tumour necrosis factor on the growth and differentiation of cultured Reed–Sternberg cells: Comparison with effects of phorbol ester and retinoic acid. *American Journal of Pathology* **136**, 181–9.

Hsu, S.M. and Jaffe, E.S. (1984a). Phenotypic expression of B lymphocytes: 1. Identification with monoclonal antibodies in normal lymphoid tissues. *American Journal of Pathology* **114**, 387–95.

Hsu, S.M. and Jaffe, E.S. (1984b). Phenotypic expression of B lymphocytes: 2. Immunoglobulin expression of germinal center cells. *American Journal of Pathology* **114**, 396–402.

Hsu, S.-M. and Jaffe, E.S. (1984c). Leu M1 and peanut agglutinin stain the neoplastic cells of Hodgkin's disease. *American Journal of Clinical Pathology* **82**, 29–32.

Hsu, S.-M. and Jaffe, E.S. (1985). Phenotypic expression of T lymphocytes in thymus and peripheral lymphoid tissues. *American Journal of Pathology* **121**, 69–78.

Hsu, S.-M., Tseng, C.K. and Hsu, P.-L. (1990). Expression of p55 (Tac) interleukin-2 receptor (Il-2R), but not p75 Il-2R, in cultured H-RS cells in tissues. *American Journal of Pathology* **136**, 735–44.

Hsu, S.-M., Yang, K. and Jaffe, E.S. (1985). Phenotypic expression of Hodgkin's and Reed-Sternberg cells in Hodgkin's disease. *American Journal of Pathology* **118**, 209–17.

Hunt, S.J., Charley, M.R. and Jegasothy, B.V. (1992). Cutaneous T-cell lymphoma – utility of antibodies to the variable regions of the human T-cell antigen receptor. *Journal of the American Academy of Dermatology* **26**, 552–8.

Hyjek, E. and Isaacson, P.G. (1988). Primary B cell lymphoma of the thyroid and its relationships to Hashimoto's thyroiditis. *Human Pathology* **19**, 1315–26.

Hyjek, E., Smith, W.J. and Isaacson, P.G. (1988). Primary B-cell lymhoma of salivary gland and its relationship to myoepithelial sialadenitis (MESA). *Human Pathology* **19**, 766–76.

Inghirami, G., Foitl, D.R., Sabichi, A., Zhu, B.Y. and Knowles, D.M. (1991). Autoantibody-associated cross-reactive idiotype-bearing human lymphocytes-B – distribution and characterization, including Ig VH gene and CD5 antigen expression. *Blood* **78**, 1503–15.

Inghirami, G., Zhu, B.Y., Chess, L. and Knowles, D.M. (1990). Flow cytometric and immunohistochemical characterization of the gamma/delta T-lymphocyte population in normal human lymphoid tissue and peripheral blood. *American Journal of Pathology* **136**, 357–67.

Isaacson, P.G. (1989). Commentary. Castleman's disease. *Histopathology* **14**, 429–32.

Isaacson, P.G. (1990). Commentary: Lymphomas of mucosa-associated lymphoid tissue [MALT]. *Histopathology* **16**, 617–19.

Isaacson, P.G., Chan, J.K.C., Tang, C. and Addis, B.J. (1990). Low grade B-cell lymphoma of mucosa-associated lymphoid tissue arising in the thymus. A thymic lymphoma mimicking myoepithelial sialadenitis. *American Journal of Surgical Pathology* **14**, 342–51.

Isaacson, P.G., Norton, A.J. and Addis, B.J. (1987). The human thymus contains a novel population of B lymphocytes. *Lancet* **2**, 1488–90.

Isaacson, P.G. and Spencer, J. (1987). Malignant lymphoma of mucosa-associated lymphoid tissue. *Histopathology* **11**, 445–62.

Isaacson, P.G., Spencer, J., O'Connor, N.T.J., Bevan, D.H., Conolly, C.E., Kirkham, N., Pollock, D.J., Wainscoat, J.S., Stein, H. and Mason, D.Y. (1985). Malignant histiocytosis of the intestine: A T-cell lymphoma. *Lancet* **2 (8457)**, 688–91.

Isaacson, P.G., Wotherspoon, A.C., Diss, T. and Pan, L.X. (1991). Follicular colonization in B-cell lymphoma of mucosa-associated lymphoid tissue. *American Journal of Surgical Pathology* **15**, 819–28.

Isaacson, P.G. and Wright, D.H. (1983). Malignant lymphoma of mucosa associated lymphoid tissue. *Cancer* **52**, 1410–16.

Jack, A.S., Boylston, A.W., Carrel, S. and Grigor, I. (1990). Cutaneous T-cell lymphoma cells employ a restricted range of T-cell antigen receptor variable region genes. *American Journal of Pathology* **136**, 17–21.

Jaffe, E.S. (1985). Surgical Pathology of the Lymph Nodes and Related Organs. WB Saunders Company, Philadelphia.

Jaffe, E.S. (1988). The morphological spectrum of T-cell lymphoma. Abstract, Society for Haematopathology Annual Meeting. *American Journal of Surgical Pathology* **12**, 158–9.

Jaffe, E.S. (1989). The elusive Reed–Sternberg cell (Editorial). *New England Journal of Medicine* **320**, 529–31.

Jaffe, E.S. (1990). The role of immunophenotypic markers in the classification of non-Hodgkin's lymphomas. *Seminars in Oncology* **17**, 11–19.

Jaffe, E.S., Bookman, M.A. and Longo, D.L. (1987). Lymphocytic lymphoma of intermediate differentiation – Mantle zone lymphoma: A distinct subtype of B-cell lymphoma. *Human Pathology* **18**, 877–80.

Jaffe, E.S., Cost, J., Fauci, A.S., Cossman, J. and Tsokos, M. (1983). Malignant lymphoma and erythrophagocytosis simulating malignant histiocytosis. *American Journal of Medicine* **75**, 741–9.

Jaffe, E.S., Gonzalez, C.L., Medeiros, L.J. and Raffeld, M. (1991). T-cell-rich B-cell lymphomas (Letter to the Editor). *American Journal of Surgical Pathology* **15**, 491–2.

Jaffe, E.S., Longo, D.L., Cossman, J., Hsu, S.-M., Arnold, A. and Korsmeyer, S.J. (1984). Diffuse B cell lymphoma with T cell predominance in patients with follicular lymphoma or 'pseudo T cell lymphoma'. *Laboratory Investigation* **50**, 27A-28A.

Jalkanen, S. (1991). Lymphocyte traffic to mucosa-associated lymphatic tissues. *Immunologic Research* **10**, 268–70.

James, S.P., Murakawa, Y., Kanof, M.E. and Berg, M. (1991). Multiple roles of Leu-8/MEL-14 in leukocyte adhesion and function. *Immunologic Research* **10**, 282–92.

Janeway, C.A. (1992). The T-cell receptor as a multicomponent signalling machine – CD4/CD8 coreceptors and CD45 in T-cell activation. *Annual Review of Immunology* **10**, 645–74.

Kadin, M.E., Agnarsson, B.A., Ellingsworth, L.R. and Newcom, S.R. (1990). Immunohistochemical evidence of a role for transforming growth factor Beta in the pathogenesis of nodular sclerosing Hodgkin's disease. *American Journal of Pathology* **136**, 1209–14.

Kadin, M.E., Muramota, L. and Said, J. (1988). Expression of T-cell antigens on Reed-Sternberg cells in a subset of patients with nodular sclerosing and mixed cellularity Hodgkin's disease. *American Journal of Pathology* **130**, 345–53.

Kadin, M.E., Nasu, K., Sako, D., Said, J. and Vonderheid, E. (1985). Lymphomatoid papulosis. A cutaneous proliferation of activated helper T-cells expressing Hodgkin's disease associated antigens. *American Journal of Pathology* **119**, 315–25.

Kamat, D., Laszewski, M.J., Kemp, J.D., Goeken, J.A., Lutz, C.T., Platz, C.E. and Dick, F.R. (1990). The diagnostic utility of immunophenotyping and immunogenotyping in the pathologic evaluation of lymphoid proliferations. *Modern Pathology* **3**, 105–12.

Kansas, G.S., Wood, G.S., Fishwild, D.M. and Engleman, E.G. (1985). Functional characterization of human lymphocyte subsets distinguished by monoclonal anti-Leu-8. *Journal of Immunology* **134**, 2995–3002.

Kant, J.A., Hubbard, S.M., Longo, D.L., Simon, R.M., DeVita, V.T. and Jaffe, E.S. (1986). The pathologic and clinical heterogeneity of lymphocyte depleted Hodgkin's disease. *Journal of Clinical Oncology* **4**, 284–94.

Kantor, A.B. (1991). The Development and Repertoire of B-1 Cells (CD5 B-Cells). *Immunology Today* **12**, 389–91.

Katzin, W.E., Linden, M.D., Fishleder, A.J. and Tubbs, R.R. (1989). Immunophenotypic and genotypic characterization of diffuse mixed non-Hodgkin's lymphomas. *American Journal of Pathology* **135**, 615–21.

Kaudewitz, P., Stein, H., Dallenbach, F., Eckert, F., Bieber, K., Burg, G. and Braun-Faulco, O. (1989). Primary and secondary cutaneous Ki-1 ($CD30^+$) anaplastic large cell lymphomas: Morphologic, immunohistologic, and clinical characteristics. *American Journal of Pathology* **135**, 359–67.

Kelly, P.M.A., Bliss, E., Morton, J.A., Burns, J. and McGee, J.O. (1988a). Monoclonal antibody EBM/11 : high specificity for human macrophages. *Journal of Clinical Pathology* **41**, 510–15.

Kelly, P.M.A., McGovern, M., Gatter, K.C., Theaker, J.M. and McGee, J.O. (1988b). EBM/11 reactivity in malignant histiocytosis. *Journal of Clinical Pathology* **41**, 1305–9.

Kernohan, N.M. and Smart, L.M. (1990). Anomalous phenotype of cutaneous T-cell infiltrates. Letter. *Journal of Pathology* **160**, 81–2.

Kimura, N., Toyonaga, B., Yoshikai, Y., Triebel, F., Debre, P., Minden, M.D. and Mak, T.W. (1986). Sequences and diversity of human T-cell receptor Beta chain variable region genes. *Journal of Experimental Medicine* **164**, 739–50.

Kinney, M.C., Glick, A.D., Stein, H. and Collins, R.D. (1990). Comparison of anaplastic large cell Ki-1 lymphomas and microvillous lymphomas in their immunologic and ultrastructural features. *American Journal of Surgical Pathology*

14, 1047–60.

Kipps, T.J., Robbins, B.A., Tefferi, A., Meisenholder, G., Banks, P. and Carson, D.A. (1990). CD5–positive B-cell malignancies frequently express cross-reactive idiotypes associated with IgM autoantibodies. *American Journal of Pathology* **136**, 809–16.

Knight, J., Laing, P., Knight, A., Adams, D. and Ling, N. (1986). Thyroid-stimulating autoantibodies usually contain only lambda-light chains: evidence for the 'forbidden clone' theory. *Journal of Clinical Endocrinology 62*, 342–7.

Knowles, D.M. (1989). Immunophenotypic and antigen receptor gene rearrangement analysis in T cell neoplasia. *American Journal of Pathology* **134**, 761–85.

Knowles, D.M., Athan, E., Ubriaco, A., McNally, L., Inghirami, G., Wieczorek, R., Finfer, M. and Jakobiec, A. (1989). Extranodal noncutaneous lymphoid hyperplasias represent a continuous spectrum of B-cell neoplasia: Demonstration by molecular genetic analysis. *Blood* **73**, 1635–45.

Knowles, D.M.I., A., N., Pelicci, P.G., Burke, J.S., Wu, A.M., Winberg, C.D., Sheibani, K. and Dalla-Favera, R. (1986). Immunoglobulin and T-cell receptor B-chain gene rearrangement analysis of Hodgkin's disease: Implications for lineage determination and differential diagnosis. *Proceedings of the National Academy of Science USA* **83**, 7942–6.

Komp, D.M. and Perry, M.C. (1991). Introduction: The histiocytic syndromes. *Seminars in Oncology* **18**, 1–2.

Koo, C.H., Mason, D.Y., Miller, R., Ben-Ezra, J., Sheibani, K. and Rappaport, H. (1990). Additional evidence that 'plasmacytoid T-cell lymphoma' associated with chronic myeloproliferative disorders is of macrophage origin. *American Journal of Clinical Pathology* **93**, 822–7.

Koopman, G., Parmentier, H.K., Schuurman, H.-J., Newman, W., Meijer, C.J. and Pals, S.T. (1991). Adhesion of human B cells to follicular dendritic cells involves both the lymphocyte function-associated antigen 1/intercellular adhesion molecule 1 and very late antigen 4/vascular cell adhesion molecule 1 pathways. *Journal of Experimental Medicine* **173**, 1297–304.

Kornstein, M.J., Wakely, P.E., Kardos, T.F. and Frable, W.J. (1990). Dendritic reticulum cells and immunophenotype in aspiration biopsies of lymph nodes: Value in the subclassification of non-Hodgkin's lymphomas. *American Journal of Clinical Pathology* **94**, 165–9.

Krajewski, A.S., Myskow, M.W., Cachia, P., Salter, D.M. and Dewar, A.E. (1988). T-cell lymphoma: morphology, immunophenotype and clinical features. Histopathology **13**, 19–41.

Krajewski, A.S., Myskow, M.W., Salter, D.M., Cunningham, D.S. and Ramage, E.R. (1989). Diagnosis of T-cell lymphoma using beta F1, anti-T-cell-receptor beta chain antibody. *Histopathology* **15**, 239–47.

Krissansen, G.W., Print, C.G., Prestidge, R.L., Hollander, D., Yuan, Q., Jiang, W.M., Jenkins, D.R., Leung, E., Mead, P., Yong, R., Ameratunga, R.V., Cerfbensussan, N. and Watson, J.D. (1992). Immunologic and structural relatedness of the integrin beta7complex and the human intraepithelial lymphocyte antigen HML-1. *FEBS Letters* **296**, 25–8.

Kruschwitz, M., Frizsche, G., Schwarting, R., Micklem, K., Mason, D.Y., Falini, B. and Stein, H. (1991). Ber-ACT8: new monoclonal antibody to the mucosa lymphocyte antigen. *Journal of Clinical Pathology* **44**, 636–45.

Kueck, B.D., Hanson, C.A., Weissman, D.E. and Bayliss, K. (1989). Primary lymph node presentation of angiocentric lymphoma associated with features of a hemophagocytic syndrome. *American Journal of Hematology* **30**, 104–11.

Kurec, A.S., Cruz, V.E., Barrett, D., Mason, D.Y. and Davey, F.R. (1990). Immunophenotyping of acute leukemias in paraffin embedded tissue sections. *American Journal of Clinical Pathology* **93**, 502–9.

Kwak, L.W., Wilson, M., Weiss, L.M., Horning, S.J., Warnke, R.A. and Dorfman, R.F. (1991). Clinical significance of morphologic subdivision in diffuse large cell lymphoma. *Cancer* **68**, 1988–93.

Lai, R., Visser, L. and Poppema, S. (1991). Tissue distribution of restricted leucocyte common antigens: A comprehensive study with protein- and carbohydrate specific CD45R antibodies. *Laboratory Investigation* **64**, 844–54.

Lamarre, L., Jacobson, J., Aisenberg, A.C. and Harris, N.L. (1989). Primary large cell lymphoma of the mediastinum: A histologic and immunophenotypic study of 29 cases. *American Journal of Surgical Pathology* **13**, 730–9.

Lanier, L.L. and Phillips, J.H. (1992). Natural killer cells. *Current Opinion in Immunology* **4**, 38–42.

Lanier, L.L., Ruitenberg, J.J. and Phillips, J.H. (1986). Human CD3 T lymphocytes that express neither CD4 nor CD8 antigens. *Journal of Experimental Medicine* **164**, 339–44.

Lardelli, P., Bookman, M.A., Sundeen, J., Longo, D.L. and Jaffe, E.S. (1990). Lymphocytic lymphoma of intermediate differentiation: Morphologic and immunophenotypic spectrum and clinical correlations. *American Journal of Surgical Pathology* **14**, 752–63.

Lavabrebertrand, T., Donadio, D., Fegueux, N., Jessueld, D., Taib, J., Charlier, D., Rousset, T., Emberger, J.M., Baldet, P. and Navarro, M. (1992). A study of 15 cases of primary mediastinal lymphoma of B-cell type. *Cancer* **69**, 2561–6.

LeBien, T.W. and McCormack, R.T. (1989). The common acute lymphoblastic leukemia antigen (CD10) – Emancipation from a functional enigma. *Blood* **73**, 625–35.

Lennert, K. and Mohri, N. (1978). Histopathology and diagnosis of non-Hodgkin's lymphomas. In Lennert, K. (ed.), *Malignant Lymphomas Other Than Hodgkin's Disease. Histology, Cytology, Ultrastructure, Immunology*, Springer-Verlag, Berlin. pp. 111–469.

Lennert, K. and Muller-Hermelink, H.K. (1975). Lymphocyten und ihre Funktionsformen-Morphologie, Organisation und immunologische Bedeutung. *Verh Anatomischen Gesellschaft* **69**, 103–22.

Lennert, K., Stein, H., Feller, A.C. and Gerdes, J. (1982). Morphology, cytochemistry, and immunohistology of T cell lymphomas. In Vitetta, E.S. (ed.), *B and T cell Tumours*, Academic Press, New York, pp. 9–28.

Leoncini, L., del Vecchio, M.T., Kraft, R., Megha, T., Barbini, P., Cevenini, G., Poggi, S., Pileri, S. and Cottier, H. (1990). Hodgkin's disease and CD30-positive anaplastic large cell lymphomas – a continuous spectrum of malignant disorders. A quantitative morphometric and immunohistologic study. *American Journal of Pathology* **137**, 1047–57.

Levine, E.G., Hanson, C.A., Jascz, W. and Peterson, B.A. (1991). True histiocytic lymphoma. Seminars in Oncology **18**, 39–49.

Li, G., Hansmann, M.-L., Zwingers, T. and Lennert, K. (1990). Primary lymphomas of the lung: morphological, immunohistochemical and clinical features. *Histopathology* **16**, 519–31.

Linden, M.D., Fishleider, A.J., Katzin, W.E. and Tubbs, R.R. (1988). Absence of B-cell and T-cell clonal expansion in nodular, lymphocyte predominant Hodgkin's disease. *Human Pathology* **19**, 591–4.

Lipford, E.H., Margolick, J.B., Longo, D.L., Fauci, A.S. and Jaffe, E.S. (1988). Angiocentric immunoproliferative lesions: A clinicopathological spectrum of post-thymic T-cell proliferations. *Blood* **72**, 1674–81.

Lipford, E.H., Smith, H.R., Pittaluga, S., Jaffe, E.S., Steinberg, A.D. and Cossman, J. (1987). Clonality of angio-immunoblastic lymphadenopathy and implications for its evolution to malignant lymphoma. *Journal of Clinical Investigation* **79**, 637–42.

Lippman, S.M., Grogan, T.M., Spier, C., Koopman, C.F., Gall, E.P., Shimm, D.S. and Durie, B.G.M. (1987). Lethal midline granuloma with a novel T-cell phenotype as found in peripheral T-cell lymphoma. *Cancer* **59**, 936–9.

Liu, Y.J., Mason, D.Y., Johnson, G.D., Abbot, S., Gregory, C.D., Hardie, D.L., Gordon, J. and Maclennan, I.C.M. (1991). Germinal center cells express bcl-2 protein after activation by signals which prevent their entry into apoptosis. *European Journal of Immunology* **21**, 1905–10.

Loftus, B., Loh, L.C., Curran, B., Henry, K. and Leader, M. (1991). Mac387 – Its non-specificity as a tumour marker or marker of histiocytes. *Histopathology* **19**, 251–5.

Loke, S.L., Ho, F., Srivastava, G., Fu, K.H., Leung, B. and Liang, R. (1992). Clonal Epstein-Barr Virus Genome in T-Cell Rich Lymphomas of B or Probable-B Lineage. *American Journal of Pathology* **140**, 981–9.

Loy, T.S., Diaz-Arias, A.A. and Perry, M.C. (1991). Familial erythrophagocytic lymphohistiocytosis. *Seminars in Oncology* **18**, 34–9.

Lukes, R.J. and Tindle, B.H. (1975). Immunoblastic lymphadenopathy, a hyperimmune entity resembling Hodgkin's disease. *New England Journal of Medicine* **292**, 1–8.

Macon, W.R., Casey, T.T., Kinney, M.C., Collins, R.D. and Cousar, J.B. (1991). Leu-22 (L60). A more sensitive marker than UCHL1 for peripheral T-cell lymphomas, particularly large-cell types. *American Journal of Clinical Pathology* **95**, 696–701.

Macon, W.R., Cousar J.B., Waldron, J.A. and Hsu S.M. (1992a). Interleukin-4 may contribute to the abundant T-cell reaction and paucity of neoplastic B-cells in T-cell rich B cell lymphomas. *American Journal of Pathology* **141**, 1031–6.

Macon, W.R., Williams, M.E., Greer, J.P., Stein, R.S., Collins, R.D. and Cousar, J.B (1992). T-Cell Rich B-Cell Lymphomas – A Clinicopathologic Study of 19 Cases. *American Journal of Surgical Pathology* **16**, 351–63.

Manconi, R., Poletti, A., Volpe, R., De Paoli, P. and Carbone, A. (1987). Mantle zone lymphoma: Additional arguments for its origin. *American Journal of Surgical Pathology* **11**, 333–4.

Martin, J.M.E., Boras, V.F., Houwen, B. and Francovich, N. (1988). Hairy cell leukemia and anti-leukocyte common antigen. *American Journal of Clinical Pathology* **90**, 412–20.

Mason, D.Y. (1987). A new look at lymphoma immunohistology. Editorial. *American Journal of Pathology* **128**, 1–4.

Mason, D.Y., Comans-Bitter, W.M., Cordell, J.L., Verhoeven, M.J. and van Dongen, J.M. (1990). Antibody L26 recognizes an intracellular epitope on the B-cell-associated CD20 antigen. *American Journal of Pathology* **136**, 1215–22.

Mason, D.Y., Cordell, J., Brown, M., Pallesen, G., Ralfkiaer, E., Rothbard, J., Crumpton, M. and Gatter, K.C. (1989). Detection of T cells in paraffin wax embedded tissue using antibodies against a peptide sequence from the CD3 antigen. *Journal of Clinical Pathology* **42**, 1194–200.

Mason, D.Y., Cordell, J.L., Tse, A.G.D., Vandongen, J.J.M., Vannoesel, C.J.M., Micklem, K., Pulford, K.A.F., Valensi, F., Comansbitter, W.M., Borst, J. and Gatter, K.C. (1991). The IgM-associated protein mb-1 as a marker of normal and neoplastic B-cells. *Journal of Immunology* **147**, 2474–82.

Mason, D.Y., Krissansen, G.W., Davey, F.R., Crumpton, M.J. and Gatter, K.C. (1988). Antisera against epitopes resistant to denaturation on T3(CD3) antigen can detect reactive and neoplastic T cells in paraffin embedded tissue biopsy specimens. *Journal of Clinical Pathology* **41**, 121–7.

Matutes, E., Brito-Babapulle, V., Swansbury, J., Ellis, J., Morilla, R., Dearden, C., Sempere, A. and Catovsky, D. (1991). Clinical and laboratory features of 78 cases of T-prolymphocytic leukaemia. *Blood* **78**, 3269.

Mcdaniel, H.L., Macpherson, B.R., Tindle, B.H. and Lunde, J.H. (1992). Lymphoproliferative Disorder of Granular Lymphocytes – A Heterogeneous Disease. *Archives of Pathology & Laboratory Medicine* **116**, 242–8.

McKenna, R.W. (1992). Lymphoproliferative Disorder of granular lymphocytes – more questions than answers. *Archives of Pathology & Laboratory Medicine* **116**, 235–7.

Medeiros, L.J. and Harris, N. (1990). Immunohistologic analysis of small lymphocytic infiltrates of the orbit and conjunctiva. *Human Pathology* **21**, 1126–31.

Medeiros, L.J. and Harris, N.L. (1989). Lymphoid infiltrates of the orbit and conjunctiva: a morphologic and immunophenotypic study of 99 cases. *American Journal of Surgical Pathology* **13**, 459–71.

Medeiros, L.J., Herrington, R.D., Gonzalez, C.L., Jaffe, E.S. and Cossman, J. (1991). My4 antibody staining of non-Hodgkin's lymphomas. *American Journal of Clinical Pathology* **95**, 363–8.

Medeiros, L.J., Kaynor, B. and Harris, N.L. (1989). Lupus lymphadenitis: Report of a case with immunologic studies on frozen sections. *Human Pathology* **20**, 295–9.

Medeiros, L.J., Peiper, S.C., Elwood, L., Yano, T., Raffeld, M. and Jaffe, E.S. (1991). Angiocentric immunoproliferative lesions – A molecular analysis of eight cases. *Human Pathology* **22**, 1150–7.

Menestrina, F., Chilosi, M., Bonetti, F., Lestani, M., Scarpa, A., Novelli, P., Doglioni, C., Todeschini, G., Ambrosetti, A. and Fiore-Donati, L. (1986). Mediastinal large-cell lymphoma of B-type, with sclerosis: histopathological and immunohistochemical study eight cases. *Histopathology* **10**, 589–600.

Micklem, K., Rigney, E., Cordell, J., Simmons, D., Stross, P., Turley, H., Seed, B. and Mason, D. (1989). A human macrophage-associated antigen (CD68) detected by six different monoclonal antibodies. *British Journal of Hematology* **73**, 6–11.

Micklem, K.J., Dong, Y., Willis, A., Pulford, K.A., Visser, L., Durkop, H., Poppema, S., Stein, H. and Mason, D.Y. (1991). HML-1 antigen on mucosa-associated T cells, activated cells, and hairy leukemic cells is a new integrin containing the beta7 subunit. *American Journal of Pathology* **139**, 1297–301.

Miettinen, M., Paljakka, P., Haveri, P. and Saxen, E. (1987). Sinus histiocytosis with massive lymphadenopathy: A nodal and extranodal proliferation of S-100 protein positive histiocytes? *American Journal of Clinical Pathology* **88**, 270–7.

Miklem, J., Stross, W. and Willis, A. (1990). Different isoforms of human FcRII distinguished by CDw32 antibodies. *Journal of Immunology* **144**, 2295–303.

Miller, J.F.A.P. (1961). Immunological function of the thymus. *Lancet* **ii**, 748–9.

Mintzer, D.M., Andreeff, M., Filippa, D.A., Jhanwar, S.C., Koziner, C. and Koziner, B. (1984). Progression of nodular poorly differentiated lymphocytic lymphoma to Burkitt's-like lymphoma. *Blood* **64**, 415.

Mirchandani, I., Palutke, M., Tabaczka, P., Goldfarb, S., Eisenberg, L. and Pak, M.S.Y. (1985). B-cell lymphomas morphologically resembling T-cell lymphomas. *Cancer* **56**, 1578–83.

Miyashita, T., Kawaguchi, H., Mizutani, S. and Tsuchida, M. (1991). Histiocytic medullary reticulosis, a lethal form of Epstein–Barr-virus-related disorder. *Lancet* **337**, 986–7.

Moller, P., Matthaei-Maurer, D.U., Hofmann, W.J., Dorken, B. and Moldenhauer, G. (1989a). Immunophenotypic similarities of mediastinal clear-cell lymphoma and sinusoidal (monocytoid) B cells. *International Journal of Cancer* **43**, 10–16.

Moller, P., Matthaei-Maurer, U. and Moldenhauer, G. (1989b). CD30 (Ki-1) antigen expression in a subset of gastric mucosal plasma cells and in a primary gastric plasmacytoma. *American Journal of Clinical Pathology* **91**, 18–23.

Moller, P., Mielke, B. and Moldenhauer, G. (1990). Monoclonal antibody HML-1 a marker for intraepithelial T cells and lymphomas derived thereof, also recognizes hairy cell leukaemia and some B-cell lymphomas. *American Journal of Pathology* **136**, 509–12.

Moller, P., Moldenhauer, G., Momberg, F., Lammier, B., Eberlein-Gonska, M., Kiesel, S. and Dorken, B. (1987). Mediastinal lymphoma of large cell type is a tumour corresponding to terminal steps of B-cell differentiation. *Blood* **69**, 1087–95.

Monda, L., Warnke, R.A. and Rosai, J. (1986). A primary lymph node malignancy with features suggestive of dendritic reticulum cell differentiation. A report of 4 cases. *American Journal of Pathology* **122**, 562–72.

Montgomery, E.A., Meis, J.M. and Frizzera, G. (1992). Rosai-Dorfman disease of soft tissue. *American Journal of Surgical Pathology* **16**, 122–9.

Mori, N., Oka, K. and Kojima, M. (1988). Immunohistochemical study of mantle zone lymphoma. *American Journal of Clinical Pathology* **89**, 143–8.

Mori, N., Oka, K., Yoda, Y., Abe, T. and Kojima, M. (1990). T-cell receptor expression in the T-cell malignancies. *American Journal of Clinical Pathology* **93**, 495–501.

Murphy, G.F., Messadi, D., Fonferko, E. and Hancock, W.W. (1986). Phenotypic transformation of macrophages to Langerhans cells in the skin. *American Journal of Pathology* **123**, 401–6.

Murray, P.G., Janmohamed, R.M.I. and Crocker, J. (1991). CD23 Expression in non-Hodgkin lymphoma – immunohistochemical demonstration using the antibody-BU38 on paraffin sections. *Journal of Pathology* **165**, 125–8.

Myhre, M.J. and Isaacson, P. (1987). Primary B-cell gastric lymphoma – a reassessment of its histogenesis. *Journal of Pathology* **152**, 1–11.

Naeim, F. (1988). Hairy cell leukemia: Characteristics of the neoplastic cells. *Human Pathology* **19**, 375–88.

Naeim, F., Hoon, D.S.B., Cheng, L., Herschman, H. and Cochran, A. (1987). Reactivity of neoplastic cells of hairy cell leukemia with antisera to S-100 protein. *American Journal of Clinical Pathology* **88**, 86–91.

Nakamine, H., Masih, A.S., Sanger, W.G., Wickert, R.S.,

Mitchell, D.W., Armitage, J.O. and Weisenburger, D.D. (1992). Richter's Syndrome with different immunoglobulin light chain types – molecular and cytogenetic features indicate a common clonal origin. *American Journal of Clinical Pathology* **97**, 656–63.

Nakamura, S., Hara, K., Suchi, T., Ito, M., Ikeda, H., Nagahama, M., Nakayama, A., Nakagawa, A., Kaneshima, H. and Asai, J. (1988). Interdigitating cell sarcoma. A morphologic, immunohistologic, and enzyme-histochemical study. *Cancer* **61**, 562–8.

Namba, K., Jaffe, E.S. and Braylan, R.C. (1977). Alkaline phosphatase-positive malignant lymphoma. A subtype of B-cell lymphomas. *American Journal of Clinical Pathology* **68**, 535.

Naumovski, L., Warnke, R. and Smith, S.D. (1990). The never-ending controversies in Hodgkin's disease. (Reply). *Blood* **75**, 1744.

Newcom, S.R., Muth, L.H. and Parker, E.T. (1990). Production of monoclonal antibodies that detect Hodgkin's high molecular weight transforming growth factor – beta. *Blood* **75**, 3434–7.

Ng, C.-S., Lam, T.-K., Hui, P.K., Ng, H.K., Szeto, S.C. and Feng, C.S. (1988). Juvenile chronic myeloid leukemia. A malignancy of S-100 protein positive histiocytes. *American Journal of Clinical Pathology* **90**, 575–82.

Ng, C.S., Chan, J.K.C., Cheng, P.N.M. and Szeto, S.C. (1986). Nasal T-cell lymphoma associated with hemophagocytic syndrome. *Cancer* **58**, 67–71.

Ng, C.S., Chan, J.K.C., Hui, P.K., Chan, W.C. and Lo, S.T.H. (1988). Application of a T cell receptor antibody beta F1 for immunophenotypic analysis of malignant lymphomas. *American Journal of Pathology* **132**, 365–71.

Ng, C.S., Chan, J.K.C., Hui, P.K. and Lau, W.H. (1989). Large B-cell lymphomas with a high content of reactive T cells. *Human Pathology* **20**, 1145–54.

Ng, C.S., Chan, J.K.C., Hui, P.K. and Lo, S.T.H. (1988). Monoclonal antibodies reactive with normal and neoplastic T cells in paraffin sections. *Human Pathology* **19**, 295–303.

Ng, C.S., Chan, J.K.C. and Lo, S.T.H. (1987a). Expression of natural killer cell markers in non-Hodgkin's lymphomas. *Human Pathology* **18**, 1257–62.

Ng, C.S., Chan, J.K.C., Lo, S.T.H. and Lo, D.S.Y. (1987b). Critical assessment of four monclonal antibodies reactive with B-cells in formalin-fixed paraffin-embedded tissues. *Histopatology* **11**, 1243–58.

Ngan, B., Picker, L.J., Medeiros, J. and Warnke, R. (1989a). Immunophenotypic diagnosis of non-Hodgkin,s lymphoma in paraffin sections. Co-expression of L60 (Leu22) and L26 antigens correlates with malignant histologic findings. *American Journal of Pathology* **91**, 579–83.

Ngan, B., Warnke, R.A. and Cleary, M.L. (1989b). Variability of immunoglobulin expression in follicular lymphoma: An immunohistologic and molecular genetic study. *American Journal of Pathology* **135**, 1139–44.

Ngan, B.-Y., Chen-Levy, Z. and Weiss, L.M. (1988a). Expression in non-Hodgkin's lymphoma of the BCL-2 protein associated with the t(14;18) chromosomal translocation. *New England Journal of Medicine* **318**, 1638–44.

Ngan, B.Y., Chen-Levy, Z., Weiss, L.M., Warnke, R.A. and Cleary, M.L. (1988b). Expression in non-Hodgkin's lymphoma of the bcl-2 protein associated with the t(14;18) chromosomal translocation. *New England Journal of Medicine* **318**, 1630–44.

Ngan, B.Y., Takagi, K., Dombrowski, A. and Dorfman, R.F. (1989). Monocytoid B-cell [para-follicular B-cell] lymphoma: a study of 20 cases. *Laboratory Investigation* **60**, 66A.

Ngan, B.Y., Warnke, R.A., Wilson, M., Takagi, K., Cleary, M.L. and Dorfman, R.F. (1991). Monocytoid B-cell lymphoma – A study of 36 cases. *Human Pathology* **22**, 409–21.

Nicholas, D.S., Harris, S. and Wright, D.H. (1990). Lymphocyte predominance Hodgkin's disease – an immunohistochemical study. *Histopathology* **16**, 157–65.

Nizze, H., Cogliatti, S.B., Von Schilling, C., Feller, A.C. and Lennert, K. (1991). Monocytoid B-cell lymphoma: morphological variants and relationship to low-grade B-cell lymphoma of the mucosa-associated lymphoid tissue. *Histopathology* **18**, 403–14.

Noorduyn, L.A., van der Valk, P., van Heerde, P., Vroom, T.M., Blok, P., Willemze, R. and Meijer, C.J.L.M. (1990). Stage is a better prognostic indicator than morphologic subtype in primary noncutaneous T-cell lymphoma. *American Journal of Clinical Pathology* **93**, 49–57.

Norton, A.J. and Isaacson, P.G. (1986). An immunocytochemical study of T-cell lymphomas using monoclonal and polyclonal antibodies effective in routinely fixed wax embedded tissues. *Histopathology* **10**, 1243–60.

Norton, A.J. and Isaacson, P.G. (1987). Detailed analysis of B-cell lymphoma using a panel of antibodies reactive in routinely fixed wax-embedded tissue. *American Journal of Pathology* **128**, 225–40.

Norton, A.J. and Isaacson, P.G. (1989a). Lymphoma phenotyping in formalin-fixed and paraffin wax-embedded tissues. I Range of antibodies and staining patterns. *Histopathology* **14**, 437–46.

Norton, A.J. and Isaacson, P.G. (1989b). Lymphoma phenotyping in formalin-fixed and paraffin wax-embedded tissues: II. Profiles of reactivity in the various tumour types. *Histopathology* **14**, 557–79.

Norton, A.J., Ramsay, A.D., Smith, S.H., Beverly, P.C.L. and Isaacson, P.G. (1986). Monoclonal antibody (UCHL1) that recognizes normal and neoplastic T cells in routinely fixed tissues. *Journal of Clinical Pathology* **39**, 399–405.

Norton, A.J., Rivas, C. and Isaacson, P.G. (1989). A comparison between monoclonal antibody MT2 and immunoglobulin staining in the differential diagnosis of follicular lymphoid proliferations in routinely fixed wax-embedded biopsies. *American Journal of Pathology* **134**, 63–70.

Nunez, G., Hockenbery, D., Mcdonnell, T.J., Sorensen, C.M. and Korsmeyer, S.J. (1991). Bcl-2 maintains B-cell memory. Nature **353**, 71–3.

O'Briain, D.S., Kennedy, M.J. and Daly, P.A. (1989). Multiple lymphomatous polyposis of the gastrointestinal tract: a clinicopathologically distinct form of non-Hodgkin's lymphoma of B-cell centrocytic type. *American Journal of Surgical Pathology* **13**, 691–9.

O'Grady, J., Blaikie, A.J., Howie, S.E., Salter, D.M. and Krajewski, A.S. (1991). Immunological analysis of the immunoreactivity of normal lymphoid cells and lymphomas with the monoclonal antibody OPD4. *Journal of Pathology* **164**, 119–25.

O'Grady, J., Krajewski, A.S. and Ramage, E.F. (1990). Demonstration of clonality in T-cell lymphoma using an anti-T-cell receptor variable region antibody panel. *Histopathology* **17**, 553–6.

O'Hara, C.J., Said, J.W. and Pinkus, G.S. (1986). Non Hodgkin's lymphoma, multilobated B-cell type: Report of nine cases with immunohistochemical and immuno-ultrastructural evidence for a follicular center cell derivation. *Human Pathology* **17**, 593.

Ohshima, K., Kikuchi, M., Eguchi, F., Kobari, S. and Tasaka, H. (1991). Virus-associated haemophagocytic syndrome with Epstein–Barr virus infection. *Virchows Archives A (Pathological Anatomy and Histopathology)* **419**, 519–22.

Ornvold, K., Carstensen, H., Junge, J., Gyhrs, A. and Ralfkiaer, E. (1992). Tumours classified as malignant histiocytosis in children are T-cell neoplasms. *Acta Pathologica Microbiologica et Immunologica Scandinavica* **100**, 558–66.

Ornvold, K., Ralfkiaer, E. and Carstensen, H. (1990). Immunohistochemical study of the abnormal cells in Langerhans cell histiocytosis (Histiocytosis X). *Virchows Archives [Anatomy]* **416**, 403–10.

Osborne, B., Butler, J. and Gresik, M. (1992). Progressive Transformation of Germinal Centres: Comparison of 23 pediatric patients to the adult population. *Modern Pathology* **5**, 135–40.

Osborne, B.M., Butler, J.J. and Pugh, W.C. (1990a). The value of immunophenotyping on paraffin sections in the identification of T-cell rich B-cell large cell lymphomas: lineage confirmed by Jh rearrangement. *American Journal of Surgical Pathology* **14**, 933–8.

Osborne, B.M., Uthman, M.O., Butler, J.J. and McLaughlin, P. (1990b). Differentiation of T-cell lymphoma from Hodgkin's disease: Mitotic rate and S-phase analysis. *American Journal of Clinical Pathology* **93**, 227–32.

Ott, M.M., Muller–Hermelink, H.K., Schmitt, B. and Feller, A.C. (1991). Chromosomal translocation detected by bcl-1 and bcl-2 rearrangement in low grade B-cell lymphomas in a European population. *Histopathology* **19**, 163–7.

Pabst, R. (1991). Lymphocyte migration to the gut – oversimplifications and controversial aspects. *Immunologic Research* **10**, 279–81.

Pallesen, G. (1990). Commentary: The diagnostic significance of the CD30 (Ki-1) antigen. *Histopathology* **16**, 409–13.

Pallesen, G. and Hamilton–Dutoit, S.J. (1988). Ki-1 (CD30) antigen is regularly expressed by tumour cells of embryonal carcinoma. *American Journal of Pathology* **133**, 446–50.

Pallesen, G. and Hamilton–Dutoit, S.J. (1990). Specificity of monoclonal antibody HML-1. *Lancet* **i**, 537.

Pallesen, G., Hamilton–Dutoit, S.J., Rowe, M. and Young, L.S. (1991). Expression of Epstein–Barr virus latent gene products in tumour cells of Hodgkin's disease. *Lancet* **337**, 320–2.

Pan, L., Diss, T.C., Cunningham, D. and Isaacson, P.G. (1989). The bcl-2 gene in primary B cell lymphoma of mucosa-associated lymphoid tissue (MALT). *American Journal of Pathology* **135**, 7–11.

Papadopoulos, K.P., Bagg, A., Bezwoda, W.R. and Mendelow, B.V. (1989). The routine diagnostic utility of immunoglobulin and T-cell receptor gene rearrangements in lymphoproliferative disorders. *American Journal of Clinical Pathology* **91**, 633–8.

Parker, C.M., Cepek, K.L., Russell, G.J., Shaw, S.K., Posnett, D.N., Schwarting, R. and Brenner, M.B. (1992). A Family of beta7 integrins on human mucosal lymphocytes. *Proceedings of the National Academy of Sciences of the United States of America* **89**, 1924–8.

Patsouris, E., Noel, H. and Lennert, K. (1988). Histological and immunohistological findings in lymphoepithelioid cell lymphoma (Lennert's lymphoma). *American Journal of Surgical Pathology* **12**, 34–350.

Patsouris, E., Noel, H. and Lennert, K. (1989a). Angioimmunoblastic lymphadenopathy-type of T-cell lymphoma with a high content of epithelioid cells. Histopathology and comparison with lymphoepithelioid cell lymphoma. *American Journal of Surgical Pathology* **13**, 262–75.

Patsouris, E., Noel, H. and Lennert, K. (1989b). Cytohistologic and immunohistochemical findings in Hodgkin's disease, mixed cellularity type, with a high content of epithelioid cells. *American Journal of Surgical Pathology* **13**, 1014–22.

Patsouris, E., Noel, H. and Lennert, K. (1990). Lymphoplasmacytic / lymphoplasmacytoid immunocytoma with a high content of epithelioid cells: histologic and immunohistochemical findings. *American Journal of Surgical Pathology* **14**, 660–70.

Paulli, M., Rosso, R., Kindl, S., Boveri, E., Marocolo, D., Chioda, C., Agostini, C., Magrini, U. and Facchetti, F. (1992). Immunophenotypic characterization of the cell infiltrate in five cases of sinus histiocytosis with massive lymphadenopathy (Rosai–Dorfman disease). *Human Pathology* **23**, 647–54.

Pavlova, Z., Parker, J.W., Taylor, C.R., Levine, A.M., Feinstein, D.I. and Lukes, R.J. (1987). Small non-cleaved follicular center cell lymphoma: Burkitt's and non-Burkitt,s variants in the US. II. Pathologic and immunologic features. *Cancer* **59**, 1892–902.

Pedersen, C., Gerstoft, J., Lundgren, J.D., Skinhoj, P., Bottzauw, J., Geisler, C., Hamiltondutoit, S.J., Thorsen, S., Lisse, I., Ralfkiaer, E. and Pallesen, G. (1991). HIV-associated lymphoma – Histopathology and association with Epstein–Barr virus genome related to clinical, immunological and prognostic features. *European Journal of Cancer* **27**, 1416–23.

Pelstring, R.J., Essell, J.H., Kurtin, P.J., Cohen, A.R. and Banks, P.M. (1991). Diversity of organ site involvement among malignant lymphomas of mucosa-associated tissues. *American Journal of Clinical Pathology* **96**, 738–45.

Peterson, L. (1991). B-cell chronic lymphocytic leukemia: new perspectives on an old disease. Society for Hematopathology Abstracts. September 1991.

Pettit, C., Zukerberg, L.R., Gray, M.H., Ferry, J.A., Rosenberg, A.E., Harmon, D.C. and Harris, N.L. (1990). Primary lymphoma of bone: A B-cell neoplasm with a high frequency of multilobated cells. *American Journal of Surgical Pathology* **14**, 329–34.

Pezella, F., Tse, A.G.D., Cordell, J.L., Pulford, K.A.F., Gatter, K.C. and Mason, D.Y. (1990). Expression of the bcl-2 oncogene protein is not specific for the 14;18 chromosomal translocation. *American Journal of Pathology* **137**, 225–32.

Pezzella, F., Jones, M., Ralfkiaer, E., Ersboll, J., Gatter, K.C. and Mason, D.Y. (1992). Evaluation of bcl-2 protein expression and 14–18 translocation as prognostic markers in follicular lymphoma. *British Journal of Cancer* **65**, 87–9.

Phillips, J.H., Hori, T., Nagler, A., Bhat, N., Spits, H. and Lanier, L.L. (1992). Ontogeny of human natural killer (NK) cells – fetal NK cells mediate cytolytic function and express cytoplasmic CD3epsilon,delta proteins. *Journal of Experimental Medicine* **175**, 1055–66.

Picker, L.J., Brenner, M.B., Michie, S. and Warnke, R.A. (1988). Expression of T cell receptor delta chains in benign and malignant T lineage lymphoproliferations. *American Journal of Pathology* **132**, 401–5.

Picker, L.J., Brenner, M.B., Weiss, L.M., Smith, S.D. and Warnke, R.A. (1987). Discordant expression of CD3 and T-cell receptor beta-chain antigens in T-lineage lymphomas. *American Journal of Pathology* **129**, 434–40.

Picker, L.J. and Butcher, E.C. (1992). Physiological and molecular mechanisms of lymphocyte homing. *Annual Review of Immunology* **10**, 561–91.

Picker, L.J., Medeiros, L.J., Weiss, L.M., Warnke, R.A. and Butcher, E.C. (1988). Expression of lymphocyte homing receptor antigen in non-Hodgkin's lymphoma. *American Journal of Pathology* **130**, 496–504.

Picker, L.J., Weiss, L.M., Medeiros, L.J., Wood, G.S. and Warnke, R.A. (1987). Immunophenotypic criteria for the diagnosis of non-Hodgkin's lymphoma. *American Journal of Pathology* **128**, 181–201.

Pileri, S., Falini, B., Delsol, G., Stein, H., Baglioni, P., Poggi, S., Martelli, M.F., Rivano, M.T., Mason, D.Y. and Stansfield, A.G. (1990). Lymphohistiocytic T-cell lymphoma (anaplastic large cell lymphoma CD30$^+$/Ki-1$^+$ with a high content of reactive histiocytes). *Histopathology* **16**, 383–91.

Pinkus, G.S. and Pinkus, J.L. (1991). Myeloperoxidase: a specific marker for myeloid cells in paraffin sections. *Modern Pathology* **4**, 733–41.

Pinkus, G.S. and Said, J.W. (1985). Hodgkin's disease, lymphocyte predominance type, nodular – a distinct entity? Unique staining profile for L & H variants of Reed–Sternberg cells defined by monclonal antibodies to leukocyte common antigen, granulocyte specific antigen, and B-cell-specific antigen. *American Journal of Pathology* **118**, 1–6.

Pinkus, G.S. and Said, J.W. (1988). Hodgkin's disease, lymphocyte predominance type, nodular – further evidence for a B cell derivation. L & H variants of Reed–Sternberg cells express L26, a pan B cell marker. *American Journal of Pathology* **133**, 211–17.

Pinkus, G.S., Thomas, P. and Said, J.W. (1985). Leu-M1 – a marker for Reed–Sternberg cells in Hodgkin's disease. An immunoperoxidase study of paraffin-embedded tissues. *American Journal of Pathology* **119**, 244–52.

Piris, M., Brown, D.C., Gatter, K.C. and Mason, D.Y. (1990). CD30 expression in non-Hodgkin's lymphoma. Histopathology **17**, 211–18.

Pittaluga, S., Raffeld, M., Lipford, E.H. and Cossman, J. (1986). 3A1 (CD7) expression precedes T beta gene rearrangements in precursor T (lymphoblastic) neoplasms. *Blood* **68**, 134–9.

Pombo de Oliveira, M.S., Jaffe, E.S. and Catovsky, D. (1989). Leukemic phase of mantle zone (intermediate) lymphoma: its characterization in 11 cases. *Journal of Clinical Pathology* **42**, 962–72.

Poppema, S. (1989). The nature of the lymphocytes surrounding Reed–Sternberg cells in nodular lymphocyte predominance and in other types of Hodgkin's disease. *American Journal of Pathology* **135**, 351–7.

Poppema, S. and Hepperle, B. (1991). Restricted V gene usage in T-cell lymphomas as detected by anti-T-cell receptor variable region reagents. *American Journal of Pathology* **138**, 1479–84.

Poppema, S., Hollema, H., Visser, L. and Vos, H. (1987). Monoclonal antibodies (MT1, MT2, MB1, MB2, MB3) reactive with leukocyte subsets in paraffin-embedded tissues. *American Journal of Pathology* **127**, 418–29.

Poppema, S., Kaiserling, E. and Lennert, K. (1979). Hodgkin's disease with lymphocyte predominance, nodular type (nodular paragranuloma) and progressively transformed germinal centres – a cytohistological study. *Histopathology* **3**, 295–308.

Poppema, S., Lai, R. and Visser, L. (1991). Monoclonal antibody OPD4 is reactive with CD45RO, but differs from UCHL1 by the absence of monocyte reactivity. *American Journal of Pathology* **139**, 725–9.

Potter, M.N., Foot, A.B.M. and Oakhill, A. (1991). Influenza A and the virus associated haemophagocytic syndrome: cluster of three cases in children with acute leukaemia. *Journal of Clinical Pathology* **44**, 297–9.

Pugh, W.C., Manning, J.T. and Butler, J.J. (1988). Paraimmunoblastic variant of small lymphocytic lymphoma/leukemia. *American Journal of Surgical Pathology* **12**, 907–17.

Pulford, K., Micklem, K., Thomas, J., Jones, M. and Mason, D.Y. (1991). A 72-kD B-cell-associated surface glycoprotein expressed at high levels in hairy cell leukaemia and plasma cell neoplasms. *Clinical and Experimental Immunology* **85**, 429–35.

Pulford, K., Ralfkiaer, E., Macdonald, S.M., Erber, W.N., Falini, B. and Gatter, K.C. (1986). A new monoclonal antibody (KB61) recognizing a novel antigen which is selectively expressed on a subpopulation of human B lymphocytes. *Immunology* **57**, 71–6.

Pulford, K.A.F., Erber, W.N., Crick , J.A., Olsson, I., Micklem, K.J., Gatter, K.C. and Mason, D.Y. (1988). Use of monoclonal antibody against human neutrophil elastase in normal and leukaemic myeloid cells. *Journal of Clinical Pathology* **41**, 853–60.

Pulford, K.A.F., Rigney, E.M., Micklem, K.J., Jones, M., Stross, W.P., Gatter, K.C. and Mason, D.Y. (1989). KP1: a new monoclonal antibody that detects a monocyte/macrophage associated antigen in routinely processed tissue sections. *Journal of Clinical Pathology* **42**, 414–21.

Radaszkiewicz, T., Hansmann, M.L. and Lennert, K. (1988). Monoclonality and polyclonality of plasma cells in Castleman's disease of the plasma cell variant. *Histopathology* **14**, 11–24.

Raghoebier, S., Kramer, M.H.H., Vankrieken, J.H.J.M., Dejong, D., Limpens, J., Kluinnelemans, J.C., Vanommen, G.J.B. and Kluin, P.M. (1991). Essential dfferences in oncogene involvement between primary nodal and extranodal large cell lymphoma. *Blood* **78**, 2680–5.

Ralfkiaer, E. (1991). Immunohistochemical markers for the diagnosis of cutaneous lymphomas. *Seminars in Diagnostic Pathology* **8**, 62–72.

Ralfkiaer, E., Delsol, G., O'Connor, N.T.J., Brandtzaeg, P., Brousset, P., Vejlsgaard, G.L. and Mason, D.Y. (1990). Malignant lymphomas of true histiocytic origin. A clinical, histological, immunophenotypic and genotypic study. *Journal of Pathology* **160**, 9–17.

Ralfkiaer, E., Pulford, K.A.F., Lauritzen, A.F., Avnstrom, S., Guldhammer, B. and Mason, D.Y. (1989). Diagnosis of acute myeloid leukaemia with the use of monoclonal anti-neutrophil elastase (NP57) reactive with routinely processed biopsy samples. *Histopathology* **14**, 637–43.

Ralfkiaer, E., Wollfsneedorff, A. and Vejlsgaard, G.L. (1991). Use of antibodies against the variable regions of the T-cell receptor alpha/beta heterodimer for the study of cutaneous T-cell lymphomas. *British Journal of Dermatology* **125**, 409–12.

Ramsay, A.D., Smith, W.J. and Isaacson, P.G. (1988). T-cell-rich B-cell lymphomas. *American Journal of Surgical Pathology* **12**, 433–43.

Rappaport, H. (1966). Tumours of the hematopoietic system. In *Atlas of Tumour Pathology*, Armed Forces Institute of Pathology, Washington DC, pp. 49–63.

Ratech, H., Burke, J.S., Blayney, D.W., Sheibani, K. and Rappaport, H. (1989). A clinicopathologic study of malignant lymphomas of the nose, paranasal sinuses, and hard palate, including cases of lethal midline granuloma. *Cancer* **64**, 2525–31.

Raziuddin, S., Malatani, T., Alsedairy, S. and Alsaigh, A.H. (1991). Peripheral T-cell lymphomas – immunophenotype, lymphokine production, and immunologic functional characteristics of the lymph-node malignant T-cells. *American Journal of Pathology* **139**, 1181–9.

Regula, D.P., Hoppe, R.T. and Weiss, L.M. (1988). Nodular and diffuse types of lymphocyte predominance Hodgkin's disease. *New England Journal of Medicine* **318**, 214–19.

Regula, D.P., Weiss, L.M., Warnke, R.A. and Dorfman, R.F. (1987). Lymphocyte predominance Hodgkin's disease: a reappraisal based upon histological and immunophenotypical findings in relapsing cases. *Histopathology* **11**, 1107–20.

Reth, M. (1992). Antigen Receptors on Lymphocytes-B. *Annual Review of Immunology* **10**, 97–121.

Rijlaarsdam, J.U., Boorsma, D.M., De Haan, P., Sampat, S. and Willemze, R. (1990). The significance of Leu 8 negative T cells in lymphoid skin infiltrates: malignant transformation, selective homing or T-cell activation? *British Journal of Dermatology* **123**, 587–93.

Risdall, R.J., McKenna, R.W. and Nesbit, M.E. (1979). Virus-associated hemophagocytic syndrome, a benign histiocytic proliferation distinct from malignant histiocytosis. *Cancer* **44**, 993–1002.

Ritz, J., Schmidt, R.E., Michon, J., Hercend, T. and Schlossman, S.F. (1988). Characterization of functional surface structures on human natural killer cells. *Advances in Immunology* **42**, 181–211.

Rivano, M.T., Falini, B., Stein, H., Canino, S., Ciani, C., gerdes, J., Ribacchi, R., Gobbi, M. and Pileri, S. (1987). Histiocytic necrotizing lymphadenitis without granulocytic infiltration (Kikuchi's lymphadenitis): morphological and immunohistochemical study of 8 cases. *Histopathology* **11**, 1013–221.

Roholl, P.J.M., Kleyne, J., Prins, M.E.F., Hooijkaas, H., Vroom, T.M. and Van Unnik, J.A.M. (1988). Immunologic marker analysis of normal and malignant histiocytes: A comparative study of monoclonal antibodies for diagnostic purposes. *American Journal of Clinical Pathology* **89**, 187–94.

Rosenberg, C.L., Wong, E., Petty, E.M., Bale, A.E., Tsujimoto, Y., Harris, N.L. and Arnold, A. (1991). PRAD1, a candidate BCL1 oncogene – mapping and expression in centrocytic lymphoma. *Proceedings of the National Academy of Sciences of the United States of America* **88**, 9638–42.

Rowlands, D.C., Hansel, T.T. and Crocker, J. (1990). Immunohistochemical determination of CD23 expression in Hodgkin's disease using paraffin sections. *Journal of Patholgy* **160**, 239–43.

Royer, H.D. and Reinherz, E.L. (1987). T lymphocytes: Ontogeny, function, and relevance to clinical disorders. Current Concepts. *New England Journal of Medicine* **317**, 1136–42.

Ruco, L.P., Gearing, A.J.H., Pigott, R., Pomponi, D., Burgio, V.L., Cafolla, A., Baiocchini, A. and Baroni, C.D. (1991). Expression of ICAM-1, VCAM-1 and ELAM-1 in angiofollicular lymph node hyperplasia (Castleman's Disease) - evidence for dysplasia of follicular dendritic reticulum cells. *Histopathology* **19**, 523–8.

Ruco, L.P., Pulford, K.A.F., Mason, D.Y., Ceccamea, A., Uccini, S., Pileri, S., Baglioni, P. and Baroni, C.D. (1989). Expression of macrophage-associated antigens in tissues involved by Langerhans' cell histiocytosis (histiocytosis X). *American Journal of Clinical Pathology* **92**, 273–9.

Ruco, L.P., Stoppacciaro, A., Barsotti, P., Vitolo, D., Mirolo, M., Cassano, A.M., Guglielmi, C., Mandelli, F., Uccini, S. and Baroni, C.D. (1984). S-100 $^+$ lymph node neoplasm. Report of a case with histological AL and immunological features intermediate between T cell lymphoma and malignant histiocytosis. *Virchows Archives [Pathology and Anatomy]* **404**, 351–8.

Said, J.W., Sassoon, A.F., Shintaku, I.P., Kurtin, P.J. and Pinkus, G.S. (1991). Absence of bcl-2 major breakpoint region and JH gene rearrangement in lymphocyte predominance Hodgkin's disease: Results of Southern blot analysis and polymerase chain reaction. *American Journal of Pathology* **138**, 261–4.

Said, J.W., Shintaku, I.P., Parekh, K. and Pinkus, G. (1990). Specific phenotyping of T-cell proliferations in formalin-fixed paraffin-embedded tissues. Use of antibodies to the T-cell receptor BF1. *American Journal of Clinical Pathology* **93**, 382–6.

Said, J.W., Shintaku, P. and Pinkus, G. (1988). Immunohistochemical staining for terminal deoxynucleotidyl transferase (TDT): An enhanced method in routinely processed formalin-fixed tissue sections. *American Journal of Clinical Pathology* **89**, 649–52.

Said, J.W., Stoll, P.N., Shintaku, P., Bindl, J.M., Butmarc, J.R. and Pinkus, G.S. (1989). Leu-22: a preferential marker for T-lymphocytes in paraffin sections. Staining profile in T- and B-cell lymphomas, Hodgkin's disease, other lymphoproliferative disorders, myeloproliferative diseases, and various neoplastic processes. *American Journal of Clinical Pathology* **91**, 542–9.

Salter, D.M., Krajewski, A.S. and Cunningham, S. (1988). Activation and differentiation antigen expression in B-cell non-Hodgkin's lymphoma. *Journal of Pathology* **154**, 209–22.

Salter, D.M., Krajewski, A.S. and Dewar, A.E. (1986). Immunophenotype analysis of malignant histiocytosis of the intestine. *Journal of Clinical Pathology* **39**, 8–15.

Salter, D.M., Krajewski, A.S., Sheehan, T., Turner, G., Cuthbert, R.J.G. and McLean, A. (1989). Prognostic significance of activation and differentiation antigen expression in B-cell non-Hodgkin's lymphoma. *Journal of Pathology* **159**, 211–20.

Sander, C.A., Jaffe, E.S., Gebhardt, F.C., Yano, T. and Medeiros, L.J. (1992). Mediastinal Lymphoblastic lymphoma with an Immature B-cell Immunophenotype. *American Journal of Surgical Pathology* **16**, 300–5.

Sander, C.A., Medeiros, L.J., Abruzzo, L.V., Horak, I.D. and Jaffe, E.S. (1991). Lymphoblastic lymphoma presenting in cutaneous sites – a clinicopathologic analysis of six cases. *Journal of the American Academy of Dermatology* **25**, 1023–31.

Sanders, M.E., Makgoba, M.W. and Shaw, S. (1988). Human naive and memory T cells: Reinterpretation of helper-inducer and suppressor-inducer subsets. *Immunology Today* **9**, 195–8.

Santamaria, M., Llamas, L., Ree, H.J., Sheibani, K., Ho, Y.S., Su, I.J. and Hsu, S.M. (1988). Expression of sialylated Leu-M1 antigen in histiocytosis X. *American Journal of Clinical Pathology* **89**, 211–16.

Schmid, C., Kirkham, N., Diss, T. and Isaacson, P.G. (1992). Splenic marginal zone cell lymphoma. *American Journal of Surgical Pathology* **16**, 455–66.

Schmid, C., Pan, L., Diss, T. and Isaacson, P.G. (1991a). Expression of B-Cell Antigens by Hodgkin's and Reed–Sternberg Cells. *American Journal of Pathology* **139**, 701–7.

Schmid, C., Sargent, C. and Isaacson, P.G. (1991b). L cells and H cells of nodular lymphocyte predominant Hodgkin's disease show immunoglobulin light-chain restriction. *American Journal of Pathology* **139**, 1281–9.

Schuurman, H.J., Van Baarlen, J., Huppes, W., Lam, B.W., Verdonck, L.F. and Van Unnik, J.A.M. (1987). Immunophenotyping of non-Hodgkin's lymphoma: lack of correlation between immunophenotype and cell morphology. *American Journal of Pathology* **129**, 140–51.

Schwarting, R., Gerdes, J., Durkop, H., Falini, B., Pileri, S. and Stein, H. (1989). Ber-H2: a new anti-Ki-1(CD30) monoclonal antibody directed at a formol-resistant epitope. *Blood* **74**, 1678–89.

Schwarting, R., Stein, H. and Wang, C.Y. (1985). The monoclonal antibodies αS-HCL 1 (αLeu-14) and αS-HCL 3 (αLeu-M5) allow the diagnosis of hairy cell leukemia. *Blood* **65**, 974–83.

Scott, R.B. and Robb-Smith, A.H.T. (1939). Histiocytic medullary reticulosis. *Lancet* **2**, 194–8.

Segal, G.H., Stoler, M.H. and Tubbs, R.R. (1992). The CD43 only phenotype – an aberrant, nonspecific immunophenotype requiring comprehensive analysis for lineage resolution. *American Journal of Clinical Pathology* **97**, 861–5.

Shamoto, M., Shinzato, M., Hosokawa, S., Kaneko, C., Hakuno, T. and Nomoto, K. (1992). Langerhans cells in the lymph node – mirror section and immunoelectron microscopic studies. *Virchows Archives B (Cell Pathology Including Molecular Pathology)* **61**, 337–41.

Sheibani, K., Battifora, H., Burke, J.S. and Rappaport, H. (1986). Leu-M1 antigen in human neoplasms. An immunohistologic study of 400 cases. *American Journal of Surgical Pathology* **10**, 227–36.

Sheibani, K., Burke, J.S., Swartz, W.G., Nadamanee, A. and Winberg, C.D. (1988). Monocytoid B cell lymphoma, clinicopathologic study of 21 cases of unique type of low grade lymphoma. *Cancer* **62**, 1531–8.

Sheibani, K., Nathwani, B.N., Winberg, C.D., Burke, J.S., Swartz, W.G., Blayney, D., Van de Velde, S., Hill, L.R. and Rappaport, H. (1987a). Antigenically defined subgroups of lymphoblastic lymphoma. Relationship to clinical presentation and biologic behaviour. *Cancer* **60**, 183–90.

Sheibani, K., Winberg, C.D., Van de Velde, S., Blayney, D.W. and Rappaport, H. (1987b). Distribution of lymphocytes with interleukin-2 receptors (Tac antigens) in reactive lymphoproliferative processes, Hodgkin's disease, and non-Hodgkin's lymphomas: An immunohistologic study of 300 cases. *American Journal of Pathology* **127**, 27–37.

Shibata, D., Hu, E., Weiss, L.M., Byrnes, R.K. and Nathwani, B.N. (1990). Detection of specific t(14;18) chromosomal translocations in fixed tissues. *Human Pathology* **21**, 199–203.

Shin, S.S., Sheibani, K., Fishleder, A., Benezra, J., Bailey, A., Koo, C.H., Burke, J.S., Tubbs, R. and Rappaport, H. (1991). Monocytoid B-cell lymphoma in patients with Sjogren's syndrome – A clinicopathologic study of 13 patients. *Human Pathology* **22**, 422–30.

Sklar, J. (1990). What can DNA rearrangements tell us about solid hematolymphoid neoplasms? *American Journal of Surgical Pathology* **14**, (Suppl.1), 16–25.

Slater, D. (1990). Clonal dermatoses: A conceptual and diagnostic dilemma. Editorial. *Journal of Pathology* **162**, 1–3.

Slater, D.N. (1987). Review article. Recent developments in cutaneous lymphoproliferative disorders. *Journal of Pathology* **153**, 5–19.

Smith, J.L., Lane, A.C., Hodges, E., Reynolds, W.M., Howell, W.M., Jones, D.B. and Janson, C.H. (1992a). T-Cell receptor variable (V) gene Usage by lymphoid populations in T-cell lymphoma. *Journal of Pathology* **166**, 109–12.

Smith, K.J., Skelton, H.G., Yeager, J., Angritt, P., Wagner, K., James, W.D., Giblin, W.J. and Lupton, G.P. (1992b). Cutaneous histopathologic, immunohistochemical, and clinical manifestations in patients with hemophagocytic syndrome. *Archives of Dermatology* **128**, 193–200.

Smith-Ravin, J., Spencer, J., Beverly, P. and Isaacson, P. (1990). Characterization of two monoclonal antibodies (UCL-4D12 and UCL-3D3) which discriminate between human mantle zone and marginal zone B cells. *Clinical and Experimental Immunology* **82**, 181–7.

Sox, H.C. (1987). Probability theory in the use of diagnostic tests. An introduction to the critical study of the literature. *Annals of Internal Medicine* **104**, 60–6.

Spencer, J., Cerf-Bensussan, N., Jarry, A., Brousse, N., Guy-Grand, D., Krajewski, A.S. and Isaacson, P.G. (1988). Enteropathy-associated T cell lymphoma (malignant histiocytosis of the intestine) is recognized by a monoclonal antibody (HML-1) that defines a membrane molecule on human mucosal lymphocytes. *American Journal of Pathology* **132**, 1–5.

Spencer, J., Choy, M., Hussell, T., Papadaki, L., Kington, J.P. and Isaacson, P.G. (1992). Properties of human thymic B-cells. *Immunology* **75**, 596–600.

Spencer, J., Diss, T.C. and Isaacson, P.G. (1988). Novel monoclonal antibodies that discriminate between mantle zone and marginal zone B-cells. *Journal of Pathology* **155**, 343A.

Spencer, J., MacDonald, T.T., Diss, T.C., Walker-Smith, J.A., Ciclitira, P.J. and Isaacson, P.G. (1989). Changes in intraepithelial lymphocyte subpopulations in coeliac disease and enteropathy associated T-cell lymphoma (malignant histiocytosis of the intestine). *Gut* **30**, 339–46.

Springer, T.A. (1990). Adhesion receptors of the immune system. *Nature* **346**, 425–34.

Stansfeld, A.G., Diebold, J., Kapanci, Y., Rilke, F., Kelenyi, G., Sundstrom, C., Lennert, K., van Unnik, J.A.M., Mioduszewska, O. and Wright, D.H. (1988). Updated Kiel classification for lymphomas. *Lancet* **1(8580)**, 292–3.

Stein, H., Dienemann, D., Sperling, M., Zeitz, M. and Riecken, E.O. (1988). Identification of a T cell lymphoma category derived from intestinal-mucosa-associated T cells. *Lancet* **ii**, 1053–4.

Stein, H., Hansmann, M.L., Lennert, K., Brandtzaeg, P. and Gatter, K.C. (1986). Reed–Sternberg and Hodgkin cells in lymphocyte predominant Hodgkin's disease of nodular subtype contain J chain. *American Journal of Clinical Pathology* **86**, 292–7.

Stein, M., Mason, D.Y., Gerdes, J., O'Connor, N., Wainscoat, J., Pallesen, G., Gatter, K.C., Falini, B., Delsol, G., Lemke, H., Schwarting, R. and Lennert, K. (1985). The expression of the Hodgkin's disease associated antigen Ki-1 in the reactive and neoplastic lymphoid tissue. Evidence that Reed–Sternberg cells and histiocytic malignancies are derived from activated lymphoid cells. *Blood* **66**, 848–58.

Strauchen, J.A. and Mandeli, J.P. (1991). Immunoglobulin expression in B-cell lymphoma. Immunohistochemical study of 345 cases. *American Journal of Clinical Pathology* **95**, 692–5.

Strickler, J.G., Medeiros, L.J., Copenhaver, C.M., Weiss, L.M. and Warnke, R.A. (1988). Intermediate lymphocytic lymphoma: An immunophenotypic study with comparison to small lymphocytic lymphoma and diffuse small cleaved cell lymphoma. *Human Pathology* **19**, 550–4.

Strickler, J.G., Schmidt, C.M. and Wick, M.R. (1990). Methods in pathology: Immunophenotype of Hairy cell leukaemia in paraffin sections. *Modern Pathology* **3**, 518–23.

Strickler, J.G., Weiss, L.M., Copenhaver, C.M., Bindl, J., McDaid, R., Buck, D. and Warnke, R.A. (1987). Monoclonal antibodies reactive in routinely processed tissue sections of malignant lymphomas, with emphasis on T-cell lymphoma. *Human Pathology* **18**, 808–14.

Stross, W.P., Warnke, R.A., Flavell, D.J., Simmons, D., Gatter, K.C. and Mason, D.Y. (1989). Molecule detected in formalin fixed tissue by antibodies MT1, DF-T1, and L60 (Leu-22) corresponds to CD43 antigen. *Journal of Clinical Pathology* **42**, 953–61.

Su, I.-J., Balk, S. and Kadin, M.E. (1988). Molecular basis for the aberrant expression of T-cell antigens in postthymic T cell malignancies. *American Journal of Pathology* **132**, 192–8.

Su, I.-J. and Kadin, M.E. (1989). Expression of growth factor/receptor genes in postthymic T cell malignancies. *American Journal of Pathology* **135**, 439–45.

Suchi, T., Lennert, K., Tu, L.Y., Kikuchi, M., Sato, E., Stansfield, A.G. and Feller, A.C. (1987). Histopathology and histochemistry of peripheral T cell lymphomas: A proposal for their classification. *Journal of Clinical Pathology* **40**, 995–1015.

Sundeen, J.T., Cossman, J. and Jaffe, E.S. (1986). Lymphocyte predominant Hodgkin's disease nodular subtype with coexistent 'large cell lymphoma'. Histologic progression or composite malignancy? *American Journal of Surgical Pathology* **12**, 599–606.

Sundeen, J.T., Longo, D.L. and Jaffe, E.S. (1992). CD5 expression in B-cell small lymphocytic malignancies – correlations with clinical presentation and sites of disease. *American Journal of Surgical Pathology* **16**, 130–37.

Suster, S. and Rywlin, A.M. (1987). A reappraisal of Richter's syndrome: Development of two phenotypically distinctive cell lines in a case of chronic lymphocytic leukemia. *Cancer* **59**, 1412–18.

Swerdlow, S.H., Habeshaw, J.A., Murray, L.J., Dhaliwal, H.S., Lister, T.A. and Stansfield, A.G. (1983). Centrocytic lymphoma: A distinct clinicopathologic and immunologic entity. A multiparameter study of 18 cases at diagnosis and relapse. *American Journal of Pathology* **113**, 181–97.

Swerdlow, S.H. and Wright, S.A. (1986). The spectrum of Leu-M1 staining in lymphoid and haemopoietic proliferations. *American Journal of Clinical Pathology* **85**, 283–8.

Tabibzadeh, S.S., Poubourdis, D., May, L. and Sehgal, P.B. (1989). Interleukin-6 immunoreactivity in human tumours. *American Journal of Pathology* **135**, 427–33.

Takagi, N., Nakamura, S., Yamamoto, K., Kunishima, K., Takagi, I., Suyama, M., Shinoda, M., Sugiura, T., Oyama, A., Suzuki, H., Koshikawa, T., Kontani, K., Ueda, R., Takahashi, T., Ariyoshi, Y. and Suchi, T. (1992). Malignant lymphoma of mucosa-associated lymphoid tissue arising in the thymus of a patient with Sjogren's syndrome – a morphologic, phenotypic, and genotypic study. *Cancer* **69**, 1347–55.

Takahashi, K., Isobe, T., Ohtsuki, Y., Sonobe, H., Yamaguchi, H. and Akagi, T. (1985). S-100 protein positive human T-lymphocyte. *American Journal of Clinical Pathology* **83**, 69–72.

Taubenberger, J.K., Jaffe, E.S. and Medeiros, L.J. (1991). Thymoma with abundant L26–positive asteroid cells – a case report with an analysis of normal thymus and thymoma specimens. *Archives of Pathology and Laboratory Medicine* **115**, 1254–7.

Tefferi, A., Zellers, R.A., Banks, P.M., Therneau, T.M. and Colgan, J.P. (1990). Clinical correlates of distinct immunophenotypic and histologic subcategories of lymphocyte-predominance Hodgkin's disease. *Journal of Clinical Oncology* **8**, 1959–65.

Therkildsen, M.H. (1986). Enzyme histochemical demonstration of hairy cell leukaemia in paraffin-embedded tissue sections. *Virchows Archives A* **408**, 505.

Thiele, H.G. (1991). Lymphocyte homing – An overview. *Immunologic Research* **10**, 261–7.

Thompson, S.D., Manzo, A.R., Pelkonen, J., Larche, M. and Hurwitz, J.L. (1991). Developmental T-Cell Receptor Gene Rearrangements – Relatedness of the alpha/beta and gamma/delta T-cell precursor. *European Journal of Immunology* **21**, 1939–50.

Timens, W., Visser, L. and Poppema, S. (1986). Nodular lymphocyte predominance type of Hodgkin's disease is a germinal center lymphoma. *Laboratory Investigation* **54**, 457–61.

Traweek, S.T., Sheibani, K., Winberg, C.D., Mena, R.R., Wu, A.M. and Rappaport, H. (1989). Monocytoid B-cell lymphoma: Its evolution and relationship to other low-grade B-cell neoplasms. *Blood* **73**, 573–8.

Trowbridge, I.S., Ostergaard, H.L. and Johnson, P. (1991). CD45–A leukocyte-specific member of the protein tyrosine phosphatase family. *Biochimica et Biophysica Acta* **1095**, 46–56.

Van den Oord, J.J., de Wolf-Peeters, C. and Desmet, V.J. (1986a). The composite nodule. A structural and functional unit of the reactive lymph node. *American Journal of Pathology* **122**, 83–91.

Van den Oord, J.J., de Wolf-Peeters, C., Pulford, K.A.F., Mason, D.Y. and Desmet, V. (1986b). Mantle zone lymphoma. Immuno- and enzymehistochemical studies on the cell of origin. *American Journal of Surgical Pathology* **10**, 780–8.

van der Valk, P. and Meijer, C.J.L.M. (1988). The non-Hodgkin's lymphomas: Old and new thinking. *Histopathology* **13**, 367.

van der Valk, P., Mullink, H., Huijgens, P.C., Tadema, T.M., Vos, W. and Meijer, C.J.L.M. (1989). Immunohistochemistry in bone marrow diagnosis: Value of a panel of monoclonal antibodies on routinely processed bone marrow biopsies. *American Journal of Surgical Pathology* **13**, 97–106.

van Krieken, J.H.J.M., Otter, R., Hermans, J., van Groningen, K., Spaander, P.J., van der Sandt, M.M., Keunig, J.F. and Kuin, P.M. (1989a). Malignant lymphoma of the gastrointestinal tract and mesentery. A clinico-pathologic study of the significance of histologic classification. *American Journal of Pathology* **135**, 281–9.

Van Krieken, J.H.J.M., Von Schilling, C., Kluin, P.M. and Lennert, K. (1989b). Splenic marginal zone lymphocytes and related cells in the lymph node: A morphologic and immunohistochemical study. *Human Pathology* **20**, 320–5.

Vannoesel, C.J.M., Brouns, G.S., Vanschijndel, G.M.W., Bende, R.J., Mason, D.Y., Borst, J. and Vanlier, R.A.W. (1992). Comparison of human B-cell antigen receptor complexes – Membrane-expressed forms of immunoglobulin (Ig)M, IgD, and IgG Are associated with structurally related heterodimers. *Journal of Experimental Medicine* **175**, 1511–19.

Vardiman, J.W., Gilewski, T.A. and Ratain, M.J. (1988). Evaluation of Leu-M5 (CD11c) in hairy cell leukemia by the alkaline phosphatase anti-alkaline phosphatase technique. *American Journal of Clinical Pathology* **90**, 250–6.

Villuendas, R., Piris, M.A., Orradre, J.L., Mollejo, M., Rodriguez, R. and Morente, M. (1991). Different bcl-2 protein expression in high-grade B-cell lymphomas derived from lymph node or mucosa-associated lymphoid tissue. *American Journal of Pathology* **139**, 989–93.

Volk, B.A., Niessner, M., Amann, B., Fauser, A.A. and Gerok, W. (1991). Expression of gammadelta lymphocytes-T derived from human intestinal biopsies. *Immunologic Research* **10**, 310–12.

Von Baarlen, J., Schuurman, H. and Van Unnik, J. (1988). Multilobated non-Hodgkin's lymphoma, a clinicopathologic entity. *Cancer* **61**, 1371–6.

Vroom, T.M., Scholte, G., Ossendorp, F. and Borst, J. (1991). Tissue distribution of human gammadelta T-cells – no evidence for general epithelial tropism. *Journal of Clinical Pathology* **44**, 1012–17.

Waldron, J.A., Leech, J.H., Glick, A.D., Flexner, J.M. and Collins, R.D. (1977). Malignant lymphoma of peripheral T-lymphocyte origin: immunologic, pathologic, and clinical features in six patients. *Cancer* **40**, 1604–17.

Walls, A.F., Jones, D.B., Williams, J.H., Church, M.K. and Holgate, S.T. (1990). Immunohistochemical identification of mast cells in formaldehyde-fixed tissue using monoclonal antibodies specific for tryptase. *Journal of Pathology* **162**, 119–26.

Warnke, R.A., Pulford, K.A.F., Pallesen, G., Ralfkiaer, E., Brown, D.C., Gatter, K.C. and Mason, D.Y. (1989). Diagnosis of myelomonocytic and macrophage neoplasms in routinely processed tissue biopsies with monoclonal antibody KP1. *American Journal of Pathology* **135**, 1089–95.

Weis, J.W., Winter, M.W., Phyliky, R.L. and Banks, P.M. (1986). Peripheral T-cell lymphomas: Histologic, immunohistologic, and clinical characterization. *Mayo Clinic Proceedings* **61**, 411–26.

Weisenburger, D., Bast, M., Perry, D., Duggan, M. and Armitage, J. (1990). Diffuse intermediate lymphocytic lymphoma: A refined definition based on comparative clinical studies. *Laboratory Investigation* **62**, 105A.

Weisenburger, D.D. (1990). B cell neoplasia, a conceptual understanding based on the normal humoral immune response. *Pathology Annual* **25**, 99–115.

Weisenburger, D.D. (1991). Non-Hodgkin's lymphomas of primary follicle/mantle zone origin. *Leukaemia* **5**(Suppl.), 26–9.

Weisenburger, D.D., Duggan, M.J., Perry, D.A., Sanger, W.G. and Armitage, J.O. (1991). Non-Hodgkin's lymphomas of mantle zone origin. *Pathology Annual* **26**, 139–58.

Weisenburger, D.D., Nathwani, B.N., Diamond, L.W., Wiberg, C.D. and Rappaport, H. (1981). Malignant lymphoma, intermediate lymphocytic type: A clinicopathologic study of 42 cases. *Cancer* **48**, 1415.

Weisenburger, D.D. and Rappaport, K.H. (1982). Mantle-zone lymphoma: A follicular variant of intermediate lymphocytic lymphoma. *Cancer* **49**, 1429.

Weisenburger, D.D., Sanger, W.G., Armitage, J.O. and Purtilo, D.T. (1987). Intermediate lymphocytic lymphoma: Immunophenotypic and cytogenetic findings. *Blood 69*, 1617–21.

Weiss, L.M., Berry, G.J., Dorfman, R.F., Banks, P., Kaiserling, E., Curtis, J., Rosai, J. and Warnke, R.A. (1990). Spindle cell neoplasms of lymph nodes of probable reticulum cell lineage:

True reticulum cell sarcoma? *American Journal of Surgical Pathology* **14**, 405–14.

Weiss, L.M., Bindl, J.M., Picozzi, V.J., Link, M.P. and Warnke, R.A. (1986). Lymphoblastic lymphoma: An immunophenotype study of 26 cases with comparison to T cell acute lymphoblastic leukemia. *Blood* **67**, 474–8.

Weiss, L.M., Crabtree, G.S., Rouse, R. and Warnke, R.A. (1985). Morphologic and immunologic characterization of 50 peripheral T cell lymphomas. *American Journal of Pathology* **118**, 316–24.

Weiss, L.M., Gaffey, M.J., Chen, Y.Y. and Frierson, H.F. (1992). Frequency of Epstein–Barr viral DNA in Western sinonasal and Waldeyer's Ring non-Hodgkin's lymphomas. *American Journal of Surgical Pathology* **16**, 156–62.

Weiss, L.M., Picker, L.J., Grogan, T.M., Warnke, R.A. and Sklar, J. (1988). Absence of beta and gamma T-cell receptor gene rearrangements in a subset of peripheral T cell lymphomas. *American Journal of Pathology* **130**, 436–42.

Weiss, L.M., Strickler, J.G., Dorfman, R.F., Horning, S., J. and Warnke, R.A. (1986). Clonal T-cell populations in angioimmunoblastic lymphadenopathy and angioimmunoblastic lymphadenopathy-like lymphoma. *American Journal of Pathology* **122**, 392–7.

Weiss, L.M., Wood, G.S. and Warnke, R.A. (1985). Immunophenotypic differences between dermatopathic lymphadenopathy and lymph node involvement in mycosis fungoides. *American Journal of Pathology* **120**, 179–85.

West, K.P. (1989). Editorial. Castleman's disease: the plot thickens. *Journal of Pathology* **157**, 191–2.

West, K.P., Warford, A., Fray, L. and Allen, M. (1986). The demonstration of B-cell, T-cell and myeloid antigens in paraffin sections. *Journal of Pathology* **150**, 89–101.

Westermann, C.D., Steele, P.E., Hurtubise, P.E., Vago, J.F. and Swerdlow, S.H. (1990). Multilobated lymphoma of B-cell type: A multiparameter investigation. *Human Pathology* **21**, 1036–40.

Wieczorek, R., Buck, D., Bindl, J. and Knowles, D.M. (1988). Monoclonal antibody Leu-22 (L60) permits the demonstration of some neoplastic T cells in routinely fixed and paraffin-embedded tissue sections. *Human Pathology* **19**, 1434.

Wieczorek, R., Burke, J.S. and Knowles, D.M.I. (1985). Leu-M1 antigen expression in T-cell neoplasia. *American Journal of Pathology* **121**, 374–80.

Williamson, J.M.S., Grigor, I., Smith, M.E.F., Holgate, C.S., Quirke, P., Bird, C.C., Alison, D.I. and Child, J.A. (1986). Cluster differentiation antigen expression, proliferative activity and clinical stage in centroblastic lymphomas. *Journal of Pathology* **150**, 51–9.

Willoughby, P.B., Jennette, J.C. and Haughton, G. (1988). Analysis of a murine B cell lymphoma, CH44, with an associated non-neoplastic T-cell population. 1. Proliferation of normal T lymphocytes is induced by a secreted product of the malignant B cells. *American Journal of Pathology* **133**, 507–15.

Witzig, T.E., Banks, P.M., Stenson, M.J., Griepp, P.R., Katzmann, J.A., Habermann, T.M., Colgan, J.P. and Gonchoroff, N.J. (1990). Rapid immunophenotyping of B-cell non-Hodgkin's lymphomas by flow cytometry. A comparison with the standard frozen section method. *American Journal of Clinical Pathology* **94**, 280–6.

Wong, K.F., Chan, J.K.C., Chan, J.C.W., Lim, W.W.L. and Wong, W.K. (1991). Dengue virus infection-associated hemophagocytic syndrome. *American Journal of Hematology* **38**, 339–40.

Wong, K.F., Chan, J.K.C., Ng, C.S., Lee, K.C., Tsang, W.Y.W. and Cheung, M.M.C. (1992). CD56 (NKH1)-positive hematolymphoid malignancies – an aggressive neoplasm featuring frequent cutaneous mucosal involvement, cytoplasmic azurophilic granules, and angiocentricity. *Human Pathology* **23**, 798–804.

Wotherspoon, A.C., Soosay, G.N., Diss, T.C. and Isaacson, P.G. (1990). Low-grade primary B-cell lymphoma of the lung. An immunohistochemical, molecular, and cytogenetic study of a single case. *American Journal of Clinical Pathology* **94**, 655–60.

Wright, D.H. (1989). Updated Kiel classification for lymphomas. Editorial. *Journal of Pathology* **157**, 283–4.

Wright, D.H. and Isaacson, P.G. (1989). Gut-associated lymphoid tumours. In Whitehead, R. (ed.), *Gastrointestinal and Oesophageal Pathology*, Churchill-Livingstone, Edinburgh, pp. 643–61.

Writing Group of the Histiocyte Society (1987). Point of view: Histiocytosis syndromes in children. *Lancet* **i**, 208–9.

Wu, A.M., Winberg, C.D., Sheibani, K., Colombero, A.M., Wallace, R.B. and Rappaport, H. (1990). Genotype and phenotype: A practical approach to the immunogenetic analysis of lymphoproliferative disorders. *Human Pathology* **21**, 1132–41.

Yamakawa, M., Matsuda, M., Imai, Y., Arai, S., Harada, K. and Sato, T. (1992). Lymph node interdigitating cell sarcoma – a case report. *American Journal of Clinical Pathology* **97**, 139–46.

Yoshino, T., Mukuzonon, H., H., A., Takahashi, K., Takeuchi, T., Kubonishi, I., Ohtsuki, Y., Motoi, M. and Akagi, T. (1989). A novel monoclonal antibody (OPD4) recognizing a helper/inducer T cell subset. Its application to paraffin-embedded tissues. *American Journal of Pathology* **134**, 1339–46.

Zukerberg, L., Medeiros, L., Ferry, J. and Harris, N. (1991a). Diffuse low grade B-cell lymphomas: identification of four major immunophenotypic subtypes [Abstract]. *Laboratory Investigation* **62**, 87A.

Zukerberg, L.R., Collins, A.B., Ferry, J.A. and Harris, N.L.

(1991b). Coexpression of CD15 and CD20 by Reed–Sternberg cells in Hodgkin's disease. *American Journal of Pathology* **139**, 475–83.

Zutter, M. (1991). Gamma-delta cells in the immune response. Editorial. *American Journal of Clinical Pathology* **95**, 761–2.

Zutter, M., Hockenbery, D., Silverman, G.A. and Korsmeyer, S.J. (1991). Immunolocalization of the Bcl-2 protein within hematopoietic neoplasms. *Blood* **78**, 1062–8.

Zutter, M.M. (1991). Immunolocalization of integrin receptors in normal lymphoid tissues. *Blood* **77**, 2231–6.

5 ◆ *Immunohistochemistry of renal diseases and tumours*

John P. Dowling

Introduction

Immunohistochemistry (IMH) of renal tissue represents a special investigative mode that is now routine practice in the assessment of diseases of the kidney; in fact it is difficult nowadays to imagine renal diagnosis without the benefit of this additional information. This chapter will discuss the IMH findings in medical (glomerular, interstitial and vascular) and surgical (neoplastic) diseases largely presented from a perspective of differential diagnosis of light microscopic features to which the application of IMH will provide staining properties assisting in differentiation of the entities. This 'pattern' approach to renal diagnosis has been suggested previously by Mostofi et al. (1971) and has formed the basis of the WHO Classification of Renal Diseases (Churg and Sobin, 1982). Although many diseases produce characteristic features allowing a diagnosis readily to be made from light microscopic appearances, many other diseases share common and often mixed features. The overlap of morphological features has made the designation of some patterns as 'basic' changes particularly difficult but the classification rests on the assessment that an individual entity possesses a 'basic' change as the main diagnostic criterion. The schema of glomerular changes outlined in this chapter is provided in Table 5.1.

Immunohistochemistry technique

The range of methods of detecting protein deposits in the kidney has increased markedly since the 1970s prior to which time usually only immunofluorescence methods were available. Immunoenzymatic techniques (immunoperoxidase, combined with avidin-biotin and alkaline phosphatase) and gold-labelled antibody techniques are available and stain both fixed and unfixed frozen tissues effectively (Allen and Dowling, 1981; Al-Nawab and Davies, 1989; Jackson et al., 1990); microwave fixation has been reported with encouraging and rapid results (Chiu and Chan, 1987) for immunofluorescence.

Individual laboratories have individual preferences based on experience and the familiarity with a technique or techniques that provide reliable results. The immunofluorescence methods using frozen tissue perhaps remain the standard reference with which other techniques are compared. Without fixation to produce antigenic changes direct immunofluorescence (DIF) using frozen tissue

Table 5.1. Classification of glomerular changes

I NORMAL/MINOR NON-SPECIFIC APPEARANCES
- A Normal/minor non-specific appearances without additional features
- B Minimal change lesion
- C IgA nephropathy
- D Thin membrane disease and Alport's syndrome (familial nephritis)
- E Silentlupus erythematosus
- F Miscellaneous

II PROLIFERATIVE AND EXUDATIVE GLOMERULONEPHRITIS

III PREDOMINANT MESANGIAL CHANGES
- A Mesangial proliferative glomerulonephritis (focal/diffuse)
  1. Diffuse mesangial proliferation with mesangial IgA deposition
     Henoch-Schönlein purpura
  2. Diffuse/focal mesangial proliferation with/without mesangial IgM deposition (non-IgA type)
  3. Mesangial proliferation in connective tissue disorders
     - 3.1 Systemic lupus erythematosus
     - 3.2 Mixed connective tissue disease/Sjögren's syndrome
     - 3.3 Rheumatoid arthritis/relapsing polychondritis
     - 3.4 Vasculitides
  4. Miscellaneous
- B Acellular Mesangial Expansion
  1. Diabetic glomerulosclerosis
  2. Renal amyloidosis
  3. Light chain nephropathy
  4. Fibrillary/immunotactoid nephropathy
  5. Idiopathic lobular glomerulonephritis
  6. Hepatic glomerulosclerosis

IV SEGMENTAL NECROSIS/CRESCENT FORMATION (FOCAL/DIFFUSE)
- A Antiglomerular basement membrane disease
- B Pauci-immune/non-immune crescentic glomerulonephritis
- C Immune complex crescentic glomerulonephritis

V GLOMERULOSCLEROSIS – SEGMENTAL/GLOBAL

VI CAPILLARY WALL CHANGES
- A Membranous (transformation) nephropathy
- B Mesangial interposition and insudative thickening
  - Type I (subendothelial) mesangiocapillary glomerulonephritis idiopathic and secondary; thrombotic microangiopathies
  - Type II (dense deposit) mesangiocapillary glomerulonephritis
  - Type III (transmural) mesangiocapillary glomerulonephritis

remains the simplest way of providing an IMH profile of renal tissue. However, the enzymatic methods, although more demanding and capricious, provide consistent results if fixation, processing and staining steps are standardized and closely monitored; variation of fixation schedules in particular as applied to biopsies from different sources is one of the main reasons for inconsistency of results using immunoenzymatic techniques. The convenience of immunoperoxidase (IMPO)-labelled permanent preparations on the fixed tissue from the same block providing sections for light microscopy with, usually, more tissue to assess, persuaded the author to use the IMPO techniques which illustrate many IMH findings in this chapter. Details of the staining methods are presented in Chapter 1. Because there are on occasions inexplicable failures of staining with IMPO, it has been the author's practice to keep a small portion of renal cortical tissue frozen from each biopsy or nephrectomy specimen to perform DIF if required. Some special features which have assisted the production of consistent results using IMPO staining are given in Table 5.2.

Table 5.2. Features of immunoperoxidase technique employed by the author

1. 'Standardized Fixation' in neutral buffered formalin for 90 min.
2. Digestion for approx. 7 min with protease.
3. Pap/Indirect staining.
4. Limited development of Dab reaction product.
5. Brief (approx. 10–30 sec.) gold salt augmentation of staining.

The IMH patterns described relate, in the main, to the use of a standard panel of antibodies made up as follows: antibodies, either monoclonal or polyclonal, to the heavy chains of IgG, IgM and IgA; monoclonal or polyclonal antibodies to the third component of complement mostly C3b or C3c deposited through the activation of the classical pathway of complement or, if seen as the sole component deposited, indicating activation of the alternate pathway of complement; monoclonal or polyclonal antibodies to C1q or C4 components of complement representing the early components activated by the classical pathway and fibrinogen representing deposition of fibrin-related antigens within various glomerular diseases. Many include routine staining with monoclonal or polyclonal antibodies to kappa and lambda light chains, properdin to suggest alternative pathway activation of complement and antibodies to IgE.

As indicated the approach to renal IMH presented here is towards a differential diagnosis of light microscopic patterns. Comments relating to aetiopathogenesis especially with respect to the 'medical' diseases are provided where this is felt appropriate but a detailed review of the extensive experimental and human literature of this aspect of renal pathology is beyond the scope of this chapter. Some excellent recent reviews pertaining to development, evolution and progression of glomerular diseases in particular are available to the reader (see Brentjens and Andres, 1989; Bruijn et al., 1989; Furness, 1991; Shah, 1991; Ballardie, 1992.)

Complement involvement in renal diseases

It may be appropriate to discuss the role of complement in the induction, resolution and perpetuation to sclerosis at this point because of the central contribution of this series of plasma proteins as a biological amplification system (Fig. 5.1). Extensive studies of both human and experimental glomerulonephritis and of interstitial nephritis indicate involvement of both the classical and alternative pathways of complement activation, the sequence of early complement proteins (C1–C4) and the protein combination activated towards the conclusion of the cascade namely the membrane attack complex (C5b–C9, (MAC)) (Biesecker, 1983). The functions of particular complement fractions relevant to the development and resolution or persistence of nephritis are presented in Table 5.3.

As the reader will note these various fragments of the complement system are found distributed in the kidney examined by IMH in a wide range of nephritic diseases, some patterns with characteristic features that are supportive of particular diagnoses. These findings are outlined in the text. The presence of ubiquitous complement participation in such a wide range of lesions argues for a role for complement in the development of glomerulonephritis in particular (Rother et al., 1991). With occasional exceptions (Hinglais et al., 1986), MAC deposition has been associated with activity in glomerulonephritis (Falk et al., 1983) and from abundant experimental evidence, has been shown to significantly influence intrinsic glomerular cells in concert with other complement components (Table 5.3) via autocrine positive feedback loops to produce sclerotic materials, particularly

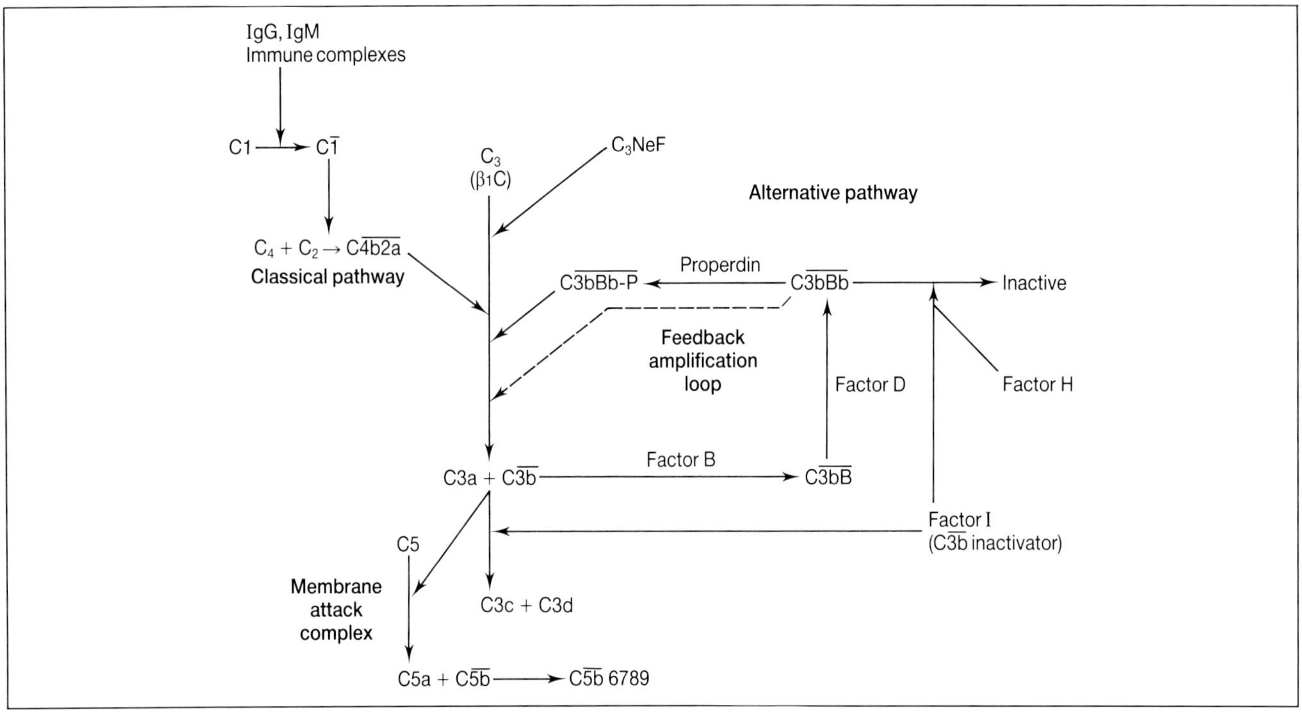

Fig. 5.1. Schema to indicate involvement of complement proteins in the cascade reactions of the classical and alternate pathways of activation and related inhibitory components.

Table 5.3. Some functions of complement relevant to nephritis

Activity	Complement production
Leucocyte mobilization	Leucocyte mobilizing factor C3a
Leucocyte activation	C5a
Immune adherence opsonization	C3b
Eicosanoid release	C3b, C5a, C5b–9
Cytokine release	C3b, C5a, C5b–9
Platelet aggregation	C3a, C5a
Immune complex	
solubilization	C3b
inhibition of formation	C4b
Modification of antibody synthesis	C3d
Erythrocyte lysis	C5b–9
cell killing	C5b–9

Source: After Rother, Hänsch and Rauterberg, 1991

collagen in progressive glomerulonephritis (summarized by Rother et al., 1991). The evidence suggests that perpetuation of leucocytic injury by MAC-stimulated leucocyte activation with oxygen radical and lysosomal release leads to persistent complement activation with further MAC generation, the activity of which is independent of specific cell receptors in contrast to other 'early' complement components.

The activation and incorporation of complement components related to immunopathogenesis of various forms of GN are reflected in many instances in the characteristic serum findings related to the concentration of these proteins with reduction in serum complement components due either to congenital or acquired complement deficiencies. Acquired deficiencies relating especially to mesangiocapillary GN are discussed in Section VI (Capillary Wall Changes) (see Table 5.22). The inherited deficiencies of complement which lack one or more complement proteins may result in the development of glomerulonephritis often mesangiocapillary in type and other extrarenal manifestations in a range of deficiencies probably related to immune complex accumulation (reviewed by Praz et al., 1984; Morgan and Walport, 1991; see Table 5.4).

Glomerular diseases

The classification of glomerular lesions outlined in this Chapter is presented in Table 5.1.

Table 5.4. Complement in nephritis: Hereditary complement deficiencies and GN

Deficiency	Relative frequency	GN patterns	IMH	Sites
1. Clq +/− LE	Infrequent	Mesangial proliferative	A, M, C3	Mesangial, capillary
		Membranous		
		Mesangiocapillary I	G, A, C3	Mesangial, capillary
2. C2	Most common	Membranous	G, M, C3, C4, Clq	Capillary
+/− LE		Proliferative	G, M, C3, C4, Clq	Mesangial, capillary
and as isolated GN		Mesangiocapillary I	G, A, M,	
		HSP – mesangial proliferative	C3	Mesangial
3. C4	Rare	Diffuse proliferative	G, A, M, C3	Mesangial
4. C3	Infrequent	Mesangial proliferative	G, C3	Mesangial, capillary
		Mesangiocapillary I	C3	
5. Cl-INH	Rare	Mesangial proliferative	G, M, C3	Mesangial, capillary
		Diffuse proliferative	G, C3, Clq	Mesangial, capillary
6. C5–C8	Rare	Membranous	G, A, M	Capillary
		Mesangiocapillary I		Mesangial, capillary
		Diffuse proliferative	G, A, M	Capillary

Notes: G = IgG; A = IgA; M = IgM; Cl-INH = Cl inhibitor

I. Normal or minor non-specific appearances

A considerable number of entities may show glomeruli that appear essentially normal or possess only a slight expansion of the mesangial matrix without evidence of hypercellularity, with no further changes seen on light microscopy. Electron microscopy may demonstrate significant findings and IMH may provide characteristic findings. The IMH findings in this group of conditions are summarized in Table 5.5.

Table 5.5. IMH of pattern I – normal or minor non-specific changes. (Summary of reported findings)

Entity	Mesangium	Loop	Other
Normal/MNSC	Negative IgM	Negative	Arteriolar C3
Minimal change	IgA, IgM, C3	IgM, C3	
IgA nephropathy	IgA, IgG, IgM, F		
Thin membrane disease/Alports*	Negative IgM, IgG, IgA, C3	Negative	Arteriolar C3
Silent lupus	IgG, IgM, IgA, C3, Clq	IgG, IgM, IgA, C3, Clq	
Light chain nephropathy		Kappa/lambda	
Anti-GBM disease		IgG	

Note: F = fibrinogen; MNSC = minor non-specific changes.
*Pattern described in some cases only

Normal/minor non-specific appearances without additional features

'Normal' transplants examined by IMH at time of implantation may show no deposits but may also demonstrate faint or light IgM mesangial staining and, on occasions, light IgA mesangial deposition (Durand et al., 1983). Nyberg et al. (1992) found similar implantation biopsy results in donated living related kidneys and that the process of graft implantation had no influence on the IMH findings; three of the past 55 implantation graft biopsies at the present author's institution have shown mesangial IgA deposition. The deposits may disappear (Silva et al., 1982).

In practice, the findings of isolated proteinuria or microscopic haematuria are common clinically. These urinary manifestations may be accompanied by very mild IgM and C3 mesangial deposition that is usually focal

(Larsen, 1979). Very few histological abnormalities are seen in biopsies from patients with constant and with transient orthostatic proteinuria in which IMH is usually negative (Dennis and Robinson, 1986). The aging kidney demonstrates an increase in the width of the glomerular basement membrane and an acellular mild expansion of the mesangial matrix; faint to light IgM mesangial staining is a frequent finding in the aged nephrosclerotic kidneys and probably represents non-specific trapping of serum protein rather than suggesting an immunological mechanism for the aging process (Zawada, 1989).

Minimal change lesion (MCL)

Some examples of this entity, characterized ultrastructurally by effaced pedicels, show IgM and less often C3 both staining faintly or lightly distributed evenly within the mesangial areas (Prasad, et al., 1977; Broyer et al., 1992) and some capillary loops (Habib et al., 1988). These usually lightly staining antibodies appear to have no influence on the outcome of the lesion which responds in the great majority of cases to corticosteroid therapy. Abnormalities of both T- and B-lymphocyte function may be demonstrated in patients with MCL and a serum factor(s) may be responsible for capillary wall alterations leading to proteinuria (Endoh et al., 1991; Broyer et al., 1992).

IgA nephropathy

A small proportion of renal biopsies from patients with IgA nephropathy (IgAN) show a slight mesangial matrix increase with minor non-specific glomerular changes (Glassock et al., 1985). Small deposits may be visible within the mesangium in some of these biopsies with a trichrome stain and similar appearances may be seen in Henoch–Schönlein purpura (Haycock, 1992). IMH shows usually even, light IgA mesangial deposits, sometimes not uniformly distributed. Small amounts of IgM and C3 and occasionally IgG and fibrinogen are found accompanying the IgA deposition (Fig. 5.2).

IgA in the mesangium is found in occasional patients with the nephrotic syndrome showing, ultrastructurally, diffuse effacement of foot processes (Rambausek et al., 1987), probably representing two relatively common disorders occurring simultaneously in the kidney; the lesion usually responds to corticosteroids. (For further discussion of IgA mesangial deposition see Section III – Mesangial Changes.)

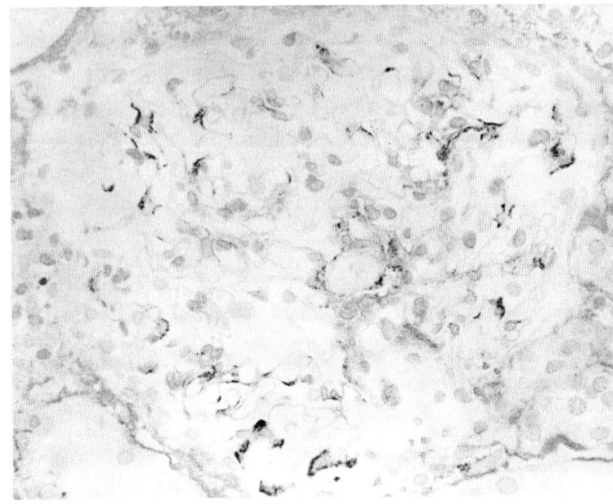

Fig. 5.2. Light IgA mesangial deposition in an implantation biopsy without evidence of glomerular proliferation. (X400)

Thin membrane nephropathy and Alport's syndrome (familial nephritis)

Diseases with basement membrane abnormalities, namely thin membrane nephropathy (TMN), both familial and sporadic (Dische et al., 1985; Tiebosch et al., 1989) and Alport's syndrome (Gubler and Habib, 1989) are commonly associated with urinary abnormalities. TMN defined by the widespread attenuation of the glomerular basement membrane, usually with normal glomerular cellularity (Yoshikawa et al., 1988), may however demonstrate mesangial proliferation and other glomerular changes (Aarons et al., 1989). IMH is characteristically negative (Perry et al., 1989) within glomeruli although slight segmental staining with IgG, IgA, IgM and C3 was described by Yoshikawa et al. (1988) in a minority of patients with a family history of haematuria; in the sporadic variety Saxena et al. (1990) noted weak granular IgM, C3 and C1q staining in a minority of cases. Some examples of TMN show C3 mesangial deposition only (Tiebosch et al., 1989). Occasionally diffuse light IgM deposition within the mesangium may be noted (Coleman et al., 1986). Arteriolar C3 deposition including involvement of the vascular pole of the glomerulus is a relatively frequent finding (Yoshikawa et al., 1988; Aarons et al, 1989).

Similar extensive attenuation of the GMB is found in some examples of Alport's syndrome (Gubler and Habib, 1989) with little or no mesangial proliferation but in other cases these same near-normal glomerular appearances are often associated with the characteristic ultrastructural lamellation of the basement membrane. Both these patterns in Alport's syndrome, which may coexist, usually demonstrate little or no immunoglobulin or complement deposition but IgM and C3 may be found in a minority of cases (Gubler and Habib, 1989). Apart from the interstitial foam cells in the 'Alport' variety of thin membrane change, which may show progressive injury, the consistent lack of the Goodpasture antigen in this form of thin membrane pathology contrasts to that of the 'benign familial/sporadic' type where the Goodpasture antigen is present although, perhaps, more weakly expressed than in the normal kidney (Savage et al. 1986; Pettersson et al., 1990). The Goodpasture epitope is located in the globular non-collagenous NCI domain of type IV collagen, the main structural component of the GBM. Further discussion related to the Goodpasture antigen is provided in the Section IV – antiglomerular basement membrane disease. The abnormality in both the thin membrane and lamellated membrane forms of Alport's syndrome of some families appears to be a defect in the production of $\alpha3$, $\alpha4$ and $\alpha5$ chains of collagen IV.

Silent lupus erythematosus

Amongst the range of patterns of 'silent' LE on renal biopsy some show minor non-specific glomerular changes (Bennett et al., 1982; Font et al., 1987) accompanied by some mesangial deposits that may or may not be visible by light microscopy; these findings may be seen in biopsies from patients with lupus erythematosus with minimal or no clinical or urinary manifestations of lupus erythematosus. Variously sited glomerular deposits are readily found on ultrastructural examination and immunohistochemistry often reveals small, predominantly mesangial deposits of IgG, IgA, IgM, C3 with small amounts of C1q evident (Cavallo et al., 1977); progression of the lesions to more serious changes does not necessarily follow (Bennett et al., 1982).

Miscellaneous

Essentially minor non-specific glomerular patterns may be found in occasional examples of renal amyloidosis associated with a nephrotic presentation (Jones et al., 1986), in light chain nephropathy (Bangerter and Murphy, 1987) and accompanied by more extensive tubular basement membrane light chain deposition and antiglomerular basement membrane glomerulonephritis with linear basement membrane staining with IgG on IMH (Carre et al., 1989).

II. Proliferative and exudative glomerulonephritis (PEGN)

PEGN known also as endocapillary glomerulonephritis represents another basic reaction pattern of the glomerulus often seen in response to a wide variety of infections but also in the context of other often systemic diseases such as lupus erythematosus (Grishman et al., 1967), mixed connective tissue disease (Eigenbrodt and Ware, 1989), Henoch–Schönlein purpura (Heaton et al., 1977), cryoglobulinaemia (Ben-Bassat et al., 1983), IgA nephropathy (Kincaid-Smith et al., 1989) vasculitis with few immune deposits (Serra et al., 1984) among other causes which include hepatitis B virus infection (Eigenbrodt and Ware, 1989; Tejani and Ingulli, 1990). The common morphological features include endocapillary proliferation, mostly of mesangial cells, and polymorphonuclear neutrophilic leucocytes and mononuclear infiltration usually global and diffuse but with segmental accentuation on occasions, protein deposits often subepithelial (the characteristic 'humps'), mesangial, intramembranous and subendothelial in distribution. Superimposed segmental lesions and crescents may be seen. Evidence of systemic deposition of immune complexes in selected organs has been detected in e.g. bacterial endocarditis with deposits in the spleen (Nast et al., 1986).

Immunohistochemical findings

The prototype of the PEGN reaction pattern is that seen following β-haemolytic group A streptococcal usually pharyngeal infection (Wannamaker, 1970). Variations of IMH pattern according to the stage of evolution of the glomerular lesion which in the vast majority of cases resolves to a normal state have been described. In the early inflammatory phase, one of three patterns of immunoglobulin and complement deposition may be found (Sorger et al., 1982, 1983) (Fig. 5.3a–c): 1. *'Starry sky'* in which IgG, IgM and/or IgA and C3 are shown as heavy granular staining of the mesangium and scattered capillary loops. 2. *'Mesangial'* where mostly C3 granular deposition within the mesangium with little capillary loop staining is seen; this pattern appears to evolve from the 'starry sky' form; and 3. *'Garland-type'* – IgG and C3

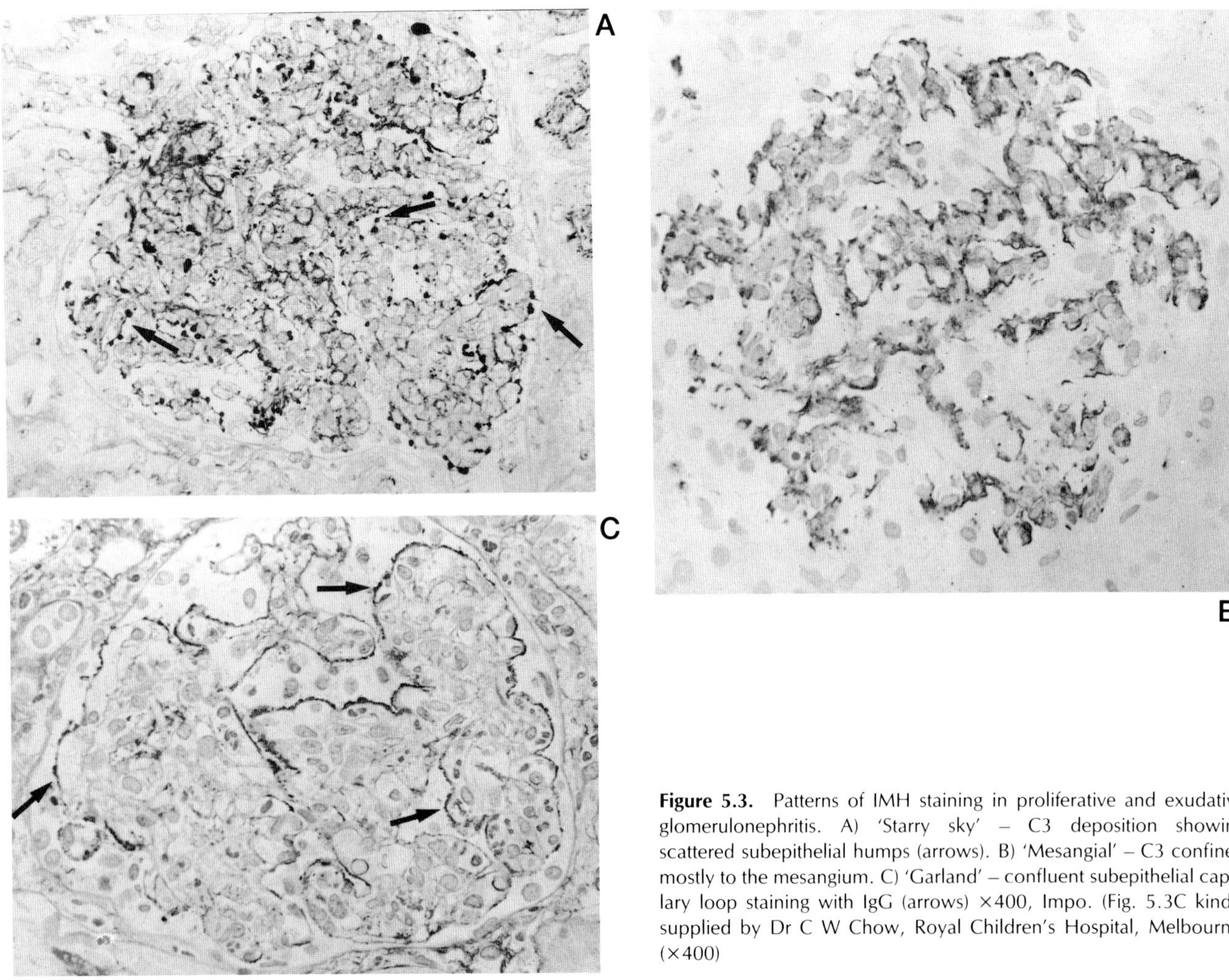

Figure 5.3. Patterns of IMH staining in proliferative and exudative glomerulonephritis. A) 'Starry sky' – C3 deposition showing scattered subepithelial humps (arrows). B) 'Mesangial' – C3 confined mostly to the mesangium. C) 'Garland' – confluent subepithelial capillary loop staining with IgG (arrows) ×400, Impo. (Fig. 5.3C kindly supplied by Dr C W Chow, Royal Children's Hospital, Melbourne) (×400)

outline several or many glomerular capillary loops with a corresponding light microscopy finding of confluent subepithelial deposits often with the characteristic 'hump' outline.

Follow-up studies relating to these three patterns (Sorger et al., 1987) suggest that persistent proteinuria in this setting is predicted by the 'garland' pattern seen in approximately 25 per cent of cases (Glassock et al., 1991) with repeat biopsies in these patients showing persisting histological abnormalities. The garland pattern shows few subendothelial deposits and the undulating outline of capillary loops may appear similar to that seen in Type I (subendothelial) mesangiocapillary GN. In the latter pattern C1q, C4 and C3 often show confluent subendothelial outline of the capillary loops and reduplication of the GBM found in some examples of PS PEGN but is usually more widespread in mesangiocapillary GN. Transformation of PS PEGN to Type I mesangiocapillary glomerulonephritis (Rodrigrez-Iturbe, 1992) or diffuse crescentic GN (Fairley et al., 1987) may be associated with the deposition of fibrin in capillary loops and in crescents (Modai et al., 1985).

The resolution of PS PEGN is usually marked by a relative loss of IMH staining but often with some persistence of C3 and/or IgG and IgM deposits within the first year following onset; deposits of IgG, IgM and C3 and, uncommonly, IgA and C1q have been found in biopsies with persistent disease taken after 18 months following onset (Rosenberg et al., 1985); these authors found small mesangial and intramembranous deposits which were seen on electron microscopy and presumably correlated with those found on IMH. There are currently several streptococcal antigens that are putatively nephritogenic namely endostreptosin, a cytoplasmic protein antigen from the supernatant of disrupted group A nephritogenic streptococci (Cronin et al., 1989), a streptokinase from streptococcus isolated from GN patients named 'nephritis strain-associated protein' that appears to deposit in glomeruli prior to complement fixation and specific antibody deposition (Peake et al., 1991); and another antigen from the supernatant of nephrogenic streptococcal cultures, a cationic protease (Batsford, 1991).

It perhaps requires emphasis that the patterns, both morphological and immunohistochemical, outlined above, may be seen with many other infections summarized by Wilson (1991) and Rodrigrez-Iturbe (1992) (Table 5.6). The reported patterns ascribed to many examples of PEGN due to many different organisms are similar to that outlined above with mesangial and variable capillary loops usually moderate to heavy granular staining with IgG, IgM and C3 with small amounts of IgA and C1q/C4 in a minority of cases. The IMH findings in PEGN are summarized in Table 5.7.

Table 5.6. Pattern II – Proliferative and exudative GN microbial antigens implicated in PEGN

Bacteria	
Streptococcus pyogenes (+), viridans (+), pneumoniae (+), αhaemolytic (+)	
Streptococcus faecalis (−)	
Staphylococcus aureus (+); albus (+)	
Treponema pallidum (+); klebsiella pneumoniae (+)	
Salmonella infection (−); yersinia enterocolitica (+)	
Brucella infection (−); leptospirosis (−)	
Myocobacterium leprae (−)	
Viruses	
Hepatitis B (+, surface Ag)	Infectious mononucleosis (+)
Varicella (+)	Rocky mountain spotted fever (+, vessels)
Mumps (+)	Coxsackie viruses (−)
Typhus (−)	Cytomegalovirus (+)
Fungi	**Parasites**
Histoplasmosis (−)	Toxoplasma gondii (+)
Trichinosis (−)	Filaria (+)
	Plasmodium falciparum (+), malariae (+)

Notes: (+) Antigen demonstrated in glomerulus
(−) Antigen not found/sought in glomerulus; Serum immune complexes with microbial antigen often demonstrated.
Source: Wilson, 1991.

Table 5.7. Pattern II – Proliferative and exudative GN IMH findings related to different causes

Cause		Mesangium	Loops
Post-Infectious:	Starry sky	IgG, C3	IgG, C3
	Mesangial	C3	
	Garland	(IgG, C3)	IgG, C3
Lupus erythematosus		IgG, IgA, IgM, C3, Clq	Similar
MCTD		IgG, C3 (IgM, IgA)	Similar
IgA nephropathy		IgA, IgM, C3	Variable
HSP		IgA, IgM, C3, F	Characteristic
Cryoglobulinaemia		IgM, IgG, C3, Clq	Similar
Vaculitides		(IgM)	–

Notes: ( ) Staining weaker, less frequently seen
– Negative
MCTD = mixed connective tissue
HSP = Henoch-Schönlein purpura

III. Predominant mesangial changes

The many functions of the mesangium composed of mesangial cells and basement membrane-like matrix provide it with a pivotal role for involvement in a great range of glomerular reactions to injury and in the related repair processes that follow injury (Kashgarian and Sterzel, 1992). It supports the glomerular capillary loops and is in continuity with the juxtaglomerular apparatus at the vascular pole of the glomerulus. The mesangial changes of proliferation, expansion of matrix, accumulation of proteins and lysis with dissolution of cells and matrix are all very commonly observed changes on optical microscopy. The mesangial patterns in the conditions outlined below represent the histological changes that usually predominate but upon which many other glomerular reactions may be superimposed, e.g. segmental necrosis/proliferation and exudation and crescent formation to mention only a few examples. The IMH findings in this diverse group of conditions are presented in Table 5.8.

Mesangial proliferative glomerulonephritis (focal/diffuse) (MPGN)

This very common alteration has been associated with many diverse aetiological agents and is found in many conditions for which the aetiological agent(s) is unknown. The proliferation is diffuse in the vast majority of instances but occasionally it may be focal and global or focal and segmental. Such changes are noted in the categories of

Table 5.8. Pattern III – Predominant mesangial changes IMH findings in mesangial proliferative glomerulonephritis

	MES	Loop
IgA nephropathy	IgA, IgM, C3	Variable
Non-IgA nephropathy	IgM, C3	Occasional
Connective tissue diseases		
Lupus erythematosus	IgG, IgM, IgA, C3, Clq	Variable
MCTD/Sjögren's syndrome	IgG, IgA, IgM, C3, Clq	Variable
Rheumatoid arthritis	IgG, C3	IgG, C3
Relapsing polychondritis	IgG, IgM, C3	
Vasculitides	±IgG, Fibrin	Fibrin
Miscellaneous		
Anti-GBM disease	IgM, C3 (L/G)	IgG
Light chain nephropathy	Variable	Kappa/ lambda
Various infections	IgG, IgM	Variable
Clq nephropathy	Clq, IgM, IgG, IgA, C3	–

Notes: L = linear; G = granular

lesion discussed below. IMH may assist considerably in distinguishing between entities with very similar histological appearances.

Diffuse mesangial proliferation with mesangial IgA deposition/Henoch–Schölein purpura

Most children or adults show mesangial proliferation of some degree with early lesions tending to show milder proliferation. In general, there is a direct correlation with the severity of glomerular change and clinical outcome (Schena, 1992). Since diffuse mesangial proliferation is the most common manifestation of IgA nephropathy (D'Amico, 1987), an outline of the immunohistochemical findings in IgA nephropathy is provided here.

IgA nephropathy (IgAN) is the commonest form of primary glomerulonephritis in many countries and is frequently associated with synpharyngitic haematuria associated with a respiratory infection (D'Amico, 1987). By outlining diffuse mesangial staining (involving most glomeruli), IMH defines this entity and the prototype pattern is usually shown as deposits evenly distributed between arborizing mesangia of individual capillary loops. IgA is deposited as either the dominant immunoglobulin or, at least, as prominently as IgG or IgM, and/or C3 (Levy et al., 1985) in the absence of systemic disease and is shown as fine or coarse granularity and/or a continuous 'streaky' outline of the mesangial areas (Silva and Hogg, 1989). Extension into peripheral (parietal) aspects of capillary walls as well as subendothelial/subepithelial deposits occurs in approximately one third of cases (Ng et al., 1984; Jennette, 1988) and is associated with more severe histological changes and a poorer outlook (Yoshimura et al., 1987) (Fig. 5.4). Jennette (1988) in reviewing IMH findings in IgAN also indicated other features of IgA commonly seen; he noted that no correlation existed between the relative intensities of IgA, IgG, IgM and the severity of glomerular disease; the presence of terminal complement (C5b–C9) components (membrane attack complex, MAC) was found consistently in biopsies and C5b–C9 positivity correlated with more severe disease; he also noted little or no C1q was deposited in the mesangium in the vast majority of cases of IgAN, a helpful differentiation from lupus glomerulonephritis; lambda light chain deposition in the mesangium was more readily found compared with kappa light chain deposition in approximately two thirds of cases. In IgAN, the amount of deposit of IgA in the mesangium shows little correlation with the severity of the histological change (Kusumoto et al., 1987). Many groups of workers have found that C3 mesangial deposition correlates with clinical activity with IgA N (D'Amico, 1987; Emancipator and Lamm, 1989). IMH and morphological differences may correlate with the mode of onset of the disease according to Suzuki et al. (1992); their group 1 patients with acute macroscopic haematuria, more severe microscopic haematuria, higher glomerular filtration rate, lower C3 serum levels and more exudative lesions had less C1q, C4 and IgM mesangial deposition than group 2 patients with insidious onset who demonstrated more mesangial proliferation, glomerular and arterial sclerosis and tubulointerstitial changes (Suzuki et al., 1992). Predominantly IgA1 subclass has been found in the mesangium by Conley et al. (1980). Polyclonal IgA antibodies of anionic polymeric type are deposited in the mesangium and studies of eluted IgA show the presence of the J chain and dimeric or larger antibodies on investigation (Sakai, 1991). The role of IgA in this disease is uncertain and has been questioned recently by Julian et al. (1991) who described four patients showing IgA deposition on a second renal biopsy after an initial biopsy had been negative on direct immunofluorescence and electron microscopy in each instance.

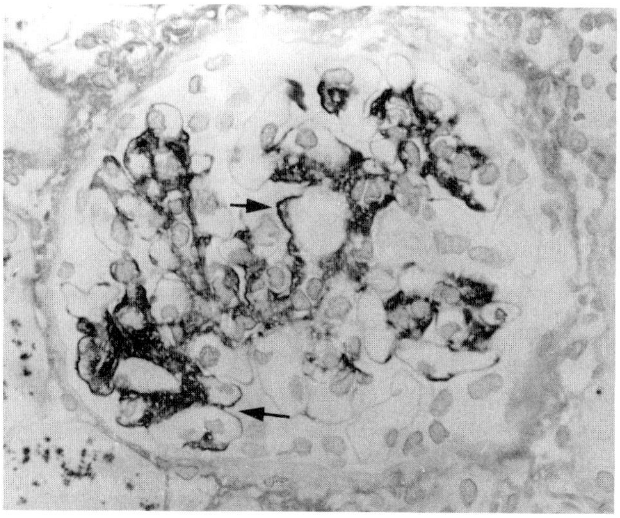

Fig. 5.4. Moderate to heavy IgA mesangial deposition with variable extension into glomerular capillary loops (arrows) in a patient with persisting haematuria and proteinuria due to IgA nephropathy (X 400)

IgA may be deposited in the mesangium and capillary loops in association with many other diseases (summarized by Silva and Hogg, 1989; Schena, 1992) (Table 5.9). The morphology described in many reports usually associated with the presence of light mesangial IgA in these diseases is very commonly described as mesangial cell proliferation, usually diffuse. Other lesions, e.g. crescents, segmental necrosis or membranous transformation, etc., are often also seen.

Table 5.9. IgA deposition in glomeruli

1. *Primary idiopathic IgAN*	
2. *Diseases with extra renal manifestations*	
Systemic lupus erythematosus	Coeliac disease
Henoch-Schönlein purpura	Dermatitis herpetiformis
Sjögrens syndrome	Ulcerative colitis
Hepatic GN	Regional enteritis
Ankylosing spondylitis	Lung diseases
Myasthenia gravis	AIDS
Various neoplasms	Cryoglobulinaemia
3. *Miscellaneous nephropathies*	
Minimal change lesion	
Focal glomerulosclerosis	
Membranous GN	
Anti GBM GN	
Follow-up to PS PEGN	

Occasional biopsies showing a membranous morphology show IgA outlining glomerular capillary loops (Emancipator and Lamm, 1989). Indeed Doi et al. (1983) and Jennette et al. (1987) have described the pattern of mixed IgAN with mesangial IgA deposition and membranous transformation with IgG granular staining along capillary walls. Similar confluent but very localized or segmental granular subepithelial staining with IgA may be found in occasional cases of IgAN (personal observation).

Henoch–Schölein purpura (HSP): The similarities and differences between Henoch–Schölein purpura and IgA nephropathy have recently been outlined by Haycock (1992). HSP is often associated with some degree of mesangial proliferation, focal or diffuse with segmental proliferative/necrotizing lesions and crescents often superimposed. The immunohistochemical findings in HSP are very similar to those of IgA nephropathy in that mesangial IgA (particularly IgA-1) is the main immunoglobulin deposited. The same variation in the intensity of mesangial IgA deposition, usually the main immunoglobulin, can be seen with a relatively lessening of mesangial staining with extension around peripheral capillary walls when proliferation and peripheral capillary loop changes including reduplication. Subepithelial deposits tend to be more numerous in HSP (Heaton et al., 1977) than in IgAN and, it has been the author's experience that fibrin is more widely and heavily distributed. The presence of IgA is accompanied by smaller amounts of either IgM and/or IgG; C3 is frequently found but C1q is usually lightly or faintly outlined.

Diffuse/focal mesangial proliferation with/without mesangial IgM deposition (non-IgA type)

This represents a relatively common diagnosis and included under this term is a variety of different entities including the recovering or persisting phase of post-infectious PEGN. Non-streptococcal respiratory infections have been shown to result in focal or diffuse mesangial proliferation in asymptomatic patients with glomerulonephritis (Smith et al., 1979). Many examples of diffuse mesangial proliferation display light to moderate uniform IgM staining accompanied by, usually, smaller amounts of C3 and little if any C1q/C4 in the mesangium. Some authors (Cohen et al., 1978; Border, 1988; and O'Donoghue et al., 1991) suggest that this combination of findings when associated with proteinuria or the nephrotic syndrome represents a separate entity, 'IgM nephropathy' distinct from minimal change lesion and focal glomerulosclerosis. However, IgM on the other hand is found in so many different circumstances within the mesangium, with or without mesangial proliferation, in patients with microscopic or macroscopic haematuria and/or in all degrees of proteinuria, with or without additional lesions such as segmental sclerosis, and transplant glomerulopathy that it is difficult to assign a precise pathogenetic significance to the finding (see Table 5.10; Fig. 5.5). Thus, others (Waldherr et al., 1978; summarized by Broyer et al., 1992) believe that such a pattern is non-specific and does not distinguish between the different entities associated with idiopathic nephrotic syndrome showing pedicel effacement and podocytic changes on electron microscopy (Border, 1988).

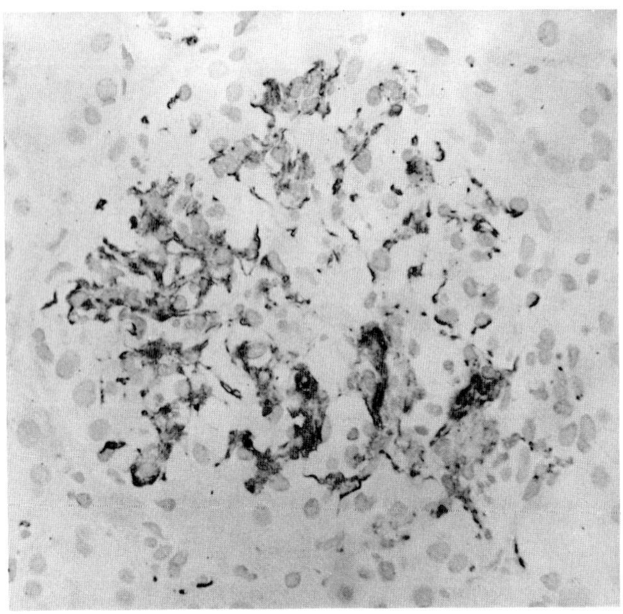

Fig. 5.5. Variable light uniform IgM mesangial deposition in a patient with nephrotic syndrome and diffuse mesangial proliferation (X400)

Mesangial proliferation in connective tissue diseases

Lupus Erythematosus (LE) of drug-induced, congenital hypocomplementaemic, 'classical' or seronegative types tends to demonstrate similar glomerular changes, regardless of aetiology; a very common manifestation is focal or diffuse mesangial proliferation (Hill, 1992). This pattern is often found in combination with other lesions and is a

Table 5.10. Pattern III – Predominant mesangial changes. Different settings of IgM mesangial staining

Entity	Strength of IgM	Mesangial proliferation
Implantation kidney	+	–
Aged kidney	+	–
Thin membrane disease	+	+/–
Minimal change lesion	+	–
Idiopathic nephrosis	+/++	+
Idiopathic focal glomerulosclerosis	+	+/–
Non-IgA mesangioproliferative glomerulonephritis	+	+/++
Cryoglobulinaemia	+/+++	+/++
Vasculitis – follow up	+	+
Hepatic glomerulosclerosis	+	–

Notes: + Light; ++ moderate; +++ heavy; – usually negative

component of the World Health Organization categories II, III and IV for LE GN (Churg and Sobin, 1982; Gladman et al., 1989). The mesangial expansion is, in part, due to protein deposits that are characteristically diffuse and evenly distributed in the mesangium. Some of these patients with mesangial proliferation have 'silent' LE with no urinary abnormalities (Font et al., 1987; Bennett et al., 1982). The typical LE IMH pattern includes immunoglobulins, IgG, IgA and IgM and complement components C3 and C1q and/or C4 and is seen in all the aetiological forms of LE indicated above. More fibrin is deposited in the mesangium and capillary loops in 'active' lesions and the early components of the classical pathway of complement represented by C1q and/or C4 tend also to correlate with activity. IgG, C3 and C1q are the most commonly found deposits (Banfi et al., 1985; Fig. 5.6). IgE is deposited more commonly in LE GN than in other lesions and may suggest a poorer outlook (Tuma et al., 1981). The mesangial staining for IgG is characteristic but the strength of staining of individual immunoglobulins varies from case to case. Some reduction in the strength of staining of these proteins is usually noted with effective therapy (Grishman et al., 1982). The focal and segmental lesions, proliferative necrotising and/or sclerosing patterns, are often highlighted by extension of the staining patterns of immunoglobulins and complement around glomerular capillary loops (Kashgarian and Hayslett, 1989). Uncommonly linear staining of the GBM unassociated with any specific histology is found and is usually shown

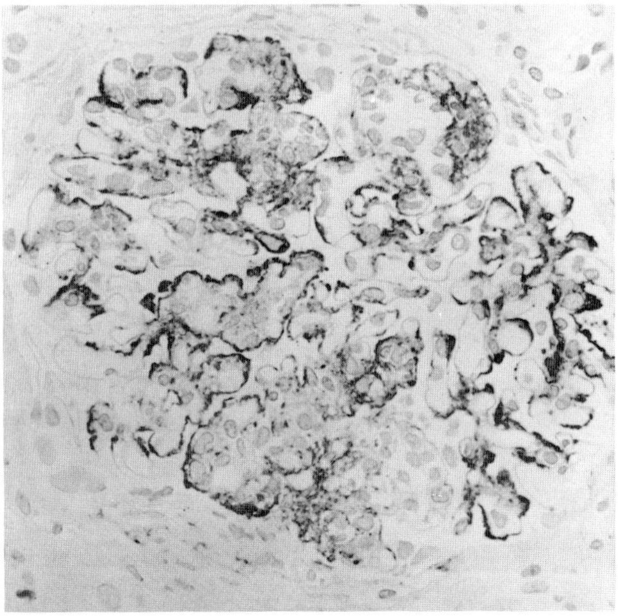

Fig. 5.6. C1q staining of capillary loops and proliferative mesangium in systemic lupus erythematosus (X400)

as IgG but other immunoglobulins may also show this pattern; the differential diagnosis of this particular change includes early membranous nephropathy with a pseudolinear pattern.

Mixed connective tissue disease (MCTD) and Sjögren's syndrome: **MCTD** commonly has renal manifestations estimated at approximately 26 per cent by Sullivan et al. (1984). Diffuse mesangial proliferation represents the most common glomerular manifestation of MCTD although other patterns of glomerulonephritis and a scleroderma-like vasculopathy as well as interstitial nephritis have been seen (summarized by Eigenbrodt and Ware, 1989).

The IMH pattern with MCTD with DMP is located in the mesangium and shows extension into capillary loops when these are involved in additional changes such as mesangiocapillary alteration. IgA is found in combination with IgG and/or IgM with IgG the most frequent immunoglobulin deposited and with less 'full house' immunoglobulin staining is found in MCTD than in LE (Eigenbrodt and Ware, 1989). Some examples of mesangial proliferative GN in MCTD also demonstrate C3, C1q and fibrin-related antigen (Kitridou et al., 1986).

In **Sjögren's Syndrome** GN is less frequent than interstitial nephritis but a variety of patterns including mesangial proliferative GN similar to those seen in LE have been described (Eigenbrodt and Ware, 1989). Proliferative changes are usually accompanied by immunoglobulin, sometimes with IgG, IgA and IgM, and C3 and/or C1q in the mesangium and glomerular capillary loops on IMH. Tubular basement membranes may be similarly stained.

Rheumatoid arthritis and relapsing polychondritis: **Rheumatoid arthritis**: Patients with rheumatoid arthritis commonly show a focal or diffuse mesangial variably proliferative GN associated with haematuria and/or proteinuria (Hordon et al., 1984; Helin et al., 1986) and with some proliferative changes associated with post-mortem findings of vasculitis (Boers et al., 1987). Although IgA is demonstrated in some patients with mesangial proliferative GN, probably related to the relatively frequent finding of raised serum IgA, mesangial deposits of IgG, IgM and C3 correlate with electron dense mesangial deposits in seven of eleven mesangial proliferative biopsies (Helin et al., 1986). It is uncertain as to whether this proliferative GN is related to rheumatoid arthritis or drug therapy. Serum estimations of rheumatoid factor, antinuclear antibodies and complement show no correlation with the extent of proliferative GN (Korpela et al., 1990).

Relapsing polychondritis: Renal manifestations are seen in approximately 25 per cent of patients (Chang-Miller et al., 1987) and consist of focal or diffuse mesangial proliferation and/or segmental necrotizing lesions; IMH shows usually faint C3 and/or IgG or IgM mainly in the mesangium. Some cases show overlap with other connective tissue diseases such as SLE, vasculitis and rheumatoid arthritis (Chang-Miller et al., 1987).

Vasculitides: The characteristic glomerular reaction pattern associated with many different vasculitides is segmental necrosis with crescent formation and varying degrees of endocapillary proliferation and leucocytic infiltration; the latter may be predominant. However, some examples of glomerular involvement in vasculitis show mild diffuse mesangial proliferation which in most cases is unassociated with significant protein deposition; diffuse mesangial light IgM and/or C3 deposition may be evident as a non-specific finding. In some examples of Wegener's granulomatosis, follow-up biopsies may more frequently show focal or diffuse mild or moderate mesangial proliferation accompanied by IMH findings of mesangial IgG and/or IgM and C3 (Weiss and Crissman, 1984). This proliferative change may be found in other forms of vasculitis, either in initial biopsies or on follow-up.

Miscellaneous

A large heterogeneous group of disorders may manifest as either focal or diffuse mesangial proliferative GN on biopsy. Some of these entities often show other forms of glomerular morphology. IMH findings contribute significantly to the differential diagnosis and selected examples of its contribution are as follows: anti-glomerular basement membrane disease with linear IgG staining (Teague et al., 1978); light chain nephropathy (Cohen, 1984); mixed essential cryoglobulinaemia with mesangial proliferation and mesangial deposits of IgM, IgG C3 and C1q and few, if any, peripheral capillary wall changes is an uncommon cause of this pattern (Frankel et al., 1992); various infective processes including Q fever (Perez-Fontan et al., 1988) with granular mesangial and capillary wall IgM and C3 staining combined with light linear IgG deposition in glomerular capillary walls in two of five patients; C1 q nephropathy (Jennette and Hipp, 1985) showing a predominance of C1q in the mesangial areas accompanied by immunoglobulins and C3 unrelated to SLE.

Acellular mesangial expansion

Selected disorders including some systemic conditions are characterized by expansion of the mesangial matrix often accompanied by variable mesangial proliferation with the matrical expansion and/or mesangial protein deposition representing the predominant change on biopsy. The IMH changes in the conditions described are presented in Table 5.11.

Diabetic glomerulosclerosis

Expansion of the mesangium due to accumulated matrix and mesangial cell proliferation is a constant feature of diabetic glomerulosclerosis and glomerular basement membrane thickening and hyalinotic arteriolopathy (Lane et al., 1990). Perhaps the more significant lesion is the diffuse and often nodular (Kimmelstiel-Wilson, KW) expansion of mesangial matrix associated with glomerulosclerosis leading to partial obliteration and reduction of relative capillary luminal area (Gellman et al., 1959). Immunohistochemistry will provide a distinction from light chain nephropathy which may closely resemble diabetic glomerulosclerosis. Immunoglobulin staining in the well-established glomerulosclerosis of diabetes mellitus, of both insulin-dependent and non-insulin-dependent types is characterized by linear light-to-moderate (rarely heavy) outline of all renal basement membranes, glomerular tubular and Bowman's membrane. IgG is the predominant immunoglobulin found (Fig. 5.7A) but IgA also has a linear outline and is accompanied often by extensive albumin basement membrane deposition; C3 may show the same linear outline but is usually light (Westberg and Michael, 1972). Both kappa and lambda light chains outline basement membranes in diabetes mellitus (personal observation). Early or mild diabetic glomerulosclerosis may show the basement membrane staining only faintly. The KW nodule often demonstrates fibrin at all stages of development accompanied by capillary loop staining for fibrin (Farquhar et al., 1972). Nodules may also show uneven staining with

Table 5.11. Pattern III – Predominant mesangial changes 2. Acellular mesangial expansion – IMH patterns

Entity	Mesangium	Loop	Comment
Diabetes mellitus	IgM (IgA)	IgG, IgA, IgM	Heavy arteriolar IgM, C3, (Clq)
Amyloidosis	IgG, IgA, IgM, C3, Clq	(IgG, IgA, IgM, Clq)	Monoclonal AA AL antibodies available
Light chain nephropathy	(Kappa/Lambda)	Kappa/lambda	TBM staining even more frequent Amyloid deposition may accompany Occasional heavy chain deposition
Fibrillary/immunotactoid nephropathy	IgG, IgM, C3, Clq	Same as MES	Sometimes small vessel deposition
Idiopathic lobular glomerulonephropathy		IgG, IgM, fibrin C3, C4	Variable sparse staining
Hepatic glomerulosclerosis	IgA, IgG, IgM, C3	(IgA, IgG, IgM)	Bacterial/food antigens may be demonstrated

Note: ( ) = staining weaker or less frequent

IgM, C3 and C1q (Fig. 5.7B). The mesangium and to a less degree, glomerular capillary loops, frequently show small, occasionally heavy deposits of IgM and C3 and less commonly IgA and C1q; the finding of mesangial IgA is an occasional diagnostic problem, difficult to interpret particularly in diabetics with cirrhosis in whom proteinuria is sometimes accompanied by haematuria. The diabetic 'fibrin caps' consisting of hyaline eosinophilic PAS-positive material staining with IgM and C3 (Tisher and Hostetter, 1989) frequently and probably represent segmental hyalinosis developing in an aneurysmal capillary loop. The extensive arteriolar hyalinosis characteristic of diabetes stains regularly with IgM and C3 and often with early complement components if 'fresh', particularly C1q. This latter finding may be helpful in distinguishing diabetic glomerulosclerosis from other glomerulosclerotic lesions but arteriolar hyaline material may also be seen in glomerulosclerosis related to light chain deposition and in renal amyloidosis with involvement of small vessels.

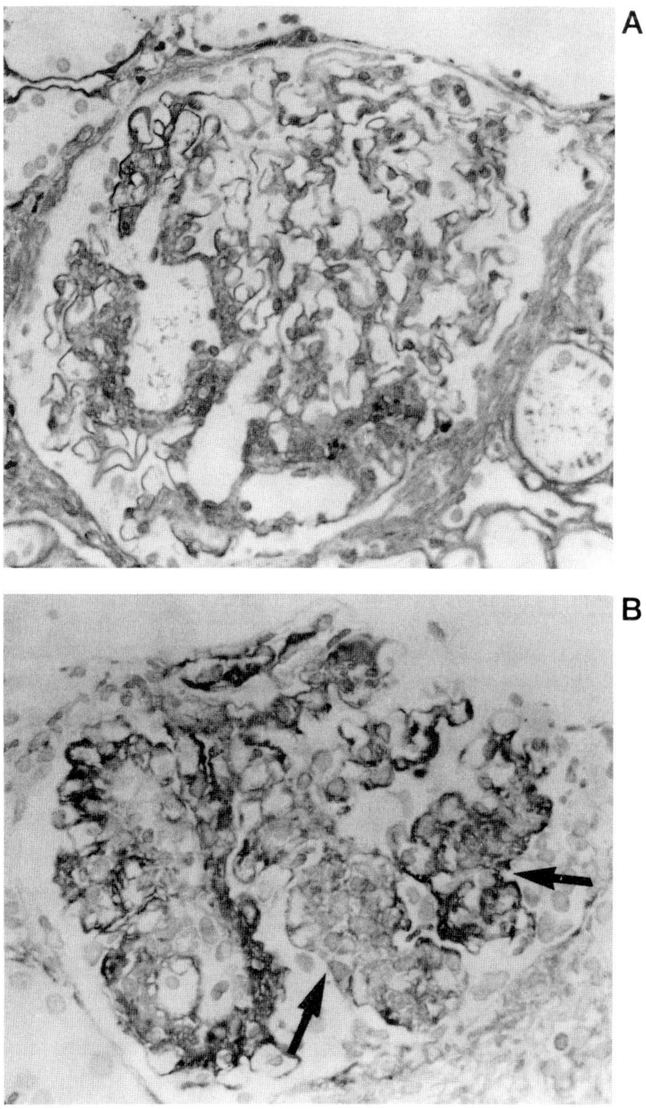

Fig. 5.7. Immunohistochemistry of early lesions of diabetic nephropathy. (A) 'Linear' staining of glomerular and tubular basement membranes with IgG. (B) Variable IgM mesangial deposition in relation to developing Kimmelstiel–Wilson nodules (arrows) (X400)

Renal amyloidosis

In recent years, different forms of the amyloid protein have been characterized and despite the diverse origins of the fibrillary material, all forms appear to follow a common final pathway through proteolytic mechanisms reducing a large circulating protein to a low molecular weight protein to polymerize to fibrils 10–12 nanometers thick with a β-pleated pattern detected by x-ray defraction (Stone, 1990). Very rarely larger amyloid fibres maybe detected (Yoshikawa et al., 1990). The systemic forms of amyloidosis that involve the kidney are classified according to the dominant amyloid protein forming fibrils (Cohen and Connors, 1987), (Table 5.12) namely (i) AL amyloid of primary (idiopathic) and myeloma-associated types with deposition of kappa and lambda light chains; (ii) AA amyloid with serum A protein deposition seen mostly with chronic inflammatory conditions and with some malignancies; (iii) AF or AE amyloid with pre-albumin or some other protein deposition in the genetic or familial forms; and (iv)

Table 5.12. Features of renal amyloidosis

Type of amyloid	Aetiology	Amyloid protein	Main renal lesion
AL amyloid	Plasma cell dyscrasias	Light chain Kappa/lambda	Glomerular and vascular
AA amyloid	Chronic inflammatory diseases Various neoplasms	SAP	Glomerular and vascular
Hereditary/ familial		Pre-albumin in many; AA	Variable involvement
Haemodialysis (H-amyloid)	Prolonged dialysis	B_2 Micro-globulin	'Amyloid calculi'

Note: SAP = serum amyloid protein

so-called H-amyloidosis with β2-microglobulin deposition in patients undergoing (haemo)dialysis (Gejyo et al. 1986). Other forms of tumour-related or senile amyloid do not appear to involve the kidney and only H-amyloid spares glomeruli, renal vessels and the interstitium (Koch, 1992); renal involvement may take the form of 2-microglobulin renal calculi (Bommer et al., 1985). Monoclonal antibodies are available to all these different types of amyloid fibril and precursor proteins.

The vast majority of examples of renal amyloidosis (RA) show acellular mesangial expansion due to the early deposition of the material in the mesangial matrix. However, accumulation of amyloid to produce large mesangial masses accompanied by extension around glomerular capillary loops is characteristic of established cases. The amount of amyloid deposited may be very slight but yet be associated with the nephrotic syndrome (Jones et al., 1986). Heavy proteinuria and/or the nephrotic syndrome are the usual manifestations of amyloid deposition.

By IMH, the mesangial and other renal deposits frequently show light staining with some or all of IgG, IgA, IgM and complement components, C3 and C1q and/or C4 and fibrinogen. The more accurate characterization of the protein(s) contributing to amyloid formation is aided by permanganate removal of congophilia considered initially to indicate AA-type amyloid (Wright et al., 1977) but is considered by others (Shirahama et al., 1985) to be less reliable in making this distinction. More recently, several groups have used monoclonal antibodies directed against specific components of the common forms of amyloidosis (Gallo et al., 1986; Nöel et al., 1987; Fitzmaurice et al., 1991) using both fresh tissue for immunofluorescence and fixed paraffin-embedded tissue for immunoenzymatic methods (Fig. 5.8). Formic acid pre-treatment of tissues may enhance amyloid immunohistochemical staining (Kitamoto et al., 1987).

Light chain nephropathy (LCN)

A characteristic pathology seen in approximately 50 per cent of cases is one of glomerulosclerosis diffusely affecting mesangial areas with, in particular, the development of mesangial nodules often combined with varying degrees of mesangial proliferation; the most constant finding in this entity, however, is tubulointerstitial damage with inflammation (Minetti, 1992). Renal involvement is the commonest manifestation of this usually systemic

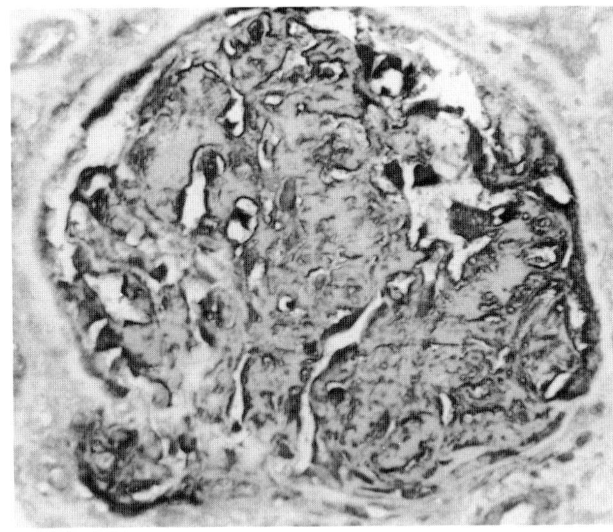

Figure 5.8. Staining of capillary loop, mesangial and arteriolar amyloid deposits with a monoclonal AA antibody in AA amyloidosis (×400)

protein deposit disease (Buxbaum, 1992) with kappa LC responsible for approximately 80 per cent of cases and lambda LC for the remainder (Gallo and Buxbaum, 1988).

Both primary idiopathic plasma cell dyscrasias and those of multiple myeloma, plasmacytosis associated with amyloidosis and the lymphocytic (often plasmacytoid) lymphomas (Buxbaum, 1992) may produce renal pathology in approximately two thirds of patients (Buxbaum, 1992; Minetti, 1992). Immunohistochemistry of haemopoietic tissue will detect a monoclonal population producing LC and occasional abnormal heavy chains that, probably, because of altered antigenicity, are sometimes undetectable in serum and urine (Minetti, 1992); it has been suggested that bone marrow immunohistochemistry detecting a disturbance of the normal 2:1 ratio of kappa:lambda plasmacyte/lymphocyte populations will provide evidence of plasma cell dysplasia if the bone marrow abnormality corresponds to the light chain found in tissue (Wolf et al., 1986). The variable glomerular morphology associated with fibrillary kappa light chain deposition in the mesangium and capillary walls has recently been outlined by Esparza et al. (1991) suggesting a link between light chain deposition and immunotactoid glomerulopathy.

The deposited light chain which has a finely to moderately granular ultrastructural morphology (Sinniah and Cohen, 1985) has an affinity for basement membranes particularly in the kidney and blood vessels in other tissues and on analysis in limited cases is of abnormal chemical composition (Buxbaum, 1992). The light chain material is negative for amyloid P component and Congo red and is periodic acid-Schiff positive. IMH with both kappa and lambda light chain stains shows deposits along all basement membranes in the kidney often in a linear outline and in most mesangial areas (Fig. 5.9). A combined pattern of deposition of light and heavy chains has also been previously described (Buxbaum, 1990).

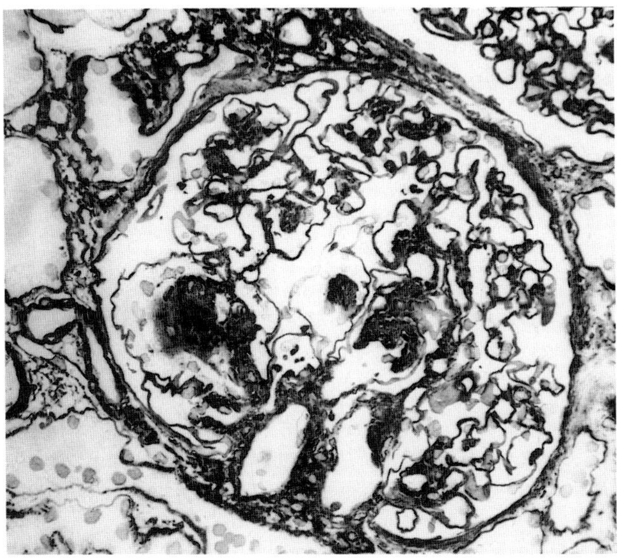

Figure 5.9. Moderate staining of capillary walls, mesangial areas including nodules, glomerular arterioles and capsular basement membranes with Kappa light chain antibody (×400m)

Fibrillary/immunotactoid nephropathy

More than a decade ago, it was suggested by Rosenmann and Eliakim (1977) that proteinaceous material that lacked congophilia could accumulate to obliterate glomeruli resulting in renal failure preceded by heavy proteinuria. This condition which was subsequently labelled 'fibrillary' or 'immunotactoid' nephritis was found to be distinct from amyloidosis and marked by a constant expansion of the mesangium with an almost equal frequency of capillary wall thickening but with variable vascular deposition (Duffy et al., 1983; Korbet et al., 1991). The lesion is diagnosed, essentially, by ultrastructural appearances which show the protein deposits are largely of fibrillary or tubular outline with a thickness greater than that seen in the standard form of amyloid i.e. greater than 12 nanometers. A comparison of the features of amyloid and immunotactoid deposits is presented in Table 5.13.

IMH consistently shows moderate-to-heavy immunoglobulin, invariably IgG, frequently IgM and less often IgA deposition accompanied always by C3 and C1q/C4 often in the mesangial capillary wall and small arterial/arteriolar sites of deposition (Korbet et al., 1991; Fig. 5.10). Both kappa and lambda light chains are usually demonstrated but in some cases only kappa light chain may be seen (Korbet et al., 1991; Esparza et al., 1991).

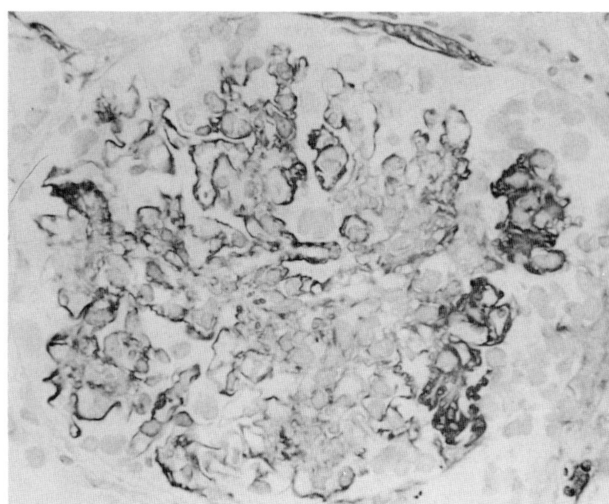

Figure 5.10. Variable staining of mesangia and capillary walls with IgG in immunotactoid nephropathy confirmed by electron microscopy (×400)

Table 5.13. Characteristics of amyloid and immunotactoid fibrils

	Fibril diameter	Congophilia	Deposit sites	IMH
Amyloid	10–12 nanometers	+	Mesangium capillary wall	AA protein/ AL-light chain/ ? other protein
Immunotactoid	Usually > 15 nm Most > 20 nm	–	Mesangium capillary wall	IgG, IgM, Kappa and lambda

Mazzucco et al. (1990) and Alpers (1992) have stressed that some patients have deposits that are distinctly microtubular on electron microscopy and that deposits in others are distinctly fibrillary; Alpers (1992) suggests that the microtubular deposits are seen in patients more likely to have disturbances of immunoglobulin production such as monoclonal gammopathy or cryoglobulinaemia in contrast to those with fibrillary deposits among whom only one patient has been described as having cryoglobulinaemia. Extra-renal deposits of the same fibrillary material were noted by Ozawa et al. (1991).

Idiopathic lobular glomerulonephritis (nodular mesangial sclerosis, Alpers and Biava, 1989)

Although possibly related to membranoproliferative (mesangiocapillary) glomerulonephritis (Mandalenakis et al., 1971) occasional biopsies may demonstrate a markedly exaggerated lobularity due to mesangial proliferation and, particularly, to increased mesangial matrix accompanied by GBM reduplication. Alpers and Biava (1989) described five patients in whom other causes of marked mesangial expansion with accentuated lobularity including mesangiocapillary GN were excluded by morphological and immunohistological studies. A paucity of deposits on electronmicroscopy was supported by immunohistochemical findings of non-specific deposition of immunoglobulin and complement with two cases showing segmental IgM, fibrinogen and both types of light chains (one showed similar deposition of C3); two cases with non-specific band-like staining of glomerular capillary loops with C3, C4, fibrinogen and albumin (one of these cases showed similar IgG and IgM staining); and one case with no significant staining demonstrated.

Hepatic glomerulosclerosis

A frequent histological pattern amidst the variety of glomerulopathies that may be associated with liver disease, particularly cirrhosis (reviewed by Eigenbrodt and Ware, 1989), is diffuse mesangial expansion with increased matrix which, in many instances, is unaccompanied by mesangial proliferation; capillary walls may be mildly to moderately uniformly thickened. 'Pure' diffuse hepatic glomerulosclerosis commonly shows mesangial deposits of IgA (Berger et al., 1978) often associated with C3 and, less often, IgG and IgM, perhaps corresponding to scattered ultrastructural mesangial deposits which are associated with electron lucent areas in the mesangial matrix. Serial biopsies have demonstrated a transition from glomerulosclerosis to a proliferative glomerulonephritis in a few patients (Nochy et al., 1976).

IV. Segmental necrosis/crescent formation (focal or diffuse)

Very localized injury to glomerular capillary loops may have severe consequences (Parfrey et al., 1985). An extremely common glomerular reaction to injury is crescent formation resulting from an accumulation of excessive cells within Bowman's space often arranged with an established substructure. This accumulation of cells may arise through different mechanisms; segmental inflammation with necrosis including rupture of the GBM with accumulation of fibrin in the related capillary loops exuding into the urinary space is a potent mechanism for this change (Bergstein, 1990). Cells may traverse Bowman's capsular membrane and emigrate as a result of interstitial periglomerular inflammation to again accumulate in the urinary space (Boucher et al., 1987). The events relating to necrosis-related crescent formation are summarized in Table 5.14.

Although spontaneous resolution of crescents is well documented, particularly with post-streptococcal glomerulonephritis (Rodriguez-Iturbe, 1992), the usual natural history, especially in the segmental necrotic-derived crescent is towards a scarring and organizing process. The inflammatory process of segmental necrosis and crescent formation may represent the basic and only pattern of glomerular injury or, in many varied glomerulonephropathies, this reaction may be superimposed on other patterns of change. Although there is some dispute as to the percentage of crescents indicating a poor outlook, the prognosis for patients with 50 per cent or more crescents in a given biopsy is poor regardless of the cause (Glassock et al., 1991). In children the outlook may not be as grave for crescentic disease in conditions unassociated with mesangiocapillary GN or 'idiopathic' diffuse crescent GN (Miller et al., 1984).

There are some IMH attributes that are common to crescents regardless of the pathomechanism of development. The cellular constituents of a crescent have been shown by glomerular culture work, experimental models and immunohistochemical labelling of cells in

Table 5.14. Events leading to crescent formation

Autoantibody/immune complex/
? cell mediated immune mechanisms

↓

PHLOGISTIC CAPILLARY WALL INJURY

↓

Endocapillary hypercellularity
Leucocytic exudation + proliferation of intrinsic cells

↓

GBM dissolution
Fibrin deposition in capillary lumen, Bowman's space

↓

Leukocytic immigration into Bowman's space
(especially if Bowman's membrane also ruptured)
Proliferation of epithelial cells

↓	↓
Fibrous repair of crescent and segmental lesion	Resolution in some cases with intact Bowman's membrane

human biopsies to be a mixture of epithelial (parietal and visceral) cells and leucocytes, mainly monocyte-macrophages (Hancock and Atkins, 1984; Boucher et al., 1987; Nolasco et al., 1987). The latter authors (Nolasco et al., 1987) demonstrated the presence of T cells suggesting cell mediated immune mechanisms involved in recruitment of monocytes to participate in crescent formation in patients with vasculitis and crescentic disease. The proportions of these different cells forming individual crescents in a particular form of crescentic GN appears to vary and the integrity of Bowman's capsular membrane influences the number of constituent mononuclear leucocytes with greater numbers found when the membrane is breached (Boucher et al., 1987). Yoshioka et al. (1987) further demonstrated collagen types IV and V, laminin and fibronectin in crescents at all stages with the epithelial cell constituents of crescents staining with cytokeratin and vimentin; these workers could demonstrate only minor monocyte-macrophage participation in crescent formation. Another constant constituent of glomerulonephritic crescents is fibrin (fibrinogen, fibrin-related antigens) derived via endothelial injury which is produced, probably, by inflammatory cell infiltration and GBM rupture (Bonsib, 1988) (Fig. 5.11A). Yoshioka et al. (1987) examined crescents from a variety of GNs and showed that the fibrinogen/fibrin-related antigens could be demonstrated in all crescentic cases. However, the crescents failed to stain with monoclonal antibody to cross-linked fibrin or von Willebrand factor (factor VIII-related antigen) suggesting that the material stained is not fibrin but fibrinogen or its degradation product. Recent work by Tipping et al. (1988) suggests that the monocyte-macrophage provides tissue pro-coagulant activity leading to fibrin deposition and crescent formation within the glomerulus. Fibrin may persist in areas of organization

A

B

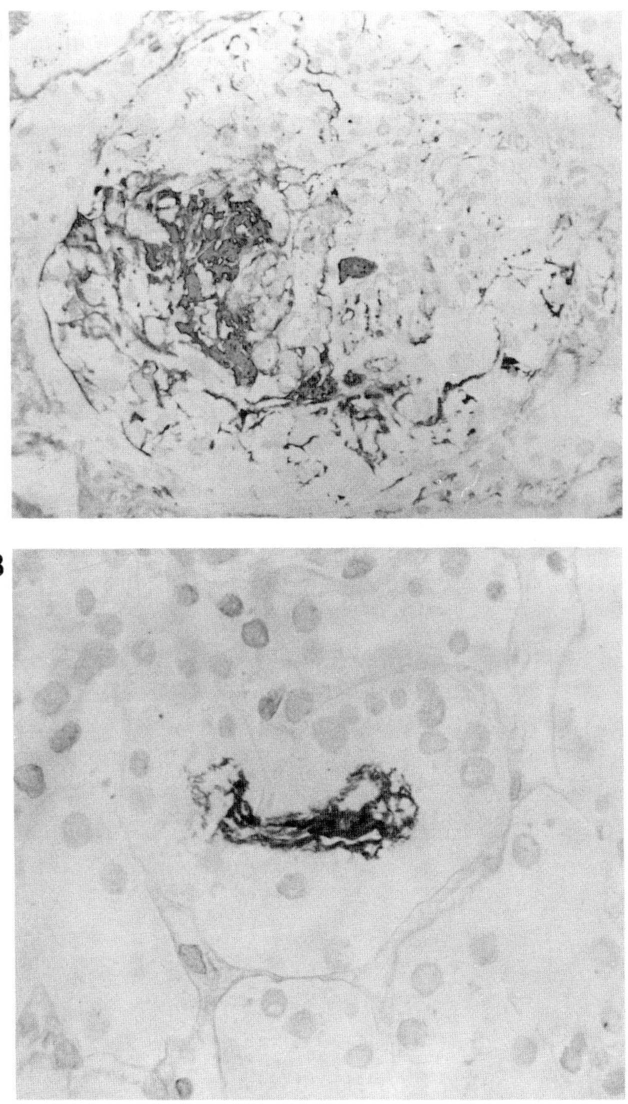

Fig. 5.11. (A) A segmental deposit of fibrinogen in glomerular capillary loops extending into Bowman's space with early crescent formation. (X400) (B)Fibrinogen staining of tubular cast in a patient with macroscopic haematuria and sparse segmental necrotizing lesions (X400)

within the affected capillary loops undergoing sclerosis and within the sclerosing crescent for a considerable time, probably weeks or months; this feature may in some instances assist in distinguishing segmental sclerotic lesions that are post-proliferative/necrotic from those that are primarily a degenerative sclerosing and/or hyalinotic process which are usually negative on IMH staining for fibrin. The limited amount of tissue available in many renal biopsies may hamper the diagnosis of focal segmental necrotizing or crescentic GN if lesions are particularly sparse; rarely early segmental necrotizing lesions may be very small and quite exquisitely involve an isolated capillary loop. In these circumstances scattered fibrin-containing casts in cortical or medullary tubules demonstrated by IMH may provide a pointer for a more exhaustive search for the glomerular necrotizing lesion(s) (Fig. 5.11B).

It is now accepted that diffuse crescentic GN (DCGN) (rapidly progressive GN) may be seen in three immunological settings in which IMH provides key diagnostic information (Couser, 1988) viz. anti-glomerular basement membrane disease (AGBMD), 'pauci-immune' or 'non-immune' crescentic glomerulonephritis, and immune complex crescentic glomerulonephritis. An outline of the immunohistochemical findings and the diseases responsible for crescentic GN follows.

Anti-glomerular basement membrane disease (AGBMD)

This autoimmune form of renal injury accounts for approximately 10–20 per cent of cases of diffuse crescentic (rapidly progressive) GN (DCGN) and maybe seen with or without accompanying lung haemorrhage (see below for discussion of findings in Goodpasture's syndrome) (Turner and Rees, 1992). Uncommonly other morphologies may be found such as diffuse mesangial proliferation or minor changes without segmental lesions (Teague et al., 1978; Carre et al., 1989).

The diagnosis of AGBMD is based on the demonstration by IMH and/or radioimmunoassay of a GBM antibody. The classic pattern on IMH is one of linear staining uniformly outlining the GBMs with IgG (IgG-1 and IgG-4) of strong intensity; in approximately 70 per cent of cases, similar confluent or interrupted staining of tubular basement membranes and Bowman's basement membrane (Turner and Rees, 1992; Fig. 5.12); the extent of TBM staining was found by Andres et al. (1978) to parallel the intensity of

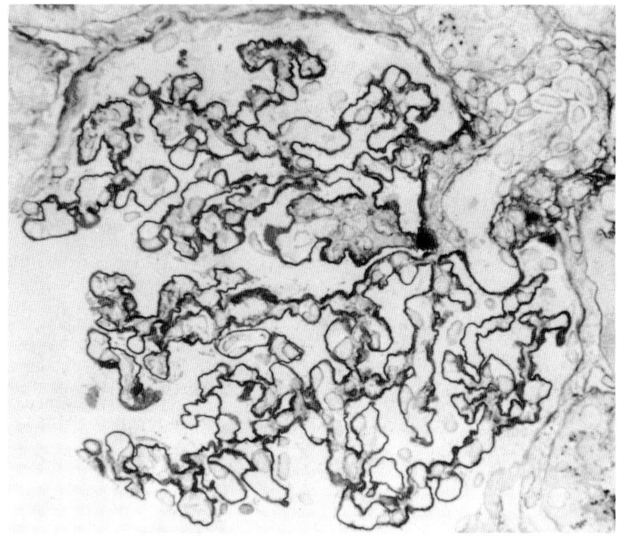

Fig. 5.12. Moderate linear staining of basement membranes with IgG in a patient with Goodpasture's syndrome (X400)

interstitial inflammation that commonly accompanies the glomerulonephritis in this lesion. The 'standard' example of AGBMD GN shows light or moderate C3 staining similarly outlining basement membranes accompanied by faint or often no IgA and irregular light IgM deposition in the mesangium and in some capillary loops, often those involved by segmental necrosis. Some variations contrasting with this pattern have been noted. Strong linear IgA has been noted on several occasions, as summarized by Gris et al. (1991). But in only two of the six cases recorded with IgA linear staining have IgA serum autoantibodies been demonstrated (Border et al., 1979; Fivush et al., 1986 and Espinosa-Meléndez et al., 1980). Similarly linear IgM cases have been described by Wilson and Dixon (1986) and Ross et al. (1986) with the latter patient also demonstrating an erythematous rash with linear IgM at the dermo-epidermal junction of lesional skin and a titre of serum IgM AGBM antibody of 1:32. Another patient with IMH-confirmed bullous pemphigoid followed by AGBMD with linear IgG on IMH was described by Davenport et al. (1987). Granularity superimposed on the linear IMH pattern with IgG and/or C3 staining (Savige et al., 1989; Cohen and Glassock, 1989) may represent combined autoimmune (linear) and immune complex (granular) injury (Fig. 5.13). The granularity of staining may only be apparent under high power examination (×400 or oil immersion).

True linear staining has been described accompanying other pathologies where its significance is uncertain

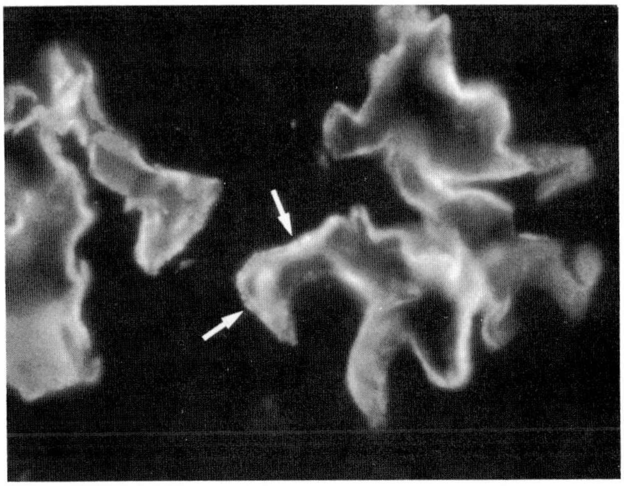

Fig. 5.13. Direct immunofluorescence outlining both linear and finely granular (arrows) staining of glomerular basement membranes in a patient with persisting proteinuria following recovery from acute renal failure due to Goodpasture's syndrome. IgG (X1000)

(see Table 5.15); in SLE (Cohen and Glassock, 1989) although a recent rare case of mesangial proliferative glomerulonephritis with linear IgG glomerular basement membrane staining in the presence of serum IgG autoantibody has been described in SLE by Richards et al., (1988); in crescentic GN thought due to vasculitis (Case Records, 1985); as a presumed incidental finding in follow-up biopsies in patients with a history of biopsy-proven PEGN (Gallo et al., 1980); and in renal transplants (Cameron and Turner, 1977) in which the linear staining does not appear to be associated with significant glomerular pathology but in which rarely a de novo autoimmune linear IgG crescentic GN may develop (Boyce et al., 1985). Linear IgG staining has been noted particularly in graft recipients with a history of Alport's syndrome (Querin et al., 1986), a small minority of whom may develop diffuse crescentic nephritis in the graft which by possessing the Goodpasture antigen excites the production of IgG autoantibody in such patients (Shah et al., 1988; Savige et al., 1989). In some instances, difficulties can be experienced with the so-called 'pseudolinear pattern' of staining seen with a uniformly developed early membranous nephropathy of either idiopathic or secondary types or in cases (see below) with superadded granular staining on a linear pattern. This difficulty can be experienced with both immuno-

Table 5.15. Pattern IV – Segmental necrosis/crescent formation linear staining of glomerular and other basement membranes

		True linear staining	
Entity	**Mesangial staining**	**Capillary wall**	**Comment**
Anti GBM disease	IgM, C3	IgG. linear Rarely IgA/IgM Linear, Granular IgG rarely superimposed	TBM linear in 70%
Systemic lupus	Variable IgG, IgA IgM, C3, Clq	IgG: linear	Very rarely significant re glomerular changes
Renal transplants	IgM, C3	IgG: linear	Usually not significant Rarely de novo DCGN Greater incidence in Alport's syndrome
		Incidental linear staining	
Post-infectious GN – on follow-up biopsy		Post-streptococcal GN	
Nail-Patella Syndrome		Chronic Q fever	
		Pseudolinear staining	
Early membranous: very finely granular IgG			
Diabetic glomerulosclerosis: All BMs – IgG, IgA, C3			
Hepatic glomerulosclerosis: GBM – IgA			
Light chain nephropathy: GBM and TBMS – Kappa or lambda LC			
Type I mesangiocapillary GN: GBM – IgG, A, C3, Clq			
Type II mesangiocapillary GN: GBM and TBMs, – C3			

fluorescence and immunoenzymatic techniques. Other entities that may require differentiation from AGBMD include the confluent outlining of glomerular capillary walls seen in type I (subendothelial) mesangiocapillary GN of varied aetiologies, light chain nephropathies, immunotactoid nephropathy and the linear staining of all diabetic basement membranes particularly with immunoglobulin and albumin. Another variation on linear GBM and TBM staining is seen when crescentic nephritis is associated with light chain linear deposition is noted by Lapenas et al. (1983) and Savige et al. (1989) with kappa and lambda light chain staining in each case respectively. The patterns associated with linear basement membrane staining and the differential diagnosis of this change are given in Table 5.15.

Extensive work in relation to the Goodpasture antigen has been summarized by Turner and Rees (1992). The 'Goodpasture antigen' is located on the non-collagenous C-terminal end of the alpha 3 chain of collagen IV, the main collagen comprising the GBM (see Section on Normal or Minor Non-Specific Appearances – Thin Membrane Nephropathy and Alport's Syndrome, page 215). The IgG linear staining of alveolar basement membranes is more likely to be seen from more centrally sited lung tissue but produces an outline that is often incomplete. Exogenous factors (Turner and Rees, 1992) such as influenza virus infection, hydrocarbons (especially organic solvents), cigarette smoke and, possibly, drugs such as penicillamine and hydralazine may act to alter or expose previously protected antigen which, because of the fixation of serum antibody to alveolar and glomerular basement membranes is presumed to be the Goodpasture antigen.

Some problems due to technical methods employed may be experienced in the interpretation of the IMH results in patients with possible AGBMD. A consistent problem is background staining with many commercial and other antisera to both whole globulin and gamma heavy chains whereby collagen in the interstitium and basement membranes is outlined. In biopsies with AGBMD showing relatively light to moderate staining, the distinction from background may be difficult. Prior absorption with collagen extracts appears to only partially improve the background staining. AGBMD is one renal disease in which IF appears to be superior to immuno-enzymatic testing which, from the author's experience, has proved quite capricious, perhaps due to a result of fixation. It has been suggested by Aguirreburyalde and Howat (1991) that neutral buffered formalin fixation may have a stronger effect on antigenicity than acidic formal saline and requires a longer digestion time. Only on one occasion can the present author recall immunoperoxidase staining on a crescentic biopsy showing strong staining with linear IgG outlining glomerular capillary walls and, on direct immunofluorescence, weak equivocal staining being evident in the same biopsy. The usual situation is the reverse. In such situations it is often very useful to have a small portion of cortex stored frozen and fresh in case the need for direct immunofluorescence arises in an urgent or difficult diagnostic situation.

Non-immune/pauci-immune segmental necrotizing GN, focal/diffuse

This category of diffuse crescentic GN (DCGN) has gained increasing recognition in recent years (Cameron, 1991) but as Cohen et al. (1981) point out the immunopathological role of small mesangial and scattered capillary loop deposits of IgM, IgG, and C3 on IMH staining is uncertain. These are now regarded as insignificant, hence the designation 'non-immune/pauci-immune'. Frequently, however, fibrinogen or fibrin-related antigen staining is the only positive immunoperoxidase pattern noted and is related to the affected capillaries and crescents which may also stain segmentally with IgM, C3 and C1q/C4. Follow-up biopsies in patients previously showing 'pauci-immune' DCGN morphology may demonstrate mesangial and less often, capillary loop IgM and C3 in particular, which may be accompanied by mild focal or diffuse mesangial proliferation (Weiss and Crissman, 1984). Cohen et al. (1981) noted the disappearance of deposits on a follow-up biopsy whilst Olsen et al. (1974) found an accumulation of immunoglobulin and complement deposits following an initial biopsy in which IMH was negative in crescentic GN. In some vasculitic diseases there is a lack of uniformity of IMH findings and although it appears that most cases of DCGN or focal CGN associated with vasculitides including Wegener's granulomatosis are negative for deposits on IMH of glomeruli (ten Berge et al., 1985; Andrassy et al., 1991) some early descriptions of the IMH in Wegener's granulomatosis (e.g. Horn et al., 1974) showed IgG staining of mesangial areas and capillary loops.

There is a recent realization that this form of pauci-immune CGN (focal/diffuse) with segmental necrosis is associated with vasculitis (Serra et al., 1984; Cameron, 1991). As summarized by Cameron (1991) so-called 'idiopathic' crescentic GN without evident immune deposits and pauci-immune crescentic GN are the same disease because of similar histology, the presence of vasculitis as the sole manifestation, the fact that some of the 'idiopathic' CGN patients subsequently develop vasculitis, that unsuspected extra-renal vasculitis may be found and anti-neutrophilic antibodies are generally positive in both sets of patients.

Almost all of the increasing number of conditions with vasculitic manifestations (Lie, 1992), may involve the kidney, usually with segmental necrosis as the main manifestation regardless of the size of the vessel involved by the main vasculitic pathological process (Cameron, 1991).

The lack of immune deposits in the kidney suggests to many that other factors such as autoimmunity and/or cell-mediated events are more important than immune complex deposition. Various forms of vasculitis involving the kidney have been associated in recent years with serological finding of antineutrophilic cytoplasmic antibodies (ANCA) providing serological markers for vasculitis and segmental necrotizing GN with crescents. Two different forms of ANCA are derived from different antigens from neutrophil lysosomes; by indirect immunofluorescence it may be determined that the C-(cytoplasmic/'classical') ANCA is directed against protease 3 (myeloblastin) and stains neutrophilic cytoplasm evenly but P-(perinuclear) ANCA stains the antigen myeloperoxidase and is distributed, due to an artefact of ethanol-related fixation in a nuclear or perinuclear pattern (Wieslander, 1991). ANCA may also be detected by an enzyme-linked immunosorbent assay (ELISA) or solid-phase assays to serve as a screening method or as a verification for indirect immunofluorescent results (Wieslander, 1991). Most ANCAs are IgG Classes I and IV but the development of Class III IgG may be related to increased activity of disease (Brouwer et al., 1991; Jayne et al., 1991). Support for the use of ANCA as a monitor of vasculitic activity has recently been provided by Pettersson and Heigl (1992).

ANCA are found in nearly all cases of Wegener's granulomatosis, usually as C-ANCA (Hoffman et al., 1992), in approximately 80 per cent of cases of idiopathic crescentic GN (Jennette and Falk, 1990) and in cases of microscopic polyarteritis without vasculitis in the kidney or elsewhere) (Cameron, 1991) and in Churg-Strauss allergic granulomatosis (Gaskin et al., 1987) as well as in some patients with AGBM-negative renal-pulmonary syndrome with lung haemorrhage (Jennette, 1991). An increasing number of diverse non-vasculitic conditions are now also known to have ANCAs usually in a minority of cases as summarized by Rees and Cameron (1992). These antibodies have proved very useful in the diagnostic process in recent years. However, they may lead to 'false-positive' interpretations of a clinical context that, without tissue providing diagnostic confirmation, may lead to an erroneous diagnosis of vasculitis (Davenport, 1992). The strength of the associations between crescentic GN, vasculitis and ANCA are presented in Table 5.16.

Crescentic glomerulonephritis related to immune complex deposition – focal or diffuse

Diverse systemic, infective and even idiopathic diseases are grouped because of the consistent finding of

Table 5.16. Pattern IV – Segmental necrosis/crescent formation: Crescentic glomerulonephritis, vasculitis and anca

	Proteinase 3	Myeloperoxidase	Indeterminate	Negative
Wegeners granulomatosis	60*	15	20	5
Microscopic polyarteritis	25	45	5	25
Primary crescentic glomerulonephritis	10	75	–	15
Polyarteritis nodosa	–	30	–	70
Churg–Strauss syndrome	–	70	–	30

Note: * Per cent of sera tested
Source: Noël *et al.*, 1992.

granular deposits on IMH of renal biopsies showing crescentic formation. In some systemic conditions, e.g. lupus erythematosus, DCGN is not infrequent but in other diseases this pattern may represent an unusual manifestation of a rare condition e.g. DCGN associated with IgA/IgG cryoglobulinaemia with IgA and IgG deposition in glomerular capillary loops (Weber et al., 1985). The reaction patterns associated with crescent formation may vary considerably with other diagnostic changes apparent on light microscopy. For instance the association of membranous transformation with crescentic glomerulonephritis may raise the possibility of lupus erythematosus or could be seen in the combined proliferative and membranous glomerulonephritis with diffuse crescentic disease described in some cases by Burkholder et al. (1970) or intramembranous confluent 'ribbon-like' deposits may point to type 2 mesangiocapillary glomerulonephritis. Crescent formation, especially focal, but sometimes diffuse, is a frequent finding in IgA nephropathy recognized by the characteristic IgA deposition in the mesangium (D'Amico, 1987). However, as stressed above, many of these different conditions may share features such as subepithelial 'humps' occurring in post-infectious glomerulonephritis, mesangiocapillary type I GN DCGN with sparse complement deposits related to subepithelial deposits (Davis et al., 1978) and diffuse crescentic GN due to bacterial endocarditis (Beaufils et al., 1976). The differentiation of these entities often relies upon salient immunohistochemical features which are outlined in Table 5.17. The staining patterns are also outlined in sections corresponding to the major morphological changes.

V. Glomerulosclerosis – segmental/global

The process of permanent partial or complete glomerular obliteration common to many forms of renal injury may result from several forms of pathological injury. These include a repair process following previous inflammatory destruction (as discussed above), an accumulation of material usually 'foreign' to the glomerulus, e.g. amyloidosis or immunotactoid material, various forms of ischaemia, virus infection, in particular HIV (Cohen and Nast, 1991), or the process of hyperfiltration related to previous severe renal damage throwing much of the 'workload' of the nephron onto the relatively few remaining glomeruli or due to a 'primary' focal glomerulosclerosis developing spontaneously or, as indicated previously, following minimal change lesion or diffuse mesangial proliferation associated with heavy proteinuria/nephrotic syndrome (Rennke and Klein, 1989). The sclerosing process (International Committee for Nomenclature and Nosology of Renal Disease (1975)) involves capillary loop collapse and adhesion to Bowman's capsular membrane, often thickened by fibrous tissue, expansion of mesangial matrix to partially or completely obliterate the capillary lumens and frequently an accumulation of so-called hyaline material derived from plasma proteins and plasma lipids within capillary loops that remain unobliterated by sclerosis and are sometimes aneurysmal. Evidence is accumulating that the lipid deposited in diseased glomeruli (Sato et al., 1991) and lipid abnormalities in the circulation may contribute to progressive glomerulosclerosis (Keane et al., 1988). IMH of material accumulating in sclerotic

Table 5.17. Pattern IV – Segmental necrosis/crescent formation/diffuse crescentic glomerulonephritis: immune complex deposition

	IgA nephropathy	HSP GN	Mesangiocapillary GN I	Mesangiocapillary GN II	Mesangiocapillary GN III	Cryoglobulinaemia
Mesangium	A, M, C3	(A)	G, C3, Clq	C3	C3(M, G, A)	(M, G, C3, Clq)
Capillary walls	M, C3(A)	A, M, C3	G, C3, Clq	C3	C3(M, G, A)	M, G, C3, Clq(A)

	Proliferative and exudative GN	Bacterial endocarditis	Systemic lupus erythematosus	Light chain nephropathy
Mesangium	G, C3, M	C3(G, M)	G, M, A, C3, Clq	(Kappa/lambda)
Capillary walls	G, C3	C3(G, M)	G, M, A, C3, Clq	Kappa/lambda

Notes: ( ) weaker/less frequent staining; A = IgA, G = IgG, M = IgM; HSP = Henoch–Schönlein purpura.

areas demonstrates that it is composed at least in part of collagen types III and IV (Morel-Maroger Striker et al., 1984).

The characteristic finding in the segmentally or globally sclerosed glomerulus is the presence on IMH of IgM and/or C3 especially relating to areas of hyalinosis (Fig. 5.14); some examples show IgA and/or IgG and/or early complement components C1q or C4 in these sclerotic areas. These proteins are located in the mesangium, in sclerotic i.e. thickened, glomerular papillary walls and in hyalinotic masses of protein. The accumulation in the post-proliferative sclerotic process is part of the repair process and is usually not progressive unless sufficient renal damage is present to induce hyperfiltration injury.

Many workers, summarized by Broyer et al. (1992), suggest immunoglobulin and complement accumulation in these lesions is a secondary or passive change due, according to Rennke and Klein (1989) to trapping of the larger molecules such as IgM and complement components as a result of charge alterations in the capillary wall (Wada et al., 1990) and the mesangium (Ueda et al., 1992); smaller molecules such as albumin appear to be excreted in the urine. The extensive deposition of IgM and/or C3 in globally and segmentally sclerotic glomeruli in severely damaged kidneys which may result from many different causes emphasises the non-specificity of the IMH changes but also suggests that progression of mesangial and capillary wall injury may result from an immunological component inducing a vicious circle of injury associated with other mechanisms such as hyperfiltration, raised capillary pressure and glomerular hypertrophy (Velosa et al., 1976; Rennke and Klein, 1989). The process of sclerosis has been associated with many different conditions (see Table 5.18, after Rennke and Klein, 1989). When lesions are clearly outlined in available tissue, characteristic IMH is easily interpreted. However, a variety of factors may

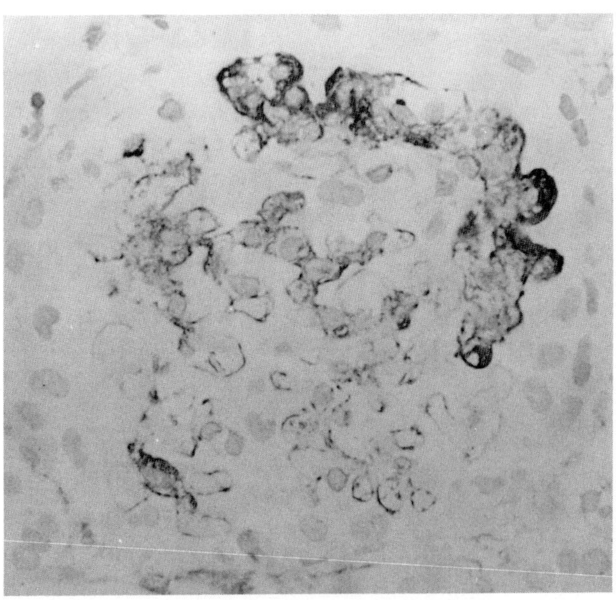

Fig. 5.14. Heavy IgM deposition in a segmental lesion from a biopsy showing idiopathic focal segmental glomerulosclerosis associated with the nephrotic syndrome (X400)

Table 5.18. Pattern V – Glomerulosclerosis: mechanisms and causes

1. *Podocytic +/− mesangial injury*
   Idiopathic focal segmental GS
   HIV-associated nephropathy
   Focal GS related to heroin

2. *Related to structural/functional adaption*
   (a) Nephron loss with hyperfiltration injury

   Unilateral renal agenesis: nephrectomy; reflux nephropathy; chronic pyelonephritis;
   Primary glomerulonephritides
   Chronic interstitial nephritis
   Papillary necrosis due to analgesic abuse
   Adult polycystic kidney disease
   Renal dysplasia
   Sickle cell disease

   (b) Normal nephron population

   Diabetic nephropathy
   Glycogen storage diseases
   Familial dysautonomia
   Morbid obesity
   Toxaemic nephropathy
   Congenital cyanotic heart defects

3. *Related to hereditary basement membrane defects*

   Alport's syndrome
   Nail-Patella syndrome
   (+/− extra renal changes)

4. *Post-proliferative/necrotizing GN lesions*

   Many different glomerulonephritides
   especially IgA GN and vasculitides

Source: Rennke and Klein, 1989

make the diagnosis of focal segmental GS difficult. Lesions may be either of a very early stage of formation or very sparse within the biopsy; they may also vary as to the location within the glomerulus i.e. situated in a perihilar or in a peripheral or 'tip' area (Howie and Brewer, 1985; Huppes et al., 1988; Thomson and Ladefoged, 1991), the latter region representing the capillary loops adjacent to the origin of the proximal convoluted tubule (Fig. 5.15). GS may also develop between these two sites. Foam cells were shown by Magil and Cohen (1989) to stain with monocyte markers and are seen through all phases of the sclerosing process, but more commonly in the early phases when monocytes are also more numerous as indicated by histochemical staining. Epithelial cells may demonstrate resorptive cytoplasmic protein droplets in the region of the sclerotic lesion; the droplets stain with albumin, the immunoglobulins including IgA, IgG and IgM and different complement components as well as fibrinogen. The droplets may be extensive in the fully developed lesion but in keeping with the epithelial injury evident in the earliest phases of this form of glomerular reaction, the droplets may highlight a lesion that is difficult to detect by optical microscopy. Non-sclerotic mesangial areas of individual glomeruli with primary segmental sclerosis may show quite variable staining with IgM, most frequently, usually of light intensity and unevenly through mesangial areas sometimes combined with IgG and/or C1q and fibrinogen, the latter uncommonly (Habib et al., 1988); staining may also extend into capillary loops. Some authors (e.g. Schwartz and Lewis, 1985) have found no staining in the non-sclerotic mesangial areas.

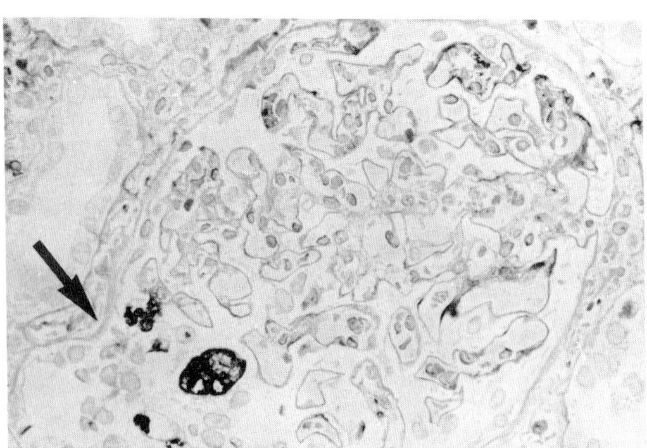

Fig. 5.15. IgM deposition at the glomerular 'tip' (near origin of proximal convoluted tubule, arrow) in an early segmental sclerotic lesion in a nephrotic patient who responded slowly to corticosteroid therapy (X400)

VI. Capillary wall changes

Glomerular capillary wall thickening may be produced in a variety of pathological processes, some of which may be apparent on light microscopy but others require IMH and electron microscopy (Seymour et al., 1983) to assist in differential diagnosis. The thickening may be produced in relatively few ways (see Table 5.19), namely, 1) protein deposits to which the membrane reacts (membranous transformation), 2) deposits which replace and expand the glomerular basement membrane (process of insudation); 3) by reduplication of glomerular basement membrane (GBM) which is related to extension of mesangial cell cytoplasm and, sometimes, nuclei around the luminal aspect and of the GBM with resulting formation of a new inner layer of GBM with or without 'subendothelial' protein deposits producing a 'tram track' or 'double contour', and, finally, 4) by synthesis of more GBM related to metabolic disease especially in diabetic nephropathy but including other conditions such as myxoedema (Naeye, 1963) or rare diseases such as lecithin: cholesterol acyltransferase deficiency (Imbasciati et al., 1986) with granular mesangial and capillary wall deposits, or possibly related to the process of sclerosis as discussed above (Section V – Glomerulosclerosis). These changes again represent a limited capacity on the part of the glomerulus to react to various forms of injury but they often demonstrate characteristic IMH patterns providing a differential diagnosis. Some patterns of capillary wall thickening, e.g. membranous transformation and mesangiocapillary-type GBM reduplication are seen in many different nephropathies often combined with other patterns of glomerular reaction. In others, IMH may identify the nature of the material producing the mural thickening more precisely.

Membranous (transformation) nephropathy

This term is applied to a staged process (Churg and Sobin, 1982) of capillary wall thickening following the formation of confluent subepithelial granular deposits, the development of GBM subepithelial projections ('spikes') and the incorporation of deposits to totally enclose them within the GBM producing an external subepithelial confluent membrane and, subsequently, in the final stages, dissolution of the deposits with residual irregularity and thickening of the GBM with some vacuolation. The prototype of this change is idiopathic membranous

Table 5.19. Pattern VI – Causes of capillary wall thickening

Process	Changes	IMH pattern
Membranous transformation	Deposit incorporation	Confluent granular
Mesangial interposition	'Subendothelial' deposit covered by new layer of GBM over luminal side	Confluent 'ribbon-like'
GBM insudative thickening	Replacement of GBM by very electron dense deposit	Confluent/interrupted 'ribbon-like'; mesangial nodules
Transmural thickening	Subendothelial, intramembranous and subepithelial deposits with ruptured and lamellated GBM.	Confluent/interrupted 'ribbon-like'; mesangial staining
Metabolic	Diabetic – increased GBM and matrix Hypothyroidism – accumulation of glycosaminoglycans Lecithin: cholesterol acyltransferase deficiency	Linear staining
Glomerulosclerosis – diverse causes	Increased GBM and matrix	–

nephropathy (IMN) in man and, in experimental animals, Heymann's nephritis, the latter greatly adding to understanding and knowledge of the underlying mechanisms of deposit formation and membrane reaction.

IMH patterns in MN are characteristic and instantly recognisable in most cases. The granular deposits show strong staining for IgG (Fig. 5.16A) and C3 characteristically but light-to-moderate IgA, IgM, C1q/C4 and fibrinogen are also frequently seen; the distribution is typically global and diffuse with an easily recognizable granularity on IMH often showing more deposits around capillary loops than are apparent on light microscopy. It is common to find IgM and, in a small number of cases, IgG mesangial deposition with IgM largely confined to the mesangium in general; a minority of idiopathic MN cases (Shearn et al., 1979) show mesangial staining and mesangial deposits on electronmicroscopy.

Some variation in staining patterns can be seen in a variety of circumstances in MN. The GBM may show extensive 'vacuolar' change relating the presence of preceding deposits (Tallqvist et al., 1979); biopsies from these patients show diffuse, usually finely granular IgG with diminution in the amount of staining when vacuolation is widespread. Similarly, staining may be less widespread than in the 'standard' MN case in some cases regarded as 'segmental membranous GN' which show IgG and C3 (Fig. 5.16B), sometimes combined with IgA and IgM; this form of MN may represent the healing phase of a previously more diffuse MN (Gaffney et al., 1982). Not infrequently only one antigen is the predominant deposit and may be either IgG or C3 and/or rarely IgA or IgM. Harrison et al. (1986) found that the presence of C3 deposition tended to be associated with the mesangial proliferation seen in some cases of IMN. It is suggested that the development of segmental sclerosis is of prognostic significance in MN in which prognostic pathological features are debated (summarized by Rosen et al., 1989; Wakai and Magil, 1992); IgM and/or C3 highlights these lesions on a background of MN staining; segmental sclerosis may represent a complication of protracted proteinuria related to the MN itself.

The association of MN with many diverse diseases and different clinical settings is a good illustration of the limited stereotypic pattern of glomerular reaction. Although many of these conditions have no clear immunological link to MN, a considerable number have been demonstrated to provide antigen and antigen-antibody complexes which appear to participate in the development of membranous transformation; the findings in relation to many of these conditions are summarized in Table 5.20. A large number of entities also associated with MN by pathomechanisms not clearly understood are presented by Alpers and Cotran (1986), Eigenbrodt and Ware (1989), Chugh and Sakhuja (1990), Wilson (1991), Zucchelli and Pasquali (1992) and Davison and Thomson (1992).

In all these categories IMH findings are essentially similar to those idiopathic MN usually demonstrating

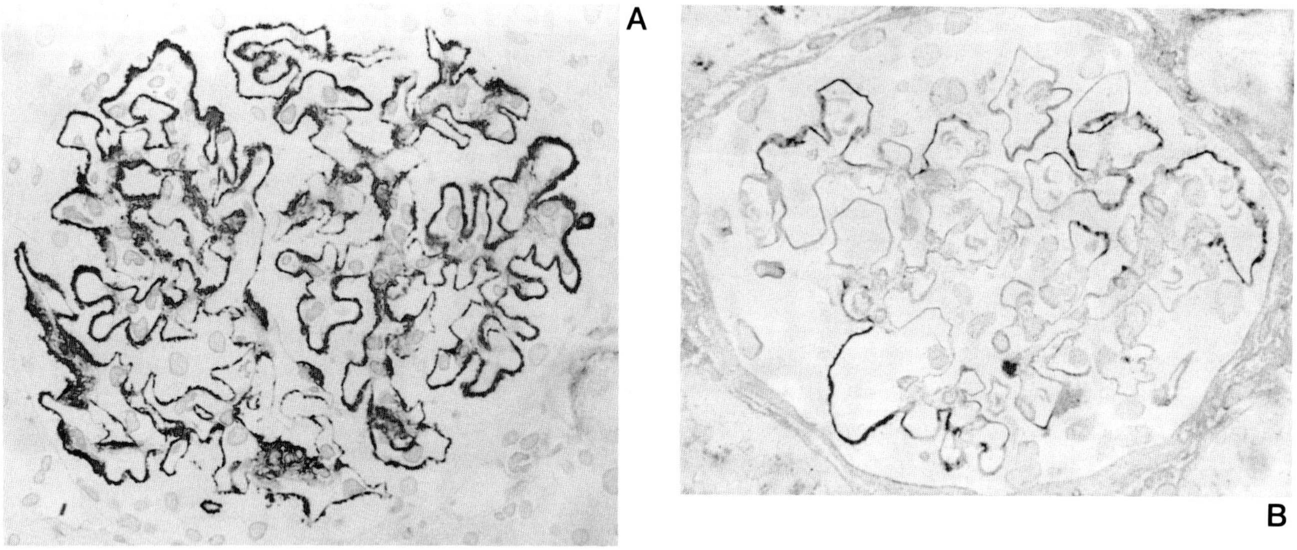

Fig. 5.16. (A) Uniform staining of capillary walls with granular IgG related to idiopathic membranous glomerulonephritis (X400). (B) Irregular fine IgG granular staining of capillary walls in a biopsy showing unevenly developed membranous glomerulonephritis (×400)

Table 5.20. Pattern VI – Capillary wall changes – Identified causes and features of membranous nephropathy

Cause	Deposit sites	Glomerular antigens	Other GNs described
1. Exogenous antigens			
Hepatitis B	Sep, Send, Mes	Surface, e antigens*	PEGN, MCGN
Syphilis	Sep, Send	Treponemal	PEGN
Leprosy	Sep, Mes	–	PEGN, DMP
Schistosomiasis	Sep, Mes	Elution of anti-Schistosomal antibody	MCGN
Filariasis	Sep	Filarial	PEGN
Hydatid	Sep	Echinococcal	–
Porcine insulin	Sep	Porcine insulin	–
2. Endogenous antigens			
Idiopathic	Sep (Mes)	(Renal tubular epithelial Ag)	
Systemic lupus erythematosus	Sep, Send, Mes	Anti-nuclear and other antibodies	Many other morphologies – often mixed
MCTD	Sep, Mes		
Rheumatoid arthritis	Sep, Mes	–	DMP, Drug-related GNs
Neoplasms			
Carcinomas, especially			
GIT, Lung	Sep	Carcinoembryonic Ag	PEGN
Melanoma	Sep	Melanoma-associated Ag(s)	
(Lymphoma)		? Immunoglobulin in products	PEGN, MCGN

Notes: Sep = Subepithelial; Send: Subendothelial; Mes: Mesangial; PEGN: Proliferative and exudative GN;
*(See Takekoshi et al., 1991); DMP: Diffuse Mesangial Proliferation; MCGN: Mesangiocapillary GN; ( ): Sometimes described

IgG and C3 granular staining around capillary loops; some minor variations may be seen even between diseases with the same aetiological background. A common problem is the differentiation between IMN and MN due to systemic lupus erythematosus. Jennette et al. (1983) contrasted idiopathic and SLE membranous nephropathy with the SLE biopsies showing IgG as the most intense immunoglobulin but C1q on occasions showed equal or greater staining intensity than IgG, segmental variation of protein deposition, some variable patterns including capillary wall IgG and IgM, heavy staining with IgG4 (without IgG1-3 deposition) no complement staining, mesangial deposits of IgA, C3, C4, C1q and/or IgM; the strong C1q staining remained the most significant differentiating feature between IMN and SLE MN. Some support for these differentiating features was provided by Schwartz et al. (1984). However other studies (e.g. that of the Southwest Pediatric Nephrology Study Group (1986)) show little if any difference between IMN and SLE MN. Often electronmicroscopic features such as endothelial tubuloreticular structures, fingerprint-like patterned deposits, more irregular outline of subepithelial deposits and microvesicular bodies are found in SLE MN as opposed to the idiopathic type but mesangial deposits, as noted above, although more common in SLE MN are also seen in the idiopathic variety (Shearn et al., 1979).

Pathogenesis of MN: The pathomechanisms relating to the development of the very characteristic IMH findings in membranous transformation may be of three types (reviewed by Zucchelli and Pasquali, 1992), viz. 1) Deposition of circulating immune complex composed of non-glomerular exogenous protein and endogenous low-affinity antibody. 2) Deposition of circulating antibody to extrinsic antigen planted in the subepithelial space due to biochemical or electrostatic affinity. 3) Deposition of circulating autoantibody reacting with an intrinsic, native glomerular antigen (the human equivalent of passive Heymann nephritis).

Mesangial interposition and insudative thickening of capillary walls (mesangiocapillary glomerulonephritides, types 1, 2 and 3)

Examples of glomerulonephritis classified as mesangiocapillary in type possess very characteristic morphological changes related especially to the peripheral capillary wall that differentiate between different forms of nephritis, namely types I (subendothelial), II (dense deposit disease, DDD) (Levy et al., 1979; Kincaid-Smith, 1987) and III (transmural) (Anders et al., 1977; Strife et al., 1977). The differentiation between these individual types of mesangiocapillary GN and other forms of GN is possible with the application of IMH and electronmicroscopy in most cases. It appears that no special pattern of immunoglobulin/complement deposition as outlined below has prognostic significance other than that reflecting the extent of renal involvement by the glomerulonephritic process. Extensive crescent formation is perhaps the most important glomerular change related to a poorer outlook (Miller et al., 1984; Schmitt et al., 1990). Morphological and IMH features of the different forms of MCGN are outlined in Table 5.21.

Table 5.21. Pattern VI – Capillary wall changes: Contrasting features of types I, II and III mesangiocapillary GNS

Type	Predominant deposits	Deposit electron density	GBM changes	IMH capillary wall	IMH Mesangial
1	Subendothelial	Moderate	Widespread Double contour	IgG, IgM, (IgA) C3, Clq	IgG, Igm (IgA) C3, Clq
2	Intramembranous	Heavy	Thickened with single or double contour	C3	C3 Nodular
3	Subendothelial Intramembranous Subepithelial	Moderate	Laminated, focal ruptures, some double contours	C3 (IgG, IgM)	C3 (IgG, IgM)

Notes: ( ) Weaker or less frequent staining

Complement in mesangiocapillary glomerulonephritis

A feature that groups these morphological patterns is the frequent finding of hypocomplementaemia (Peters and Williams, 1974; Herbert et al., 1991) present in approximately 80 per cent of all cases (West, 1992). This is due, at least in part, to different complement activating factors (Varade et al., 1990; Tanuma et al., 1990) which correlate with morphological sub-types. These protein activating factors are IgG autoantibodies, the C3 nephritic factors (C3 nefs). In type II MCGN (dense deposit disease), the C3 nephritic factor activating the amplification of complement (known as NFII or NFa, West, 1992) is frequently found and results in reduced serum C3 with normal serum C5. Another form of C3 nephritic factor, slowly activating C3 and the terminal pathway of complement (known as NFt, West, 1992) is consistently associated with the common finding of C5 and C7-9 serum reduction in type III MCGN. The hypocomplementaemia of type I MCGN appears to be a combination of immune complex C-activation and feedback loop amplification, possibly via C4 nef (Tanuma et al., 1989) and terminal pathway C3 nefs with characteristic classical pathway activation combined with low serum levels of C6, C7 and/or C9 (Zwirner et al., 1989; Varade et al., 1990). These authors also found C8 depressed in all hypocomplementaemic states and Clardy et al. (1989) showed that C5 activation and reduction in serum in type III MCGN was as profound as that in acute proliferative GN and type I MCGN but serological differentiation was suggested by greater activation of C7–C9 in type III MCGN compared with the two other forms of GN. These findings (summarized by West, 1992) accord with those of Tanuma et al. (1990) who have described two forms of C3 nephritic factor,

Table 5.22. Acquired hypocomplementaemia and glomerulonephritis

GN	Frequency of hypocomplementaemia	C components reduced	Mechanism of reduction			Correlation with activity
			Classical pathway	Alternate pathway	Complement synthesis	
MCGN I	Approx 50% of cases	C3, Clq, C5a, Cq Properdin	Immune complex activation Nf_t, C4Nf			Poor
MCGN II	Approx 80% of cases	C3, Factor B, Properdin (C5 – Normal)		NfII	Possibly decreased	Poor
MCGN III	Approx 50% of cases	C3, C5, C7–9		Nf_t		Poor
Systemic lupus erythematosus	Majority with proliferative GN	C4, Clq, C3	Immune complex Activation		Decreased	Usually rapid return to normal with adequate therapy
Proliferative and exudative (Post-infectious) GN	Almost all cases	C4 (early phases) C3 (all phases)	Immune complex activation	Also activated	Decreased	Usually rapid return to normal
Cryoglobulinaemia (mixed essential)	Majority cases	C4, Clq (C3 less reduced)	Immune complex activation			Poor
Thrombotic microangiopathies	Approx 50%	C3 (C4)	Toxins/microbes activate	Damaged endothelium		Reduced during activity
Cholesterol embolism	All active cases	C3 (C4)		Activated by emboli		Reduced during embolization
Sepsis with shock	Almost all cases	C3, C4		Proteolytic inactivation by plasma Cl inhibitor		Reduced by infection

Note: ( ) = less frequently lowered

viz. one properdin-dependent and the other, properdin-independent in MCGN, types I and II and in partial lipodystrophy, a disease associated with both these types of MCGN. Although the correlation between the finding of hypocomplementaemia and glomerular inflammation and a deterioration in glomerular morphology was considered poor in varying types of MCGN treated with alternate day corticosteroids (McEnery et al., 1986; Bennett et al., 1989) loss of haematuria was associated with morphological improvement. Ohi and co-workers (Ohi and Tanuma, 1992; Ohi et al., 1992a) suggest that better correlation between the finding of various forms of nephritic factors including C4 nephritic factor in both hypocomplementaemic and non-hypocomplementaemic sera from MCGN (I and II) patients and disease activity is possible, especially if C3 and C5 (the latter measurement relating to MAC concentration) serum measurements are undertaken.

The relationship between acquired hypocomplementaemia and various glomerulonephritides is given in Table 5.22.

Type 1, Subendothelial mesangiocapillary (membranoproliferative) glomerulonephritis (MCGNI), idiopathic and secondary

Usually diffuse, sometimes focal the main morphological glomerular feature in this entity is formation of a 'double contour' or 'tram-track' due to replication of the capillary basement membrane by the process of mesangial interposition associated with subendothelial protein deposits which are formed prior to the mesangial response (Jones, 1977; Zamarovic and Churg, 1984). The deposits are characteristically found in the capillary loops and often in mesangial areas. Confluently or sometimes with an interrupted pattern they outline the subendothelial aspect of the GBM and are enclosed by a new layer of replicated membrane over the luminal aspect of the deposit. Although usually coarse, deposits may be fine imparting a pseudolinear pattern to the IMH. The usual findings on IMH indicate the presence of moderate to strong staining with immunoglobulins IgG and/or IgM, occasionally IgA the latter seen especially in the secondary forms (see below), and usually moderate to heavy deposition of complement and early complement components, especially C1q and C4 (Fig. 5.17); some examples of type I MCGN may show C3 deposition as the predominant finding (Yoshikawa et al., 1988). Exacerbations of activity of type I MCGN of idiopathic type may be accompanied by predominantly C3 capillary wall and mesangial staining (personal observation). The pattern with heavy immunoglobulin and complement deposition characterizing the IMH of the idiopathic form of type I MCGN is seen in a large number of secondary forms; the characteristic IMH findings are summarized in Table 5.23

Some more detailed comments relating to the IMH of several entities producing type I MCGN changes as listed in Table 5.23, namely cryoglobulinaemia, lupus MCGN, chronic liver disease-related MCGN and chronic transplant glomerulopathy are presented below.

Cryoglobulinaemia: The mixed forms of cryglobulinaemia in which a monoclonal (type II) and a polyclonal (type III) anti-immunoglobulin, acting as a rheumatoid factor, usually IgM, reacts with a serum antibody, usually IgG to form immune complexes which precipitate on cooling; the pure monoclonal cryoglobulins (type I) are not usually associated with GN (Cordonnier et al., 1987). The morphology of the mixed monoclonal (type II) cryoglobulin nephritis is usually that of the subendothelial form of mesangiocapillary GN, so-called 'cryoglobulinaemic glomerulonephritis' in which endocapillary monocyte-macrophages are often prominent (Cordonnier et al., 1987). Other patterns of GN are more commonly seen with the polyclonal form of mixed

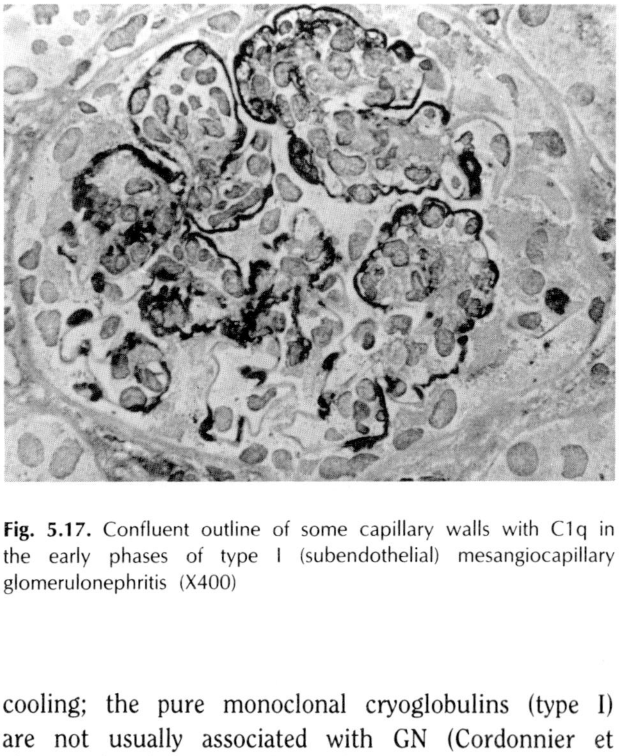

Fig. 5.17. Confluent outline of some capillary walls with C1q in the early phases of type I (subendothelial) mesangiocapillary glomerulonephritis (X400)

Table 5.23. Pattern VI – Capillary wall changes: IMH findings in type 1 mesangiocapillary GNS

Cause	Capillary wall staining	Comment
Idiopathic	IgG C3 Clq (IgA, IgM)	Clq often strong; usually weak in PEGN
Lupus erythematosus	IgG IgA IgM C3 Clq	Heavy mesangial and capillary staining
Congenital complement deficiencies	IgG IgM IgA C3 Clq	Only traces or no deposit of missing components
Cryoglobulinaemia (mixed essential)	IgM IgG C3 Clq	Vascular deposits may stain
Shunt nephritis, bacterial endocarditis	C3 (IgG IgM)	C3 often predominates
IgAN Henoch-Schönlein purpura	IgA IgM C3 Fib	Patterns are essentially similar
Chronic infections – schistosomiasis, Quartan malaria, Q fever	IgM C3	Quartan-malaria – pattern may resemble type III MCGN
Sickle cell nephropathy	IgG IgM C3 Clq	Other GNs also described
Heroin nephropathy	IgM IgG C3	Focal glomerulosclerosis and amyloidosis more characteristically seen
Light chain nephropathy	Kappa or Lambda Light chain	Occasionally combined with heavy chain deposition
Neoplasms–leukaemia, lymphoma	IgG IgM C3	Paraprotein may be deposited
Chronic transplant glomerulopathy	IgM IgG C3	Deposits usually inconspicuous on microscopy

Note: ( ) =Weaker or less frequent staining

cryoglobulinaemia (type III) (Cordonnier et al., 1987). 'Cryoglobulinaemic GN' shows extensive bright IgG and/or IgM, and C3 and C1q/C4 staining of capillary loops and the mesangium. Capillary luminal precipitates in approximately 50 per cent of cases (D'Amico et al., 1989), and arteriolar and small arterial deposits are outlined especially by the immunoglobulins. Confirmation that the deposits in the glomeruli are indeed the precipitated cryoglobulins is provided by the use of monoclonal antibodies directed against rheumatoid factors and by electromicroscopy showing tubular/crystalline deposits (D'Amico et al., 1989). This form of cryoglobulinaemic GN has also produced a pattern of nodular mesangial expansion with variable endocapillary proliferation (D'Amico et al., 1989).

Lupus mesangiocapillary GN: The development of severe proliferative lupus nephritis with extensive membrane reduplication is usually accompanied by marked proliferative and exudative changes with extensive glomerular deposits including subendothelial wire loops (Hill, 1992). Superimposed segmental necrosis and crescents are common. Unusual examples with extensive reduplication may feature heavy mesangial and subendothelial protein deposits with only slight proliferation and exudation; these features still indicate of a poorer outlook (Schwartz et al., 1984). If this mesangiocapillary pattern of 'diffuse proliferative type' is combined with diffuse membranous transformation (Schwartz et al., 1989) prognosis appears particularly poor. These more severe forms of LEGN usually show confluent and granular capillary loop and mesangial IgG, IgM and IgA with decreasing order of strength of staining, with C1q the heaviest complement component, often accompanied by moderate to heavy C3 and C4 (Hill,

1992). Hyaline thrombi and 'lupus vasculitis' are most commonly found in the severe proliferative forms of LEGN.

Chronic liver disease-related mesangiocapillary GN: The development of a pattern of type I MCGN in chronic liver disease is an uncommon but well recognized complication, seen especially in those with established cirrhosis and/or chronic hepatitis virus infection (Newell, 1987). The lesion is associated with circulating immune complexes and, in contrast to idiopathic IgA nephropathy with IgA1 glomerular deposition (Sakai, 1991), IgA2 staining of the mesangium characteristically extending along glomerular capillary walls in association with reduplication may be seen in the liver-related examples (Newell, 1987). Some examples of MCGN in liver disease may show IgG and/or IgM as the predominant immunoglobulin-deposited; varying mesangial and capillary wall staining with C3, C1q and/or C4 is found in most examples (Newell, 1987). The resolution of renal morphology and clinical manifestations in a patient with type I MCGN showing abundant IgA, IgM, IgG and complement in the mesangium and capillary loops after liver transplantation for cirrhosis, reported by Ghabra et al., (1991) is strong support for the role of the liver in the development of this lesion.

Chronic transplant glomerulopathy: A sometimes difficult differentiation lies between recurrent or de novo mesangiocapillary glomerulonephritis in transplants and chronic transplant glomerulopathy which is probably due to chronic, particularly vascular, rejection; it is generally held (Cameron and Turner, 1977; Mathew, 1988) that deposits are absent in the biopsies of transplants on light microscopy and electronmicroscopy although this may not always be so (Zhang et al., 1988). Most cases of recurrent or de novo mesangiocapillary glomerulonephritis in transplants have a characteristic pattern of immunoglobulin and complement deposition and deposits are readily seen subendothelially. However immunohistochemistry shows moderate to heavy IgM, lighter IgG, C3 and C1q/C4 outlining glomerular capillary walls and mesangium in the well-developed chronic rejection-related variety of mesangiocapillary reduplication transplant glomerulopathy, and if heavy, they may correspond to subendothelial deposits usually seen by electronmicroscopy (Olsen, 1992) and, on occasions, by light microscopy.

Thrombotic microangiopathies (TMA): Another group of conditions with variable but often extensive reduplication of glomerular basement membranes showing endothelial injury indicated by ultrastructural swelling of endothelial cytoplasm with or without vascular alterations are the TMAs (Habib and Levy, 1983; Zamarovic and Churg, 1984) (see Vascular Immunohistochemistry; and Table 5.26 for causes of TMA). In the entities grouped as TMA, IgM, sometimes IgG and IgA, C3 and C1q and fibrinogen or fibrin-related antigens outline capillary walls and sometimes the mesangium on immunohistochemistry (Fig. 5.18). It is likely that the deposits demonstrated on immunohistochemistry are secondary to the endothelial injury and, in general, deposits are not as heavy as those seen by optical microscopy or IMH as those of MCGN type I. Rarely thrombotic microangiopathy may complicate different forms of GN (de Chadarévian et al., 1980; Stave and Croker 1984; Loirat et al., 1984).

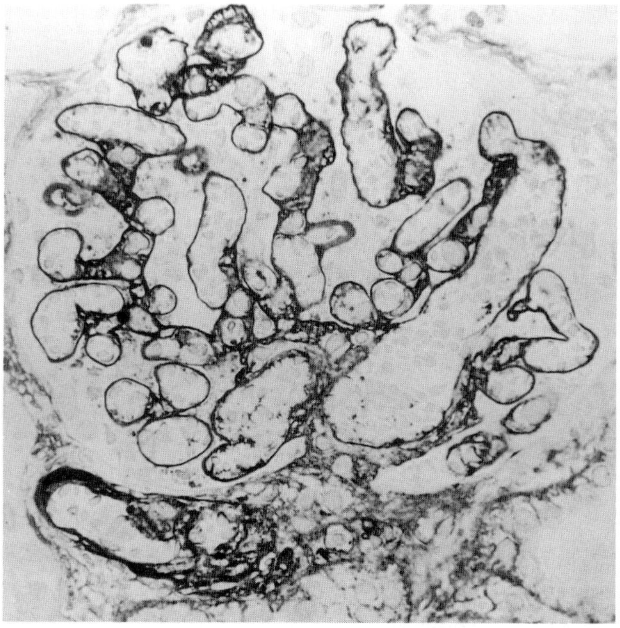

Fig. 5.18. Global outline of capillary walls and a glomerular arteriole with IgM in thrombotic microangiopathy (X400)

Type II (dense deposit) mesangiocapillary GN

Dense deposit disease (DDD) is defined by an accumulation of very electron-dense material in renal basement membranes, especially the GBM, and the mesangium but often extending to Bowman's basement and tubular basement membranes (Kashtan et al., 1990); the deposition is accompanied by very variable endocapillary and/or extracapillary cellular proliferation and leucocytic accumulation with these later changes often associated with intercurrent infections (Bennett et al., 1989). The material related to the basement membranes is moderately to intensely periodic acid-schiff-positive after digestion with diastase and stains with thioflavine-T (Churg et al., 1979) and is markedly osmiophilic. The dense deposits selectively stained with the lectin, wheat germ agglutinin, or its succinylated derivative (Nevins, 1985; Onetti Muda et al., 1988) indicating the presence of internally linked N-acetylglucosamine; the deposits of type I MCGN are negative when stained with wheat germ agglutinin (Nevins, 1985). The osmiophilic component of the DD is extractable with lipid solvents and may consist in part of unsaturated fatty acids (Onetti Muda et al., 1988). Ultrastructural argyrophilia of the DD may be helpful in differentiating the material from other types of dense deposits (Anders et al., 1977; Strife et al., 1977; Dowling and Mathews, 1987). The findings and the differential diagnostic features of insudative capillary wall thickening are given in Table 5.24.

Table 5.24. Pattern VI – Capillary wall changes differential causes of GBM Insudative thickening

Entity	Deposit ultrastructure	IMH
Dense deposit disease	Non-granular	C3
Light chain nephropathy	Granular Occasionally fibrillary Occasionally non-granular	Kappa or lambda LC
Fibrillary/immuno-tactoid nephropathy	Fibrillary or tubular	IgG, IgM kappa and lambda LC
DDD Simulants		
1. Granular dense deposits	Granular	C3, IgM
2. Heparin-injection – related deposits	Amorphous	C3, IgM IgM IgG C3

Note: LC = light chain

The predominant finding in DDD on IMH is moderate to heavy C3 deposition outlining material according to the distribution of the dense deposit in the kidney (Habib et al., 1973; Fig. 5.19). Rarely, C3 deposition may precede the accumulation of the dense deposit seen on light microscopy (Sato et al., 1987). Within the glomerulus in addition to the undulating ribbon-like pattern characteristic features of C3 deposition may be seen, namely, a 'tram-track' double layered appearance of the intramembranous material and mesangial 'rings' in which C3 staining outlines dense deposits with a nodular morphology these being embedded within the mesangial matrix (Kim et al., 1979; Sibley and Kim, 1984). Such peripheral staining of heavy intramatrical deposits has been rarely noted by the author with C3 staining in other lesions e.g. type I mesangiocapillary disease and IgA nephropathy. Occasional examples of dense deposit disease evolve from proliferative GN without distinguishing features (Taguchi and Bohle, 1989) or rarely following a post-infectious lesion with typical morphology and granular immunoglobulin and complement on IMH (Habib et al., 1975) or in association with other infections (Eddy et al., 1984). Immunoglobulin deposition in the typical DDD is a very minor component on IMH. Small deposits of IgM in the mesangium and around glomerular capillary loops are common and occasionally IgG and IgA may also be seen (Kim et al., 1979; Southwest Pediatric Nephrology Study Group, 1985; Salinas-Madrigal and Torlani, 1988). The peripheral pattern of C3 staining in relation to the deposits suggests that this component does not form the bulk of the material accumulated (Cameron et al., 1983; Nevins, 1985; Onetti Muda et al., 1988). The form of C3 deposits may be granular, globular or 'linear' with the latter usually confluent and sometimes interrupted (Habib et al., 1975; Lamb et al., 1977). The DD material is rarely found in other organs e.g. spleen (Ormos et al., 1979).

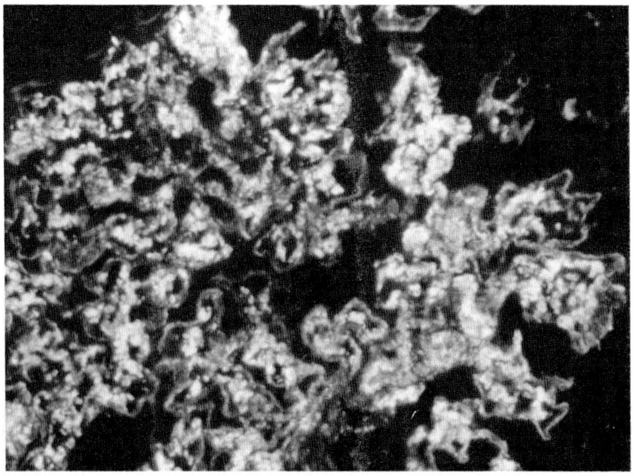

Fig. 5.19. Moderate confluent capillary wall and nodular 'mesangial ring' staining in type II mesangiocapillary glomerulonephritis (dense deposit disease) (X400, direct immunofluorescence)

In the differential diagnosis of insudative GBM thickening, similar patterns may be seen with other substances of either unknown origin (King et al., 1978; Mampaso et al., 1983) but staining irregularly with C3 and IgM or deposited light chains (Sinniah and Cohen, 1985; Minetti, 1992) may produce similar light microscopic patterns and the marked electron density of dense deposit disease. The very electron dense light chains are either finely or coarsely granular under EM (Sinniah and Cohen, 1985) and can be differentiated too by IMH for light chains. The deposits described by Mampaso et al. (1983) and King et al. (1978) showed little affinity for C3 and appear to have been neither DD or a light chain. Yamase et al. (1988) reported irregular intramembranous and intramatrical deposits with negative immunofluorescence in a patient receiving heparin injections adding to the patterns that may mimic dense deposit disease. DDD with C3 staining may be widespread even in those patients with a more benign course (Klein, 1983) and occasionally may resolve, at least in part, when the DD are found more in the lamina rara interna than the GBM lamina densa (McEnery and McAdams, 1988). The almost inevitable recurrence of DDD in renal transplants (Mathew, 1988) was initially felt to have only a mild effect on renal transplant function but more recently it has been realised that the graft may be hastened in its demise (Eddy et al., 1984; Mathew 1988). IMH features in this setting are similar to those in non-transplant kidneys but some may show additional deposition in the mesangium and capillary loops related to transplant glomerulopathy particularly IgM and C1q staining of the mesangium and capillary walls.

Type III (transmural) mesangiocapillary glomerulonephritis

Sufficient morphological immunohistochemical and complement-related serological differences have been documented to suggest that there is a distinct form of mesangiocapillary GN to be differentiated from type I subendothelial and DDD (type II) mesangiocapillary GN (Anders et al., 1977; Strife et al.; 1977, Strife et al., 1984). These groups of workers described variable endocapillary proliferation with the distinguishing features of transmural capillary wall deposits related to focally laminated and ruptured basal laminae and localized membranous transformation; the cases described by Burkholder et al. (1970) showed more extensive and regular MT and extensive proliferation. Morphological distinction between types II and III mesangiocapillary GNs rests not only in the marked electron density of type II deposits but also in the differences concerning the siting of the deposition and the GBM reaction to the material. However it is widely believed that Anders-Strife type III MCGN is related morphologically and, perhaps, immunologically and genetically to the subendothelial variety (Jackson et al., 1987). Most examples of type III MCGN morphology are idiopathic but this pattern appears to be associated with quartan malarial infection (Chugh and Sakhuja, 1990).

In addition to serological differences (see above) and the probable inhibition of immune complex solubilization, which is considered important in the development of both types I and III MCGN (Welch et al., 1988), IMH in type III is marked by the constant finding of moderate to strong C3 capillary loop and usually mesangial deposition (Fig. 5.20) with variable but frequent deposition of IgM, IgG and IgA and properdin (Strife et al., 1977 and Strife et al., 1984); immunoglobulins are more readily found compared with type II MCGN but are often not as confluent and as extensive as in the subendothelial (type I) variety of MCGN. Considerable difficulty may be found in differentiating type III MCGN with numerous subepithelial deposits and membranous transformation in some loops and membranous nepropathy with coarse deposits, and complex capillary wall morphology (Mrozowicz-Picken

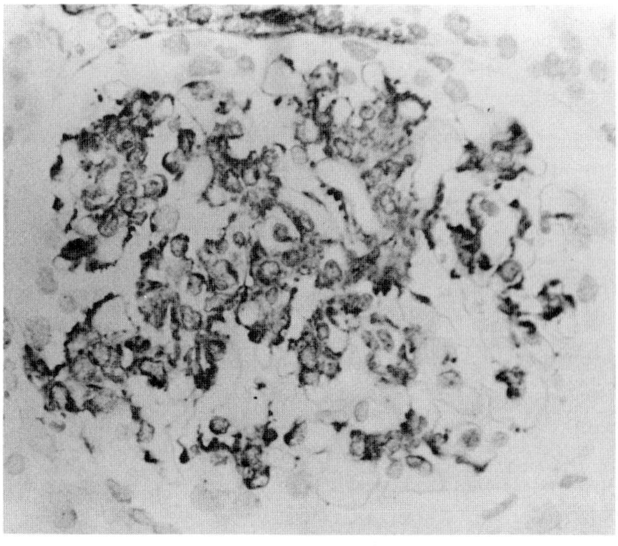

Fig. 5.20. C3 deposition in the mesangium and some glomerular capillary walls in type III (transmural) mesangiocapillary glomerulonephritis (X400)

and Wrzolkowa, 1980); ultrastructural evidence of lamellation and rupture of GBM may provide evidence for type III MCGN, but IMH may appear essentially similar in both conditions. It is probable that type III MCGN has a more indolent course compared with type I MCGN (Strife et al., 1984).

Interstitial diseases

As suggested by Neilson (1989) three patterns of histological injury in tubulointerstitial nephritis (TIN) may be noted, namely (1) with a mixed polymorphonuclear (eosinophil and neutrophilic) and mononuclear leucocyte component unassociated with positive immunohistochemistry; (2) tubulointerstitial inflammation of mononuclear leucocytes with immune complexes related to tubular basement membranes; and (3) mononuclear leucocyte infiltration with linear tubular basement membrane, IgG and complement deposition – so called 'anti-tubular basement membrane disease'. Extensive experimental studies, reviewed by Wilson (1991a) indicate that there is a variety of nephritogenic antigens capable of exciting both humoral and cell-mediated immune responses resulting in tubulointerstitial injury; these studies also demonstrate that mechanisms such as molecular mimicry, cross-reactive antigens, trapped or planted antigens may also be factors in the development of interstitial inflammatory disease. Lehman et al. (1975) were among the first to appreciate that a variety of extra-glomerular tubulointerstitial deposits were found in a different interstitial diseases including the interstitial component of various forms of glomerulonephritis and in renal transplants. For the immunological forms of TIN, the IMH patterns and related diseases have been summarized by Mujais and Quintanilla (1988). A summary of IMH staining in interstitial diseases is given in Table 5.25.

Immune complex deposition

Granular staining with IgG and/or IgM and C3 is a common finding in a wide range of conditions with interstitial inflammation and tubular injury. Many primary and secondary forms of GN show patchy IMH staining particularly when interstitial changes are extensive. In some GN conditions the interstitial IMH is characteristic and parallels that of the glomeruli; SLE with deposits of IgG, IgA, IgM, C3 and C1q/C4; some examples of mixed essential cryoglobulinaemia show IgG, IgM and complement components; some examples of Sjögren's syndrome with circulating anti-TBM antibody staining may demonstrate granular IgM deposition which may also be seen in shunt nephritis and in other glomerulonephritides. The contribution of these deposits in TI injury is debated but on current evidence it appears unlikely that they either initiate or sustain the damage (see below).

Table 5.25. IMH patterns in interstitial diseases

1. GRANULAR Ig and C STAINING OF TBM
   - Many forms of primary and secondary (systemic) GN – C3 + Clq, IgM
     - LE GN – IgG, M, A, C3, Clq
     - Cryoglobulinaemia – IgG, IgM, C3, Clq
     - Sjögren's syndrome – IgM, IgG, C3
     - Shunt nephritis – IgM, C3
   - Interstitial rejection, especially chronic – C3, IgM
   - Chronic interstitial nephritis (various causes) – C3, IgM, IgG
   - 'Non-immunological interstitial disease', e.g.
     - Endemic Balkan Nephropathy – C3, IgM
2. LINEAR TBM STAINING
   - Antiglomerular basement membrane disease
   - Primary idiopathic, interstitial nephritis
     - Chronic idiopathic interstitial nephritis
   - Membranous nephropathy
   - Methicillin acute interstitial nephritis (rare)
   - Phenyloin-induced interstitial nephritis
   - Systemic lupus erythematosus

   - Post-streptococcal GN
   - Renal oxalosis after jejuno-ileal by-pass
3. DIFFERENTIAL DIAGNOSES
   - Light chain nephropathy
   - Dense deposit disease

Linear tubular basement membrane deposition

Although approximately 70 per cent of patients with glomerulonephritis due to anti-GBM disease show TBM linear IgG deposition this appears to correlate poorly with the development of tubulointerstitial injury in this disease (Andres et al., 1978). Similar staining has been noted with methicillin-induced acute interstitial nephritis (Mujais and Quintanilla, 1988) although the vast majority of cases due to this drug and other antibiotics and drugs are negative on IMH. A primary idiopathic form of autoimmune-type interstitial nephritis has been described (Neilson, 1989). Recently the target antigen involved in examples of tubulointerstitial nephritis in two patients was identified by Fliger et al. (1987) as a M58,000 component antigen unique to the tubular basement membrane. A form of chronic tubulointerstitial nephritis, associated with a wide range of non-glomerulonephritic disorders, showed linear C3 and IgG or IgM TBM staining in a small minority of cases (Eknoyan et al., 1990). Similar linear staining with IgG has also been noted in renal allografts (see below), membranous nephropathy, lupus erythematosus, post-streptococcal glomerulonephritis, in renal oxalosis after jejuno-ileal bypass and also with phenytoin (reviewed by Mujais and Quintanilla, 1988). The differential diagnosis of linear TBM staining extends to light chain nephropathy in which TIN changes are even more characteristic than the glomerular lesions (Cohen, 1984; see Glomerular Changes, section III, B3); kappa or lambda light chain deposition may be solely manifest as a TIN and produce severe renal injury with marked tubular atrophy, interstitial fibrosis and impaired renal function; as with the glomerular lesions, gammopathy is not found in a significant minority. Lockwood (1991) suggests that other aspects of autoimmunity may play a role in IN; 4 patients under his care developed interstitial nephritis, verified by biopsy, and ANCA.

Cell-mediated immune injury

This appears to be responsible for much interstitial injury whether associated with glomerulonephritis or various forms of TIN due to toxin-/drug-related or infective interstitial injury. Microbial antigens causing tubular injury and/or interstitial nephritis with a lymphocytic infiltrate may be identified in the kidney by the use of IMH; e.g. Kang et al., (1990) have demonstrated the envelope glycoprotein of the Hanta virus, the cause of the haemorrhagic fever renal syndrome in many countries, in tubular epithelial cells in 50 per cent of their patients in Korea; and the accumulation of leptospiral antigen in renal interstitium and epithelium, demonstrated by IMPO using a polyclonal antibody (Alves et al., 1987) suggests that at least in part the manifestations of this disease are due to endothelial damage. It has been suggested that even a rare condition such as medullary cystic disease may be of autoimmune cell-mediated origin (Kelly and Neilson, 1987). Several recent studies of a range of interstitial inflammatory lesions (Boucher et al., 1986; Alexopoulos et al., 1989; Sabadini et al., 1988; summarized by Cameron, 1988) reveal that T lymphocytes form the majority of the infiltrate combined with varying numbers of monocyte-macrophages and B lymphocytes in a wide variety of interstitial diseases both 'primary' and of secondary type. In some glomerulonephritides the cell type appears to correlate with subsequent renal impairment; e.g. in IgA nephropathy the presence of increased T cells, mainly CD8+, suggested the subsequent development of impairment (Sabadini et al., 1988); Alexopoulos et al. (1989) showed that progressive impairment in membranous nephropathy was associated with the increased numbers of interstitial T cells and monocyte-macrophages in the first biopsy. Perhaps IMH may assist in the differentiation between granulomatous drug-related TIN and sarcoidal granulomas; it has been suggested (Kenouch and Mery, 1992) that the latter stain with angiotensin converting enzyme antibodies to distinguish sarcoidosis from other forms of epithelioid granuloma.

Evidence suggests that TI damage is an important predictor of prognosis (Bohle et al., 1990), and that non-humoral immune events are involved in many forms of renal interstitial injury. There is accumulating evidence (summarized by D'Amico, 1991) that persistent proteinuria may be directly responsible for some of this injury, and indirectly induce damage via cell-mediated immune events. A direct relationship between the development of cell-mediated (? and other) immune injury to the TI tissues and fibrosis is suggested by the studies of Müller et al. (1991); these workers have demonstrated, by IMH and cell culture of renal biopsies, that the numbers of T lymphocytes, the main cell type found in the interstitium correlate directly with deteriorating renal function; they also noted that in GN abnormal expression of HLA-DQ/-DP molecules, often concomitant with aberrant expression of the intercellular adhesion molecule (ICAM-I), was present on proximal tubular epithelium which probably thus has an antigen presenting function; their cultures revealed increased fibroblast proliferation, collagen III and V synthesis and response to cytokine in tissue from biopsies with renal interstitial fibrosis (Müller et al., 1991).

Vascular immunohistochemistry

Vascular IMH is very commonly positive due to the development of nephrosclerosis often seen as a background to many renal diseases; C3 often accompanied by IgM is a very frequent finding that highlights small arterial and arteriolar sclerosis/hyalinosis in this setting. The appearances are essentially non-specific but the thrombotic microangiopathies and some relatively uncommon vasculopathies provide characteristic IMH patterns.

Thrombotic microangiopathy (TMA)

The renal changes noted in this group of conditions effect small arteries and arterioles in most cases and frequently show extensive glomerular changes including crescent formation. Glomerular involvement is seen commonly as a form of 'endotheliosis'. Some examples of TMA may show pathology confined to the glomeruli (Churg et al., 1989) (see Glomerular Changes, Section VI, Changes in Capillary Walls) and Bohle et al. (1985) suggest that the syndrome may develop even without vascular or glomerular changes. A wide range of aetiological factors (Kaplan et al., 1990) is responsible for the TMAs and the common mechanism for all of them appears to be related to endothelial injury perhaps due to activated neutrophils degrading fibronectin (Forsyth et al., 1989) and involvement of the coagulation/fibrinolysis system (Kincaid-Smith, 1975; Lian, 1987; Kaplan et al., 1990). There is little support currently for the suggestion that immune complexes play a role in the vascular injury although a complement-dependent cytotoxic antibody reacting with endothelial cells has been described in some patients with thrombocytopenic purpura (Wall and Harker, 1980) and in children with the haemolytic uraemic syndrome (Leung et al., 1988). The prognosis in lesions with 'primary' TMA is worse if the vascular proliferative changes and extent of involvement are more marked (Morel-Maroger et al., 1979). The conditions associated with TMA are listed in Table 5.26.

As noted with respect to the glomerular capillary wall changes in TMA, the vascular (arteriolar and small arterial) staining is remarkably similar regardless of the precipitating factor(s) or the disease producing the condition. These associations may be grouped under the following headings – drugs and toxins, post-partum renal failure syndrome, transplantation of bone marrow or solid organs, viral, bacterial or other microbial infections, hereditary-familial settings, malignancy, malignant hypertension, connective tissue diseases including scleroderma (Donohoe, 1992), anti-cardiolipin antibody syndrome with or without lupus erythematosus (Kincaid-Smith et al., 1988; D'Agati et al., 1990; Mackworth-Young, 1990) and mixed connective tissue disease showing scleroderma-like vascular changes (summarized by Churg et al., 1989). Even rare vasculopathies such as Kohlmeier-Degos' disease may produce a similar vascular reaction in the kidney (Bjorck et al., 1984).

Table 5.26. Causes of thrombotic microangiopathy

Classic haemolytic-uraemic syndrome
Post infectious
Shigella dysenteriae 1
Streptococcus pneumoniae
Salmonella typhi
E. Coli, verotoxin-producing forms
Viruses
Hereditary and recurrent forms
Abnormalities of complement
Mostly persistently low serum C3
Accompanying other, often systemic, diseases
Systemic sclerosis, mixed connective tissue disease
Lupus anticoagulant with or without systemic lupus erythematosus
Malignant hypertension
Superimposed on glomerulonephritis of various types
Rejection-related in transplants
Post-partum renal failure
Irradiation
Drugs
Antimetabolites – mitomycin, cisplatin, daunorubicin, cytospine, arabinoside, etc.
Cyclosporine A, penicillamine, oral contraceptives, metronidazole
Toxins
Carbon monoxide, bee sting, arsenic, sulfonamide, iodine

IMH vascular findings in TMA are very stereotypic in that staining usually shows luminal and mural moderate-to-bright deposition of fibrinogen, IgM, C3 and C1q/C4 (Fig. 5.21); occasionally IgA and/or IgG are noted but in general do not appear to have any aetiological connotations.

Glomerular IMH patterns of mesangial and capillary wall staining with the same antibodies to those found in the vessels are frequently seen.

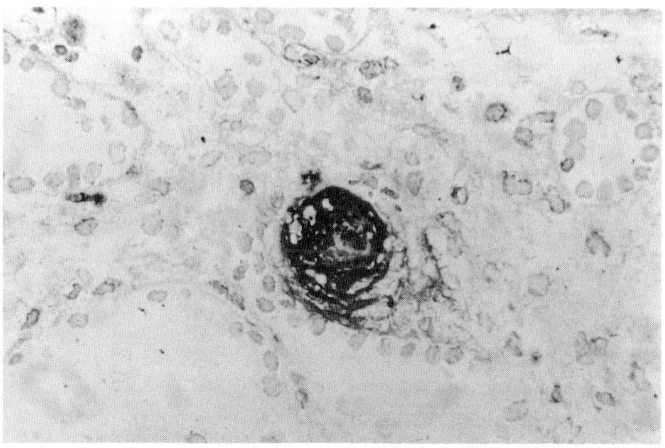

Fig. 5.21. Vascular staining with fibrinogen in thrombotic microangiopathy related to lupus anticoagulant (X400)

Vasculopathies

Some uncommon vascular lesions occasionally associated with distinct clinical syndromes, may show IMH changes of diagnostic help.

Light chain vasculopathy

Both kappa and lambda light chains may be separately deposited in crystalline form in the vessels of multiple organs with the kidneys involved as a constant finding and associated with renal failure (Peng et al., 1988; Stone et al., 1989).

Cryoglobulinaemia

In addition to the glomerulonephritic and vasculitic manifestations, cryoglobulinaemia, especially mixed essential cryoglobulinaemia, may show eosinophilic vascular thrombotic 'plugs' associated with a variable vascular and inflammatory reaction within the kidney or additional organs (Cordonnier et al., 1987; D'Amico et al., 1989); the intraluminal thrombi stain strongly with the constituent cryoglobulin(s) usually IgG and/or IgM, occasionally IgA; complement components and fibrinogen may lightly stain the material particularly peripherally.

Cyclosporine (CyA) arteriolopathy

In clinical transplantation a quite characteristic vasculopathy related to CyA was recognized by Mihatsch et al. (1983) that affected arterioles and small arteries and was marked by a mucoid degenerative change involving the endothelium accompanied by muscle cell necrosis without inflammation; subsequently sclerotic expansion of the wall with nodular PAS-positive hyalinosis of endothelium and replacement of smooth muscle cells developed; vascular lumens were partially or completely obliterated in some instances. The IMH of this lesion shows heavy IgM and/or C1q and/or C3 with only approximately 20 per cent of cases showing fibrin deposition (Mihatsch et al., 1988; Fig. 5.22A). Verani et al. (1984) showed that biopsies with either CyA toxicity or rejection or both patterns combined may show similar staining patterns of arteriolar IgM, C3 and/or IgA deposition. At autopsy similar arteriolar changes are seen in some other CyA-treated heart and bone marrow transplants more often found in the latter group (Nizze et al., 1988) and in non-transplant patients e.g. diabetics treated with CyA (Mihatsch et al. 1991). The changes found in all these different clinical settings relating to the use of CyA are dose-dependent. The prediction of CyA vasculopathy from CyA blood levels shows only moderate positive correlation; some patients appear to be particularly sensitive to low levels of the drug (Mihatsch et al., 1988). In chronic CyA vasculopathy, the IMH nodular pattern helps in distinction from hypertensive or recurrent diabetic hyalinosis which shows IgM and/or C3 and/or C1q solid intimal/endothelial masses as a characteristic (Fig. 5.22B). Reduction or cessation of CyA in patients with the arteriolopathy will at least partially reverse the vascular damage in many of these patients as recently demonstrated by Versluis et al. (1988) and Morozumi et al. (1992). The new immunosuppressant, FK506, appears to be safer than CyA with respect to the development of vascular pathology (Demetris et al., 1990).

'Lupus Vasculitis'

A lesion very similar morphologically and on IMH to TMA is so-called 'lupus vasculitis' (Bhathena et al., 1981; Grishman and Venkataseshan, 1988), with some subtle distinct features related to the deposits which expand the arterolar and small arterial endothelial and intimal layers respectively; the 'fibrinoid' deposits show duller

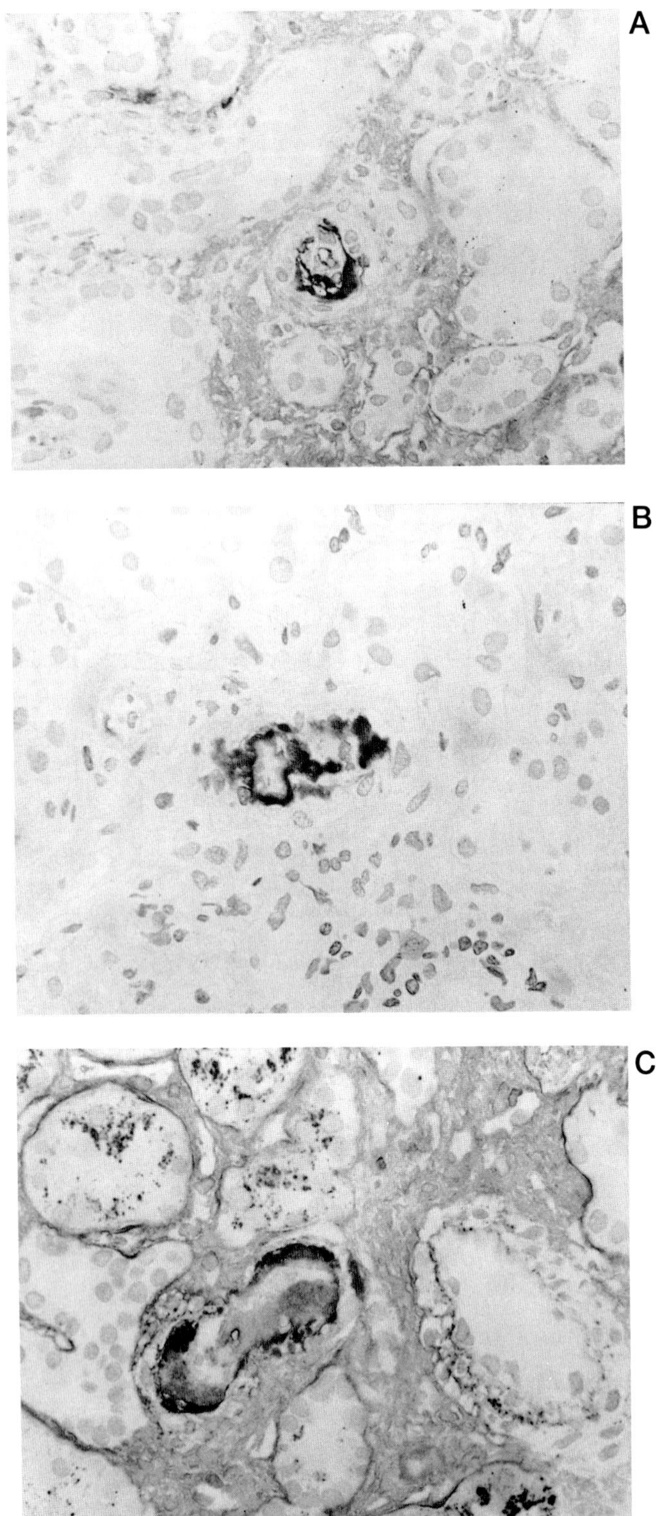

Fig. 5.22. (A)C1q deposition in acute Cyclosporine A arteriolopathy. (B)IgM staining of a hyalinotic arteriole in chronic Cyclosporine A toxicity. (C)Small arterial subendothelial staining with IgG in 'lupus vasculitis'; the adjacent artery shows minimal staining (X400)

eosinophilic staining compared with true 'vasculitic' fibrinoid, are clumped rather than hyaline and are limited by a membrane frequently and are less fibrillar than fibrin on electron microscopy; no inflammation accompanies the change but occasional examples show haematoxylin bodies. The material deposited stains with the immunoglobulins G,A and M (all 3 are characteristic of this lesion) C3 and fibrin, the latter two deposits staining variably (Fig. 5.22C).

Kohlmeier–Degos' disease (malignant atrophic papulosis) may involve the kidney but in one autopsy example (Bjorck et al., 1984) IMH was negative. The more frequently involved skin and intestinal tissues demonstrate, usually, vascular fibrinogen and, on occasions, IgM staining in this disease (Degos, 1979).

Renal neoplasms

In many instances the diagnosis of a renal neoplasm is a straightforward exercise not requiring special immunohistochemistry; the clinical and histological details are characteristic for the entity in a given patient. However, immunohistochemistry may often offer considerable diagnostic assistance in situations where the amount of tissue processed is small, e.g. fine needle aspirate/needle biopsy or, possibly, the lesion may have a pattern requiring differential diagnostic consideration. The immunohistochemical attributes presented below are applied to renal tumours from a differential diagnostic viewpoint. The antigenic staining patterns and information regarding the proposed histogenesis of many of these lesions has recently been reviewed (Wick et al., 1990; Mackay et al., 1987). The histological classification of renal cell carcinoma (RCC) has recently been expanded by Thoenes et al., (1986) (Table 5.27); some of the subtypes that they outline are included in the differential diagnostic approach presented here. The different neoplasms and relevant IMH findings are summarized in Table 5.28.

Clear cell neoplasms

In most cases, the clinical setting will provide an indication of the diagnosis of the clear cell lesion – clear cell sarcoma appears only to occur in childhood and RCC with a clear cell pattern is rare in the first two decades of life (Medeiros and Weiss, 1990). Clear cell

Table 5.27. Classification of renal cell carcinoma

Clear cell
Chromophobe
Chromophilic (Granular)
Basophilic
Eosinophilic
Duophilic (Baso- and Eosinophilic)
Mixed
Spindle-Shaped/Pleomorphic
Others

Source: Thoenes et al., 1986; 1988

RCC has been shown by a number of authors (reviewed by Wick et al., 1990) to possess cytokeratin (especially types 8 and 18) and/or epithelial membrane antigen with the majority of cases also showing vimentin staining. On occasions, epithelial membrane antigen may prove a better marker than cytokeratin for RCC (Pinkus et al., 1986). Cytokeratin (CK) and vimentin (V) are both markers found in the developing kidney, but CK without V is noted in the mature kidney (Oosterwijk et al., 1990). Combined CK and V are also present in a variety of carcinomas, including those from lung, liver, and adrenal cortex, and also in non-seminomatous germ cell tumours, all of which may possess a clear cell pattern (Wick et al., 1990). However adreno-cortical carcinomas do not stain with epithelial membrane antigen (Pinkus and Kurtin, 1985). Takashi et al. (1988) found that S100, particularly of $\alpha\alpha$ subunit composition stained the majority of RCCs.

The clear/transparent cell form of chromophobe RCC described by Thoenes et al. (1986) shows in addition to positive Hale's colloidal iron staining, CK but not V IMH staining; ultrastructure shows that the cells of chromophobe RCC contain many cytoplasmic microvesicles 150–300 nm in diameter (Thoenes et al., 1988). In contrast, clear cell sarcoma of childhood stains with V consistently (Fig. 5.23) and CK and epithelial membrane antigen are uniformly negative (Wick et al., 1990). The clear cell sarcoma probably arises from a primitive mesanchymal cell and shows lectin staining patterns similar to the blastema and stroma of Wilm's tumour (Webber et al., 1992). The rare clear cell variant of Wilm's tumour of which only two examples in a seven-month-old boy and a two-year-old girl respectively have been described (Glick et al., 1981; Edwards and Chatten, 1985) but immunohistochemical findings have not been outlined.

Table 5.28. IMH Differentiation of renal neoplasms

	Cytokeratin	Vimentin	EMA	CEA	S100
Clear cell type					
RCC-usual type	+ (MW8 & 18)	+	+		+(α0)
Chromophobe (colloidal iron +)	+	–	–		
Clear cell sarcoma	–	+	–		–
Extra renal neoplasms					
adrenocortical carcinoma	+	+	(+)	–	
lung	+	–	(+)	(+)	
Eosinophilic cell type					
RCC – granular eosinophil	+	+			
Oncocytoma	+	–			
Chromophobe with eosinophilic cells (colloidal iron +)	+	–			
Spindle cell type					
Sarcomatoid RCC	+ (LMW)	+	(+)		(+)
Sarcomatoid transitional cell carcinoma	+ (HMW)	(+)	–		+

Notes: ( ) = some cases stain positively; + = most cases positive; – = usually negative; L/H MW = low/high molecular weight

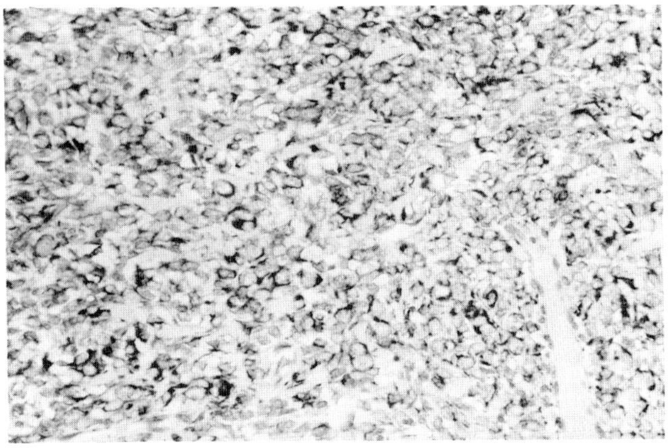

Fig. 5.23. Vimentin staining in clear cell sarcoma of childhood (× 400, Impo). (Kindly supplied by Dr C W Chow, Royal Children's Hospital, Melbourne.)

Eosinophil cell types of renal cell carcinoma

Several different neoplasms may have eosinophilic cells composing part or all of the cell population (Engel and Horn, 1991). These eosinophilic cells often form part of the histology of RCC often mixed with clear cells but oncocytic RCC or oncocytoma is composed of a uniform population of granular eosinophilic cells shown by electron microscopy to be laden with mitochondria. This neoplasm has a more favourable prognosis than clear cell RCC and stains only with CK and not V (Van Krieken et al., 1988). Using a series of monoclonal antibodies reacting to proximal and distal tubular epithelium, Van Krieken et al. (1988) also presented evidence of a distal tubular origin for the renal oncocytoma; this view differs from that of Zerban et al. (1987) who suggested an origin from the collecting duct for the oncocytoma. A more recently recognized variant of the colloidal iron-positive chromophobe RCC is also composed of eosinophilic cells (Thoenes et al., 1988) and stains only with CK (especially subtype 18) but not V, a similar staining pattern to that of renal oncocytoma and the pale chromophobe RCC.

Spindle cell neoplasms

Sarcomatoid RCC with its characteristic undifferentiated, often spindle cell histology, may be mistaken for various sarcomas, e.g. malignant fibrous histiocystoma leiomyosarcoma and fibrosarcoma if more typical clear/eosinophilic cells are not represented. Most examples of sarcomatoid RCC show CK (Fig. 5.24) and V staining but EMA is infrequently found (Fleming et al., 1985). In contrast, poorly differentiated (histological grade 3) or anaplastic sarcomatoid transitional cell carcinoma of the pelvicalyceal system may invade renal parenchyma and express cytokeratins of high molecular weights (57–60 kD) that are not seen or stain weakly in sarcomatoid RCC (Lofton et al., 1989). CEA is also found in most sarcomatoid transitional cell carcinomas but not sarcomatoid RCCs with occasional exceptions (Harris et al., 1989). For RCC, the expression of V is found more frequently in higher grade tumours with a poorer prognosis (Donhuijsen and Schulz, 1989). Takashi et al. (1988) also noted that one of two sarcomatoid RCCs was positive using both α and β forms of S100. Deletion or inappropriate expression of any of the range of ABH blood group isoantigens, Lewis (a) and Lewis (b) and Thomsen-Friedenreich (T) antigens carries an indication of poorer outlook as expressed by recurrence or invasion of the renal parenchyma by sarcomatoid transitional cell carcinomas (Wick et al., 1985). Other forms of soft tissue sarcoma with spindle cell patterns that may involve the kidney may be differentiated by IMH, the details of which are provided in Chapter 2.

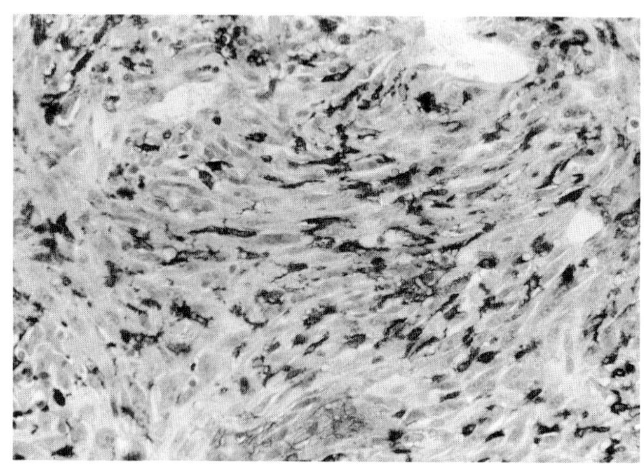

Fig. 5.24. Cytokeratin positivity in sarcomatoid renal cell carcinoma (X400)

Rhabdoid tumour and rhabdoid simulators

Rhabdoid tumour of the kidney (RTK) is characterized by hyaline perinuclear inclusions composed of whorled aggregates of intermediate filaments seen on ultrastructure that consistently stain with V (Fig. 5.25). Extensive review of this neoplasm in children by Weeks et al. (1989) revealed a variety of histological patterns described as classical, epithelioid, sclerosing, lymphomatoid, histiocytoid, spindled and vascular; these authors showed that of 11 neoplasms stained with V, seven of 11 showed EMA decoration and non-specific staining of cytoplasmic inclusions; other markers which stained some RTKs in this study were desmin, myoglobin, neurofilament and antichymotrypsin (Weeks et al., 1989). These results are in accord with those of many authors reviewed by Schmidt et al. (1989) who also found some RTKs to be S100-positive and suggest that RTKs may have heterogeneous origins.

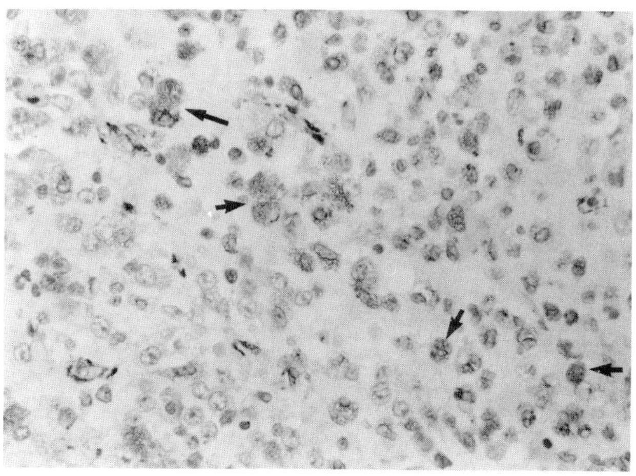

Fig. 5.25. Rhabdoid neoplasm of kidney showing light cytoplasmic vimentin staining of some cells (arrows) (X400, Impo). (Kindly supplied by C W Chow, Royal Children's Hospital, Melbourne).

The experience of Weeks et al. (1991) led them to indicate that RTK may be simulated by a wide diversity of renal neoplasms, the differentiation of which may be assisted by IMH; the distinguishing features of these simulators are as follows: Wilm's tumour, most of favourable histology, showing IMH evidence of myogenous development; highly cellular congenital mesoblastic nephroma without filamentous cytoplasmic inclusions on IMH or electronmicroscopy; various forms of RCC, usually found in older patients, may have similar IMH to RTK but often possess evidence of tubular formation in contrast to RTK; renal rhabdomyosarcoma and smooth muscle neoplasms, leiomyosarcoma and angiomyolipoma, may demonstrate rhabdoid patterns and will be differentiated by IMH and electronmicroscopy with evidence of myogenic differentiation; neuroepithelial tumours mostly provide evidence of neural marking with positive neurone-specific enolase; and, finally, malignant lymphoma may be mistaken for RTK but marks with leucocyte-common antigen and other leucocytic antigens (Weeks et al., 1991).

Special forms of primary renal cell carcinoma

Although the origin of RCC and its variants (see below) still requires clarification it is apparent that several uncommon/rare forms of primary renal carcinoma exist and that they possess unique features.

Small cell carcinoma: Capella et al. (1984) first described an example of primary neuroendocrine carcinoma and subsequent confirmation of its existence was provided by Tetu et al. (1987) who outlined three cases with typical 'small cell' histology and keratin staining in two of the neoplasms with neurone-specific enolase evident in the third. Cell of origin of these neoplasms and of renal carcinoid tumours is currently uncertain (Someren et al., 1989) and although neuroendocrine cells are not found in the normal kidney they are described in pelvic epithelium undergoing intestinal metaplasia (Salm, 1969).

Collecting duct carcinoma: There are sufficiently distinctive features such as tubulopapillary patterns with nests of clear cells, infiltrating tubules with a dense desmoplastic stroma, mucin staining and immunohistochemistry showing high molecular weight cytokeratins and peanut agglutinins to separate this neoplasm from other renal carcinomas; these distinguishing features were described by Kennedy et al. (1990) who described six cases of collecting duct carcinoma. Further examples were described by Rumpelt et al. (1991) who presented an immunohistochemical pattern for this lesion showing cytokeratins 13 and 19, and Ulex europeus A-I that help separate these neoplasms from other RCCs.

Additional aspects of immunohistochemistry of renal carcinoma

A more detailed examination of the CK expression by various forms of RCC was carried out by Priz et al. (1987). Clear cell carcinomas were found to express mostly CK Nos.

8/18, eosinophilic-granular and basophilic chromophilic carcinomas commonly stained with CK Nos. 7 and 19; chromophobe cell carcinomas usually stained with CKs 8/18 and sometimes with CK 7.

The weight of evidence following IMH staining with monoclonal antibodies of developing foetal kidney and RCC of clear and granular type, favours an origin of these neoplasms from the proximal convoluted tubule (reviewed by Wick et al, 1990). Both the chromophobe variants of RCC (pale and eosinophilic cell types), described by Thoenes et al. (1986) and oncocytomas stain with lectins which mark distal aspects of nephrons particularly collecting ducts and which in the normal kidney show strict compartmentalization of saccharide moieties in the tubules (Ortmann et al., 1991). The origin of the chromophobe RCC and renal oncocytoma from the collecting duct is further supported by staining of both neoplasms with antibody to carbonic anhydrase and EMA with the chromophobe RCC showing exclusive staining with a polyclonal antibody to the anion exchanger band 3, a HCO3 exchange protein found in the basolateral membrane of intercalated cells of the collecting ducts (Störkel et al., 1989).

The *prognosis of RCC* is related to clinical staging of the local and/or distal spread of the carcinoma. The cytological grading supported by flow cytometry studies particularly with respect to RCC with eosinophilic cells (Baretton et al., 1991) independently of other variables appears to predict outcome. IMH using V and CK antibodies demonstrated consistent CK staining but the presence of V correlates with greater cytological abnormalities (Donhuijsen and Schultz, 1989; Dierick et al., 1991). Similar findings were noted by Medeiros et al. (1988). Ki-67, a nuclear cell proliferation marker staining frozen but not formalin-fixed paraffin-embedded tissue (Gerdes et al., 1984) stained an increasing proportion of proliferating cells with a rise in the histological grade associated with an increase in nuclear DNA content on flow cytometry indicating that this marker may be used as a supportive prognostic guide in RCC (Baretton et al., 1991); other proliferation nuclear markers such as PC10 may also demonstrate similar features and can be used on formalin-fixed paraffin embedded tissue (Hall et al., 1990).

Staining of specialized renal antigens

Another facet of RCC that may be helpful in differential diagnosis is the ability of primary and metastatic RCC tumours to produce antigens of renal origin that assist in identifying the lesion as renal (Table 5.29). These products may be divided into 'intrinsic renal antigens' such as angiotensin-converting enzyme (Takada et al., 1985), renin (Tomita et al., 1987; Corvol, 1989), Tamm-Horsfall glycoprotein (Gaulier et al., 1990) and villin a brush border glycoprotein which also marks other tissues and adenocarcinomas but is not found in IMH of chromophobe RCC (Moll et al., 1987), erythropoietin (Waldmann et al., 1968) and proximal renal tubular surface membrane antigens in both primary and secondary RCC (Yoshida et al., 1986). Other 'shared' antigens found in RCC and other neoplasms include S100 (Takashi et al., 1988), α-1-antitrypsin and α-1-antichymotrypsin (Fleming and Gibson, 1986), two different enolase enzymes (Haimoto et al., 1988) and pre-albumin (Ang et al., 1991).

Table 5.29. Specialized antigens demonstrated in renal neoplasms

Angiotensin converting enzyme
Renin
Tamm–Horsfall glycoprotein
Villin
Erythropoietin
S100-α
α 1 antitrypsin
α 1 antichymotrypsin
Enolase enzymes
Pre-albumin
Proximal renal tubular surface Ags

Histogenesis of renal cell carcinoma.

The cell of origin of RCC has been investigated with both polyclonal and monoclonal antibodies raised to various tubular antigens. Initial studies (Wallace and Nairn, 1972) and the bulk of IMH staining evidence (reviewed by Wick et al., 1990) suggest an origin of the clear and granular eosinophilic cell types from the proximal convoluted tubular cell. However recently Droz et al. (1990) using a series of monoclonal markers related to nephron development namely CK, V, CD24, CALLA/CD10, villin, CD26 and HLA class I and HLA class II molecules found in various segments of the mature nephron. The patterns of staining of a series of 28 RCCs, classified according to the criteria of Thoenes et al. (1986) suggested an origin from cells with blastemic potential and that clear cell tumours by staining with CD26, CALLA and villin differentiate towards the proximal tubular cell type. The basophilic small cuboidal cell type of RCC stained with CD24 which is consistently found on blastemic cells but they did not stain with villin, CD26 or CALLA; these findings pointed to a histogenesis from 'primitive' or distal tubular cells. These concepts support the histogenetic proposals of Cohen et al. (1988). Störkel et al. (1989) suggest that IMH staining patterns and morphological changes point to an origin of the chromophobe form of RCC from the intercalated cells of the collecting duct.

Special neoplasms

Wilm's tumour (WT)

WT or nephroblastoma is, in most instances, a diagnosis readily made but IMH may be helpful in some situations and may provide clues to directions of differentiation. Wick et al. (1990) have presented extensive data on the staining of the usual blastema, epithelial and stromal components of WT. In summary, Wick et al. (1990) found that the blastema consistently stained focally with V but was negative for CK although this antigen may be induced by in vitro culture. The stromal element shows consistent V staining too, but desmin, myoglobin and neurone-specific enolase may be outlined. S100, glial fibrillary acidic protein and NSE indicating neural differentiation have been noted in some cases by Magee et al. (1987). The epithelial elements of WT suggesting tubular differentiation were found by Wick et al. (1990) to stain uniformly with epithelial membrane antigen, CK in most cases and variable co-expression with V and CK, blood group isoantigens, leu-7 and CEA were also found. Their finding of leu-7 staining raised the possibility of neuroendocrine differentiation within the epithelial elements. Further support for epithelial differentiation in WT is found with staining for laminin and collagen IV which demonstrate formation of cellular basement membranes, as outlined by Kumar et al. (1986).

Congenital mesoblastic nephroma of infancy

Described initially as a separate entity by Bolande et al. (1967). This neoplasma presents in the majority of instances before three months of age and is regarded as a neoplasm separate from Wilm's tumour. An essentially benign lesion that is unilateral it is composed of bundles of plump and spindle-shaped fibroblasts and myofibroblasts in the main, forming a solid tumour (Sotelo-Avila, 1989). Neoplasms with dense cellularity and mitoses may infiltrate the renal pelvis or perirenal tissue and contain areas of haemorrhage and necrosis and are regarded as *atypical mesoblastic nephromas* (Joshi et al., 1986). Immunohistochemical findings have been reviewed by Wick et al. (1990) who also studied 11 cases, six of which were of conventional type while the remaining five showed at least one atypical feature; nine of the 11 neoplasms showed staining for desmin, muscle-specific actin or both and all expressed V but CK, epithelial membrane antigen, myoglobin and neural determinants were all negative. This study and that of Kumar et al. (1985) suggest a predominantly smooth muscle or myofibroblastic origin for mesoblastic nephroma.

Juxtaglomerular cell tumour

This benign neoplasm is a rare but curable cause of hypertension caused by hypersecretion of renin. The neoplasm composed of sheets of uniform round and/or oval cells separated by avascular spaces may resemble haemangiopericytoma but the demonstration of renin production in both active and inactive forms by the cells of a juxtaglomerular cell tumour distinguishes the lesion from an haemangiopericytoma (Corvol et al., 1989). Erythropoietic secretion may be associated with the juxtaglomerular cell tumour (Remynse et al., 1989).

Angiomyolipoma

This neoplasm which has a strong association with tuberose sclerosis whereby approximately 80 per cent of tuberose sclerosis patients develop angiomyolipoma may be bilateral in this condition and other neoplasms and haematomas may also be found associated with tuberose sclerosis. Confusion between angiomyolipoma and RCC may arise because both neoplasms may be large, may breach the renal capsule and show marked nuclear atypia (Wick et al., 1990). Occasionally angiomyolipoma and RCC may coexist in the kidney of patients with tuberose sclerosis (Graves and Barnes, 1986). IMH with desmin and actin stain the smooth muscle component and epithelial markers are negative in angiomyolipoma (Wick et al., 1990).

References

Aarons, I., Smith, P.S., Davies, R.A., Woodroffe, A.J. and Clarkson, A.R. (1989) Thin membrane nephropathy: A clinico-pathological study. *Clinical Nephrology* **32**, 151–8.

Aguirreburyalde, A. and Howat. A.J. (1991) Immuno-alkaline phosphatase technique in renal pathology. *Journal of Clinical Pathology* **44**, 175.

Alexopoulos, E., Seron, D., Hartley, R.B., Nolasco, F. and Cameron, J.S. (1989) Immune mechanisms in idiopathic membranous nephropathy: the role of the interstitial infiltrates. *American Journal of Kidney Diseases* **13**, 404–12.

Allen, D.E. and Dowling, J.P. (Editors) (1981) *Techniques for Nephropathology*. CRC Press, Boca Raton, pp. 1–117.

Al-Nawab, M.D. and Davies, D.R. (1989) Light and electron microscopic demonstration of extracellular immunoglobulin deposition in renal tissue. *Journal of Clinical Pathology* **42**, 1104–8.

Alpers, C.E. And Cotran, R.S. (1986) Neoplasia and glomerular injury. *Kidney International* **30**, 465–73.

Alpers, C.E. and Biava, C.G. (1989) Idiopathic lobular glomerulonephritis (nodular mesangial sclerosis): A distinct diagnostic entity. *Clinical Nephrology* **32**, 68–74.

Alpers, C.E. (1992) Immunotactoid (microtubular) glomerulopathy: An entity distinct from fibrillary glomerulonephritis? *American Journal of Kidney Diseases* **19**, 185–91.

Alves, V.A.F., Vianna, M.R., Yasuda, P.H. and De Brito, T., (1987) Detection of leptospiral antigen in the human liver and kidney using an immunoperoxidase staining procedure. *Journal of Pathology* **151**, 125–31.

Anders, D., Agricola, B., Sippel, M. and Thoenes, W. (1977) Basement membrane changes on membranoproliferative glomerulonephritis. II. Characterization of a third type by silver impregnation of ultrathin sections. *Virchows Archives A, (Pathological Anatomy and Histology)* **376**, 1–19.

Andrassy, K., Erb, A., Koderisch, J., Waldherr, R. and Ritz, E. (1991) Wegener's granulomatosis with renal involvement: patient survival and correlations between initial renal function, renal histology, therapy and renal outcome. *Clinical Nephrology* **35**, 139–47.

Andres, G.A., Brentjens, J., Kohl, T.R., Anthone, R., Anthone, S., Baliah, T., and Montes, M., Mookerjee, B.K., Prezyyna, A., Sepulueda, M., Venuto, R. and Elwood, C. (1978) Histology of tubulointerstitial nephritis associated with antibodies to renal basement membrane. *Kidney International* **13**, 480–91.

Ang, L.C., Debowski, T. and Michalski, R. (1991) Immunolocalization of pre- albumin (transthyretin) in renal cell carcinoma. *Histopathology* **18**, 565–8.

Ballardie, F.W. (ed.) (1992) *Autoimmunity in Nephritis*. Harwood Academic, Berkshire, pp. 1–310.

Banfi, G., Mazzucco, G., Di Belgiojoso, G.B., Bosisio, M.B., Stratta, P., Confalonieri, R., Ferrario, F., Imbasciati, E. and Monga, G. (1985) Morphological parameters in lupus nephritis. Their relevance for classification and relationship with clinical and histological findings and outcome. *Quarterly Journal of Medicine* **55**, 153–68.

Bangerter, A.R. and Murphy, W.M. (1987) Kappa light chain nephropathy. A pathologic study. *Virchows Archivs A Pathological Anatomy* **410**, 531–9.

Baretton, G., Kuhlmann, B., Krech, R. and LŒ hrs, U. (1991) Intratumoral heterogeneity of nuclear DNA – content and proliferation in clear cell type carcinomas of the kidney. *Virchows Archiv B Cell Pathology* **61**, 57–63.

Batsford, S.R. (1991) Cationic antigens as mediators of inflammation. *Acta Pathologica Microbiologica Immunologica Scandinavia* **99**, 1–9.

Beaufils, H., Morel-Maroger, L., Sraer, J-D., Kanfer, A., Kourilsky, O. and Richet, G. (1976) Acute renal failure of glomerular origin during visceral abscesses. *New England Journal of Medicine* **295**, 185–9.

Ben-Bassat, M., Boner, G., Rosenfeld, J., Pick, A.I., Kahana, M., Hazah, B. and Hochman, B. (1983) The clinico-pathologic features of cryoglobulinemic nephropathy. *American Journal of Clinical Pathology* **79**, 147–56.

Bennett, W.M., Fassett, F.G., Walker, R.G., Fairley, K.F., D'Apice, A.J.F. and Kincaid-Smith, P. (1989). Mesangiocapillary glomerulonephritis type II (Dense Deposit disease): clinical features of progressive disease. *American Journal of Kidney Diseases* **13**, 469–76.

Bennett, W.M., Bardana, E.J., Norman, D.J. and Houghton, D.C. (1982) Natural history of 'silent' lupus nephritis. *American Journal of Kidney Diseases* **1**, 359–63.

Berger, J., Yaneva, H. and Nabarra, B. (1978) Glomerular changes in patients with cirrhosis of the liver. *Advances in Nephrology* **7**, 3–14.

Bergstein, J.M. (1990) Glomerular fibrin deposition and removal. *Pediatric Nephrology* **4**, 78–87.

Bhathena, D.B., Sobel, B.J. and Migdal, S.D. (1981) Non-inflammatory renal microangiopathy of systemic lupus erythematosus ('lupus vasculitis'). *American Journal of Nephrology* **1**, 144–59.

Biesecker, G. (1983) Biology of disease. Membrane attack complex of complement as a pathologic mediator. *Laboratory Investigation* **49**, 237–49.

Bjorck, S., Johansson, S.L. and Aurell, M. (1984) Acute renal failure caused by a rapidly progressive arterio-occlusive syndrome: Kohlmeier–Degos' disease. *Scandinavian Journal of Urology and Nephrology* **18**, 343–6.

Boers, M., Croonen, A.M., Dijkmans, B.A.C., Breedvelt, F.C., Eulderrink, F., Cats, A. and Weening, J.J. (1987) Renal findings in rheumatoid arthritis: clinical aspects of 132 necropsies. *Annals of Rheumatic Diseases* **46**, 658–63.

Bohle, A., Grabensee, B., Fischer, R., Berg, E. and Klust, H. (1985) On four cases of hemolytic-uremic syndrome without microangiopathy. *Clinical Nephrology* **24**, 88–92.

Bohle, A., Mackensen-Haen, S., Von Gise, H., Grund, K-E., Wehrmann, M., Batz, C.L., Bogenschütz, O. Schmitt, H., Nagy J., Muller, C. and Müller, G. (1990). The consequences of tubulointerstitial changes for renal function in glomerulopathies. A morphometric and cytological analysis. *Pathology Research and Practice* **186**, 135–44.

Bolande, R.P., Brough, A.J. and Izant, R.J.J. (1967) Congenital mesoblastic nephroma of infancy. *Pediatrics* **400**, 272–8.

Bommer, J., Waldherr, R. and Ritz, E. (1985) Kidney lesions in uraemic patients and beta-2 microglobulin derived amyloid. (Letter). *Lancet* **ii**, 1437–8.

Bonsib, S.M. (1988) Glomerular basement membrane necrosis and crescent organization. *Kidney International* **33**, 966–74.

Border, W., Baehler, R. and Bathena, D. (1979) IgA anti-basement membrane nephritis with pulmonary haemorrhage. *Annals of Internal Medicine* **91**, 21–5.

Border, W.A. (1988). Nephrology forum: distinguishing minimal-change disease from mesangial disorders. *Kidney International* **34**, 419–34.

Boucher, A., Droz, D., Edafer, E. and Noël, L-H. (1986) Characterization of mononuclear cell subsets in renal cellular interstitial infiltrates. *Kidney International* **29**, 1043–9.

Boucher, A., Droz, C., Adafer, E. and Noël, L-H., (1987) Relationship between the integrity of Bowman's capsule and the composition of cellular crescents in human crescentic glomerulonephritis. *Laboratory Investigation* **56**, 526–33.

Boyce, N., Holdsworth, S., Atkins, R. and Dowling, J.P. (1985) De novo anti-GBM-antibody-induced glomerulonephritis in a renal transplant. *Clinical Nephrology* **23**, 148–53.

Brentjens, J. and Andres, G.A. (1989) Interaction of antibodies with renal cell surface antigens. *Kidney International* **35**, 954–68.

Brouwer, E., Cohen Tervaert, J.W., Horst, G., Huitema, M.G., Van Der Giessen, M., Limburg, P.C. and Kallenberg, C.G.M. (1991) Predominance of IgG1 and IgG4 subclasses of anti-neutrophil cytoplasmic autoantibodies (ANCA) in patients with Wegener's granulomatosis and clinically related disorders. *Clinical and Experimental Immunology* **83**, 379–86.

Broyer, M., Meyrier, A., Niaudet, P. and Habib, R. (1992) Minimal changes and focal segmental glomerular sclerosis. In Cameron, S., Davison, A.M., Grünfeld, J-P., Kerr, D. and Ritz, E. (eds), *Oxford Textbook of Clinical Nephrology, Volume 1*. Oxford Medical, Oxford, pp. 298–339.

Bruijn, J.A., Hoedemaeker, P.J. and Fleuren, G.J. (1989) Pathogenesis of anti- basement membrane glomerulopathy and immune-complex glomerulonephritis: dichotomy dissolved. *Laboratory Investigation* **61**, 480–8.

Burkholder, P.M., Marchand, A. and Krueger R.P. (1970) Mixed membranous and proliferative glomerulonephritis. A correlative light, immunofluorscence, and electron microscope study. *Laboratory Investigation* **23** 459–79.

Buxbaum, J. (1992) Mechanisms of disease: monoclonal immunoglobulin deposition; amyloidosis, light chain deposition disease, and light and heavy chain deposition disease. *Hematology/Oncology Clinics of North America* **6**, 323–46.

Buxbaum, J.N., Chuba, J.V., Hellman, G.C., Solomon, A. and Gallo, G.R. (1990) Monoclonal immunoglobulin deposition disease: light chain and light and heavy chain amyloidosis. *Annals of Internal Medicine* **112**, 455–64.

Cameron, J.S., Turner, D.R., Heaton, J., Williams, D.G., Ogg, C.S., Chantler, C., Haycock, G., and Hicks, J. (1983) Idiopathic mesangiocapillary glomerulonephritis comparison of type I and II in children and adults and long term prognosis. *American Journal of Medicine* **74**, 175–92.

Cameron, J.S. and Turner, D.R. (1977) Recurrent glomerulonephritis in allograted kidneys. *Clinical Nephrology* **7**, 47–54.

Cameron, J.S. (1988) Allergic interstitial nephritis: clinical features and pathogenesis. *Quarterly Journal of Medicine* **66**, 97–115.

Cameron, J.S. (1991) New horizons in renal vasculitis. *Klinische Wochenschrift* **69**, 536–51.

Capella, C., Eusebi, V. and Rosai. J. (1984) Primary oat cell carcinoma of the kidney. *American Journal of Surgical Pathology* **8**, 855–61.

Carre, Ph., Lloveras, J.J., Didier, A., Gorguet, B., Orfila, C., Durand, D. and Leophonte, P. (1989) Goodpasture's syndrome with normal renal function. *European Respiratory Journal* **2**, 911–15.

Case Records of the Massachusetts General Hospital. (1985) Case 16–1985. *New England Journal of Medicine* **312**, 1042–52.

Cavallo, T., Cameron, W.R. and Lapenas, D. (1977) Immunopathology of early and clinically silent lupus nephropathy. *American Journal of Pathology* **87**, 1–8.

Chang-Miller, A., Okamura, M., Torres, V.E., Michet, C.J., Wagoner, R.D., Donadio, J.V.Jr., Offord, K.P. and Holley, K.E. (1987) Renal involvement in relapsing polychondritis. *Medicine (Baltimore)* **66**, 202–17.

Chiu, K.Y. and Chan, K.W. (1987) Rapid immunfluorescence staining of human renal biopsy specimens using microwave irradiation. *Journal of Clinical Pathology* **40**, 689–92.

Chugh, K.S. and Sakhuja, V. (1990) Glomerular diseases in the tropics. *American Journal of Nephrology* **10**, 437–50.

Churg, J., Duffy, J.L. and Bernstein, J. (1979) Identification of dense deposit disease. *Archives of Pathology and Laboratory Medicine* **103**, 67–72.

Churg, J. and Sobin, L.H. (1982) In collaboration with pathologists and nephrologists in 14 countries. *Renal Disease Classification and Atlas of Glomerular Diseases*.

Iagku-Shoin, Tokyo, pp. 1–359.

Churg, J., Goldstein, M.H. and Bernstein, J. (1989) Thrombotic microangiopathy including hemolytic-uremic syndrome, thrombotic thrombocytopenic purpura, and post-partum renal failure. In Tisher, C.C. and Brenner, B.M. (eds), *Renal Pathology with Clinical and Functional Correlations, Volume 2*. Lippincott, Philadelphia, pp. 1081–113.

Clardy, C.W., Forristal, J., Strife, C.F. and West, C.D. (1989) Serum terminal complement component levels in hypocomplementemic glomerulonephritides. *Clinical Immunology and Immunopathology* **50**, 307–20.

Cohen, A.H., Border., W.A. and Glassock, R. (1978) Nephrotic syndrome with glomerular mesangial IgM deposits. *Laboratory Investigation* **38**, 610–19.

Cohen, A.H., Border, W.A., Shankel, E. and Glassock, R.J. (1981) Crescentic glomerulonephritis: Immune vs. non-immune mechanisms. *American Journal of Nephrology* **1**, 78–83.

Cohen, A.H. (1984) Pathology of light chain nephropathies. In Robinson, R.R. (ed.) *Nephrology, Volume II. Proceedings of the IXth International Congress of Nephrology*. Springer-Verlag, New York, pp. 895–904.

Cohen, A.H. and Glassock, R.J. (1989) Anti-GBM glomerulonephritis including Goodpasture's syndrome. In Tisher, C.C. and Brenner, B.M. (eds), *Renal Pathology, with Clinical and Functional Correlations, Volume 1*. Lippincott, Philadelphia, pp. 494–521.

Cohen, A.H and Nast, C.C. (1991) Pathology of the kidneys. In Nash, G. and Said, J.W. (eds), *The Pathology of AIDS, Major Problems in Pathology Volume 26*. Saunders, Philadelphia, pp. 130–47.

Cohen, A.S. and Connors, L.H. (1987) Invited review: The pathogenesis and biochemistry of amyloidosis. *Journal of Pathology* **151**, 1–10.

Cohen, C., McCue, P.A. and Derose, P.B. (1988) Histogenesis of renal cell carcinoma and renal oncocytoma. An immunohistochemical study. *Cancer* **62**, 1946–51.

Coleman, M., Haynes, W.D.G., Dimopoulos, P., Barratt, L.J. and Jarvis, L.R. (1986) Glomerular basement membrane abnormalities associated with apparently idiopathic hematuria: ultrastructural morphometric analysis. *Human Pathology* **17**, 1022–30.

Conley, M.E., Cooper, M.D. and Michael, A.F. (1980) Selective deposition of IgA1 in IgA nephropathy, anaphylactoid purpura nephritis and systemic lupus erythematosus. *Journal of Clinical Investigation* **66**, 1432–6.

Cordonnier, D.J., Renversez, J.C., Vialtel, P. and Dechelette, E. (1987) The kidney in mixed cryoglobulinaemias. *Springer Seminars in Immunopathology* **9**, 395–415.

Corvol, P., Pinet, F., Galen, F.X., Plouin, P.F., Chateilier, G., Pagny, J.Y., Corvol, M.T. and Menard, J. (1989) Seven lessons from seven renin-secreting tumours. In Laragh, J.H., Brenner, B.M. and Kaplan, N.M. (eds), *Endocrine Mechanisms in Hypertension*. Raven Press, New York, pp. 189–99.

Couser, W.G. (1988) Rapidly progressive glomerulonephritis: classification, pathogenetic mechanisms, and therapy. *American Journal of Kidney Diseases* **11**, 449–64.

Cronin, W., Deol, H. Azadegan, A. and Lange, K. (1989) Endostreptosin: isolation of the probable immunogen of acute post-streptococcal glomerulonephrits (PSGN). *Clinical and Experimental Immunology* **76**, 198–203.

D'Agati, V., Kunis, C., William, G. and Appel, G.B. (1990) Anti-cardiolipin antibody and renal disease: A report of three cases. *Journal of the American Society of Nephrology* **I**, 777–84.

D'Amico G. (1987). The commonest glomerulonephritis in the world: IgA nephropathy. *Quarterly Journal of Medicine* **64**, 709–27.

D'Amico, G., Colasanti, G., Ferrario, F. and Sinico, R.A. (1989) Renal involvement in essential mixed cryglobulinemia. *Kidney International* **35**, 1004–14.

D'Amico, G. (1991) The clinical role of proteinuria. *American Journal of Kidney Diseases* **17**, Suppl. 1, 48–52.

Davenport, A., Verbov, J.L. and Goldsmith, H.J. (1987) Circulating anti-skin basement membrane zone antibodies in a patient with Goodpasture's syndrome. *British Journal of Dermatology* **117**, 125–7.

Davenport, A. (1992) 'False positive' perinuclear and cytoplasmic anti-neutrophilic cytoplasmic antibody results leading to misdiagnosis of Wegener's granulomatosis and/or microscopic polyarteritis. *Clinical Nephrology* **37**, 124–30.

Davis, C.A., McEnery, P.T., Maby, S., McAdams, A.J. and West, C.D. (1978) Observations on the evolution of idiopathic rapidly progressive glomerulonephritis. *Clinical Nephrology* **9**, 91–101.

Davison, A.M. and Thomson, D. (1992) Malignancy-associated glomerular disease. In Cameron, S., Davison, A.M., Grünfeld, J-P., Kerr, D. and Ritz, E. (eds), *Oxford Textbook of Nephrology, Volume 1*. Oxford Medical, Oxford, pp. 475–86.

de Chadarévian, J-P., Goodyer, P.R. and Kaplan, B.S. (1980) Acute glomerulonephritis and hemolytic uremic syndrome. *Canadian Medical Association Journal* **123**, 391–3.

Degos R. (1979) Malignant atrophic papulosis. (Review) *British Journal of Dermatology* **100**, 21–35.

Demetris, A.J., Fung, J.J., Todo, S., Banner, B., Zerbe, T., Sysyn, G. and Starzl, T.E. (1990) Pathological observations in human allograft recipients treated with FK506. *Transplant Proceedings* **22**, Suppl. 1, 25–34.

Dennis, V.W. and Robinson, R.R. (1986) Clinical proteinuria. *Advances in Internal Medicine* **31**, 243–63.

Dierick, A-M., Praet, M., Roels, H., Verbeeck, P., Robyns, L.

and Oosterlinck, W. (1991) Vimentin expression of renal cell carcinoma in relation to DNA content and histological grading: A combined light microscopic, immuno--cytochemical and cytophotometrical analysis. *Histopathology* **18**, 315–22.

Dische, F.E., Weston, M.J. and Parsons, V. (1985) Abnormally thin glomerular basement membrane associated with hematuria proteinuria or renal failure in adults. *American Journal of Nephrology* **5**, 103–9.

Doi, T., Kanatsu, K., Nagai, H., Kohrogi, N. and Hamashima, Y. (1983) An overlapping syndrome of IgA nephropathy and membranous nephropathy? *Nephron* **35**, 24–30.

Donhuijsen, K. and Schulz, S., (1989) Prognostic significance of vimentin positivity in formalin-fixed renal cell carcinomas. *Pathology Research and Practice* **184**, 287–91.

Donohoe, J.F. (1992) Nephrology forum. Scleroderma and the kidney. *Kidney International* **41**, 462–77.

Dowling, J.P. and Mathews, D.C. (1987) Silver methenamine impregnation: A useful adjunct to renal electron microscopy. *Pathology* **19**, 410–14.

Droz, D., Zachar, D., Charbit, L., Gogusev, J., Chrétien, Y. and Iris, L. (1990) Expression of the human nephron differentiation molecules in renal cell carcinomas. *American Journal of Pathology* **137**, 895–905.

Duffy, J.L., Khurana, E., Susin, M., Gomez-Leon, G. and Churg, J. (1983) Fibrillary renal deposits and nephritis. *American Journal of Pathology* **113**, 279–90.

Durand, D., Segonds, A., Orfila, C., Degroc, G., Bories, P., Giraud, P. and Suc, J.M. (1983) Transplant biopsies and short-term outcome of cadaveric renal allografts. *Advances in Nephrology* **12**, 309–30.

Eddy, A., Sibley, R., Mauer, S.M. and Kim, Y. (1984) Renal allograft failure due to recurrent dense intramembranous deposit disease. *Clinical Nephrology* **21**, 305–13.

Edwards, O. and Chatten, J. (1985) Hydropic cell variant (clear cell variant) of Wilm's tumor. *Archives of Pathology and Laboratory Medicine* **109**, 956–8.

Eigenbrodt, E.H. and Ware, A.J. (1989) Renal involvement in hepatic disease, rheumatoid arthritis, Sjögren's syndrome, and mixed connective tissue disease. In Tisher, C.C. and Brenner, B.M. (eds), *Renal Pathology with Clinical and Functional Correlations, Volume 1*. B.M. Lippincott, Philadelphia, pp. 522–47.

Eknoyan, G., McDonald, M.A., Appel, D. and Truong, L.D. (1990) Chronic tubulointerstitial nephritis: Correlations between structural and functional findings. *Kidney International* **38**, 736–43.

Emancipator, S.N. and Lamm, M.E. (1989) IgA nephropathy: pathogenesis of the most common form of glomerulonephritis. *Laboratory Investigation* **60**, 168–83.

Endoh, M., Miyazaki, M., Suga, T., Miura, M., Nomoto, Y. and Sakai, H. (1991) Rheumatoid factors in patients with minimal change nephrotic syndrome. *Clinical Nephrology* **35**, 93–7.

Engel, U. and Horn, T. (1991) Eosinophilic renal cell tumours. A study of tumour heterogeneity with special emphasis on oncocytes. *Scandinavian Journal of Urology and Nephrology* **25**, 297–301.

Esparza, A.R., Chazan, J.A., Nayak, R.N. and Cavallo, T. (1991) Fibrillary (immunotactoid) glomerulopathy – a possible role for kappa light chain in its etiology and/or pathogenesis. *American Journal of Surgical Pathology* **15**, 632–43.

Espinosa-Meléndez, E., Forbes, R.D., Hollomby, D., Ahuja, J. and Katz, M.G. (1980) Goodpasture's syndrome treated with plasmapheresis. *Archives of Internal Medicine* **140**, 542–3.

Fairley, C., Mathews, D.C. and Becker, G.J. (1987) Rapid development of diffuse crescents in post-streptococcal glomerulonephritis. *Clinical Nephrology* **28**, 256–60.

Falk, R.J., Dalmasso, A.P., Kim, Y., Tsai, C.H., Scheinman, J.E., Gewurz, H. and Michael, A.F. (1983) Neo-antigen of the polymerized ninth component of complement. Characterization of a monoclonal antibody and immunohistochemical localization in renal disease. *Journal of Clinical Investigation* **72**, 560–73.

Farquhar, A., MacDonald, M.K. and Ireland, J.T. (1972) The role of fibrin deposition in diabetic glomerulosclerosis: A light electron and immunofluorescence microscopy study. *Journal of Clinical Pathology* **25**, 657–67.

Fitzmaurice, R.J., Bartley, C. McClure, J. and Ackrill, P. (1991) Immunohistological characterization of amyloid deposits in renal biopsy specimens. *Journal of Clinical Pathology* **44**, 200–4.

Fivush, B., Melvin, T., Solez, K. and McLean, R. (1986) Idiopathic linear glomerular IgA deposition. *Archives of Pathology and Laboratory Medicine* **110**, 1189–91.

Fleming, S., Lindop, G.B.M. and Gibson, A.A.M. (1985) The distribution of epithelial membrane antigen in the kidney and its tumours. *Histopathology* **9**, 729–39.

Fleming, S. and Gibson, A.A.M. (1986) Proteinase inhibitors in the kidney and its tumours. *Histopathology* **10**, 1303–13.

Fliger, F.D., Wieslander, J., Brentjens, J.R., Andres, G.A. and Butkowski, R.J. (1987) Identification of a target antigen in human anti-tubular basement membrane nephritis. *Kidney International* **31**, 800–7.

Font, J., Torras, A., Cervera, R., Darnell, A., Revert, L. and Ingelmo, M. (1987) Silent renal disease in systemic lupus erythematosus. *Clinical Nephrology* **27**, 283–8.

Forsyth, K.D., Simpson, A.C., Fitzpatrick, M.M. Barratt, T.M., and Levinsky, R.J. (1989) Neutrophil-mediated endothelial injury in haemolytic uraemic syndrome. *Lancet* **ii**, 411–14.

Frankel, A.H., Singer, D.R.J., Winnearls, C.G., Evans, D.J., Rees, A.J. and Pusey, C.D. (1992) Type II essential mixed cryoglobulinaemia: presentation, treatment and outcome in 13 patients. *Quarterly Journal of Medicine* **82**, 101–24.

Furness, P. (1991) The formation and fate of glomerular immune complex deposits. *Journal of Pathology* **164**, 195–202.

Gaffney, E.F., Alexander, R.W. and Donnelly, W.H. (1982) Segmental membranous glomerulonephritis. *Archives of Pathology and Laboratory Medicine* **106**, 409–12.

Gallo, G.R., Feiner, H.D., Steele, J.M.Jr., Schacht, R.G., Gluck, M.C. and Baldwin, D.S. (1980) Role of intrarenal vascular sclerosis in progression of post-streptococcal glomerulonephritis. *Clinical Nephrology* **13**, 49–57.

Gallo, G.R., Feiner, H.D., Chuba, J.V., Beneck, D., Marion, P. and Cohen, D.H. (1986) Characterization of tissue amyloid by immunofluorescence microscopy. *Clinical Immunology and Immunopathology* **39**, 479–90.

Gallo, G. and Buxbaum, J. (1988) Monoclonal immunoglobulin deposition disease: immunopathological aspects of renal involvement. In Minetti, L., d'Amico, G. and Ponticelli, C. (eds), *The Kidney in Plasma Cell Dyscrasias*. Kluwer, Dordrecht, pp. 171–81.

Gaskin, G., Clutterbuck, E.J. and Pusey, C.D. (1987) Renal disease in the Churg–Strauss syndrome. *Contributions to Nephrology* **94**, 58–65.

Gaulier, A., Lucas, G. and Ronco, P. (1990) Tamm Horsfall protein expression by a small renal cell carcinoma presenting with metastases. *Histopathology* **17**, 451–5.

Gejyo, F., Odani, S., Yamada, T., Homma, W.N., Saito, H., Suzuki, Y., Nakagawa, Y., Kobayashi, H., Maruyama, Y., Hirasawa, Y., Suzuki, M. and Arakawa, M. (1986) β2-microglobulin: A new form of amyloid protein associated with chronic hemodialysis. *Kidney International* **30**, 385–90.

Gellman, D.D., Pirani, C.L., Soothill, J.F., Meuhrcke, R.C. and Kark, R.M. (1959) Diabetic nephropathy: A clinical and pathological study based on renal biopsies. *Medicine (Baltimore)* **38**, 321–67.

Gerdes, J., Lemke, H., Baisch, H., Wacker, H., Schwab, U. and Stein, H. (1984) Cell cycle analysis of a cell-proliferation associated human nuclear antigen defined by the monoclonal antibody Ki-67. *Journal of Immunology* **133**, 1710–15.

Ghabra, N. Pirano, B., Greenberg, A and Banner, B. (1991). Resolution of cirrhotic glomerulonephritis following successful liver transplantation. *Clinical Nephrology* **35**, 6–9.

Gladman, D.D., Urowitz, M.B., Cole, E., Ritchie, S., Chang, C.H. and Churg, J. (1989) Kidney biopsy in SLE. I. A clinical-morphological evaluation. *Quarterly Journal of Medicine* **73**, 1125–33.

Glassock, R.J., Kurokawa, K., Yoshida, M., Sakai, O., Okada, M., Shigematsu, H., Ohno, J. and Sakai, H. (1985) IgA nephropathy in Japan. *American Journal of Nephrology* **5**, 127–37.

Glassock, R., Adler, S.G., Ward, H.J. and Cohen A.H. (1991) Primary glomerular diseases. In Brenner, B.M. and Rector, F.C. (eds), *The Kidney (4th edn) Volume 1*. Saunders, Philadelphia, pp. 1182–279.

Glick, A.D., Heung, N.K., Tham, K.J. et al. (1981) Unusual clear cell tumor of the kidney of infancy. *American Journal of Surgical Pathology* **5**, 581–7.

Graves, N. and Barnes, W.F. (1986) Renal cell carcinoma and angiomyolipoma in tuberous sclerosis. Case report. *Journal of Urology* **135**, 122–3.

Gris, P., Pirson, Y., Hamels, J., Baerman, J-P., Quoidbach, A. and Demol, L. (1991) Anti-glomerular basement membrane nephritis induced by IgA1 antibodies. *Nephron* **58**, 418–24.

Grishman, E., Porush, J.C., Rosen, S.M. and Churg, J. (1967) Lupus nephritis with organized deposits in the kidney. *Laboratory Investigation* **16**, 717–22.

Grishman, E., Gerber, J.A. and Churg, J. (1982) Patterns of renal injury in systemic lupus erythematosus: Light and immunofluorescence microscopic observations. *American Journal of Kidney Diseases* **2**, Suppl.1, 135–41.

Grishman, E. and Venkataseshan, V.S. (1988) Vascular lesions in lupus nephritis. *Modern Pathology* **1**, 235–41.

Gubler, M.C. and Habib, R. (1989) Alport's syndrome – hereditary nephritis. In Holliday, M.A., Barratt, T.M. and Vernier, R.L. (eds), *Pediatric Nephrology*, (2nd edn). Williams and Wilkins, Baltimore, pp. 470–6.

Habib, R., Kleinknecht, C., Gubler, M.C. and Levy, M. (1973) Idiopathic membranoproliferative glomerulonephritis in children. Report of 105 cases. *Clinical Nephrology* **1**, 194–214.

Habib, R., Gubler, M.C., Loirat, C., Ben-Maiz, H. and Levy, M. (1975) Dense deposit disease, a variant of membranoproliferative glomerulonephritis. *Kidney International* **7**, 204–15.

Habib, R. and Levy, M. (1983) The hemolytic-uremic syndrome. In Rosen, S. (ed.), *Pathology of Glomerular Disease, Volume 1, Contemporary Issues in Surgical Pathology*. Churchill Livingstone, New York, pp. 239–47.

Habib, R., Girardin, E., Gagnodoux, M.F., Hinglais, N., Levy, M. and Broyer, M. (1988) Immunopathological findings in idiopathic nephrosis: clinical significance of glomerular 'immune deposits'. *Pediatric Nephrology* **2**, 402–8.

Haimoto, H., Takashi, M., Koshikawa, T., Asai, J. and Kato, K. (1986) Enolase isozymes in renal tubules and renal cell carcinoma. *American Journal of Pathology* **124**, 488–95.

Hall, P.A., Levison, D.A., Woods, A.L., Uy, C.C-W., Kellock, D.B., Watkins, J.A., Barnes, D.M., Gillett, C.E., Camplejohn, R., Dover, R., Waseem, N.H. and Lane, D.P. (1990) Proliferating cell nuclear antigen (PCNA) immunolocalization in paraffin sections: An index of cell proliferation with evidence of deregulated expression in some neoplasms. *Journal of Pathology* **162**, 285–94.

Hancock, W.W. and Atkins, R.C. (1984) Cellular composition of crescents in human rapidly progressive glomerulonephritis identified by using monoclonal antibodies. *American Journal of Nephrology* **4**, 177–81.

Harris, S.C., Hird, P.M. and Shortland, J.R. (1989) Immunohistochemistry and lectin histochemistry in sarcomatoid renal cell carcinoma: A comparison with classical renal cell carcinoma. *Histopathology* **15**, 607–16.

Harrison, D.J., Thomson, D. and MacDonald, M.K. (1986) Membranous glomerulonephritis. *Journal of Clinical Pathology* **39**, 167–71.

Haycock, G.B. (1992) The nephritis of Henoch–Schönlein purpura. In Cameron, J.S. Davison, A.M. Grünfeld, J-P, Kerr, D. and Ritz, E. *Oxford Textbook of Clinical Nephrology Volume 1*. Oxford Medical Publications, Oxford, pp. 595–612.

Heaton, J.M., Turner, D.R. and Cameron, J.S. (1977) Localization of glomerular 'deposits' in Henoch–Schönlein nephritis. *Histopathology* **1**, 93–104.

Helin, H., Korpela, M., Mustonen, J. and Pasternack, A. (1986) Mild mesangial glomerulopathy – a frequent finding in rheumatoid arthritis patients with hematuria or proteinura. *Nephron* **42**, 224–30.

Herbert, L.A., Cosio, F.G. and Neff, J.C. (1991) Diagnostic significance of hypocomplementemia. *Kidney International* **39**, 811–21.

Hill, G.S. (1992) Systemic lupus erythematosus and mixed connective-tissue disease. In *Pathology of the Kidney, (4th edn), Volume 2*. Heptinstall, R.H. Little Brown, Boston, pp. 871–951.

Hinglais, N., Kazatchkine, M.D., Bhakdi, S., Appay, M.-D., Mandat, C., Grossetete, J. and Bariety, J. (1986) Immunohistochemical study of the C5b-9 complex of complement in human kidneys. *Kidney International* **30**, 399–410.

Hoffman, G.S., Kerr, G.S., Leavitt, R.Y., Hallahan, C.W., Lebovics, R.S., Travis, W.D., Rottem, M. and Fauci, A.S. (1992) Wegener's granulomatosis: An analysis of 158 patients. *Annals of Internal Medicine* **116**, 488–98.

Hordon, L.D., Sellars, L., Morley, A.R., Wilkinson, R., Thompson, M. and Griffiths, I.D. (1984) Haematuria in rheumatoid arthritis: An association with mesangial glomerulonephritis. *Annals of the Rheumatic Diseases* **43**, 440–3.

Horn, R.G., Fauce, A.S., Rosenthal, A.S. and Wolf, S.M. (1974) Renal biopsy pathology in Wegener's granulomatosis. *American Journal of Pathology* **74**, 423–40.

Howie, A.J. and Brewer, D.B. (1985) Further studies on the glomerular tip lesion: Early and late stages and life table analysis. *Journal of Pathology* **147**, 245–55.

Huppes, W., Hené, R.J. and Kooiker, D.J. (1988) A distinct entity or not? Author's reply. *Journal of Pathology* **154**, 353.

Imbasciati, E., Paties, C., Scarpioni, L. and Mihatsch, M.J. (1986) Renal lesions in familial lecithin-cholesterol acyltransferase deficiency. Ultrastructural heterogeneity of glomerular changes. *American Journal of Nephrology* **6**, 66–70.

International Committee for Nomenclature and Nosology of Renal Disease (1975) *A Handbook of Kidney Nomenclature and Nosology. Criteria for Diagnosis, including Laboratory Procedures*. Little, Brown, Boston, pp. 3–80.

Jackson, E.L., McAdams, A.J.J., Strife, C.G., Forristal, J., Welch, T.R. and West, D.C. (1987) Differences between membranoproliferative glomerulonephritis types I and III in clinical presentation, glomerular morphology and complement perturbation. *American Journal of Kidney Diseases* **9**, 115–20.

Jackson, R., Holme, E.R., Phimister, G.M., Kennedy, A. and McLay, A.L.C. (1990) Immuno-alkaline phosphatase technique applied to paraffix wax embedded tissues in diagnostic renal pathology. *Journal of Clinical Pathology* **43**, 665–70.

Jayne, S.R.W., Weetman, A.P. and Lockwood, C.M. (1991) IgG subclass distribution of autoantibodies to neutrophil cytoplasmic antigens in systemic vasculitis. *Clinical and Experimental Immunology* **84**, 476–81.

Jennette, J.C., Iskandar, S.S. and Dalldorf, F.G. (1983) Pathologic differentiation between lupus and non-lupus membranous glomerulopathy. *Kidney International* **24**, 377–85.

Jennette, J.C. and Hipp, D.G. (1985) Clq nephropathy: A distinct pathologic entity usually causing nephrotic syndrome. *American Journal of Kidney Diseases* **6**, 103–10.

Jennette, J.C., Newman, W.J. and Diaz-Buxo, J.A. (1987) Overlapping IgA and membranous nephropathy. *American Journal of Clinical Pathology* **88**, 74–8.

Jennette, J.C. (1988) The immunohistology of IgA nephropathy. *American Journal of Kidney Diseases* **12**, 348–52.

Jennette, J.C. and Falk, J.J. (1990) Anti-neutrophilic cytoplasmic autoantibodies and associated diseases: A review. *American Journal of Kidney Diseases* **15**, 517–29.

Jennette, J.C. (1991) Anti-neutrophilic cytoplasmic autoantibody-associated diseases: A pathologist's perspective. *American Journal of Kidney Diseases* **18**, 164–70.

Jones, B.A., Shapiro, H.S., Rosenberg, B.F. and Bernstein, J. (1986) Minimal renal amyloidosis with nephrotic syndrome. *Archives of Pathology and Laboratory Medicine* **110**, 889–92.

Jones, D.B. (1977) Membranoproliferative glomerulonephritis: one or many diseases? *Archives of Pathology and Laboratory Medicine* **101**, 457–61.

Joshi, V.V., Kasznica, J. and Walters, T.R. (1986) Atypical mesoblastic nephroma. Pathological characterization of a potentially aggressive variant of conventional congenital mesoblastic nephroma. *Archives of Pathology and Laboratory Medicine* **110**, 100–6.

Julian, B.A., Cannon, V.R., Waldo, F.B. and Egido, J. (1991)

Macroscopic hematuria and proteinuria preceding renal IgA deposition in patients with IgA nephropathy. *American Journal of Kidney Diseases* **17**, 472–9.

Kang, E.T., Yoon, H.J., Han, J.S., Kim, S., Lee, J.S., Kim, Y.I., Hall, W., Dalrymple, J.M. and Peters, C.J. (1990) Demonstration of envelope glycoprotein (EG) of hantaan virus (HV) in Korean haemorrhagic fever (KHF) kidney with monoclonal antibodies (MoAb). *Abstracts of the XIth International Congress of Nephrology, Tokyo*, 13A.

Kaplan, B.S., Cleary, T.G. and Obrig, T.G. (1990) Recent advances in understanding the pathogenesis of the hemolytic uremic syndromes. *Pediatric Nephrology* **4**, 276–83.

Kashgarian, M. and Hayslett, J.P. (1989) Renal involvement in systemic lupus erythematosus. In Tisher, C.C. and Brenner, B.M. (eds), *Renal Pathology with Clinical and Functional Correlations, Volume 1*. J.P. Lippincott, Philadelphia, pp. 380–408.

Kashgarian, M. and Sterzel, R.B. (1992) The pathobiology of the mesangium. *Kidney International* **41**, 524–9.

Kashtan, C.E., Burke, B., Burch, G., Fisker, S.G. and Kim, Y. (1990) Dense intramembranous deposit disease: A clinical comparison of histological types. *Clinical Nephrology* **33**, 1–6.

Keane, W.F., Kasiske, B.L. and O'Donnell, M.P. (1988) Lipids and progressive glomerulosclerosis. *American Journal of Nephrology* **8**, 261–71.

Kelly, C.J. and Neilson, E.G. (1987) Medullary cystic disease: An inherited form of autoiummune interstitial nephritis? *American Journal of Kidney Diseases* **10**, 389–95.

Kennedy, S.M., Merino, M.J., Lineham, W.M. Roberts, J.R., Robertson, C.N. and Neumann, R.D. (1990) Collecting duct carcinoma of the kidney. *Human Pathology* **21**, 449–56.

Kenouch, S. and Mery J-Ph. (1992) Sarcoidosis. In Cameron, S., Davison, A.M., Grünfeld, J-P., Kerr, D. and Ritz, E. (eds), *Oxford Textbook of Clinical Nephrology Vol 1*. Oxford Medical, Oxford, pp. 576–82.

Kim, Y., Vernier, R.L., Fish, A.J. and Michael, A.F. (1979) Immunofluorescence of dense deposit disease. The presence of railroad tracks and mesangial rings. *Laboratory Investigation* **40**, 474–80.

Kincaid-Smith, P. (1975) Participation of intravascular coagulation in the pathogenesis of glomerular and vascular lesions. *Kidney International* **7**, 242–53.

Kincaid-Smith, P. (1987) Part I. Normal structure and classification of idiopathic glomerulonephritis. In Kincaid-Smith, P. and Whitworth, J.A. (eds), *The Kidney, a Clinicopathological Study*, 2nd edn. Blackwell, Oxford, pp. 49–56.

Kincaid-Smith, P., Fairley, K.F. and Kloss, M. (1988) Lupus anti-coagulant associated with thrombotic microangiopathy and pregnancy-related renal failure. *Quarterly Journal of Medicine* **69**, 795–815.

Kincaid-Smith, P., Nicholls, K. and Birchall, I. (1989) Polymorphs infiltrate glomeruli in mesangial IgA glomerulonephritis. *Kidney International* **36**, 1108–12.

King, J.T., Valenzuela, R., McCormack, L.J. and Osborne, D.G. (1978) Granular dense deposit disease. *Laboratory Investigation* **39**, 591–6.

Kitamoto, T., Ogomori, K., Tateishi, J. and Prusiner, S.B. (1987) Formic acid pre-treatment enhances immunostaining of cerebral and systemic amyloids. *Laboratory Investigation* **57**, 230–6.

Kitridou, R.C., Akmal, M., Turkel, S.B., Ehresmann, G.R., Quismorio, F.P.Jr. and Massary, S.G. (1986) Renal involvement in mixed connective tissue disease: A longitudinal clinicopathological study. *Seminars in Arthritis and Rheumatism* **16**, 135–45.

Klein, M., Poucell, S., Arbus, G.S., McGraw, M., Rance, C.P., Yoon, S-J. and Baumal, R. (1983) Characteristics of a benign sub-type of dense deposit disease: comparison with the progressive form of this disease. *Clinical Nephrology* **20**, 163–71.

Koch, K.M. (1992) Nephrology forum: dialysis-related amyloidosis. *Kidney International* **41**, 1416–29.

Korbet, S.M., Schwartz, M.M. and Lewis, E.J. (1991) Immunotactoid glomerulopathy. *American Journal of Kidney Diseases* **17**, 247–57.

Korpela, M., Mustonen, J., Helin, H. and Pasternack, A. (1990) Immunological comparison of patients with rheumatoid arthritis with and without nephropathy. *Annals of the Rheumatic Diseases* **49**, 214–18.

Kumar, S., Marsden, H.B., Carr, T. and Kordet, R. (1985) Mesoblastic nephroma contains fibronectin but lacks laminin. *Journal of Clinical Pathology* **38**, 507–11.

Kumar, S., Carr, T., Marsden, H.B. and Calabuig-Grespo, M.C. (1986) Study of childhood renal tumours using antisera to fibronectin, laminin, and epithelial membrane antigen. *Journal of Clinical Pathology* **39**, 51–7.

Kusumoto, Y., Takebayashi, S., Taguchi, T., Harada, T. and Naito, S. (1987) Long-term prognosis and prognostic indices of IgA nephropathy in juvenile and in adult Japanese. *Clinical Nephrology* **28**, 118–24.

Lamb, V., Tischer, C.C., McCoy, R.C. and Robinson, R.R. (1977) Membranoproliferative glomerulonephritis with dense intramembranous deposits. *Laboratory Investigation* **36**, 607–17.

Lane, P.H., Steffes, M.W. and Mauer, S.M. (1990) Renal histologic changes in diabetes mellitus. *Seminars in Nephrology* **10**, 254–9.

Lapenas, D.J., Drewry, S.J., Luke, R.L. and Leeberg, D.A. (1983) Crescentic light chain glomerulopathy. Report of a case. *Archives of Pathology and Laboratory Medicine* **107**, 319–23.

Larsen, S. (1979) Glomerular immune deposits in kidneys from patients with no clinical or light microscopic evidence of glomerulonephritis. *Acta Pathologica Microbiologica Scandinavica Section A.* **87**, 313–19.

Lehman, D.H., Wilson C.B. and Dixon, F.J. (1975) Extraglomerular immunoglobulin deposits in human nephritis. *The American Journal of Medicine* **58**, 765–86.

Leung, D.Y.M., Moake, J.L., Havens, P.L., Kim, M. and Pober, J.S. (1988) Lytic anti-endothelial cell antibodies in haemolytic-uraemic syndrome. *Lancet* **ii**, 183–6.

Levy, M., Gubler, M.C. and Habib, R. (1979) New concepts on membranoproliferative glomerulonephritis. In Kincaid-Smith, P., D'Apice, A.J.F. and Atkins, R.C. (eds), *Progress in Glomerulonephritis*. Wiley and Sons, New York, pp. 177–205.

Levy, M., Gonzalez-Burchard, G., Broyer, M., Dommergues, J-P., Foulard, M., Sorez, J-P. and Habib, R. (1985) Berger's disease in children. *Medicine (Baltimore)* **64**, 157–80.

Lian, E.G.Y. (1987) Pathogenesis of thrombotic thrombocytopenic purpura. *Seminars in Hematology* **24**, 82–100.

Lie, J.T. (1992) Vasculitis, 1815 to 1991: classification and diagnostic specificity. *Journal of Rheumatology* **19**, 83–9.

Lockwood, C.M. (1991) Anti-neutrophil cytoplasmic autoantibodies: the nephrologists' perspective. *American Journal of Kidney Diseases* **18**, 171–4.

Lofton, S.A., Gown, A.M., Vogel, A.M. and Krieger, J.N. (1989) Differential diagnosis of genitourinary tumors using monoclonal antibodies to intermediate filament proteins. *Urology* **33**, 433–9.

Loirat, C., Sonsino, E., Moreno, A.V., Pillion, G., Mercier, J.C., Beaufils, F. and Mathieu, H. (1984) Hemolytic uremic syndrome: An analysis of the natural history and prognostic features. *Acta Paediatrica Scandinavica* **73**, 505–14.

McEnery, P.T., McAdams, A.J. and West, C.D. (1986) The effect of prednisone in a high-dose, alternative-day regimen on the natural history of idiopathic membranoproliferative glomerulonephritis. *Medicine (Baltimore)* **64**, 401–24.

McEnery, P.T. and McAdams, A.J. (1988) Regression of membranoproliferative type II (dense deposit disease): observations in six children. *American Journal of Kidney Diseases* **12**, 138–46.

MacKay, B., Ordonez, N.G., Khoursand, J. and Bennington, J.L. (1987) The ultrastructure and immunohistochemistry of renal cell carcinoma. *Ultrastructural Pathology* **11**, 483–502.

Mackworth-Young, C. (1990) Antiphospholipid antibodies: more than just a disease marker? *Immunology Today* **11**, 60–5.

Magee, F., Mah, R., Taylor, G.P. and Dimmick, J.E. (1987) Neural differentiation in Wilm's tumour. *Human Pathology* **18**, 33–7.

Magil, A.B. and Cohen, A.H. (1989) Monocytes and focal glomerulosclerosis. *Laboratory Investigation* **61**, 404–9.

Mampaso, F., Leyva-Lobian, F., Martinez-Montero, J.C., Gonzalo, A., Bellas, C., Moneo, I. and Junquera, E. (1983) Mesangial proliferative glomerulonephritis with unusual intramembranous granular dense deposits. *Clinical Nephrology* **19**, 92–8.

Mandalenakis, N., Mendoza, N., Pirani, C.L. and Pollak, V.E. (1971) Lobular glomerulonephritis and membranoproliferative glomerulonephritis. *Medicine (Baltimore)* **50**, 319–54.

Mathew, T.H. (1988) Recurrence of disease following renal transplantation. *American Journal of Kidney Diseases* **12**, 85–96.

Mazzucco, G., Casanova, S., Donini, U., Rollino, C., Zucchelli, P., Piccoli, G. and Monga, G. (1990) Glomerulonephritis with organized deposits: A new clinicopathological entity? Light-electron microscopic and immunofluorescence study of 12 cases. *American Journal of Nephrology* **10**, 21–30.

Medeiros, L.J. Michie, S.A., Johnson, D.E., Warnke, E.A. and Weiss, L.M. (1988) An immunoperoxidase study of renal cell carcinomas: Correlation with nuclear grade, cell type, and histologic pattern. *Human Pathology* **19**, 980–7.

Medeiros, L.J. and Weiss, L.M. (1990) Renal adenocarcinoma. In Eble, J.N. (ed.), *Tumors and Tumor-Like Conditions of the Kidneys and Ureters*. Churchill Livingstone, New York, pp. 35–70.

Mihatsch, M.J., Thiel, G., Spichtin, H.P., Oberholzer, M., Branner, F.P., Harder, F., Olivieri, V., Bremer, R., Ryffel, B., Stöcklin, E., Torhorst, J., Gudat, F., Zollinger, H.U. and Lörtscher, R. (1983) Morphological findings in kidney transplants after treatment with cyclosporin. *Transplantation Proceedings* **15**, 2821–53.

Mihatsch, M.J., Thiel, G. and Ryffel, B. (1988) Morphological diagnosis of cyclosporine A nephrotoxicity. *Seminars in Diagnostic Pathology* **5**, 105–21.

Mihatsch, M.J. and Helmchen, U. (in collaboration with 8 other authors) (1991) Kidney biopsy findings in cyclosporine treated patients with insulin-dependent diabetes mellitus. *Klinische Wochenschrift* **69**, 354–9.

Miller, M., Baumal, R., Poucells, S. and Steele, B.T. (1984) Incidence and prognostic importance of glomerular crescents in renal diseases of childhood. *American Journal of Nephrology* **4**, 244–7.

Minetti, L. (1992) Kidney involvement in plasma cell dyscrasias. In Cameron, J.S., Davison, A.M., Grünfeld, J-P., Kerr, D. and Ritz, E., *Oxford Textbook of Clinical Nephrology Volume 1*. Oxford Medical, Oxford, pp. 562–76.

Modai, D., Pik, A., Behar, M., Eidelman, A., Averbukh, Z., Weissgarten, J., Gabizon, D. and Rosenmann, E. (1985) Biopsy proven evolution of post-streptococcal glomerulonephritis to rapidly progressive glomerulonephritis of a post-infectious type. *Clinical Nephrology* **23**, 198–202.

Moll, R., Robine, S., Dudouet, B. and Louvard, D. (1987) Villin: A cytoskeletal protein and a differentiation marker expressed in some human adenocarcinomas. *Virchows Archiv B Cell Pathology* **54**, 155–69.

Morel-Maroger, L., Kanfer, A., Solez, K., Sraer, J.D. and Richet,

G. (1979) Prognostic importance of vascular lesions in acute renal failure with microangiopathic hemolytic anemia (haemolytic uremic syndrome): Clinicopathological study of 20 adults. *Kidney International* **15**, 548–58.

Morel-Maroger Striker, L., Killen, P.D., Chi, E. and Striker G.E. (1984) The composition of glomerulosclerosis. I. Studies in focal sclerosis, crescentic glomerulonephritis, and membranoproliferative glomerulonephritis. *Laboratory Investigation* **51**, 181–92.

Morgan, B.P., and Walport, M.J. (1991) Complement deficiency and disease. *Immunology Today* **12**, 301–6.

Morozumi, K., Thiel, G., Albert, F.W., Banfi, G., Gudat, F. and Mihatsch, M.J. (1992) Studies on morphological outcome of cyclosporine-associated arteriolopathy after discontinuation of cyclosporine in renal allografts. *Clinical Nephrology* **38**, 1–8.

Mostofi, F.K., Antonovych, T.T. and Limas, E. (1971) Patterns of glomerular reaction to injury. A teaching syllabus. *Human Pathology* **2**, 233–52.

Mrozowicz-Picken, M. and Wrzolkowa, T. (1980) Mesangiocapillary glomerulonephritis in children – electron microscopic studies. *International Journal of Pediatric Nephrology* **1**, 204–10.

Mujais, S.K. and Quintanilla, A. (1988) Chronic tubulointerstitial nephritis: Saga of the ubiquitous. *Seminars in Nephrology* **8**, 4–10.

Müller, G.A., Markovic-Lipkovski, J. and Rodemann, H.P., (1991). The progression of renal diseases: On the pathogenesis of renal interstitial fibrosis. *Klinische Wochenschrift* **69**, 576–86.

Naeye, R.L. (1963) Capillary and venous lesions in myxedema. *Laboratory Investigation* **12**, 465–70.

Nast, C.A., Colodro, I.H. and Cohen, A.H. (1986) Splenic immune deposits in bacterial endocarditis. *Clinical Immunology and Immunopathology* **40**, 209–13.

Neilson, E.G. (1989) Pathogenesis and therapy of interstitial nephritis. *Kidney International* **35**, 1257–70.

Nevins, T.E., (1985) Lectin binding in membranoproliferative glomerulonephritis. *American Journal of Pathology* **118**, 325–30.

Newell, G.C., (1987) Cirrhotic glomerulonephritis: Incidence, morphology, clinical features and pathogenesis. *American Journal of Kidney Diseases* **9**, 183–90.

Ng, W.L., Chan, K.W., Yeung, C.K. and Kwan, S. (1984) Peripheral glomerular capillary wall lesions in IgA nephropathy and their implications. *Pathology* **16**, 324–30.

Nizze, H., Mihatsch, M.J., Zollinger, H.U., Brocheriou, C., Gokel, J.M., Henry, K., Sloane, J.P. and Stovin, P.G. (1988) Cyclosporine-associated nephropathy in patients with heart and bone marrow transplants. *Clinical Nephrology* **30**, 248–60.

Nochy, D., Callard, P., Bellon, B., Bariety, J. and Druet, P. (1976) Association of overt glomerulonephritis and liver disease: A study of 34 patients. *Clinical Nephrology* **6**, 422–7.

Noël, L-H., Droz, D. and Ganeval, D. (1987) Immunohistochemical characterization of renal amyloidosis. *American Journal of Clinical Pathology* **87**, 756–61.

Noël, L.F., Geffriaud, D.C., Chauveau, D., Houhou, S., Landais, P., Khiraoui, F., Nusbaum, P., Gouarin, C., O'Donohue, D., Halbwachs-Mecarelli, L., Grünfeld, J.P. et Lesavre, P. (1992) Anticorps anticytoplasme des neutrophiles (ANCA): Associations cliniques et aspects immunologiques. In Funck-Brentano, J.L., Bach, J.F., Kreis, H. et Grünfeld, J.P. Flammarion (eds), *Actualités Néphrologiques Jean Hamburger*. Paris, pp. 223–53.

Nolasco, F.E.B., Cameron, J.S., Hartley, B., Coelino, A., Hildreth, G. and Reuben, R. (1987) Intraglomerular T cells and monocytes in nephritis: Study with monoclonal antibodies. *Kidney International* **31**, 1160–7.

Nyberg, G., Hedman, L., Blohme, T. and Svalander, C. (1992) Morphological findings in baseline kidney biopsies from living related donors. *Transplantation Proceedings* **24**, 355–6.

O'Donohue, D.J., Lawler, W., Hunt, L.P., Acheson, E.J. and Mallick, N.P. (1991) IgM associated primary diffuse mesangial proliferative glomerulonephritis: Natural history and prognostic indicators. *Quarterly Journal of Medicine* **79**, 333–50.

Ohi, H. and Tanuma, Y. (1992) Does nephritic factor relate to the disease activity in hypocomplementemic membranoproliferative glomerulonephritis. *Nephron* **62**, 116.

Ohi, H., Watanabe, S., Fujita, T. and Yasugi, T (1992a) Significance of C3 nephritic factor (C3 NeF) in non-hypocomplementaemic serum with membranoproliferative glomerulonephritis (MPGN). *Clinical and Experimental Immunology* **89**, 479–84.

Olsen, T.S., Petersen, V.P. and Hansen, H.S. (1974) Immunofluorescence studies of extracapillary glomerulonephritis. *Acta Pathologica Microbiologica Scandinavica, Section*, **A 249**, Suppl.20–8.

Olsen, T.S. (1992) Pathology of allograft rejection. In Burdick, J.F., Racusen, L.C., Solez, K. and Williams, G.M., *Kidney Transplant Rejection, Diagnosis and Treatment*, 2nd edn. Marcel Dekker, New York, pp. 333–57.

Onetti Muda, A., Barsotti, P. and Marinozzi, V. (1988) Ultrastructural histochemical investigations of 'dense deposit disease'. Pathogenetic approach to a special type of mesangiocapillary glomerulonephritis. *Virchows Archiv A Pathological Anatomy* **413**, 529–37.

Oosterwijk, E., Van Muijen, G.N.P., Oosterwijk-Wakka, J.C. et al. (1990) Expression of intermediate-sized filaments in developing and adult human kidney and in renal cell carcinoma. *Journal of Histochemistry and Cytochemistry* **38**, 385–92.

Ormos, J., Magori, A., Sonkodo, S. and Strizmann, K. (1979) Type II membranoproliferative glomerulonephritis with electron dense basement membrane alteration in the spleen. *Archives of Pathology and Laboratory Medicine* **103**, 265–6.

Ortmann, M., Vierbuchen, M. and Fischer, R. (1991) Sialylated glycoconjugates in chromophobe cell renal carcinoma compared with other renal cell tumors. *Virchows Archives (B, Cell Pathology)* **61**, 123–32.

Ozawa, K., Yamabe, H., Fukushi, K., Osawa, H., Chiba, N., Miyata, M., Seino, S., Inuma, H., Sasaki, T., Yoshikawa, S. and Onodera, K. (1991) Case report of amyloidosis-like glomerulopathy with hepatic involvement. *Nephron* **58**, 347–50.

Parfrey, P.S., Hutchinson, T.A., Jothy, S., Cramer, B.C., Matin, J., Hanley, J.A. and Seely, J.F. (1985) The spectrum of diseases associated with necrotizing glomerulonephritis and its prognosis. *American Journal of Kidney Diseases* **6**, 387–96.

Peake, P.W., Pussell, B.A., Karplus, T.E., Riley, E.H. and Charlesworth, J.A. (1991) Post-streptococcal glomerulonephritis: Studies on the interaction between nephritis strain-associated protein (NSAP), complement and the glomerulus. *Acta Pathologica et Microbiologica Scandinavica* **99**, 460–6.

Peng, S-K., French, W.J., Cohen, A.H. and Fausel, R.E. (1988) Light chain cardiomyopathy associated with small-vessel disease. *Archives of Pathology and Laboratory Medicine* **112**, 844–6.

Perez-Fontan, M., Huarie, E., Tellez, A., Rodriquez-Carmona, A., Picazo, M.L. and Martinez-Ara, J. (1988) Glomerular nephropathy associated with chronic Q fever. *American Journal of Kidney Diseases* **11**, 298–306.

Perry, G.J., George, C.R.P., Field, M., Collett, P.V., Kalowski, S., Wyndham, R.N., Newland, R.C., Lin, B.P.C., Kneale, L.L. and Lawrence, J.R. (1989) Thin membrane nephropathy – a common cause of glomerular haematuria. *Medical Journal of Australia* **151**, 638–42.

Peters, D.K. and Williams, D.G. (1974) Complement and mesangiocapillary glomerulonephritis: Role of complement deficiency in the pathogenesis of nephritis. *Nephron* **13**, 189–97.

Pettersson, E., Törnroth, T. and Wieslander, J. (1990) Abnormally thin glomerular basement membrane and the Goodpasture epitope. *Clinical Nephrology* **33**, 105–9.

Pettersson, E. and Heigl, Z. (1992) Anti-neutrophil cytoplasmic antibody (CANCA and PANCA) titers in relation to disease activity in patients with necrotizing vasculitis: A longitudinal study. *Clinical Nephrology* **37**, 219–28.

Pinkus, G.S. and Kurtin, P.J. (1985) Epithelial membrane antigen – a diagnostic discriminant in surgical pathology. *Human Pathology* **16**, 929–40.

Pinkus, G.S., Etheridge, C.L. and O'Connor, E.M. (1986) Are keratin proteins a better tumor marker than epithelial membrane antigen? *American Journal of Clinical Pathology* **85**, 269–77.

Prasad, D.R., Zimmerman, S.W. and Burkholder, P.M. (1977) Immunohistological features of minimal change nephrotic syndrome. *Archives of Pathology and Laboratory Medicine* **101**, 345–9.

Praz, F., Halbwachs, L. and Lesavre, P. (1984) Genetic aspects of complement and glomerulonephritis. *Advances in Nephrology* **13**, 271–96.

Priz, S., Moll, R., Störkel, S. and Thoenes, W. (1987) Expression of intermediate filament proteins in subtypes of renal cell carcinomas and in renal oncocytomas. Distinction of two classes of renal cell tumours. *Laboratory Investigation* **56**, 642–53.

Querin, S., Noël, L.H., Grünfeld, J-P., Droz, D., Mathieu, P. and Berger, J. (1986) Linear glomerular IgG fixation in renal allografts: Incidence and significance in Alport's syndrome. *Clinical Nephrology* **25**, 134–40.

Rambausek, M., Waldherr, R., Rauterberg, W., Andrassy, K. and Ritz, E. (1987) Mesangial IgA nephropathy and idiopathic nephrotic syndrome. *Nephron* **47**, 190–3.

Rees, A.J. and Cameron, J.S. (1992) Crescentic glomerulonephritis. In Cameron, J.S., Davison, A.M., Grünfeld, J-P., Kerr, D. and Ritz, E.(eds), *Oxford Textbook of Clinical Nephrology, Volume 1*. Oxford Medical, Oxford, pp. 418–38.

Remynse, L.C., Begun, F.P., Jacobs, S.C. and Lawson, R.K. (1989) Juxtaglomerular cell tumor with elevation of serum erythropoietin. *Journal of Urology* **142**, 1560–2.

Rennke, H.G. and Klein, P.S. (1989) Pathogenesis and significance of non-primary focal and segmental glomerulosclerosis. *American Journal of Kidney Diseases* **13**, 443–56.

Richards, N.T., Lueck, C., Davies, D.R., Jones, N.F., Alkhader, A. and Coode, P. (1988) Anti-glomerular membrane antibody and linear glomerular immunofluorescence in a patient with systemic lupus erythematosus. *Clinical Nephrology* **30**, 115–16.

Rodriguez-Iturbe, B. (1992) Acute endocapillary glomerulonephritis. In Cameron, J.S., Davison, A.M., Grünfeld, J-P., Kerr, D. and Ritz, E. (eds), *Oxford Textbook of Clinical Nephrology, Volume 1*. Oxford University Press, Oxford pp. 405–17.

Rosen, S., Törnroth, T. and Bernard, D.B., (1989) Membranous glomerulonephritis. In Tisher, C.C. and Brenner, S.M. (eds), *Renal Pathology with Clinical and Functional Correlations, Volume 1*. Lippincott, Philadelphia, pp. 196–227.

Rosenberg, H.G., Vial, S.U., Pomeroy, J., Figueroa, S., Donoso, P.L. and Carranza, C. (1985) Acute glomerulonephritis in children. An evolutive morphologic and immunologic study of the glomerular inflammation. *Pathology Research and Practice* **180**, 633–45.

Rosenmann, E. and Eliakim, M. (1977) Nephrotic syndrome associated with amyloid-like glomerular deposits. *Nephron* **18**, 301–8.

Ross, J.B., Cohen, A.D. and Ghose, T. (1985) Goodpasture's syndrome associated with skin involvement. *Archives of Dermatology* **121**, 1442–4.

Rother, K., Hänsch, G.M. and Rauterberg, E.W. (1991) Complement in inflammation: Induction of nephritides and progress to chronicity. *International Archives of Allergy and Applied Immunology* **94**, 23–37.

Rumpelt, H.J., Storkel, S., Moll, R., Scharfe, T. and Thoenes, W. (1991) Bellini duct carcinoma: Further evidence for this rare variant of renal cell carcinoma. *Histopathology* **18**, 115–22.

Sabadini, E., Castiglione, A., Colasanti, G., Ferrario, F., Civardi, R., Fellin, G. and D'Amico, G. (1988) Characterization of interstitial infiltrating cells in Berger's disease. *American Journal of Kidney Diseases* **12**, 307–15.

Sakai, H. (1991) IgA nephropathy: Recent views on pathogenesis and treatment. In Hatano, M. (ed.), *Nephrology Proceedings of the XIth International Congress of Nephrology*. Springer-Verlag, Tokyo, pp. 62–76.

Salinas-Madrigal, L. and Torlani, A.S. (1988) Morphologic diagnosis of proteinuria – nephrotic syndrome. *Seminars in Diagnostic Pathology* **5**, 38–62.

Salm, R. (1969) Combined intestinal and squamous metaplasia of the renal pelvis. *Journal of Clinical Pathology* **22**, 187–91.

Sato, H., Saito, T., Seino, J., Ootaka, T., Kyogoku, Y., Furuyana, T. and Yoshinaga, K. (1987) Dense deposit disease: Its possible pathogenesis suggested by an observation of a patient. *Clinical Nephrology* **27**, 41–5.

Sato, H., Suzuki, S., Kobayashi, H., Ogino, S., Inomata, A. and Arakawa, M. (1991) Immunohistochemical localization of apolipoproteins in the glomeruli in renal disease: Specifically apo B and apo E. *Clinical Nephrology* **36**, 127–33.

Savage, C.O.S., Pusey, C.D., Kershaw, M.J., Cashman, S.J., Harrison, P., Hartley, B., Turner, D.R., Cameron, J.S., Evans, D.J. and Lockwood, C.M. (1986) The Goodpasture antigen in Alport's syndrome: Studies with a monoclonal antibody. *Kidney International* **30**, 107–12.

Savige, J., Yeung, S.P., Bierre, A.R. and Kincaid-Smith, P. (1989) Lambda-light-chain-mediated anti-GBM disease. *Nephron* **52**, 144–8.

Savige, J.A., Mavrova, L. and Kincaid-Smith, P. (1989) Inhibitable anti-GBM antibody activity after renal transplantation in Alport's syndrome. *Transplantation* **48**, 704–5.

Savige, J.A., Dowling, J.P. and Kincaid-Smith, P. (1989) Superimposed glomerular immune complexes in anti-glomerular basement membrane disease. *American Journal of Kidney Diseases* **14**, 145–53.

Saxena, S., Davies, D.J. and Kirsner, R.L.G. (1990) Thin basement membranes in minimally abnormal glomeruli. *Journal of Clinical Pathology* **43**, 32–8.

Schena, F.P. (1992) IgA nephropathies. In Cameron, J.S., Davison, A.M., Grünfeld, H-P., Kerr, D. and Ritz, E. (eds), *Oxford Textbook of Clinical Nephrology, Volume 1*. Oxford Medical, Oxford, pp. 339–69.

Schmidt, D., Levschner, I., Harms, D., Sprenger, E. and Schäfer, H-J. (1989) Malignant rhabdoid tumor. A morphological and flow cytometric study. *Pathology Research and Practice* **184**, 202–10.

Schmitt, H., Bohle, A., Reineke, T., Mayer-Eischberger, D. and Vogl, W. (1990) Long-term prognosis of membranoproliferative glomerulonephritis type I. Significance of clinical and morphological parameters: An investigation of 220 cases. *Nephron* **55**, 242–50.

Schwartz, M.M., Kawala, K., Robert, J.L., Humes, C. and Lewis, E.J. (1984) Clinical and pathological features of membranous glomerulonephritis of systemic lupus erythematosus. *American Journal of Nephrology* **4**, 301–11.

Schwartz, M.M. and Lewis, E.J. (1985) Focal segmental glomerular sclerosis: The cellular lesion. *Kidney International* **28**, 968–74.

Schwartz, M.M., Lan, S-P., Bonsib, S.M., Gephardt, G.N., Sharma, H.M. and the Lupus Nephritis Collaborative Study Group. (1989) Clinical outcome of three discrete histological patterns of injury in severe lupus glomerulonephritis. *American Journal of Kidney Diseases* **13**, 273–83.

Serra, A., Cameron, J.S., Turner, D.R., Hartley, B., Ogg, C.S., Neild, G.H., Williams, D.G., Taube, D., Brown, C.B. and Hicks, J.A. (1984) Vasculitis affecting the kidney: Presentation, histopathology and long-term outcome. *Quarterly Journal of Medicine* **53**, 165–80.

Seymour, A.E., Canny, A. and Spargo, B.H. (1983) Thickening of glomerular capillary walls: A guide to differential diagnosis of electron microscopy. *Ultrastructural Pathology* **4**, 123–43.

Shah, B., First, M.R., Mendoza, N.C., Clyne, D.H., Alexander, J.W. and Weiss, M.A. (1988) Alport's syndrome: Risk of glomerulonephritis induced by anti-glomerular basement membrane antibody after transplantation. *Nephron* **30**, 34–8.

Shah, S.V. (Editor) (1991) Mechanisms of glomerular injury. *Seminars in Nephrology* **11**, 259–372.

Shearn, M.A., Biava, C. and Hopper J.Jr. (1979) Mesangial deposits (by electron microscopy) in idiopathic membranous glomerulonephritis. *New England Journal of Medicine* **301**, 212.

Shirahama, T., Skinner, J., Cohen, A.S., Gejyo, F., Arakawa, M., Suzuki, M. and Hirasawa, Y. (1985) Histochemical and immunohistochemical characterization of amyloid associated with chronic hemodialysis as B2–microglobulin. *Laboratory*

Investigation **53**, 705–9.

Sibley, R.K. and Kim, Y. (1984) Dense intramembranous deposit disease: New pathological features. *Kidney International* **25**, 660–70.

Silva, F.G., Chander, P., Pirani, C.L. and Hardy, M.A. (1982) Disappearance of glomerular mesangial IgA deposits after renal allograft transplantation. (Letter) *Transplantation* **33**, 214–16.

Silva, F.G. and Hogg, R.J. (1989) IgA nephropathy. In Tisher, C.C. and Brenner, B.M. (eds), *Renal Pathology and Clinical and Functional Correlations, Volume 1*. Lippincott, Philadelphia, pp. 434–93.

Sinniah, R. and Cohen, A.H. (1985) Glomerular capillary aneurysms in light chain nephropathy: An ultrastructural proposal of pathogenesis. *American Journal of Pathology* **118**, 298–305.

Smith, M.C., Cooke, J.H., Zimmerman, D.M., Bird, J.J., Feaster, B.L., Morrison, R.E. and Reimann, B.E.F. (1979) Asymptomatic glomerulonephritis after non-streptococcal upper respiratory infections. *Annals of Internal Medicine* **91**, 697–702.

Someren, A., Zaatari, G.S., Campbell, W.G. Jr., Parrott, T., White, J.M. Jr., Baumgartner, B.R., Atkinson, G.O. Jr., Graham, S.D. Jr., Woodard, J.R., Chezmar, J.L., Wyly, J.B., Fekete, P.S. and Hertzler, G. (1989) The kidney. In Someren, A. (ed.), *Urologic Pathology with Clinical and Radiologic Correlations*. Macmillan, New York, p. 214.

Sorger, K., Gessler, M., Hübner, F.K., Köhler, H., Schulz, W., Stühlinger, W., Thoenes, G.H. and Thoenes, W. (1982) Subtypes of acute post-infectious glomerulonephritis. Synopsis of clinical and pathological studies. *Clinical Nephrology* **17**, 1–14.

Sorger, K., Balun, J., Hübner, F.K., Köhler, H., Olbing, H., Schulz, W., Seybold, D., Thoenes, G.H. and Thoenes, W. (1983) The garland type of acute post-infectious glomerulonephritis: Morphological characteristics and follow-up studies. *Clinical Nephrology* **20**, 17–26.

Sorger, K., Gessler, M., Hübner, F.K., Köhler, H., Olbing, H., Schulz, W., Thoenes, G.H. and Thoenes, W. (1987) Follow-up studies of three subtypes of acute post-infectious glomerulonephritis ascertained by renal biopsy. *Clinical Nephrology* **27**, 111–24.

Sotelo-Avila, C. (1989) Nephroblastoma and other pediatric renal cancers. In Eble, J.N. (ed.), *Tumors and Tumor-Like Conditions of the Kidneys and Ureters*. Churchill Livingstone, New York, pp. 94–9.

Southwest Pediatric Nephrology Study Group (1985) Dense deposit disease in children: Prognostic value of clinical and pathological indicators. *American Journal of Kidney Diseases* **6**, 161–9.

Southwest Pediatric Nephrology Study Group (1986) Comparison of idiopathic and systemic lupus erythematosus-associated membranous glomerulopathy in children. *American Journal of Kidney Diseases* **7**, 115–24.

Stave, G.M. and Croker, B.P. (1984) Thrombotic microangiopathy in anti-glomerular basement membrane glomerulonephritis. *Archives of Pathology and Laboratory Medicine* **108**, 747–51.

Stone, G.C., Wall, B.A., Oppliger, I.R., Wener, M.H., Jolly, S.L., Aguirre, A., Dwyer, R. and Simkin, P.A. (1989) A vasculopathy with deposition of lambda light chain crystals. *Annals of Internal Medicine* **110**, 275–8.

Stone, M.J. (1990) Amyloidosis: A final common pathway for protein deposition in tissues. *Blood* **75**, 531–45.

Störkel, S., Steart, P.V., Drenckhahn, D. and Thoenes, W. (1989) The human · chromophobe cell renal carcinoma: Its probable relation to intercalated cells of the collecting duct. *Virchows Archiv B Cell Pathology* **56**, 237–45.

Strife, C.F., McEnery, P.T., McAdams, A.J. and West, C.D. (1977) Membranoproliferative glomerulonephritis with disruption of the glomerular basement membrane. *Clinical Nephrology* **7**, 65–72.

Strife, C.F., Jackson, E.C. and McAdams, A.J. (1984) Type III membranoproliferative glomerulonephritis: Long-term clinical and morphological evaluation. *Clinical Nephrology* **21**, 323–34.

Sullivan, W.D., Hurst, D.J. and Harmon, C.E. (1984) A prospective evaluation emphasizing pulmonary involvement in patients with mixed connective tissue disease. *Medicine (Baltimore)* **63**, 92–107.

Suzuki, S., Sato, H., Kobayashi, H., Takayama, R., Maruyama, Y., Ogino, S., Ueno, H., Inomata, A., Nishi, S., Saito, T., In, H. and Arakawa, M (1992) Comparative study of IgA nephropathy with acute and insidious onset. *American Journal of Nephrology* **12**, 22–8.

Taguchi, T. and Bohle, A. (1989) Evaluation of change with time of glomerular morphology in membrane proliferative glomerulonephritis: A serial biopsy study of 33 cases. *Clinical Nephrology* **31**, 297–306.

Takada, Y., Hiwada, K., Yokoyama, M., Ochi, K., Takeuchi, M. and Kokubu, T. (1985) Angiotensin converting enzyme – a possible histological indicator for human renal cell carcinoma. *Cancer* **56**, 130–33.

Takashi, M., Haimoto, H., Murase, T., Mitsuya, H. and Kato, K. (1988) An immunohistochemical and immunohistochemical study of S100 protein in renal cell carcinoma. *Cancer* **61**, 889–95.

Takekoshi, Y., Tochimaru, H., Nagata, Y. and Itami, N. (1991) Immunopathogenetic mechanisms of hepatitis B virus-related glomerulopathy. *Kidney International* **40**, Suppl. 1, S.34–S.39.

Tallqvist, G., Törnroth, T., Vanttinen, T. and Pasternack, A. (1979) Vacuolization of the glomerular basement membrane. *Acta Pathologica Microbiologica Scandinavica Section A*, **87**,

411–19.

Tanuma, Y., Ohi, H., Watanabe, S., Seki, M. and Hatano, M. (1989) C3 nephritic factor and C4 nephritic factor in the serum of two patients with hypocomplementaemic membranopliferative glomerulonephritis. *Clinical and Experimental Immunology* **76**, 82–5.

Tanuma, Y., Ohi, H. and Hatano, M. (1990) Two types of C3 nephritic factor: Properdin-dependent C3NeF and properdin-independent C3NeF. *Clinical Immunology and Immunopathology* **56**, 226–38.

Teague, C.A., Doak, P.B., Simpson, I.J., Rainer, S.P. and Herdson, P.B. (1978) Goodpasture's syndrome: An analysis of 29 cases. *Kidney International* **13**, 492–504.

Tejani, A. and Ingulli, E. (1990) Post-streptococcal glomerulonephritis. Current clinical and pathological concepts. *Nephron* **55**, 1–5.

ten Berge, I.J.M., Wilmink, J.M., Meyer, C.J.L.M., Surachno, J., ten Veen, K.H., Balk, T.G. and Schellenkens, P.Th.A. (1985) Clinical and immunological follow-up of patients with severe renal disease in Wegener's granulomatosis. *American Journal of Nephrology* **5**, 21–9.

Tetu, B., Ro, J.Y., Ayala, A.G., Ordonez, N.G. and Johnson, D.E. (1987) Small cell carcinoma of the kidney. A clinicopathological, immunhistochemical and ultrastructural study. *Cancer* **60**, 1809–14.

Thoenes, W., Störkel, S.T. and Rumpelt, H.J. (1986) Histopathology and classification of renal cell tumors, (adenomas, oncocytomas and carcinomas) - the basic cytological and histopathological elements and their use for diagnostics. *Pathology Research and Practice* **181**, 125–43.

Thoenes, W., Störkel, S.T., Rumpelt, H.J., Moll, R., Baum, H.P. and Werner, S. (1988) Chromophobe cell renal carcinoma and its variants – a report on 32 cases. *Journal of Pathology* **155**, 227–87.

Thomson, O.F. and Ladefoged, J. (1991) Glomerular tip lesions in renal biopsies with focal segmental IgM. *Acta Pathologica, Microbiologica et Immunologica Scandinavica* **99**, 836–43.

Tiebosch, A.T.M.G, Frederik, P.M., Van Breda, Vriesman, P.J.C., Mooy, J.M.V., Van Rie, H., Van De Wiel, T.W.M., Wolters, J. and Zeppenfeldt, E. (1989) Thin basement membrane nephropathy in adults with persistent hematuria. *New England Journal of Medicine* **320**, 14–18.

Tipping, P.G., Dowling, J.P. and Holdsworth, S.R. (1988) Glomerular procoagulant activity in human proliferative glomerulonephritis. *Journal of Clinical Investigation* **81**, 119–25.

Tisher, C.C. and Hostetter, T.H. (1989) Diabetic nephropathy. In Tisher, C.C. and Brenner, B.M. (eds), *Renal Pathology with Clinical and Functional Correlations, Volume 2*. Lippincott, Philadelphia, pp. 1309–34.

Tomita, T., Poisner, A. and Inagami, T. (1987) Immunohistochemical localization of renin in renal tumors. *American Journal of Pathology* **126**, 73–80.

Tuma, S.N., Llach, F., Sostrin, S., Dubois, E.L. and Massry, S.G. (1981) Glomerular IgE deposits in patients with lupus nephritis. *American Journal of Nephrology* **1**, 31–6.

Turner, N. and Rees, A.J. (1992) Anti-glomerular basement membrane disease. In Cameron, S., Davison, A., Grünfeld, J-P., Kerr, D. and Ritz, E. (eds), *Oxford Textbook of Clinical Nephrology, Volume 1*. Oxford Medical Publishers, Oxford, pp. 438–56.

Ueda, Y., Ono, Y., Sagiya, A., Kanaya, H. and Iidaka, K. (1992) Mesangial anionic sites are decreased in human focal glomerular sclerosis. *Clinical Nephrology* **37**, 280–4.

Van Krieken, J.H.J.M., Oosterwijk, E., Lycklama, A., Nijeholt, A.A.B. and Ruiter, D.J. (1988) Renal oncocytoma – a report of two cases with immunohistochemical evaluation. *Human Pathology* **19**, 460–4.

Varade, W.S., Forristal, J. and West, C.D. (1990) Patterns of complement activation in idiopathic membranoproliferative glomerulonephritis, types I, II and III. *American Journal of Kidney Diseases* **16**, 196–206.

Velosa, J., Miller, K. and Michael, A.F. (1976) Immunopathology of the end-stage kidney. Immunoglobulin and complement component deposition in non-immune disease. *American Journal of Pathology* **84**, 149–62.

Verani, R.R., Flechner, S.M., Van Buren, C.T. and Kahan, B.D. (1984) Acute cellular rejection or cyclosporine A nephrotoxicity? A review of transplant renal biopsies. *American Journal of Kidney Diseases* **4**, 185–91.

Versluis, D.J., Ten Kate, F.J.W., Wenting, G.J., Jeekel, J. and Weimar, W. (1988) Histological lesions associated with cyclosporin: Incidence and reversibility in one year old kidney transplants. *Journal of Clinical Pathology* **41**, 498–503.

Wada, N., Ueda, Y., Iidaka, K., Inage, Z., Kikkawa, Y. and Katagawa, T. (1990) Portion of basement membrane with decreased negative charge in various glomerulonephritides. *Clinical Nephrology* **34**, 9–16.

Wakai, S. and Magil, A.B. (1992) Focal glomerulosclerosis in idiopathic membranous glomerulonephritis. *Kidney International* **41**, 428–34.

Waldherr, R., Gubler, M., Levy, M., Broyer, M. and Habib, R. (1978) The significance of pure diffuse mesangial proliferation in idiopathic nephrotic syndrome. *Clinical Nephrology* **10**, 171–9.

Waldmann, T.A., Rosse, W.F. and Swarm, R.L. (1968) The erythropoietic-stimulating factors produced by tumors. *Annals of the New York Academy of Science* **149**, 509–15.

Wall, R.T. and Harker, L.A. (1980) The endothelium and thrombosis. *Annual Review of Medicine* **31**, 361–71.

Wallace, A.C. and Nairn, R.C. (1972) Renal tubular antigens in kidney tumors. *Cancer* **29**, 977–81.

Wannamaker, L.W. (1970) Differences between streptococcal infections of the throat and of the skin. *New England Journal of Medicine* **282**, 23–30; 78–85.

Webber, B.L., Parkham, D.M., Drake, L.G. and Wilimas, J.A. (1992) Renal tumors in childhood. In *Pathology Annual Volume 27, Pt. 2*. Appleton and Lange, Norwalk, pp. 191–232.

Weber, M., Köhler, H., Fries, J., Thoenes, W. and Meyer Zum Büschenfelde, K-H. (1985) Rapidly progressive glomerulonephritis in IgA/IgG cryoglobulinaemia. *Nephron* **41**, 258–61.

Weeks, D.A., Beckwith, J.B., Merau, G.W. and Luckey, D.W. (1989) Rhabdoid tumor of kidney: A report of 111 cases from the national Wilm's tumor study pathology center. *American Journal of Surgical Pathology* **13**, 439–58.

Weeks, D.A., Beckwith, J.B., Mierau, G.W. and Zuppan, C.W. (1991) Renal neoplasms mimicking rhabdoid tumor of kidney. A report from the national Wilm's Tumor Study Pathology Center. *American Journal of Surgical Pathology* **15**, 1042–54.

Weiss, M.A. and Crissman, J.D. (1984) Renal biopsy findings in Wegener's granulomatosis. Segmental necrotizing glomerulonephritis with glomerular thrombosis. *Human Pathology* **15**, 943–56.

Welch, T.R., Kleesattel, A. and Beischel, I. (1988) Inhibition of immune complex solubilization by sera of patients with membranoproliferative glomerulonephritis. *Clinical and Experimental Immunology* **72**, 103–7.

West, C.D., (1992) Invited review. Idiopathic membranoproliferative glomerulonephritis in childhood. *Pediatric Nephrology* **6**, 96–103.

Westberg, N.G. and Michael, A.F. (1972) Immunohistopathology of diabetic glomerulosclerosis. *Diabetes* **21**, 163–74.

Wick, M.R., Perrone, T.L. and Burke, B. (1985) Sarcomatoid transitional cell carcinomas of the renal pelvis. An ultrastructural and immunohistochemical study. *Archives of Pathology and Laboratory Medicine* **109**, 55–8.

Wick, M.R., Cherwitz, D.L., Manivel, J.C. and Sibley, R. (1990) Immunohistochemical findings in tumors of the kidney. In Eble, J.N. (ed.), *Tumors and Tumor-Like Conditions of the Kidneys and Ureters*. Churchill Livingstone, New York, pp. 207–46.

Wieslander, J. (1991) How are anti-neutrophil cytoplasmic autoantibodies detected? *American Journal of Kidney Diseases* **18**, 154–8.

Wilson, C.B. and Dixon, F.J. (1986) The renal response to immunological injury. In Brenner, B.M. and Rector, F.C. (eds), *The Kidney, Volume 1* (3rd edn) Saunders, Philadelphia, pp. 800–89.

Wilson, C.B. (1991) The renal response to immunological injury. In Brenner, B.M. and Rector, F.C. (eds), *The Kidney Volume 1* (4th edn). Saunders, Philadelphia, pp. 1062–181.

Wilson, C.B. (1991a) Nephritogenic tubulointerstitial antigens. *Kidney International* **39**, 501–17.

Wolf, B.C., Kumar, A. and Vera, J.C. (1986) Bone marrow morphology and immunology in systemic amyloidosis. *American Journal of Clinical Pathology* **86**, 84–8.

Wright, J.R., Calkins, E. and Humphrey, R.L. (1977) Potassium permanganate reaction in amyloidosis, a histologic method to assist in differentiating forms of this disease. *Laboratory Investigation* **36**, 274–81.

Yamase, H.T., Gillies, C. and Kaplan, A.A. (1988) Glomerular spherical electron dense deposits in a patient undergoing long-term regional heparinization. *American Journal of Kidney Diseases* **12**, 227–32.

Yoshida, S.O., Imam, A., Olson, C.A. and Taylor, C.R. (1986) Proximal renal tubular surface membrane antigens identified in primary and metastatic renal cell carcinomas. *Archives of Pathology and Laboratory Medicine* **110**, 825–32.

Yoshikawa, N., Yoshiara, S., Yoshiya, K., Matsuo, T., Matsuyama, S. and Okada, S. (1988) Focal and diffuse membranoproliferative glomerulonephritis in children. *American Journal of Nephrology* **8**, 102–7.

Yoshikawa, N., Matsuyama, S., Iijima, K., Maehara, K., Okada, S. and Matsuo T. (1988) Benign familial hematuria. *Archives of Pathology and Laboratory Medicine* **112**, 794–7.

Yoshikawa, Y., Truong, L.D., Nattioli, C. and Cartwright, J.Jr. (1990) Renal amyloidosis characterized by abnormally thick fibres. *Human Pathology* **21**, 868–71.

Yoshimura, M., Kida, H., Abe, T., Takeda, S-I., Katagiri, M. and Hattori, N. (1987) Significance of IgA deposits on the glomerular capillary walls in IgA nephropathy. *American Journal of Kidney Diseases* **9**, 404–9.

Yoshioka, K., Takemura, T., Akano, N., Miyamoto, H., Iseki, T. and Maki, S. (1987) Cellular and non-cellular compositions of crescents in human glomerulonephritis. *Kidney International* **32**, 284–91.

Zamarovic, D. and Churg, J. (1984) Idiopathic and secondary mesangiocapillary glomerulonephritis. *Nephron* **38**, 145–53.

Zawada, E.T. Jr. (1989) The aging kidney. In Massry S.G. and Glassock R.J. (eds), *Textbook of Nephrology Volume 2*. Williams and Wilkins, Baltimore, pp. 996–1002.

Zerban, G., Nogueira, E., Riedasch, G. and Bannasch, P. (1987) Renal oncocytoma: Origin from the collecting duct. *Virchow Archivs Cell Pathology* **52**, 375–87.

Zhang, P., Rao, K.V. and Anderson, W.R. (1988) An ultrastructural study of the membranoproliferative variant of transplant glomerulopathy. *Ultrastructural Pathology* **12**, 185–94.

Zucchelli, P. and Pasquali, S. (1992) Membranous nepthropathy. In Cameron, S., Davison, A.M., Grünfeld, J-P., Kerr, D., and Ritz, E. (eds), *Oxford Textbook of Clinical Nephrology, Volume 1*. Oxford Medical, Oxford, pp. 371–88.

Zwirner, J., Felber, E., Herzog, V., Riethmüller, G. and Feucht, H.E. (1989) Classical pathway of complement activation in normal and diseased human glomeruli. *Kidney International* **36**, 1069–77.

6 ◆ *Immunohistochemistry of cutaneous tumours*

Paul E. Swanson and Mark R. Wick

Introduction

The skin is a complex microenvironment. The normal structures of the epidermis, dermis and cutaneous adnexae are incredibly diverse in design, and the myriad histologically defined entities that occupy this tissue compartment are no less heterogeneous. Much as any other organ, the skin may harbour lesions that require the surgical pathologist to rely on lessons learned elsewhere. Foremost among such lesions are those of the lymphoreticular and mesenchymal tissues. Inasmuch as the complex diagnostic and immunohistochemical issues framed by these tumours have been covered in considerable detail elsewhere in this text, our comments pertaining to these particular topics will be limited in scope, stressing tumours peculiar to the skin and their differential diagnoses. More important to the present discussion, perhaps, are those lessons that can be learned through primary study of the epithelial components of the skin and their tumours. Hence, the ensuing discussion will initially emphasize the immunohistochemical attributes of epidermal and cutaneous adnexal epithelial neoplasms, and tumours exhibiting melanocytic differentiation.

Throughout this chapter, we will place greater importance on antigenic profiles obtained in routinely processed (formalin- or alcohol-fixed) tissues using commercially available reagents. Aspects of cell function and differentiation that rely on molecular diagnostic or immunohistochemical study using novel or privately held reagents will be discussed only in brief, rather than allowing the narrative to detract from the diagnostic emphasis of this text. Special topics in the immunohistochemical analysis of cutaneous disease will be summarized at the conclusion of this chapter.

Epithelial tumours of the skin

Because of the diversity of normally differentiated epidermal and adnexal epithelial elements in skin, the categorization of cutaneous epithelial tumours is confounded by a confusing list of rare or 'previously undescribed' patterns of epidermal or adnexal differentiation. From a more pragmatic viewpoint, however, the diagnostic applications of immunohistochemistry require that only five basic patterns of epithelial differentiation be recognized: epidermal, sudoriferous, sebaceous, pilar and endocrine.

Epidermal tumours

Tumours that show differentiation towards cells of the epidermis are the most common epithelial neoplasms of skin. The most important of these are squamous cell carcinoma and basal cell carcinoma.

Squamous cell carcinoma (SCC) is typically a tumour composed of relatively uniform keratinizing polygonal cells, and as such, poses few diagnostic challenges in this histologic form. However, several microscopic subtypes of SCC have been described, each of which may occasionally mimic both glandular and mesenchymal neoplasms in skin. These include adenoid (acantholytic), pleomorphic, small-cell, and spindle-cell forms (Lever and Schaumberg-Lever, 1989; Manivel et al., 1985; Nappi et al., 1989; Wick and Coffin, 1985; Wick and Schiethauer, 1985; Zarbo et al., 1986). Because of these latter variants, an understanding of the immunohistologic attributes of SCC is important to the differential diagnosis of cutaneous tumours in general. Fortunately, all forms of SCC show similar antigenic profiles, with minor exceptions.

SCC contains an abundance of cytokeratin intermediate filament proteins that range from 40 to 68 kD in molecular weight (Battifora, 1984; Penneys et al., 1983; van Muijen et al., 1991). The cells of those neoplasms that are well-differentiated synthesize high-molecular weight cytokeratin (CK); in contrast, more poorly differentiated tumours express low molecular weight keratin peptides. The concomitant expression of both cytokeratins and vimentin characterizes spindle-cell, pleomorphic and some acantholytic squamous carcinomas (Nappi et al., 1989; Zarbo et al., 1986).

Other epithelial determinants displayed in SCC include epithelial membrane antigen (EMA). Although variable amounts of this glycoprotein are encountered in most examples of SCC (Kuwano et al., 1985; Pinkus and Kurtin, 1985), we have observed that diffuse EMA-reactivity is usually only a feature of poorly differentiated tumours (Broders' grades 3 and 4) (Fig. 6.1). Carcinoembryonic antigen (CEA) staining has been described, but in our experience, such reactivity is generally lacking in SCC.

All squamous carcinomas of the skin lack S100 protein, salivary amylase (SA), neuron-specific enolase (NSE), LeuM1 (CD15), and Leu7 (CD57) (Wick and Kaye, 1986). Further, reactivity with HMB-45 is not evident (Gown et al., 1986), while desmin and muscle-specific isoforms of actin are absent in spindle-cell forms of these neoplasms. These latter observations have obvious bearing on the immuno-

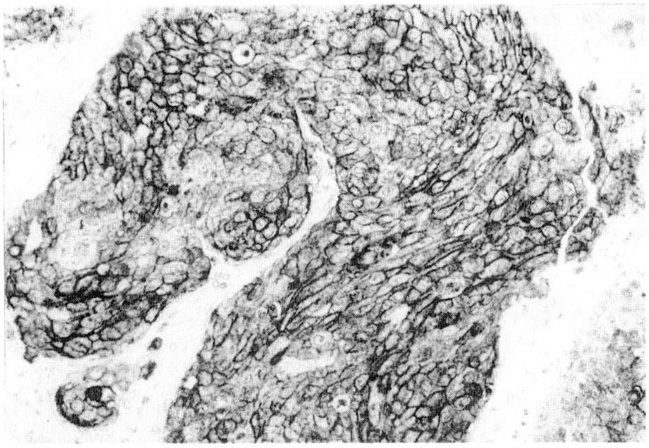

Figure 6.1. Epithelial membrane antigen in squamous cell carcinoma. Membrane-based reactivity is accentuated in poorly differentiated tumours.

histologic diagnosis of malignant cutaneous neoplasms, as illustrated in Tables 6.1 and 6.2.

Unfortunately, there are no well-characterized substances that exclusively define epidermal differentiation. Substances associated with epidermal keratinization, such as filaggrin and involucrin (Dale et al., 1987; Hashimoto et al., 1987; Klein-Szanto et al., 1984; Said et al., 1984; Smoller et al., 1986), are preferentially expressed in SCC, and as such have been touted as markers of malignancy among keratinocytic proliferations (Reed et al., 1990). Such claims, however, have invariably proven unfounded; indeed, we contend that no well-characterized marker has reliably separated benign cutaneous (or extracutaneous) neoplasms from histologically similar malignant tumours. This point is of particular relevence to fillagrins and involucrin, since both have more recently been detected in both keratoacanthomas and a variety of benign keratinocytic proliferations (Klein-Szanto et al., 1984; Kvedar et al., 1986; Murphy et al., 1984). And while they may distinguish SCC from basal cell carcinomas, they cannot separate SCC from tumours of cutaneous adnexae (Hashimoto et al., 1987; Kanitakis et al., 1986; Tokura et al., 1989), particularly those of the pilar apparatus. Hence, while these determinants may

Table 6.1. Immunophenotype of spindled and pleomorphic cutaneous neoplasms

Tumour	VIM	DES	MSA	S100	Leu7	CK	EMA	F8	UEA	ENZ
Fibrosarcoma	+	0	0	0	0	0	0	0	0	+/−
Malignant fibrous histiocytoma	+	r	+/−	0	0	0(a)	0	0	0	+
Atypical fibroxanthoma	+	0	+/−	0	0	0	0	0	0	+
Dermatofibrosarcoma protuberans	+	0	r	0	0	0	0	0	0	+/−
Leiomyosarcoma	+	+	+	+/−	+/−	0(a)	0	0	0	+/−(b)
Malignant peripheral nerve sheath tumour	+	r	r	+	0(a)	0	0	0	0	+/−
Angiosarcoma	+	0	0	0	0	0(a)	0	+/−	+	+/−
Kaposi's sarcoma	+	0	0	0	0	0	0	r(c)	r(c)	+/−
Spindle cell squamous carcinoma	+/−	0	0	0(d)	0	+	+	0	0	+/−
Spindle cell malignant melanoma										

Notes:
+ = at least 50 per cent of cases positive
+/− = between 10 and 50 per cent of cases positive
r = rare reactivity reported
a = we consider reported instances of CK-reactivity spurious (see text)
b = negative for AAT and AACT, but may express cathepsin B
c = our experience only; others report more frequent reactivity
d = HMB-45 negative; however, pleomorphic melanomas are HMB-45 positive

Abbreviations: VIM – vimentin; DES – desmin; MSA – muscle specific actin; CK – cytokeratin; EMA – epithelial membrane antigen; F8 – factor VIII-related antigen; UEA – *Ulex europaeus* agglutinin; ENZ – proteolytic enzymes

Table 6.2. Immunophenotype of epithelioid cutaneous neoplasms

Tumour	VIM	HMB	S100	Leu7	MSA/DES	UEA	CK	EMA	CEA	CD15	LCA
Leiomyosarcoma	+	0	(a)	(a)	+	0	0(b)	0	0	+/−	0
Malignant peripheral nerve sheath tumour	+	0	+	+	r	0	0(b)	0(c)	0(c)	0	0
Angiosarcoma	+	0	0	0	0	+	0(b)	0	0	0	0
Epithelioid haemangioendothelioma	+	0	0	0	0	+/−	0(b)	0	0	0	0
Epithelioid sarcoma	+	0	r	0	0	+	+	+	r	0	0
Squamous cell carcinoma	0	0	0	0	0	0	+	+	0	0	0
Eccrine carcinoma	0	0	+/−	r	0	0	+	+	+	+	0
Sebaceous carcinoma	0	0	0	0	0	0	+	+	0	+	0
Malignant melanoma	+	+	+	+/−	0	0	0(b)	0	0	0	0
Malignant lymphoma	+	0	0	0	0	0	0	+/−	0	+/−	+

Notes: + = at least 50 per cent of cases positive
+/− = between 10 and 50 per cent of cases positive
r = rare reactivity reported
a = untested in epithelioid leiomyosarcoma of skin
b = we consider reported instances of CK-reactivity spurious (see text)
c = reactivity for CK, EMA and CEA has been reported in glandular foci of MPNST
Abbreviations: VIM – vimentin; HMB – HMB-45; DES – desmin; MSA – muscle specific actin; UEA – *Ulex europaeus* agglutinin; CK – cytokeratin; EMA – epithelial membrane antigen; CEA – carcinoembryonic antigen; CD15 – LeuM1 antigen; LCA – leucocyte common antigen (CD45).

enhance our understanding of the neoplastic keratinocyte, they have proven less useful as diagnostic aids.

Basal cell carcinoma (BCC), like SCC, has several distinctive variants, all of which invoke dissimilar differential diagnoses. Among the better recognized subtypes are the morpheaform, adenoid, clear cell, keratotic, and 'metatypical' forms of BCC (Lever and Schaumberg-Lever, 1989; Starink et al., 1990).

In general, basal cell carcinoma is devoid of complex patterns of antigenic expression. Like SCC, this tumour displays cytoplasmic reactivity for cytokeratin (CK) polypeptides; however, in all instances, these intermediate filaments are under 50 kiloDaltons (kD) in molecular weight (Shimizu et al., 1989; van Muijen et al., 1984). In contrast to SCC, EMA is not observed in any variant of pure BCC (George et al., 1989a; Heyderman et al., 1984; Pinkus and Kurtin, 1985; Wick and Swanson, 1986).

Occasional examples of BCC display reactivity with HMB-45 (Gown et al., 1986). Similarly, a few lesion studied in our laboratory exhibited staining for endocrine-associated peptides, including NSE and chromogranin (CG) (George et al., 1989a). It should be pointed out, however, that most analyses of BCC fail to confirm our observations (Gu et al., 1983; Lloyd and Wilson, 1983; Sibley and Dahl, 1985; Wilson and Lloyd, 1984). The apparent ability of BCC to express these specialized determinants has been used to support the premise that the cells of BCC recapitulate the properties of epidermal 'stem' cells. However, the absence of vimentin (Caselitz et al., 1983; Miettinen et al., 1983c), CEA (Heyderman et al., 1984; Kariniemi et al, 1984; Penneys, 1984; Penneys et al., 1982b, 1983; Wick, 1988), S100 protein (Cohen et al., 1990; Egan et al., 1986; Springall et al., 1983; Stefansson et al., 1982), Leu7 (CD57) (Perentes and Rubinstein, 1985), LeuM1 (CD15) (Sheibani et al., 1986a), and SA (Swanson et al., 1987a; Wick and Swanson, 1986), suggest that the stem cell hypothesis is not generally applicable to this tumour. Similarly, cells of BCC fail to exhibit immunoreactivity for the EPM-1 antigen (Klingel et al., 1990), a high molecular weight glycoprotein that is expressed by fetal basal epidermal cells. Nonetheless, BCC with additional patterns of differentiation, such as 'eccrine' epithelioma (Sanchez and Winkelmann, 1982), 'apocrine' epithelioma (Sakamoto et al., 1985), and 'basosebaceous' epithelioma (Rulon and Helwig, 1974), may demonstrate positivity for EMA, CEA, or SA in histologically divergent areas.

Sudoriferous tumours

The eccrine and apocrine glandular adnexae comprise the sudoriferous structures of skin. The proliferative lesions of these structures are histologically diverse (Wick and Coffin, 1985), but maintain certain immunohistologic features in common. All of these neoplasms demonstrate CK-reactivity, and the potential for expression of CEA, EMA, LeuM1, and SA (Swanson et al., 1987a) (Fig. 6.2). The last three of these substances are seen in varying proportions of sweat gland adenomas and carcinomas. EMA is more often observed in malignant sudoriferous neoplasms than in benign ones; indeed, certain benign lesions of the eccrine sweat gland, including spiradenoma and cylindroma, are typically devoid of this determinant (Lever and Schaumberg-Lever, 1989). In contrast, CEA, LeuM1, and SA may be detected in roughly 70–80 per cent of all eccrine and apocrine tumours (Heyderman et al., 1984; Kariniemi et al., 1984; Mazoujian et al., 1984; Nickoloff et al., 1986; Penneys et al., 1982a, b; Swanson et al., 1987a; Wick and Swanson, 1986), regardless of their biological potentials. This profile proves useful in the separation of sudoriferous neoplasms from other cutaneous glandular and epidermal neoplasms, as will become evident shortly. It has also been instrumental in verifying the presence of sudoriferous differentiation in occasional examples of lymphoepithelioma-like carcinoma of the skin, a poorly differentiated tumour showing histologic similarites with nasopharyngeal 'lymphoepithelioma' (Wick et al., 1991). Similar comments apply to the detection of sudoriferous differentiation in mixed adnexal carcinomas of the skin (Nakhleh et al., 1990b).

Immunophenotypic differences between eccrine and apocrine neoplasms may occasionally be exploited to diagnostic advantage. For instance, eccrine carcinomas express S100 protein in almost 50 per cent of cases, whereas apocrine carcinomas, including extramammary Paget's disease (EPD), are generally S100-negative (Wick and Kaye, 1986). Conversely, gross cystic disease fluid protein-15 (GCDFP-15) is a glycoprotein that is rather selectively expressed by apocrine cells and neoplasms (Mazoujian, 1988; Mazoujian and Margolis, 1987; Mazoujian et al., 1984). This marker represents a discriminant by which EPD, superficial spreading malignant melanoma, and Pagetoid Bowen's disease (intraepidermal squamous carcinoma) may be separated, since GCDFP-15 is present only in the first of these three tumours (Mazoujian et al., 1984) (Fig. 6.3). In contrast, Bowen's disease is alone in its expression of high-molecular weight keratin (as is typical of other low grade SCC); further,

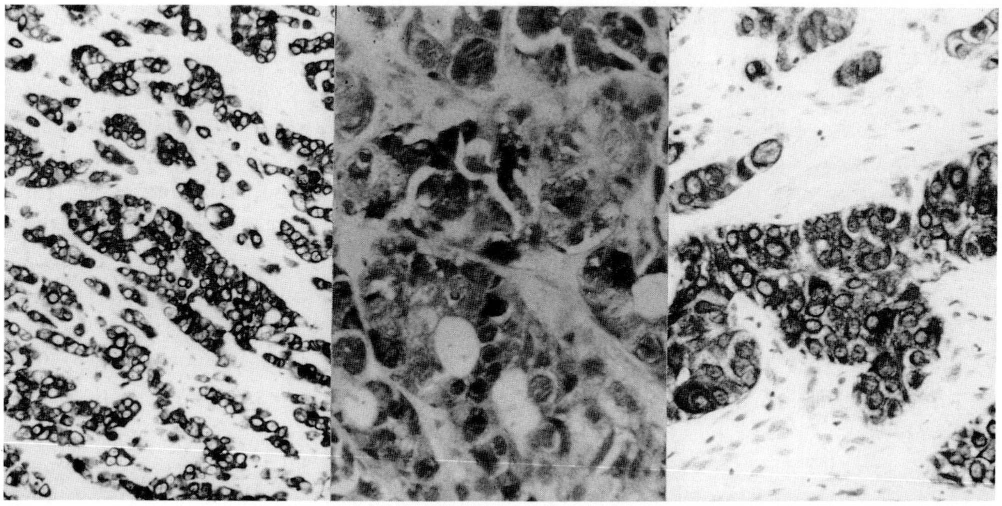

Fig. 6.2. Immunophenotype of eccrine carcinoma. Most examples are diffusely reactive for cytokeratin (left). Fewer than half of eccrine ductal carcinomans stain positively for S100 protein (middle), whereas the majority are positive for LeuM1 (CD15) (right).

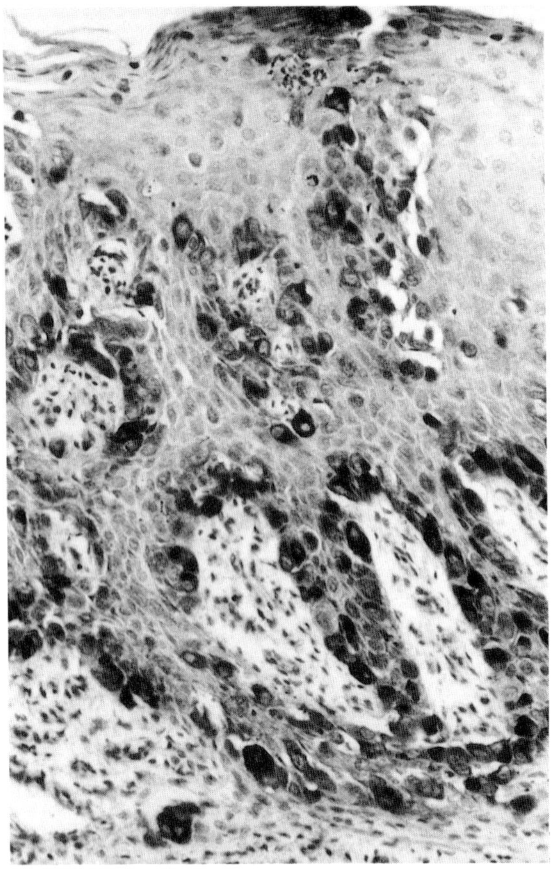

Fig. 6.3. Gross cystic disease fluid protein-15 in extrammammary Paget's disease. Intraepidermal apocrine carcinoma cells are strongly reactive.

only melanoma is reactive with HMB-45 and antibodies to S100 protein, among this group of lesions (Gown et al., 1986; Mazoujian et al., 1984; Reed et al., 1990).

GCDFP-15 is not absolutely specific for apocrine cells; 1 of 22 eccrine carcinomas studied in our laboratory was also reactive (Swanson et al., 1987a). However, the selectivity of this determinant has proven useful in the evaluation of some benign sudoriferous lesions. For example, although sporadic GCDFP-15 staining in encountered in a variety of benign sweat gland tumours, it is consistently displayed in tumours of known apocrine differentiation (Mazoujian, 1988). The apparent exception has been that of benign mixed tumour (chondroid syringoma), a tumour previously considered to be eccrine in nature. The uniformity of GCDFP-15 in tubular components of the latter tumour have led to its recent reevaluation as an apocrine neoplasm (Hassab-El-Naby et al., 1989; Mazoujian, 1988). Other gross cystic disease fluid proteins, including GCDFP-24 and zinc alpha-2-glycoprotein, are less selective markers in this context (Mazoujian, 1990).

Several papers have described the selective expression of specific cytokeratin peptides and other cellular determinants in eccrine tumours. Antibodies to these substances, including EKH5, EKH6 and SKH1 (Aiba et al., 1983; Hashimoto et al., 1983; Kanitakis et al., 1983; Suzuki et al., 1989) may indeed show a preference for eccrine tumours, but the lack of systematic study of cutaneous and extracutaneous neoplasms leaves most such observations unsubstantiated. The same comments apply to the use of antibodies to ferritin (Penneys and Zlatkiss, 1990). For the moment, we are resigned to question the validity of such claims.

Sebaceous tumours

Although it is a glandular adnexal structure, the sebaceous gland is topographically and ontogenetically related to the hair sheath. Hence, antigenic similarities between the isthmus of the outer hair sheath and the germinative basaloid cells of the sebaceous gland are not unexpected. Similarly, the occasional admixture of basosebaceous and hair sheath elements (as in superficial epithelioma with sebaceous differentiation and 'sebaceoma') is understandable (Wick and Swanson, 1991). The common expression of both high and low molecular weight species of cytokeratin in pilar and sebaceous, but not eccrine or apocrine, tumours also points to similar patterns of cellular differentiation (Heyderman et al., 1984). In addition, the architectural features of both benign and malignant sebaceous neoplasms bear more of a resemblance to pilar neoplasms than to sudoriferous tumours. It follows from these observations that many of the antigens associated with sweat gland tumours (including S100 protein and CEA) are absent in sebaceous neoplasms.

Reactivity for EMA and related substances is often obtained in sebaceous tumours (Tsubura et al., 1987; Wick and Swanson, 1991); the former of these is typically displayed in a manner unique to these neoplasms. In both benign and malignant sebaceous proliferations, the characteristic microvesicular or 'bubbly' cytoplasmic profile of the mature sebocyte is often maintained. EMA staining in these cells is similarly evocative of non-neoplastic sebaceous epithelium, in that these cytoplasmic lipid vesicles are clearly rimmed by EMA-reactivity (Fig. 6.4). Even in poorly differentiated sebaceous carcinomas, EMA stains may highlight otherwise inapparent cytoplasmic complexity (Wick and Swanson, 1991).

The only other diagnostically relevant determinant shared by sebaceous and sweat gland neoplasms is LeuM1 (CD15). We have identified this marker in 18 of 36 examples of sebaceous carcinoma (Wick and Swanson, 1991) (Fig. 6.5). Despite the proclivity for both eccrine and sebaceous neoplasms to express CD15, an antibody panel directed at EMA, SA, S100 protein, and CEA will allow for a separation between these tumours in most instances (see Table 6.2).

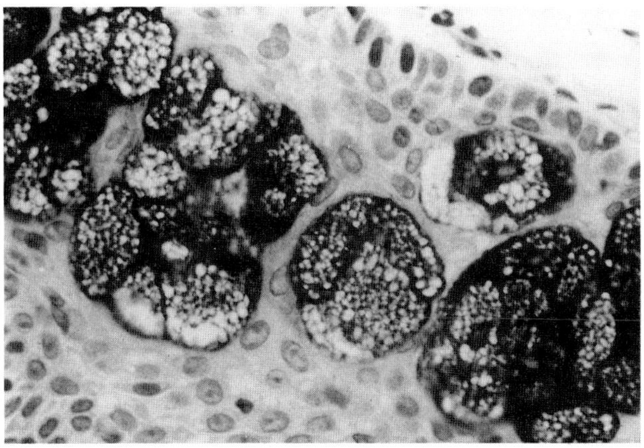

Fig. 6.4 Epithelial membrane antigen in normal sebaceous epithelium. Intracytoplasmic vacuoles are highlighted, a pattern that is recapitulated in sebaceous neoplasms.

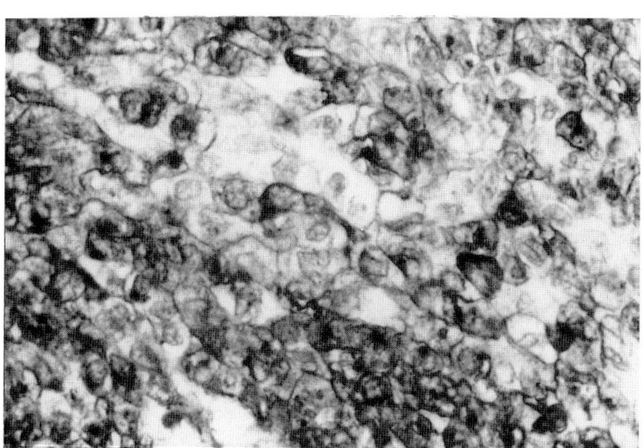

Fig. 6.5 LeuM1 (CD15) in sebaceous carcinoma. Heterogenous membrane and cytoplasmic staining typifies the majority of sebaceous carcinomas.

To date, specific markers of sebaceous differentiation have not been characterized. In two studies, specific labelling of sebaceous neoplasms with biotinylated concanavalin-A lectin has been described, to the exclusion of other epithelial cutaneous tumours (Kindblom et al., 1982; von Kuster et al., 1986); unfortunately, we have been unable to reproduce these findings. More recent studies have suggested that reactivity for immunoglobulin A, lipase, the milk fat globule-associated (ovarian carcinoma-associated) sebaceous antigen OV-2 and the OKM5 (CD36) antigen may be selective for sebaceous lesions (Allen et al., 1991; Grossniklaus et al., 1990; Jimenez-Acosta et al., 1990; Latham et al., 1989; Layton et al., 1990; Lisby et al., 1990; Metze et al., 1989; Zhao et al., 1991). However, such analyses await corroboration.

Pilar tumours

The multiplicity of diagnoses assigned to benign pilar tumours (Headington, 1976) bespeaks the protean manifestations of trichogenic differentiation. Unfortunately, most commercially available antibodies fail to select among the various patterns of pilar differentiation including germinal matrix, cortex, inner hair sheath, outer hair sheath and infundibulum. Indeed, using the antibody reagents commonly applied to cutaneous epithelial tumours, the antigenic profiles of all benign pilar tumours are similar. They generally contain cytokeratin polypeptides over 50 kD in molecular weight (Broelaert et al., 1990; Manivel et al., 1986; van Muijen et al., 1984), but (with the exception of occasional proliferating pilar tumours) are EMA-negative (Manivel et al., 1986). CEA, S100, SA, LeuM1, NSE, the HMB 45 antigen, and GCDFP-15 are not detected in these tumours. The immunophenotype of pilar adenomas is thus similar to that of BCC (Wick and Kaye, 1986; Wick and Swanson, 1991).

More detailed evaluations of pilar and epidermal neoplasms by various authors have identified patterns of keratin peptide expression that characterize selected groups of pilar lesions (Ito et al., 1986a, 1986b; Lynch et al., 1986). The most intriguing finding from these investigations is that 'hard keratins' recognized by the antibodies AE12 and AE13 are selectively expressed in cells exhibiting matrical differentiation. Pilomatrixoma, as the prototypical matrical neoplasm, is diffusely reactive with AE13 (Fig. 6.6), whereas diminutive or abortive

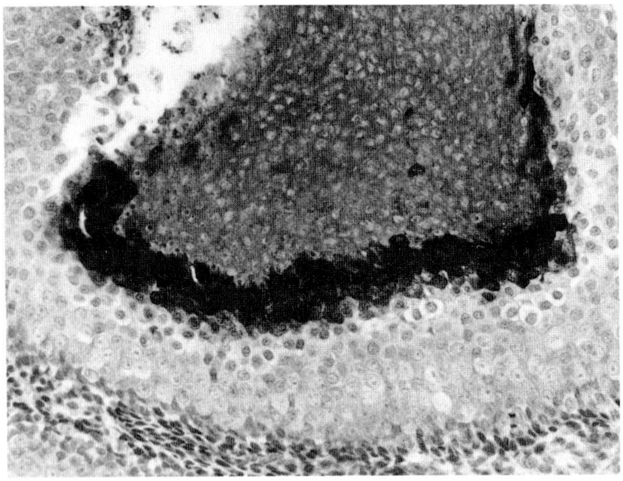

Fig. 6.6. AE13 reactivity in pilomatrixoma. Cortical differentiation from matrical cells is highlighted by AE13.

hair follicles represent the only reactive population in trichofolliculoma (Swanson et al., 1988b). Tumours with trichilemmal patterns of differentiation, such as proliferating pilar tumour and tricholemmoma, are AE13-negative, but may instead be labelled with AE14. This latter reagent is a monoclonal antibody that recognizes both a cortical sulphur-containing moiety and a low molecular weight cytokeratin (Swanson et al., 1988b) (Fig. 6.7). The latter substance is typically expressed by most adnexal epithelia and epidermal basal cells (Swanson et al., 1988b), and as such is not as useful a marker as AE13. Interestingly, occasional small keratotic cysts in desmoplastic trichoepithelioma are AE13 positive, whereas examples of the usual form of trichoepithelioma are uniformly negative with this antibody. It is this reproducible pattern of follicular reactivity with AE13 that led us to conclude that AE13 staining in the small keratin cysts of microcystic adnexal carcinoma is indicative of mixed pilar/eccrine differentiation in this tumour (Wick et al., 1990).

The expression of keratin associated proteins labelled by the antibodies HKN5, HKN6 and HKN7 (Ito et al., 1986a, 1986b), and the anti-human hair keratin (HHK) antibody (Tateyama et al., 1992) may also be indicative of specialized patterns of pilar differentiation. Substances recognized by HKN6/7 are found only cuticular, cortical and inner hair sheath cells, whereas HKN5 also labels a cellular component of the outer hair sheath. Pilomatrixomas typically express the HKN6/7 and HHK antigens; the latter is also present in malignant

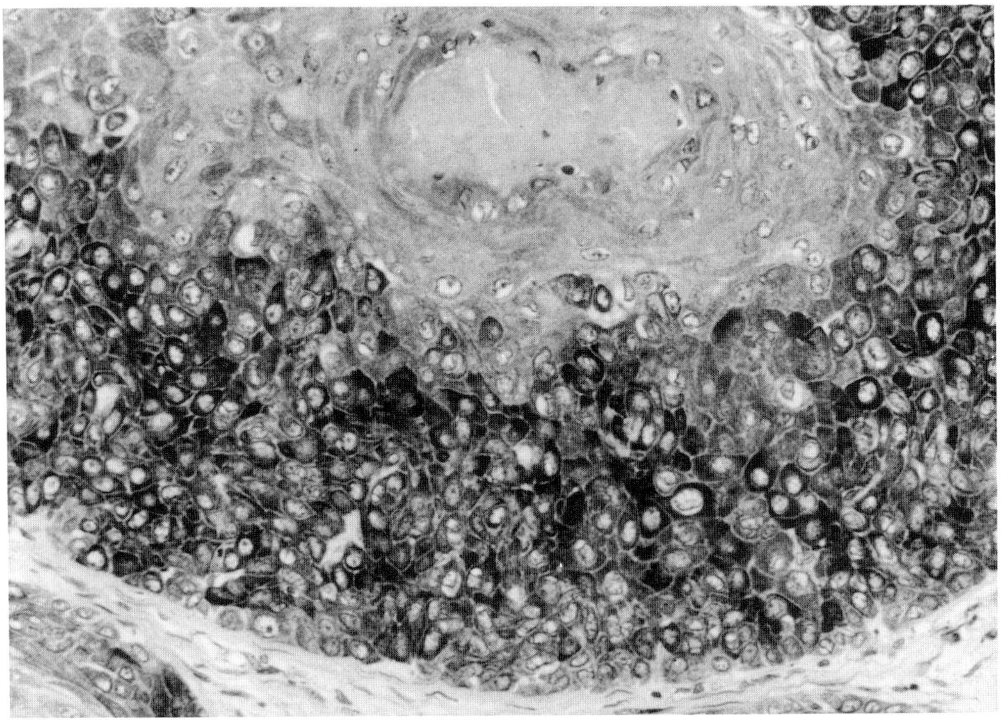

Fig. 6.7. AE14 reactivity in proliferating pilar tumour. A mosaic pattern of cytoplasmic reactivity for AE14 is evident.

pilomatrixoma, whereas the former have not been tested in this tumour (Tateyama et al., 1992). In contrast, most other pilar tumours, BCC and epidermal proliferations do not contain these substances. The expression of HKN5 is shared by pilar tumours and BCC, but is not seen in seborrheic keratoses. Hence, the detection of HKN5, 6 and 7 in some examples of the 'Borst-Jadassohn' type of intraepidermal epithelioma suggests that such lesions may have pilar characteristics (Ito et al., 1988).

With malignant transformation, the immunophenotypes of pilar neoplasms become somewhat more complex. Pilar carcinomas (squamous carcinoma-like neoplasms arising in proliferating pilar tumours – Amaral et al., 1984) often display EMA (Wick and Coffin, 1985), and trichilemmal carcinoma (a tumour with architectural and cytologic similarities to tricholemmoma) has the potential to express both CEA and S100 protein, although such reactivity is generally focal (Wick and Swanson, 1991). No other commonly studied antigens, with the obvious exception of cytokeratins, are shared by pilar and sudoriferous neoplasms.

Endocrine tumours

Originally described in 1972 under the designation of 'trabecular carcinoma of the skin' (Toker, 1972) (a tumour also known as 'Merkel cell carcinoma'), primary cutaneous neuroendocrine carcinoma (PCNC) remains the object of extensive biochemical and immunohistochemical study. After its recognition as a distinct nosologic entity, some authors postulated that PCNC displayed neurotactile differentiation, emulating 'Merkel' cells of the normal skin and oral mucosa (Sibley et al., 1980; Warner et al., 1983). Subsequent studies have failed to substantiate or negate this hypothesis definitively. Normal Merkel cells are reactive for cytokeratin, NSE, met-enkephalin, vasoactive intestinal polypeptide (VIP), and blood group antigen Pr(h), but in general appear to lack the ability to synthesize other endocrine determinants (Wick and Scheithauer, 1985). In contrast, CK, neurofilament protein, Leu7, LeuM1, EMA, NSE, CG, calcitonin, somatostatin, adrenocorticotrophic hormone, VIP, pancreatic polypeptide, and substance P are typically encountered in PCNC (Gu et al., 1983; Miettinen et al., 1983a; Sibley and Dahl, 1985; Wick and Kaye, 1986; Wick et al., 1986a; Wick and Scheithauer, 1985; Wick et al., 1983).

The authors of the original study, in keeping with the proposed diagnosis of 'trabecular carcinoma' (Toker, 1972), suggested that PCNC was closely related to sudoriferous carcinomas, a claim repeated in later reports (Heenan et al, 1990). However, despite having studied more than 65 cases, we have not to date shown reactivity in PCNC for CEA, S100 protein, SA, or GCDFP-15, among those determinants commonly expressed in eccrine or apocrine carcinomas.

Because of its capacity for diffuse or medullary patterns of growth, and because of it uniform, occasionally dyscohesive small cell population, PCNC is often mistaken for lymphoma cutis (Wick and Scheithauer, 1985). As should become evident later in this chapter, this problem is readily resolved by immunohistochemcal analyses (also see Table 6.3). Whereas lymphoma is reactive for CD45 (leukocyte common antigen), PCNC contains low molecular weight cytokeratin peptides. Moreover, these latter intermediate filaments are often clustered in the perinuclear cytoplasm, yielding a characteristic 'dot' of chromogenic precipitate (Battifora and Silva, 1986; Sibley and Dahl, 1985; Szadowska et al., 1989; Wick et al., 1986a) (Fig. 6.8).

No one group of histologic features can reliably distinguish PCNC from metastatic small cell neuroendocrine carcinoma from pulmonary or (less commonly) other

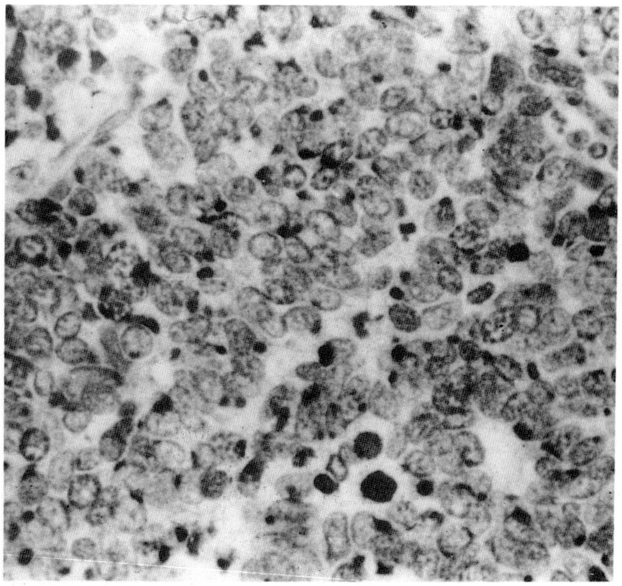

Fig. 6.8. Cytokeratin in primary cutaneous neuroendocrine carcinoma. Cytokeratin reactivity is characteristically perinuclear, imparting a 'dot-like' pattern of immunostaining.

sites. Nonetheless, a battery of antibodies to CEA, met-enkephalin, leu-enkephalin, beta-endorphin, and bombesin is useful in this context, since bronchogenic small cell carcinoma typically displays at least one of these determinants (Wick, 1988; Wick et al., 1985). Conversely, the novel intestinal cytoskeletal protein IT (cytokeratin 20) may be selectively expressed by PCNC, when compared with immunohistochemically negative pulmonary neuroendocrine carcinomas (Moll et al., 1992). In practical terms, the absence of CEA reactivity is provocative evidence that a small cell neuroendocrine carcinoma is primary in skin. However, attention to clinical findings, including careful follow-up, is necessary in most cases before metastasis can be excluded with certainty (Wick and Swanson, 1991).

Tumours of the cutaneous melanocytic system

Melanocytic neoplasms of the skin provide the surgical pathologist with perplexing, and at times, seemingly insoluable histologic challenges. This comment is most relevant to the accurate diagosis of malignant melanoma, particularly when extracutaneous manifestations of this disease are encountered. However, we cannot readily dismiss the problems occasionally posed by the benign melanocytic proliferations in skin, since these lesions may occasionally be mistaken for variants of malignant melanoma. Unfortunately, immunohistochemistry is unlikely to resolve these latter problems. Rather, the diagnostic advantage offered by immunohistochemistry is better suited to the former of these challenges. Nevertheless, the immunophenotypic features of benign melanocytic proliferations are important as an introduction to this group of cellular proliferations.

Naevi

Naevi, despite their proximity to, and often obligate association with, the epidermis, are not truly epithelial, and thus uniformly lack CK and EMA. The latter of these determinants has purportedly been observed in spindled areas of neurotized naevi (Cramer, 1990), but we consider such reactivity to be spurious. In contrast, nevus cells contain the intermediate filament vimentin (Miettinen et al., 1983c; Stefansson et al., 1982); S100 protein and NSE expression also typifies most examples (Stafensson et al., 1982). The so-called 'Spitz' nevus is unusual among benign melanocytic proliferations in that fewer than 50 per cent of such tumours express these latter two determinants (Palazzo and Duray, 1989).

Few readers should be unaware of the antibody HMB-45. In their original description of this monoclonal reagent, Gown and colleagues suggested that this premelanosome-associated glycoprotein was a marker for cell activation or proliferation (Gown et al., 1986). However, recent studies by Smoller and associates have demonstrated that the HMB-45 antigen is not associated with cell proliferation (Smoller et al., 1989), but instead is an inducible substance whose expression may be modulated by components of supplemented growth media that include epidermal growth factor (Smoller et al., 1991). Although initial studies indicated that only a small proportion of benign naevi express the HMB-45 antigen (Gown et al., 1986), subsequent analyses suggest that reproducible subtypes of naevi are likely to contain this determinant, including junctional naevi, dysplastic naevi and blue naevi (Ahmed et al., 1991; Palazzo and Duray, 1989; Sun et al., 1990; Wood and Tron, 1991).

Staining heterogeneity among benign nevocellular proliferations is also revealed by the application of Leu7 (CD57), an antibody that labels natural killer cells, various endocrine and neuroectodemal tumours, and several different soft tissue neoplasms (Swanson et al., 1987b). In our experience, fewer than 50 per cent of naevi are reactive for this determinant. Other endocrine and specialized epithelial determinants, including CEA, SA, LeuM1, and CG, are absent in nevocellular proliferations.

In maturing dermal naevi, spindled areas (neurotization) may dominate. In some instances, such lesions may be difficult to distinguish from dermal neurofibromas. However, these lesions differ in their ability to express Factor XIIIa. Whereas both neurofibromas and neurotized melanocytic naevi are S100 reactive (Gray et al., 1990b; Gray et al., 1990c), only the former of these lesions stains for Factor XIIIa (Gray et al., 1990c; Ushigome et al., 1986).

The separation of benign naevi from cutaneous glomus tumours may be complicated by a peculiar pseudoangiomatous pattern that dominates occasional examples of the former lesions. However, the routine reactivty of glomus tumours for muscle-specific isoforms of actin, together with the absence of these filamentous proteins in most naevi (Kaye and Dehner, 1991), should resolve matters, as will staining for vascular-associated determinants (see below).

In recent analyses by Puches et al. (1991) and Smolle et al. (1990a), tubulin peptides were detected in the majority of benign and malignant melanocytic lesions. Although these findings may contribute to our understanding of the cytoskeleton of these cells, they appear to have no immediate diagnostic application, since tubulin may also be detected in several mesenchymal and epithelial tumours of skin.

Malignant melanoma

The ability of malignant melanomas to assume virtually any morphological pattern of growth is well known (Nakhleh et al., 1990a). Nonetheless, failure to consider malignant melanoma in the differential diagnosis of polygonal, spindled or pleomorphic cell neoplasms of skin and extracutaneous sites continues to contribute to the misdiagnosis of this neoplasm. For those who have failed to heed the admonition 'always consider melanoma in the differential diagnosis', perhaps a rational approach to immunohistochemical analysis can make up for the occasional lapse of judgement.

Like naevi, melanomas uniformly stain for vimentin to the exclusion of other intermediate filament proteins (Caselitz et al., 1983; Miettinen et al., 1983c). Epithelial membrane antigen is also absent (Pinkus and Kurtin, 1985), although spurious reactivity may occasionally be encountered adjacent to areas of necrosis. We do not report these tumours as positive, because such lesions are not uniformly reactive; further, staining in these areas is exclusively cytoplasmic, a pattern which we have associated with non-specific reactivity in other non-epithelial malignancies (Swanson et al., 1989).

Virtually all melanomas, regardless of histologic type, are immunoreactive for S100 protein (Drier et al., 1987; From et al., 1983; Kahn et al., 1983; Ordonez et al., 1988; Springall et al., 1983; Stefansson et al., 1982) (Fig. 6.9); in our experience, less than 1 per cent (3/345 cases) fail to express this antigen. These tumours are also commonly positive for neuron-specific enolase.

The most specific commercially available marker of melanocytic differentiation, as already alluded to, is the HMB-45 antigen. In the differential diagnosis of anaplastic, polygonal cell or small cell neoplasms, reactivity with

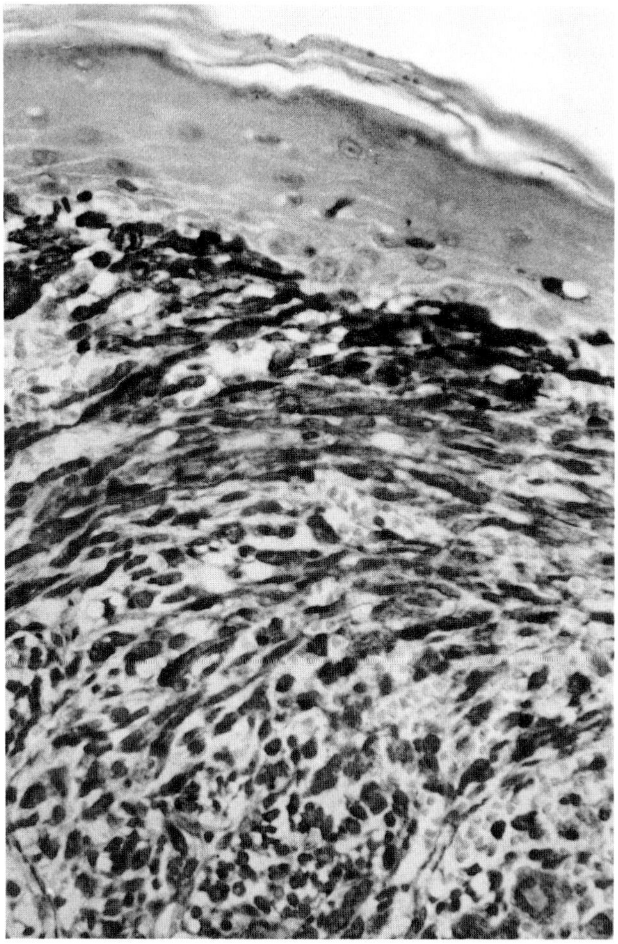

Fig. 6.9. S100 protein in spindle cell malignant melanoma. Since most examples are HMB-45 negative, diffuse reactivity for S100 remains the only reliable marker of melanocytic differentiation in this lesion.

HMB-45 is essentially diagnostic of melanoma (Gown et al., 1986; Nakhleh et al., 1990a; Ordonez et al., 1988; Wick et al., 1988) (Fig. 6.10). The only practical problem with this antibody is its general lack of reactivity with spindled-desmoplastic forms of melanoma (Gown et al., 1986; Ordonez et al., 1988; Wick et al., 1988). We have failed to detect HMB-45 reactivity in each of 18 such neoplasms.

To date, few other antibodies to melanoma-associated determinants have become routinely available (Mackie et al., 1984). As Smoller has recently reviewed (Smoller, 1991), a variety of antibodies that are potentially applicable to the diagnosis of HMB-45 negative melanomas have been described, but few of them are reactive in formalin-fixed tissues. Of those that have demonstrable

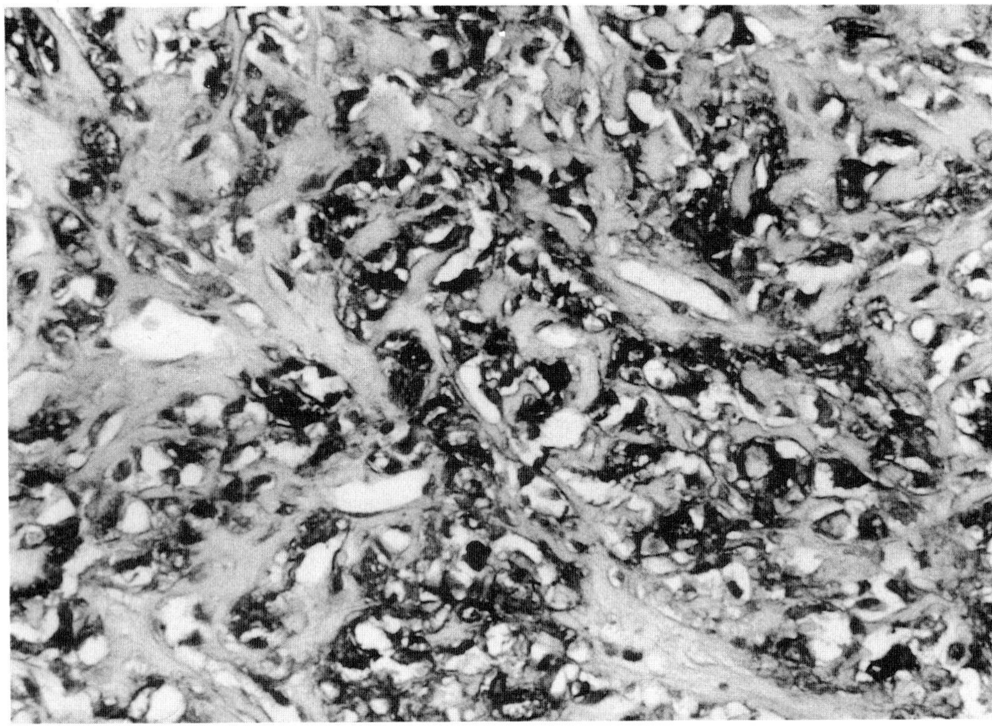

Fig. 6.10. HMB-45 reactivity in malignant melanoma. HMB-45 labels polygonal cells in this example of malignant melanoma.

reactivity in such materials, MEL1-5 labels a cytoplasmic determinant prevalent only in heavily pigmented cells, whereas NKI/C3 (a sensitive marker for melanocytic differentiation) may stain a considerable number of non-melanocytic lesions. As a result, neither is likely to have diagnostic applications. In contrast, cytoplasmic antigens recognized by the antibodies 2-139-1 (Imam et al., 1986; White et al., 1991), 6-26-3 (Imam et al., 1986) and HMSA-2 (Maeda et al., 1989) are apparently expressed exclusively by melanocytic elements. Whether such reagents might contribute to the differential diagnosis of spindle melanomas awaits their commercialization and further characterization.

Other determinants, including CEA, SA, LeuM1, and CG, are absent in malignant melanomas (Penneys et al., 1982b; Sheibani et al., 1986a; Wick, 1988; Wick and Kaye, 1986; Wilson and Lloyd, 1984). Leu7 antigen, although purportedly a sensitive marker of melanocytic differentiation, has been detected in fewer than 20 per cent of melanomas in our laboratory.

Beta-2-microglobulin and the Class II histocompatibility antigens HLA-DR, DQ and DP, have been detected in malignant melanoma (Takata et al., 1989; van Vreeswijk et al., 1988; Wilson et al., 1984). Since benign naevi may also exhibit these determinants in some instances (Takata et al., 1989), neither HLA-DR nor beta-2-microglobulin can be considered a marker of malignancy. The prevalence of cells containing histocompatibility antigens in earlier or thin melanomas and inflamed halo naevi suggests that these antigens may be involved in target recognition by lymphocytes, and thus may modulate the clinical behaviour of these lesions. This suggestion, however, is not uniformly supported by other recent analyses (Swanson and Wick, 1990; Wilson et al., 1984).

While many considerations will mould an immunohistochemical approach to the difficult cutaneous or extracutaneous neoplasm, the foregoing should emphasize that any immunophenotypic panel is not complete without the inclusion of antibodies to vimentin and S100 protein. The former is critical for two reasons: 1) it should always be reactive with ubiquitous endothelial and mesenchymal elements, establishing the adequacy of tissue fixation for immunohistochemistry; 2) the presence of this peptide in neoplastic cells, to the exclusion of other intermediate filaments, provides evidence of a non-epithelial pattern of differentiation. Of course, melanoma is not the only tumour in skin that is immunoreactive for vimentin to the exclusion of other intermediate filaments, but this result alone should prompt the pathologist to consider melanoma as a likely alternative, even if such a diagnosis was not initially considered during histologic examination.

S100 protein reactivity, in the context described above, may be presumptive evidence of melanocytic differentiation, but it must be remembered that eccrine carcinomas, including histologically 'undifferentiated' examples, may also express this substance (Swanson et al., 1987a). These observations illustrate that an incomplete immunohistochemical panel designed to 'confirm' the diagnosis of malignant melanoma may be just as inappropriate as one's failure to consider melanoma among the diagnostic alternatives.

Cutaneous lymphohaematopoietic disorders

Given the histologic diversity of T-cell and B-cell lymphoid and histiocytic proliferations of skin, a detailed discussion of each condition is well beyond the scope of this review. Histopathologic criteria for the separation of benign and malignant lymphoreticular processes, while not without limitations, are widely applicable to lesions of skin, but definitive separation of cell lineage in several of these disorders is often difficult or impossible when only histologic and clinical attributes are considered. Hence, as in other anatomic sites, the immunophenotypic evaluation of cutaneous lymphoreticular infiltrates is often invaluable to the surgical pathologist. As this latter topic has been discussed in detail elsewhere in this volume, our discussion will emphasize only a few aspects of immunophenotypic study that are of special importance to the skin.

Lymphoma and leukaemia cutis

Despite recent advances in the development of lineage selective markers that label routinely fixed tissues, cutaneous haematologic infiltrates are still best studied through the use of cryostat sections or cell-suspension preparations, since most specialized haematopoietic antigens do not survive routine tissue processing techniques (Banks, 1985). Nonetheless, we must emphasize that a small but effective arsenal of monoclonal and polyclonal antibodies to various lymphoid and histiocyte/monocyte selective antigens is applicable in most settings (Faure et al., 1990; Norton and Isaacson, 1989a, b; Ralfkiaer, 1991; Rest and Horn, 1991). Most importantly, virtually all examples of lymphoma and leukaemia cutis are reactive for CD45 (leukocyte common antigen, LCA) in paraffin sections (Battifora and Silva, 1986; Kurtin and Pinkus, 1985; Wick et al., 1986a, 1987a), an attribute of considerable utility when histologically similar non-haematologic cellular proliferations must be excluded (see Tables 6.2 and 6.3). In addition, several lineage selective reagents may be employed to advantage, including UCHL-1 (CD45RO), MT1 (CD43) and polyclonal anti-CD3 as effective T-cell markers; 4KB5, MB1 and MT2 (CD45R), L26 (CD20), LN1 (CDw75), LN2 [(CD74); HLA Class II invariant chain]; also labels Reed–Sternberg cells) and MB2 as B-cell markers; KP1 and EMB11 (CD68), MAC 387 (L1 antigen), HAM56 and various proteolytic enzymes (such as cathepsin B, alpha-1-antitrypsin, alpha-1-antichymotrypsin and lysozyme) as histiocyte/monocyte markers; and BerH2 (CD30; Ki-1), LeuM1 (CD15), and EMA as selective markers in anaplastic T-cell proliferations and Reed–Sternberg cells (Epstein et al., 1984; Faure et al., 1990; Hyder and Schnitzer, 1986; Norton and Isaacson, 1989a, b; Norton et al., 1986; Ralfkiaer, 1991; Rest and Horn, 1991). Of the foregoing markers, L26 (CD20) and UCHL-1 (CD45RO) are most closely restricted to lymphoid lineages, whereas CD43 antibodies often label both B-cell and immature myeloid proliferations. The latter attribute is noteworthy; cutaneous myelomonocytic infiltrates are typically MT1 positive, while only weakly reactive for CD45.

One important limitation of immunophenotypic analysis on routinely fixed paraffin sections is that the markers just described are 'pan-lineage' markers that, for the most part, do not recognize differences between benign reactive infiltrates and malignant lymphoreticular proliferations (Faure et al., 1990; Ralfkiaer, 1991; Rest and Horn, 1991; Rijlaarsdam and Wilemze, 1991; Smolle et al., 1990b). The literature is replete with clinicopathologic analyses that depict the fundamental histologic differences between the classic T-cell and B-cell cutaneous lymphomas and the benign lesions that histologically or clinically mimic them (the so-called 'pseudolymphomas'), but the separation of benign and malignant tumours is not always facilitated by such a traditional approach. Rather, this separation is more readily demonstrated by the immunocytochemical analysis of cryostat sections and cell suspensions.

Although the presence of functionally and immunophenotypically mature lymphoid follicles (containing follicular dendritic cells polytypic for light chains) and a mixed inflammatory infiltrate often distinguish a benign cutaneous B-cell infiltrate from generally monomorphic B-cell lymphomas, the detection of a monotypic B-cell population is a more reliable marker of malignancy. Since most cutaneous B-cell malignancies express cell surface or cytoplasmic immunoglobulins, monotypia for immunoglobin light chains (kappa or lambda) may be a valuable observation. Most commercially available anti-kappa and anti-lambda reagents work poorly in fixed tissue, but may be both sensitive and specific in adequately prepared frozen sections and cell suspensions. Genotypic evidence of clonal heavy or light chain immunoglobulin gene rearrangements in cutaneous B-cell lymphomas confirm these immunophenotypic findings.

Lineage specific immunophenotypic markers of T-cell monoclonal proliferations are not as yet characterized. However, subtle alterations in broad T-cell selective immunophenotypic panels have been described that may be helpful in selected cases. Cutaneous T-cell lymphomas (CTCL) characteristically express 'aberrant' phenotypes, manifest either as the absence of the pan-T cell markers CD2, CD3 and CD5, or the concordant expression (or loss) of both CD4 and CD8. Neither result is detected in mature reactive T-cell populations (Ralfkiaer, 1991; Rijlaarsdam and Wilemze, 1991; Smolle et al., 1990b). Unfortunately, most low grade CTCLs fail to exhibit aberrant phenotypes, making these attributes of limited value in the separation of such lymphomas from reactive infiltrates (Ralfkiaer, 1991; Rijlaarsdam and Wilemze, 1991). More definitive evidence of T-cell neoplasia may be deduced from genotypic analyses confirming clonal rearrangement of the T-cell receptor (Griesser et al., 1990).

Certain aberrant B-cell phenotypes may also be of diagnostic value. The most important example is the expression of the T-cell marker CD5 in the B-cell small cell infiltrates that typify chronic lymphocytic leukaemia (Ralfkiaer, 1991).

In the rest of this section, we will consider three diagnostic settings in which lymphoid infiltrates in the skin may be the source of consternation or confusion. Further discussion of the immunohistology of other cutaneous haematopoietic neoplasms is available elsewhere (Banks, 1985; Foon and Todd 1986; Knowles, 1985; Norton and Isaacson, 1989a).

Langerhans' cell histiocytosis (histiocytosis X)

Langerhans' cell histiocytosis (LCH), like many of the more typical benign and malignant T-cell and B-cell infiltrates of skin, is often diagnosed readily when clinicopathologic features are analysed. Typically an affliction of children, cutaneous LCH often presents as a multifocal macular or papular eruption consisting of vaguely defined or nodular infiltrates of histiocytoid cells with characteristically folded or grooved nuclei. Often, these children have a prior history of LCH involving extracutaneous sites. Nevertheless, in some instances, LCH may present as a solitary lesion, without prior clinical evidence of Langerhan's cell infiltrates; further confusion may be added by cases that arise in adults. In each of these latter circumstances (and particularly in the adult patients), the differential diagnosis may include lymphoma cutis, malignant melanoma, and poorly differentiated epithelial and mesenchymal lesions of skin.

Regardless of its clinical presentation in skin, LCH displays a consistent immunophenotype. As is typical of the normal intraepidermal Langerhan's cell, the constituent cells of LCH are often reactive for S100 protein (Rowden et al., 1983) and HLA-DR antigens (Taylor et al., 1983). This phenotype is readily obtained in routinely fixed tissues, although the latter of these substances is usually best displayed in cryostat preparations (Wick et al., 1987a). Such a profile is presumptive evidence of LCH (if LCA reactivity is detected (Taylor et al., 1983), and other determinants such as cytokeratin, EMA and HMB-45 are absent) (Hui et al., 1987; Rowden et al., 1983; Springall et al., 1983; Taylor et al., 1983; Wilson et al., 1984), since S100 reactivity is otherwise limited to the very few examples of non-LCH histiocytic proliferations, including lymphomas differentiating as dendritic reticulum cells and the extranodal cutaneous infiltrates of sinus histiocytosis with massive lymphadenopathy.

Definitive evidence of Langerhan's cell differentiation requires detection of CD1 (OKT6) reactivity (Fithian et al., 1981; Knowles, 1985; Murphy et al., 1981) or the ultrastructural demonstration of Birbeck granules. While ultrastructural examination may be performed on paraffin-embedded tissues in lieu of optimally fixed tissues samples (although with predictably suboptimal results), the former requires the use of fresh or frozen tissues (Banks, 1985). Hence, in cases where neither clinical or histologic attributes allow a certain diagnosis of LCH, or when routine tissue fixation has not adequately preserved S100 protein, additional tissue may need to be obtained. Ideally, representative samples of the original biopsy specimen should be collected fresh and stored in a low temperature freezer.

Diagnostic difficulties are uncommonly posed by other cutaneous histiocytoses that affect children, among them the so-called 'congenital self-healing reticulohistiocytosis' (Davaris et al., 1991; Kapila et al., 1985) and 'benign cephalic histocytosis' (Gianotti et al., 1986). The former of these is a proliferation of Langerhan's cells, and shares all immunophenotypic and ultrastructural attributes with LCH (Davaris et al., 1991; Kapila et al., 1985). In fact, many regard this limited cutaneous eruption as a localized form of LCH. Benign cephalic histiocytosis (BCH) is also comprised of S100-positive histiocytes, but shares few other attributes with LCH. The infiltrates of BCH are generally less expansive, are well-circumscribed, and are limited to superficial dermis. Further, they lack the cytologic features of the Langerhan's cell. Accordingly, they are CD-1 negative and lack Birbeck granules (Gianotti et al., 1986).

Intravascular lymphomatosis (malignant angioendotheliomatosis)

Intravascular lymphomatosis (IL) is a unique disorder that commonly presents clinically as violaceous cutaneous nodules and plaques. Microscopically, it is characterized by an intravascular proliferation of large, non-cohesive, cytologically malignant cells that are often enmeshed in fibrin-platelet thrombi. Dermal venules and capillaries are most commonly involved (Wick et al., 1986b).

Because of these histologic features, IL was initially thought to represent an endothelial neoplasm. Early reports detailing the presence of focal Factor VIII-related antigen (FVIIIrag)-reactivity in the neoplastic elements of IL added support for this premise (Fulling and Gersell, 1983; Kermarec et al., 1984). It was later shown, however, that the FVIIIrag-positivity seen in IL is observed only in cells that are entrapped in fibrin thrombi (Wick et al., 1986b). They neither bind *Ulex europaeus* I agglutinin (UEA) nor express other endothelial-selective determinants; hence, we have concluded that FVIIIrag-reactivity in this tumour is due to passive adsorption of soluble antigen, rather than being a reflection of endothelial differentiation (Wick et al., 1986b). These matters aside, IL has in recent years been the source of endless 'novel' determinations of its actual lymphoid nature (see Wick and Mills, 1991). Given its history, it is important to note that Bhawan et al. (1985) were the first to demonstrate diffuse CD45-reactivity in this disorder, an observation that explained an association which they had noted previously between IL and extravascular malignant lymphoma in the same patients. Subsequently, a variety of investigators have reproduced these findings, and have further shown that IL is, in fact, an angiotropic large-cell lymphoma (Burgdorf et al., 1981; Carroll et al., 1986; Mori et al., 1985; Shiebani et al., 1986b; Wick et al., 1986b; Wrotnowski et al., 1985). Most examples are B-cell tumours, but T-cell differentiation has also been seen in this neoplasm (Sheibani et al., 1986b; Wick and Mills, 1991).

'Pseudo-pseudolymphomas'

Among all lymphohaematopoietic lesions of skin, those that present as recurrent and recrudescent eruptions may be the source of considerable diagnostic consternation. Two such lesions, the so-called 'regressing atypical histiocytosis' and lymphomatoid papulosis, historically were considered benign cutaneous lesions, but careful clinical evaluation and immunophenotypic analyses have demonstrated that these atypical infiltrates once thought to be mimics of cutaneous lymphoma ('pseudolymphoma') are in fact clinically malignant diseases. As such, these two entities might wistfully be thought of as 'pseudo-pseudolymphomas'.

In 1982, Flynn et al. (1982) described two cases of a distinctive lesion of the skin, composed of large, anaplastic, pleomorphic lymphoid cells. Despite the appearance of this dermal and subcutaneous infiltrate, each patient so afflicted initially followed a favourable clinical course; cutaneous lesions regressed spontaneously, and patients enjoyed a relatively long period during which they were 'disease-free'. The disease was given the name 'regressing atypical histiocytosis' (RAH) to emphasize its apparently indolent, if not benign, nature. Unfortunately, these and other patients with RAH subsequently developed an aggressive cutaneous and extracutaneous lymphoid proliferation with the phenotypic characteristics of 'malignant histiocytosis', 'true histiocytic lymphoma' and anaplastic T-cell lymphoma (Turner et al., 1984; Weiss et al., 1985).

Immunohistochemically, the cells of RAH in its initial and subsequent manifestations are reactive for CD45, CD43, CD45RO, LN2, cathepsin B, and EMA, among markers reactive in paraffin sections. This 'mixed' phenotype would support the interpretation of these lesions as either T-cell or histiocytic neoplasms. However, detailed imunophenotypic, flow cytometric and genotypic analyses of the original cases described by Flynn et al. (1982) have demonstrated a more consistent histiocytic profile (Hanson et al., 1989).

Lymphomatoid papulosis (LP), in contrast to RAH, follows a more persistently indolent course, and as such is still not uniformly accepted as a malignant disease. LP may arise on any cutaneous or orogenital mucosal surface, although axial sites are most common. The typical lesion of LP is a small papule that may undergo central haemorrhage and necrosis before healing spontaneously. Some lesions may persist indefinately, and local or distant recurrence is common (Kaudewitz and Burg, 1991; Kerl and Smolle, 1990).

Histologically, LP is a deep and superficial perivascular infiltrate that is often accompanied by a lichenoid component in the superfical dermis. The overlying epidermis is often spongiotic and parakeratotic. The infiltrate of LP is mixed, and lymphocytes are usually uniform, small lymphocytic in appearance. The minority of lymphoid cells have atypical cytologic features; in some cases, these cells may be multinucleated or contain atypical mitotic spindles. The latter are more prevalent in active lesions, whereas resolving or healing lesions contain few, if any, atypical elements (Kaudewitz and Burg, 1991). Less commonly, atypical elements may form tumoural nodules or sheets; in such cases, despite characteristic clinical features of LP, a diagnosis of anaplastic T-cell lymphoma may be entertained (Kaudewitz and Burg, 1991; Kerl and Smolle, 1990).

The latter attribute of LP is considered by many to be vital to the interpretation of LP as a malignant (albeit low grade) T-cell lymphoma. Immunophenotypic analyses of LP support this latter view, since in many instances of LP, the aberrant phenotype typical of high grade T-cell lymphoma may be detected. Further, a significant number of LP cases may be reactive with BerH2 (anti-CD30 (Ki-1)) (Kaudewitz and Burg, 1991), another attribute of anaplastic T-cell lymphoma (Banerjee et al., 1991; Beljaards et al., 1989; Ralfkiaer et al., 1989). While it is possible that the latter reflects only a state of activation in an atypical, but benign T-cell population, the variable detection of monoclonal T-cell receptor rearrangements in LP is cause for careful consideration by those unwilling to classify this disorder as malignant (Griesser et al., 1990). Such rearrangements are uncommon in benign reactive T-cell infiltrates. Interestingly, the one instance of a T-cell receptor rearrangement among ten cases of LP studied by Griesser et al. (1990) was detected in a case that subsequently evolved into a pleomorphic Ki-1 reactive T-cell lymphoma. The inconstant association of LP with the subsequent or concurrent development of immunophenotypicaly similar CD30+ T-cell lymphomas is also well known.

Mesenchymal tumours of the skin

Patterns of mesenchymal differentiation in cutaneous neoplasms are no less diverse than those encountered in deeper soft tissues (Enzinger and Weiss, 1989; Kaye and Swanson, 1991). Fibroblastic or myofibroblastic, 'fibrohistiocytic', muscular, neural and vascular elements may comprise both benign and malignant cutaneous mesenchymnal proliferations. Of course, our ability to list these patterns belies the diagnostic difficulties posed by soft tissue tumours in skin. Indeed, as is also true in deep soft tissues, the histologic evaluation of these mesenchymal neoplasms often fails to reveal unequivocal diagnostic information. Hence, immunohistochemistry has proven to be of considerable value in this context. As illustrated in Tables 6.1, 6.2 and 6.3, the diagnostic separation of the various spindled-polygonal cell, epithelioid cell and small cell lesions of skin is facilitated in many settings by immunohistochemical analysis. While the tables conceptually stand alone, the following discussion is provided to elaborate on points of particular importance to our understanding of these various mesenchymal proliferations.

Fibroblastic/myofibroblastic neoplasms

In general, tumours showing pure fibroblastic or myofibroblastic differentiation are uncommon. Only three cutaneous neoplastic proliferations consistently display only fibroblastic or myofibroblastic features – recurring digital fibroma (digital fibromatosis (Bhawan et al., 1979; Enzinger and Weiss, 1989; Visona et al., 1987)), cutaneous fibrosarcoma (Manivel et al., 1985), and congenital superficial 'haemangiopericytoma' (Swanson and Dehner,

Table 6.3. Immunophenotype of small cell cutaneous neoplasms

Tumour	VIM	CK	EMA	CEA	S100	HMB	DES	MSA	SNP	Leu7	LCA
Squamous cell carcinoma	0	+	+	0	0	0	0	0	0	0	0
Eccrine carcinoma	0	+	+	+	+/−	0	0	0	0	r	0
Primary cutaneous neuroendocrine carcinoma	0	+(a)	+	0	0	0	0	0	+	+	0
Metastatic neuroendocrine carcinoma	0	+	+	+	+/−	0	0	0	+	+	0
Malignant melanoma	+	0(b)	0	0	+	+	0	0	0	+/−	0
Malignant lymphoma	+	0	0	0	0	0	0	0	0	0	+
Rhabdomyosarcoma(c)	+	0	0	0	0	0	+	+	0	+/−	0
Primitive peripheral neuroectodermal tumour(c)	+	0	0	0	0	0	0	0	+	+/−	0
Extraskeletal Ewing's sarcoma(c)	+	0(b)	0	0	0	0	0	0	r	+/−	0

Notes:
+ = at least 50 per cent of cases positive
+/− = between 10 and 50 per cent of cases positive
r = rare reactivity reported
a = 'dot-like' perinuclear staining pattern
b = we consider reported instances of CK-reactivity spurious (see text)
c = cutaneous lesions anecdotally reported.

Abbreviations: VIM – vimentin; CK – cytokeratin; EMA – epithelial membrane antigen; CEA – carcinoembryonic antigen; HMB – HMB-45; DES – desmin; MSA – muscle specific actin; SNP – synaptophysin; LCA – leucocyte common antigen (CD45).

1991). The first of these tumours typically occurs on the hands of children; in many instances, it is multifocal. Ultrastructural analysis has shown that digital fibroma (DF) consists of myofibroblasts (Bhawan et al., 1979; Enzinger and Weiss, 1989); accordingly, DF displays uniform reactivity for vimentin and muscle-specific isoforms of actin. In our experience, desmin may be detected as well, although our data are not supported by other authors (Schurch et al., 1984). Our results should not be unexpected, however, since the ultrastructural and biochemical attributes of myofibroblast contractile elements are essentialy identical to those of the smooth muscle cell. Notably, the peculiar intracytoplasmic inclusions that are present in DF correspond to aggregates of immunodetectible actin filaments (Enzinger and Weiss, 1989).

Fibrosarcoma of the skin has been reported in association with burn scars, surgical scars, smallpox vaccinations, and other injection sites (Enzinger and Weiss, 1989; Flotte et al., 1984). This exceedingly uncommon neoplasm consists exclusively of fibroblastic elements, and thus stains only for vimentin, to the exclusion of the many mesenchyme-associated deteminants that may be associated with non-fibroblastic patterns of differentiation (see Table 6.1).

Congenital haemangiopericytoma (so named because of the peculiar vascular pattern that supports this spindled cell tumour of dermis and subcutis in young children) is a lesion that none the less shares clinical and histologic features with the myofibromatoses that afflict this same age population (Enzinger and Weiss, 1989). Unlike true haemangiopericytomas, which often fail to stain for muscle-specific actin, congenital haemangiopericytomas are often diffusely reactive for this myogenic (myofibroblastic) determinant (Swanson and Dehner, 1991).

'Fibrohistiocytic' neoplasms

The concept that such tumours as atypical fibroxanthoma (AFX), malignant fibrous histiocytoma (MFH), and dermatofibrosarcoma protuberans (DFSP) display 'fibrohistiocytic' cellular features (that is, morphologic, functional, and phenotypic characteristics of both fibroblasts and histiocytes) is proving less tenable, as more detailed immunohistochemical analyses of these lesions are reported. Although there is some disagreement on this point (Sieber et al., 1990; Strauchen and Dimitriu-Bona, 1986; Wood et al., 1986), the minority of these lesions express specialized haematopoietic determinants (Holden, 1989; Lloyd and Wilson, 1983). The latter include CD45/leukocyte common antigen (LCA), CD4, CD11c, CD14, CD16, CD18, CD36 (OKM5), CD43 (MT1), CD56 and CD68 (KP1) all of which may be displayed by bone marrow-derived monocytes and histocytes (Mechterscheimer, 1991; Turner et al., 1984; Wood et al., 1986). The presence of HLA-DR in MFH has been substantiated in a handful of reports (Sieber et al., 1990; Strauchen and Dimitriu-Bona, 1986; Swanson and Wick, 1990) (Fig. 6.11), but analyses of various soft tissue malignancies reveals that the expression of this histocompatibility antigen complex is not limited to tumour cells differentiating as histiocytes (Mechterscheimer et al., 1990; Swanson and Wick, 1990).

Similarly, cellular proteases such as alpha-1-antichymotrypsin (AACT), alpha-1-antitrypsin (AAT), and cathepsin-B (CB), while typical of the cellular constituents of histiocytes, are regularly present not only in AFX, MFH and DFSP (Crocker et al., 1984; DuBoulay 1982; Kindblom et al., 1982; Manivel et al., 1985; Roholl et al., 1985; Wood et al., 1986) (Fig. 6.12), but in most other spindled cell tumours in skin as well (Leader et al., 1987; Silvis et al., 1988). The exception appears to be leiomyosarcoma, in which we have not detected AACT or AAT (Silvis et al., 1988). MAC 387, an antibody to a cytoplasmic determinant (the L1 antigen) that is characteristic of functionally mature monocytes and macrophages, also frequently labels multinucleated, and, less commonly, spindled elements in MFH, AFX and DFSP. However, recent studies indicate that with the exception of squamous cell carcinoma and malignant melanoma, MAC 387 also labels virtually every other type of neoplasm in skin (Loftus et al., 1991). Finally,

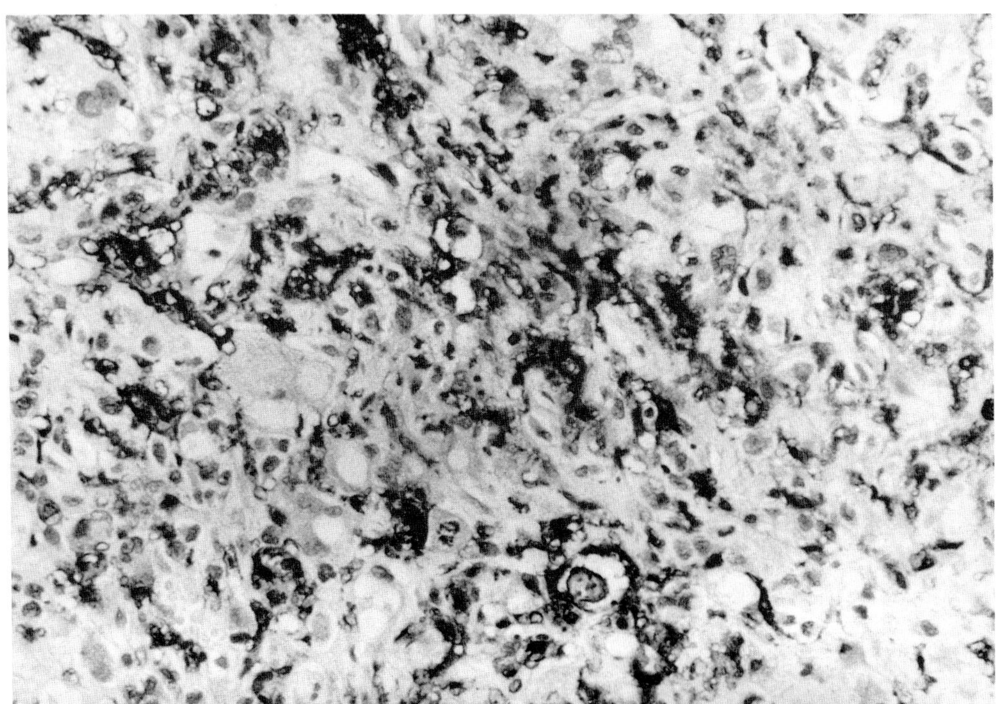

Fig. 6.11. HLA-DR in malignant fibrous histiocytoma. Both spindled and pleomorphic elements in malignant fibrous histiocytoma may be reactive.

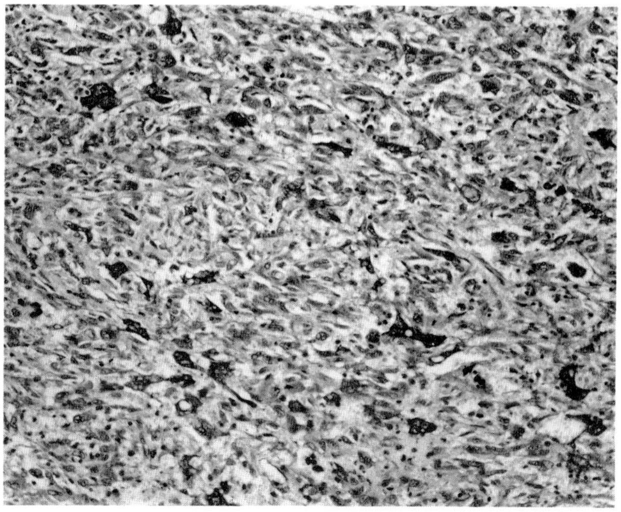

Fig. 6.12. Alpha-1-antichymotrypsin in malignant fibrous histiocytoma. Multinucleated giant cells stain preferentially for this proteolytic enzyme.

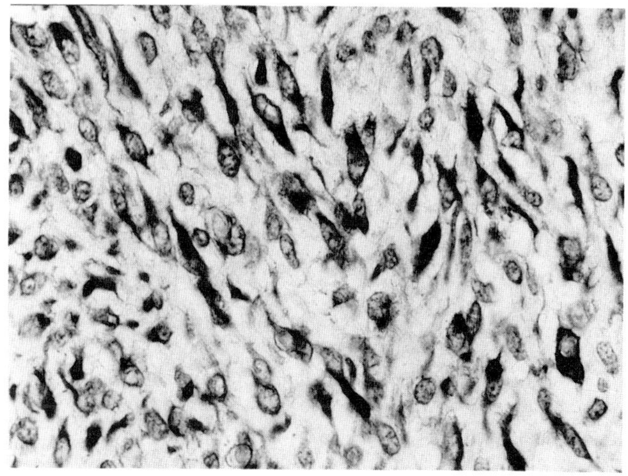

Fig. 6.13. Muscle-specific actin in malignant fibrous histiocytoma. Area of staining like that illustrated here are uncommon. In most examples, staining is either focal or absent.

immunoreactivity for Factor XIIIa, a coagulation factor also expressed by fibroblasts and non-fibroblastic stromal elements (Nemeth and Penneys, 1989), is encountered in many examples of MFH, but is also occasionally encountered in other sarcomas, granular cell tumours, and neurofibromas (Cerio et al., 1990; Gray et al., 1990c; Nemes and Thomazy, 1988; Nemeth and Penneys, 1989).

The most consistent finding in MFH, AFX and DFSP is diffuse reactivity for vimentin (Hirose et al., 1989; Lautier et al., 1990; Pettinato et al., 1990; Ricci et al., 1988). Muscle-specific actins have also been detected in these neoplasms (Fig. 6.13), albeit sparingly in most cases (Hirose et al., 1989; Pettinato et al., 1990; Ricci et al., 1988), while focal desmin reactivity may also be obtained in MFH (Wick and Kaye, 1986). Ultrastructural evidence of myofibroblastic elements in MFH has also been reported (Martorelli et al., 1989).

The aforementioned data suggest that MFH, AFX and DFSP are largely fibroblastic or myofibroblastic in nature. However, not even this general pattern can adequately define the nature of each example of MFH. Indeed, recent studies of cultured cells from MFH explanted in nude mice have shown the potential for both myogenic and nerve sheath differentiation in some instances (Roholl et al., 1988). It is likely, therefore, that MFH, among the 'fibrohistiocytic' tumours of skin and soft tissue, is not a unified entity, but instead a common final pathway of differentiation for several different mesenchymal neoplasms, a concept first espoused by Brooks (1986). In this context, it is interesting that DFSP is purported to have arisen as the recurrence of the clinically benign mesenchymal (?myofibroblastic) proliferation of skin in children and young adults that is known as 'giant cell fibroblastoma' (Alguacil-Garcia, 1991; Dymock et al., 1987; Fletcher 1988; Schmookler et al., 1989).

Standing in stark contrast to the malignant tumours just discussed are the benign cutaneous 'fibrohistiocytic' tumours. From the fairly common dermatofibroma to the less often encountered and recently described lesions such as storiform and plexiform fibrohistiocytic tumours (Enzinger and Weiss, 1989; Enzinger and Zhang, 1988), a mixed (myo)fibroblastic and histiocytic proliferation is commonly verified by immunohistochemical analysis (Fletcher 1990; Smith et al., 1991; Soini 1990). Indeed, spindled and multinucleated elements in most such benign lesions of skin are reactive with MAC387 and HAM56 (a novel histiomonocytic marker) (Cerio et al., 1990; Fletcher 1990). Further, it is these tumours among lesions of skin (along with the angiomatoid variant of MFH, occasional examples of granular cell tumour, and malignant melanoma (Facchetti et al., 1991; Smith et al., 1991)) that are reproducibly reactive for CD68 (detected with the monoclonal antibody KP1) (Fletcher 1990; Smith et al., 1991). While it is plausible to conclude that malignant degeneration in such cell populations may be associated with the loss of 'histiocytic' markers, it may be more reasonable to assume that there is no necessary relationship between the benign and malignant 'fibrohistiocytic' tumours in skin.

Smooth muscle tumours

Comparative ultrastructural and immunohistochemical studies of cutaneous and extracutaneous leiomyomas and leiomyosarcomas have revealed few notable differences. Most, if not all, such tumours are diffusely labelled by antibodies to vimentin and muscle specific actins (Miettinen et al., 1982; Swanson et al., 1987b; Wick and Kaye, 1986). The latter determinant has been touted by others as the most sensitive marker of smooth muscle differentiation among the muscle-associated determinants commonly studied in routine practice (Azumi et al., 1988; Tsukuda et al., 1987). However, desmin reactivity is also an expected attribute of these tumours (Azumi et al., 1988; Swanson et al, 1988a). In our experience, in fact, virtually all smooth muscle neoplasms, both benign and malignant, will harbour detectible quantities of these intermediate filament peptides (Swanson et al., 1988a) (Fig. 6.14).

Cutaneous leiomyosarcomas appear to differ from their extracutaneous relatives in that more than 30 per cent of dermal-based lesions are S100 protein reactive (Fig. 6.15), while a similar number of subcuticular tumours are labeled by Leu7 (Swanson et al., 1988a). We have speculated that the former of these findings is predicted from the presence of S100 protein in pilar musculature, whereas the detection of Leu7 antigen in vascular smooth muscle may relate to the latter. Apart from such fanciful histogenetic ruminations, these observations are more germain to the diagnostic separation of cutaneous leioyosarcomas from peripheral neurogenic tumours and spindled melanocytic neoplasms. As Tables 6.1 and 6.2 emphasize, however, the paucity of myogenic markers in the latter tumours minimizes the likelihood of misdiagnosis when only immunopheotypic characteristics are considered. Focal expression of desmin in malignant peripheral nerve sheath tumours may rarely be problematic (Swanson et al., 1987b), but the concordance of S100 and Leu 7 reactivity in such lesions (seen in about one-third of nerve sheath sarcomas (Wick et al., 1987b), but not in LMS) may be helpful. The occasional presence of muscle-specific actin or desmin reactivity in MFH, and the expression of Cathepsin B in LMS may rarely complicate the separation

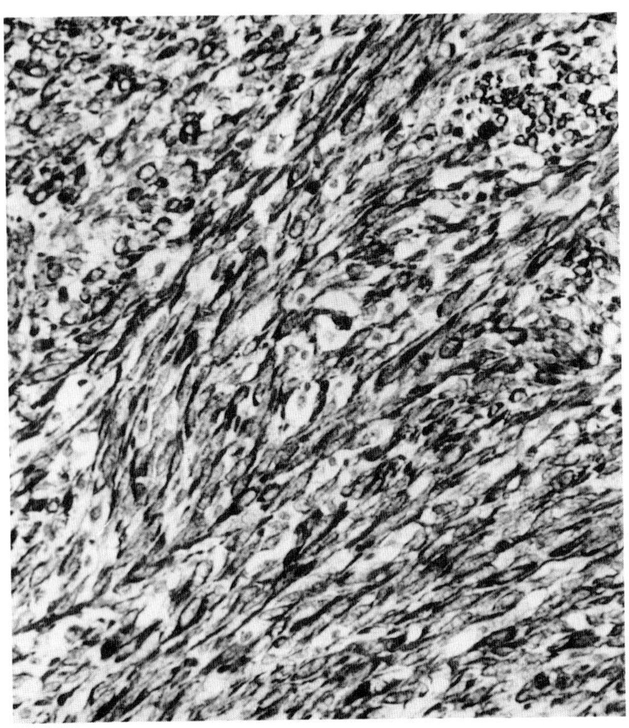

Fig. 6.14. Desmin in leiomyosarcoma. Most examples of cutaneous leiomyosarcoma are diffusely reactive for this intermediate filament.

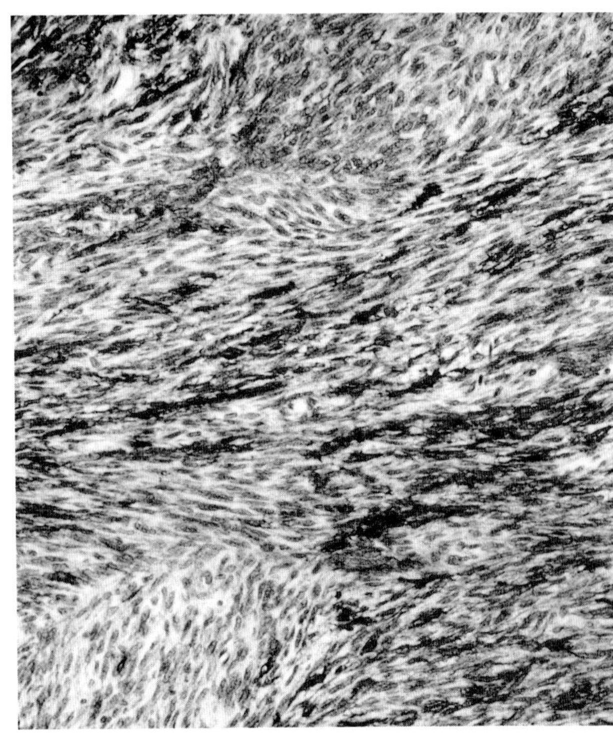

Fig. 6.15. S100 protein in leiomyosarcoma. Focal reactivity characterizes dermal-based leiomyosarcomas.

of these two sarcomas (Miettinen et al., 1982). Notably, however, the distribution of these myogenic markers in MFH is rarely anything but focal, in contrast to their diffuse distribution in LMS.

Glomangiomas and glomangiosarcomas are neoplasms that are related to tumours of smooth muscle, in that they exhibit feature of specialized perivascular smooth muscle cells (pericytes) (Enzinger and Weiss, 1989). However, they differ from other smooth muscle tumours in that they lack desmin-positivity. It has been suggested that glomangiocellular tumours should be classified as vascular tumours; however, their uniform lack of Factor VIII-related antigen and binding sites for *Ulex europaeus* agglutinin I (UEA), together with evidence of pericytic differentiation, make such an hypothesis untenable (Burgdorf et al., 1981; Miettinen et al., 1983; Mukai and Rosai, 1984; Mukai et al., 1980; Ordonez and Batsakis, 1984).

Nerve sheath tumours

The most common cutaneous (and extracutaneous) nerve sheath tumour is the neurofibroma; often, such tumours in skin are multiple and occur in the setting of von Recklinghausen's neurofibromatosis (Enzinger and Weiss, 1989; Manivel et al., 1985; Sharma et al., 1990). Cutaneous malignant peripheral nerve sheath tumours are considerably less common (Enzinger and Weiss, 1989; George et al., 1989b). Most such lesions arise primarily in dermal or subcutaneous tissues, although secondary involvement by direct extension from deeper lesions may also occur (Mogollon et al., 1984).

The immunophenotypic attributes that typify most forms of peripheral nerve sheath tumours (PNST) include staining for vimentin, S100 protein (Fig. 6.16) and Leu7 (CD57) antigen (Fig. 6.17) (Gallagher and Helwig, 1980; George et al. 1989b; Kahn et al., 1983; Manivel et al., 1985; Miettinen et al., 1982; Perentes and Rubinstein, 1985; Sharma et al., 1990; Stefannson et al., 1982; Swanson et al., 1987b). We have also shown that reactivity for myelin basic protein (MBP) is common in both benign and malignant PNST (Swanson et al., 1987b; Wick et al., 1987b), despite earlier reports to the contrary (Clark et al., 1985). The contribution of differences in antibody reagents and staining techniques to this apparent discrepancy is supported is supported by the positive results obtained by various authors (Mogollon et al., 1984; Penney et al., 1984)

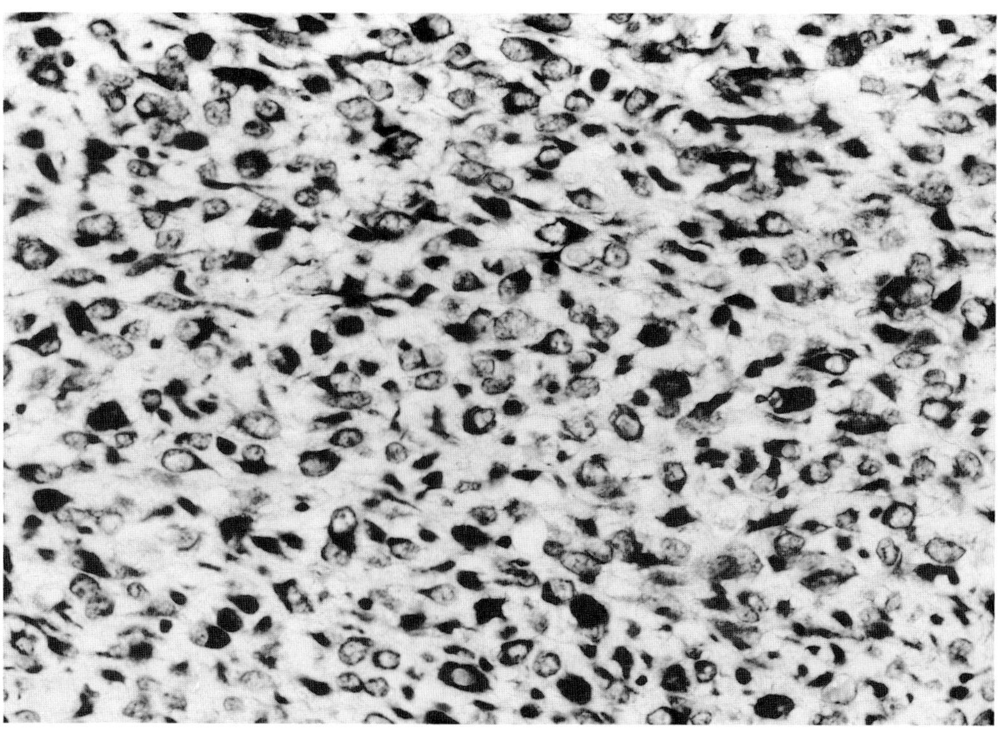

Fig. 6.16. S100 protein in malignant peripheral nerve sheath tumour. Pleomorphic malignant peripheral nerve sheath tumours are usually reactive.

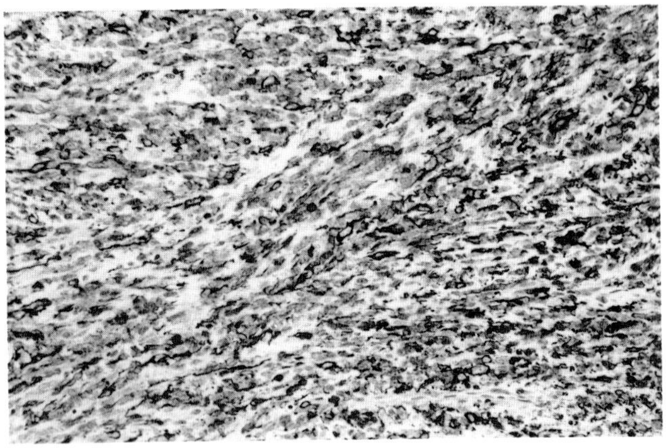

Fig. 6.17. Leu7 (CD57) in malignant peripheral nerve sheath tumour. The majority of lesions are reactive for this myelin-associated substance.

using similar methodologies. The detection of S100, Leu7 antigen and MBP, alone or in combination, provides the basis for the reliable identification of PNST (Wick et al., 1987b).

A variety of other determinants have been detected in certain examples of PNST, including glial fibrillary acidic protein, neuron specific enolase and neural cell adhesion molecules (distinct from the Leu7 antigen) (Gray et al., 1989; Stanton et al., 1987), but none have contributed consistently to the accurate diagnosis of malignant PNST in skin.

It is commonly accepted that most examples of granular cell tumour of the skin display Schwann cell differentiation (Penneys et al., 1984; Stefansson and Wollman, 1982), although few examples of leiomyoma, haemangioma and basal cell carcinoma, among other tumour types, have been comprised largely of granular cells (LeBoit et al., 1991). Accordingly, most granular cell tumours display reactivity for S100 protein (Stefansson and Wollman, 1982), Leu7 (Smolle et al, 1985), or myelin basic protein (Penneys et al., 1984; Smolle et al., 1985). GCT also shares with neurofibroma (but not neurilemmoma) the apparent expression of Factor XIIIa (Cerio et al., 1990). Malignant granular tumours of skin are exceedingly rare, but like their benign counterparts are presumed to exhibit nerve sheath differentiation. However, we have studied two such lesions that contained neither S100 protein, Leu7 antigen nor MBP (LeBoit et al., 1991). Instead, one tumour expressed only NSE and vimentin, while the second had an immunophenotype that more closely resembled the malignant 'fibrohistiocytic' tumours described above.

Vascular neoplasms

Benign tumours showing endothelial differentiation (haemangiomas) are the most common vascular neoplasms of skin; such lesions may afflict patients of any age. Malignant endothelial or vessel-associated neoplasms are considerably less common, and usually afflict adults older than 50 years of age (Enzinger and Weiss, 1989). The latter neoplasms include Kaposi's sarcoma, angiosarcoma, and epithelioid haemangioendothelioma (Snover and Rosai, 1985).

Haemangiomas are readily identified in most instances, although occasional examples are composed of a solid proliferation of spindled cells (as in some capillary haemangiomas in young children) or epithelioid (histiocytoid) tumour cells, with little overt vasogenesis (Enzinger and Weiss, 1989; Gonzalez-Crussi and Reyes-Mugica, 1991). In such cases, immunostaining for Factor VIII-related antigen (FVIIIrag) or binding of *Ulex europaeus* agglutinin I (UEA) may be helpful. The latter stain is more sensitive than FVIIIrag (Little et al., 1986; Ordonez and Batsakis, 1984); more than 80 per cent of haemangiomas will bind UEA, wheras fewer than 50 per cent may contain detectible amounts of FVIIIrag. In addition, the latter is not consistently displayed in lesions comprised of lymphatic type endothelium, in contrast to UEA. Of course, since UEA recognizes a terminal fucosyl residue present on the H antigen (ABO blood type O) that may also be secreted by certain epithelial cell populations, this marker is of relatively low specificity for endothelial differentiation, compared to FVIIIrag (Little et al., 1986; Ordonez and Batsakis, 1984). Nevertheless, the exclusion of epithelial differentiation by the use of immunostains for cytokeratin and EMA enhances the diagnostic utility of UEA.

The tumour cells of angiosarcomas are less consistently labelled with UEA and antibodies to FVIIIrag, compared with benign vascular lesions (Little et al., 1986; Miettinen et al., 1983; Miettinen et al., 1983b; Mukai and Rosai, 1984; Ordonez and Batsakis, 1984; Perez et al., 1986; Snover and Rosai, 1985). Even so, in poorly differentiated solid or spindle-cell angiosarcomas (Perez et al, 1986; Wick and Kaye, 1986), FVIIIrag reactivity may be encountered in approximately 30 per cent, while 75 per cent of such lesions bind UEA. Cutaneous angiosarcomas in the Stewart–Treves syndrome (Miettinen et al, 1983b) are no different than sporadic examples in the skin of the head and neck (Perez et al., 1986), in this respect. Similar comments apply to the evaluation of epithelioid angiosarcomas and the low grade vascular neoplasm epithelioid haemangioendothelioma (Enzinger and Weiss, 1989; Weiss and Enzinger, 1982).

In recent years, a number of reagents have been developed that have been described as similar in specificity, but considerably improved in sensitivity for endothelial differentiation, compared to anti-FVIIIrag. Most notable among them are antibodies to thrombomodulin (TM) (Maruyama et al., 1985; Yonezawa et al., 1987), an endothelial product with an effect that is antagonistic to FVIIIrag. In published reports, this marker has been detected in virtually all vascular tumours studied, including haemangiomas, angiosarcomas and epithelioid haemangioendotheliomas. Unfortunately, certain non-endothelial tumours may also be immunoreactive for TM, including squamous cell carcinomas and trophoblastic tumours (Maruyama et al., 1985). The potential confusion of acantholytic variants of the former tumour with epithelioid angiosarcoma in skin highlights the interpretative pitfalls that TM might engender.

A variety of monoclonal antibodies to other endothelial-associated determinants have been discussed, few of which have proved particularly useful or popular as diagnostic reagents. One such antibody, 'PAL-E' (Schlingemann et al., 1985), is reactive only with frozen tissue, a trait that limits its utility in routine pathology practice. Two others, EN-4 and BW200 (Alles and Bosslet, 1986; Swanson and Wick, 1991), have not been made commercially available, despite their apparent selectivity for endothelial determinants in frozen and fixed tissues, respectively. A number of other antibodies have been shown to label neoplastic and non-neoplastic endothelial cells, but are of dimished utility, owing to their ability to bind non-endothelial populations as well. Among these, the antibodies E92, OKM1, OKM5 and HC-1 (Holden et al., 1986; Kaplan et al., 1983; Posnett et al., 1984; Rutgers et al., 1986; Swanson and Wick, 1991) label various haematolymphoid and mesenchymal tissues, in addition to endothelium. Finally, antibodies to ABO blood group isoantigens, while sensitive markers for endothelial cells when used together as an isoantigen 'cocktail', suffer the same drawback as UEA – binding of epithelial cell populations (Berry and Amerigo, 1983; Feigl et al., 1976; Little et al., 1986).

The most recently introduced 'endothelial marker' is CD34, an antigen corresponding to a 110 kD glycoprotein human progenitor cell antigen that is recognized by several different monoclonal antibodies, among them My10 (Traweek et al., 1991) and QBend/10 (Fletcher et al., 1991a). Despite its initial use as a marker of immature haematopoietic elements in bone marrow, CD34 has more recently been found in normal endothelial cells and periadnexal cutaneous mesenchymal cells. The former of these attributes is reflected in its exquisite sensitivity for normal and reactive, as well as benign and malignant endothelial cells (Cohen et al., 1991; Traweek et al., 1991; Fletcher et al., 1991a) (Fig. 6.18). Unfortunately, like the other markers described before it, CD34 suffers a specificity problem, in that such diverse tumours as epithelioid sarcoma, leiomyosarcoma, and neurofibroma may also be labelled. In our recent analysis of epithelioid soft tissue

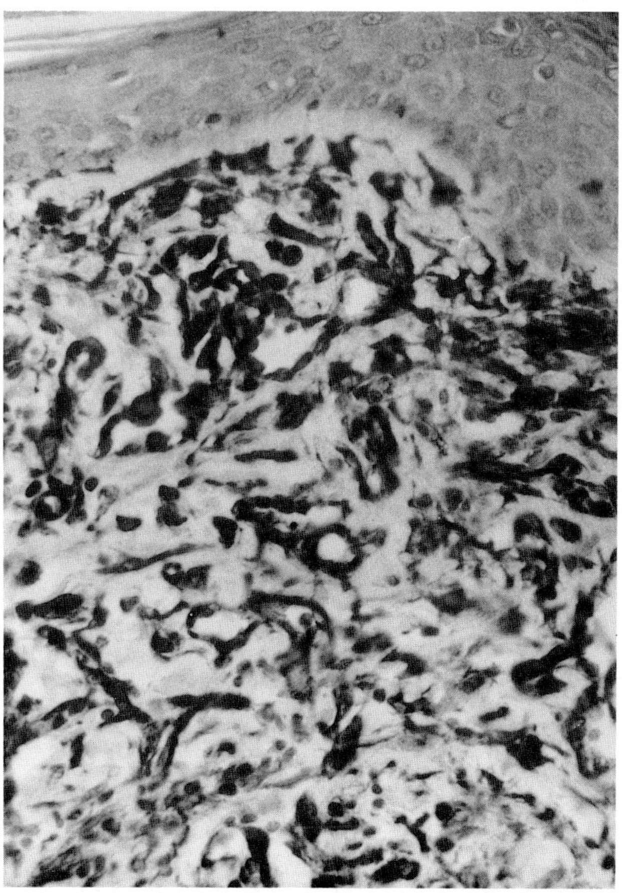

Fig. 6.18. CD34 in angiosarcoma. This example of angiosarcoma in the scalp is diffusely reactive for CD34.

sarcomas, a differential diagnosis in which FVIIIrag negative epitheioid angiosarcomas may be difficult to recognize, still other tumour types, including epithelioid malignant PNST, epithelioid leiomyosarcomas, MIFH and clear cell sarcomas were occasionally CD34-reactive (Swanson and Sirgi, 1992). Our concurrent observation that only epithelioid angiosarcoma, among these latter soft tissue tumours, is reactive with the anti-tumour associated glycoprotein (TAG) antibody B72.3 (Fig. 6.19), requires further study (Swanson and Sirgi, 1992).

In contrast to the well-documented endothelial tumours described above, the putative endothelial nature of both epidemic and endemic forms of Kaposi's sarcoma (KS) has been the subject of speculation and study since the original description of this lesion (Kaposi, 1872). In addition, there is considerable controversy regarding whether KS is truly a neoplasm, rather than a reactive mesenchymal proliferation (Snover and Rosai, 1985). Immunohistochemistry, unfortunately, has been incapable of solving either of these problems, although the issue of endothelial differentiation has been studied at length.

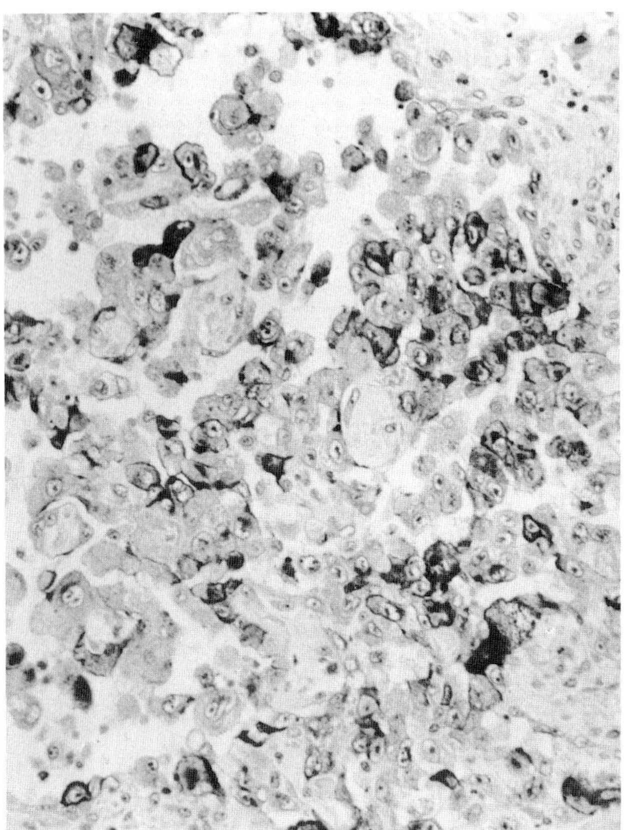

Fig. 6.19. B72.3 reactivity in epithelioid angiosarcoma. Staining for the tumour associated glycoprotein is limited to epithelioid angiosarcomas, among the epithelioid malignancies of soft tissue.

Most such investigations have proven inconclusive when considered as a single body of evidence (Wick, 1991a). While some investigators have detected FVIIIrag-positivity or UEA binding in the spindle cells of KS (Flotte et al, 1984; Guarda et al., 1981; Holden, 1989; Modlin et al., 1983; Nadji et al., 1981; Ordonez and Batsakis, 1984; Taylor et al., 1983), others have consistently failed to do so (Beckstead et al., 1985; Burgdorf et al., 1981; Dorfman 1986; Russell-Jones et al., 1986). In our laboratory, KS is rarely positive with either reagent, although UEA binding is somewhat more common. Among the other aforementioned endothelial-selective reagents, OKM-5 or anti-E92 have been detected in examples of spindle-cell KS, using cryostat sections (Rutgers et al., 1986). Similarly, CD34 reactivity is reported to be uniformly present in KS (Cohen et al., 1991; Kraffert et al., 1991), although in our experience, fewer than half of such lesions are positive. Such results presumably support the notion of endothelial differentiation in KS, but the lack of specificity displayed by these reagents leaves such conclusions in doubt.

Similar issues are raised by the recently described entity spindle-cell haemangioendothelioma (SCH), although the histologic appearance of SCH is sufficient evidence of at least partial endothelial differentiation (Fletcher et al., 1991b; Scott and Rosai, 1988; Weiss and Enzinger, 1986). These tumours, usually solitary nodules in the dermis and subcutaneous tissue of young adults, are composed of KS-like spindled elements admixed with an endothelial proliferation indistinguishable from capillary and cavernous haemangiomas. While the latter are typically reactive for FVIIIrag and bind UEA, the spindled elements are usually negative for both. Epithelioid areas in some examples of SCH have been taken as evidence that this lesion is related to epithelioid haemangioendothelioma and is thus best regarded as a low grade endothelial malignancy. However, recent ultrastructural analyses have documented rudimentary endothelial features in some spindled elements, and have found a variably prominent smooth muscle component in overtly vasogenic areas, together with evidence of old and organizing thrombi, suggesting a reactive, as opposed to a neoplastic, origin (Fletcher et al., 1991b; Imayama et al., 1992).

The persistent similarities between SCH and KS, together with the clinical manifestations of AIDS-asociated KS, have led to further speculation regarding the possible reactive nature of the latter lesion as well. While we continue to regard KS as a malignant neoplasm of putative endothelial differentiation, the issue remains unresolved. From a practical perspective, one should not be dissuaded from a diagnosis of KS if a dermal or subcuticular spindle cell lesion is FVIIIrag or UEA negative (Swanson and Wick, 1991). Coexpression of vimentin and CD34, to the exclusion of nerve sheath- or smooth muscle-associated antigens, should be considered supportive evidence for this diagnosis.

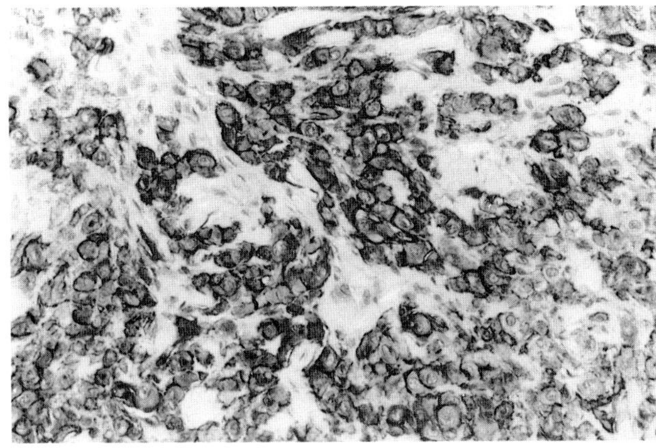

Fig. 6.20. Epithelial membrane antigen in epithelioid sarcoma. Distinct membrane-based reactivity typifies over 70 per cent of epithelioid sarcomas.

Epithelioid sarcoma

Epithelioid sarcoma (ES) is an unusual polygonal-cell neoplasm of the dermis and subcutis (Chase et al., 1984; Enzinger and Weiss, 1989) that may assume various microscopic appearances (Enzinger and Weiss, 1989; Manivel et al., 1987) that result in its confusion with other lesions of skin. When predominantly growing in a solid pattern, ES may be mistaken for metastatic carcinoma or malignant melanoma; a granulomatoid pattern of growth, with palisading of neoplastic cells around areas of necrosis, may impart a similarity to necrobiotic granulomas (rheumatoid nodules; deep granuloma annulare); pseudoangiomatous areas in ES, when predominant, may make the histologic separation of this tumour from epithelioid haemangioendothelioma quite difficult (Enzinger and Weiss, 1989; Manivel et al., 1987; Wick and Manivel, 1986).

The immunophenotypic characteristics of ES generally facilitate its accurate diagnosis in the second of the settings just described, but may further complicate its separation from metastatic carcinomas. Among epithelioid mesenchymal tumours of superficial soft tissues, only ES is consistently immunoreactive for CK (Battifora, 1984; Chase et al., 1984; Manivel et al., 1985; Manivel et al., 1987); this attribute is shared by synovial sarcomas, but these latter lesions are more typically situated in the deeper soft tissues (Enzinger and Weiss, 1989; Salisbury and Isaacson, 1985). The immunophenotypic overlap between ES and metastatic carcinoma is accentuated by the detection of EMA in at least 70 per cent of examples of ES (Fig. 6.20). Indeed, the exclusion of metastatic carcinoma is virtually impossible on immunohistological grounds. In contrast, the separation of ES from malignant melanoma is generally secure, since fewer than 15 per cent of ES are S100 protein reactive, and no examples of ES to date have stained for HMB-45.

With respect to the separation of ES from epithelioid haemangioendothelioma (EH), the presence of UEA binding in over 50 per cent of ES cases is problematic (Wick and Manivel, 1987). Similarly, the common expression of CD34 antigens in ES may complicate this differential diagnosis (Traweek et al., 1991). Recent reports of CK-like reactivity in various vascular tumours (Eusebi et al., 1990; Fletcher et al., 1991a; Gray et al., 1990a), including EH (Gray et al., 1990a), may further contribute to confusion in this setting. More will be made of the latter point at the end of the chapter, but while we have not encountered CK-positivity in EH or other vascular lesions and consider such reports as examples of spurious staining, it is likely that others will continue to regard CK-reactivity with some concern. Hence, for those unwilling to accept CK-negativity as the expected result in EH, the absence of Factor VIII-related antigen reactivity in ES will none the less provide corroborative evidence that this EMA-reactive lesion can be accurately separated from vascular tumours as a group.

Small round cell tumours

The infiltration of dermis and subcutis by small neoplastic cells may conceivably indicate the presence of peripheral neuroectodermal tumour (PNET), extraskeletal Ewing's sarcoma (ES) or rhabdomyosarcoma (RMS). Such tumours constitute an exceedingly minute minority of the small cell tumours of skin, the more common of which are malignant lymphoma, Merkel cell carcinoma (primary cutaneous neuroendocrine carcinoma), and small cell malignant melanoma, in that order. Although their occurrence in skin is at best anecdotal, the histologic and immunophenotypic attributes of such tumours have mirrored those encountered in the more usual anatomic sites (Chang et al., 1990; Jacinto et al., 1991; Patterson and Maygardern, 1986). RMS predictably expresses the myogenic determinants desmin and muscle-specific actin, while PNET and ES stain variably for Leu7, NSE, and synaptophysin (Swanson and Dehner, 1991). None of these tumours are typically reactive for either cytokeratin, CD45 (leucocyte common antigen) or HMB-45, making the immunophenotypic confusion of histologically enigmatic cases less likely (Table 6.3).

Special topics in cutaneous immunohistochemistry

Cytokeratin expression in non-epithelial neoplasms

As stressed in the foregoing discussion, immunoreactivity for cytokeratin is a consistent and reliable marker of epithelial differentiation. However, as we alluded to earlier, the recent literature is replete with reports of 'unexpected' or 'aberrant' reactivity for these intermediate filaments in a variety of non-epithelial tumours (Swanson, 1991), including leiomyosarcoma (Gown et al., 1988; Miettinen, 1988), malignant peripheral nerve sheath tumours (Gray et al., 1989; Miettinen, 1990), malignant fibrous histiocytoma (Miettinen and Soini, 1989), epithelioid angiosarcoma (Eusebi et al., 1990; Fletcher et al., 1991a; Gray et al., 1990a), epithelioid haemangioendothelioma (Gray et al, 1990a) and malignant melanoma (Miettinen and Franssila, 1989; Om et al., 1991; Zarbo et al., 1990). In most cases, reactivity for low molecular weight keratin moieties has been described.

What should we make of these reports? There is biochemical evidence (obtained from immunoblot studies of two-dimensional electrophoretic studies) that smooth muscle tumours and malignant melanoma may contain variable. amounts of these keratin moieties (Gown et al., 1988; Zarbo et al., 1990). However, even in frozen sections, the immunohistochemical detection of keratins is uncommon in non-uterine leiomyosarcomas (Swanson, 1991), and, in our experience, is an event as yet unobserved in malignant melanoma (Swanson, 1990). While these filaments might be detected more readily by increasing the sensitivity of the detection method, such manipulations have the potential of altering the specificity of routine immunohistochemical stains, yielding a bewildering array of unexpected results. We have noted, for example, that when cytokeratin-negative sarcomas (defined by reactivity with well-characterized anti-CK reagents at diagnostically optimal titers in an established, controlled detection system) are stained with higher concentrations of the same antibodies, the majority exhibit 'unexpected' staining.

To date, we have detected aberrant cytokeratin positivity in only two of 286 malignant 'non-epithelial' and non-leiomyogenous soft tissue sarcomas (Swanson, 1990). As a result, we suspect that most reported instances of unexpected staining are spurious. None the less, we are aware that other laboratories have been 'more successful' at reproducing aberrant keratin reactivity under 'diagnostic' staining conditions. Our recommendation at this time is that the interpretion of cytokeratin results be predicated not on the literature experience, but on one's own experience with carefullly controlled methodology, together with a rational and careful histopathologic examination of the case under study (Swanson, 1991).

Oestrogen and progesterone receptor proteins

Oestrogen receptor related substances are commonly expressed in normal keratinocytes and in both reactive and neoplastic keratinocytic proliferations (Kanitakis et al., 1989). As a general rule, however, normal sudoriferous epithelia do not express these hormone receptor moieties. By extension, the apparent lack of these receptors in neoplastic proliferations of sweat glands has been touted as a means of separating eccrine caricnomas from histologically similar metastatic deposits of mammary carcinoma (Lloveras et al., 1991). Our recent analyses have shown, however, that oestrogen receptor protein immunoreactivity is common in certain benign apocrine neoplasms of skin (especially hidradenoma papilliferum), as well as low grade eccrine carcinomas (Swanson et al., 1991) (Fig. 6.21). Progesterone receptor proteins may also be present in some examples of eccrine carcinoma (Voytek et al., 1991). The relationship of these observations to the prognosis of eccrine lesions is unclear, although the detection of oestrogen receptor protein (ERP) in predominantly low grade lesions suggests that reactivity for this receptor may not have any independent prognostic value. Interestingly, no example of either apocrine carcinoma or extramammary Paget's disease has stained for ERP (Lloveras et al., 1991; Swanson et al., 1991).

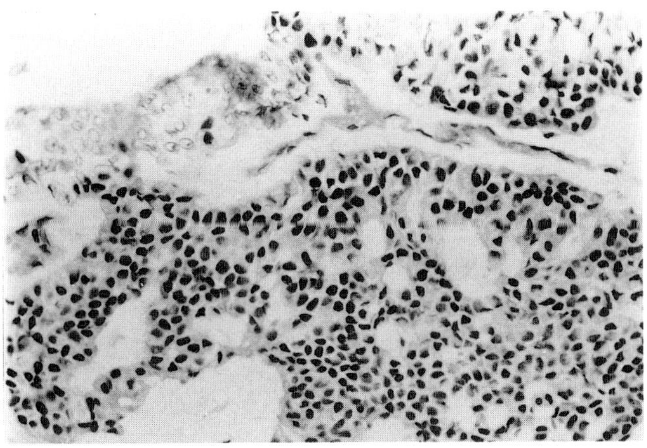

Fig. 6.21. Estrogen receptor protein in eccrine carcinoma. Diffuse nuclear reactivity is seen in this example of low grade eccrine ductal carcinoma.

Study of oestrogen receptor content is probably of no value in the evaluation of malignant melanoma. Despite earlier reports to the contrary (Delarve et al., 1987), oestrogen receptors are either not expressed or are not immunodetectible in melanocytic tumours (Cohen et al., 1990; Flowers et al., 1987).

The extracellular matrix

The expression of matrical proteins, the interaction of neoplastic cells with this matrical environment and the homing of haematopoietic elements to sites of neoplastic proliferation, through the activity of integrins and other cell-adhesion moieties, are the subject of ongoing investigations (Lee, 1988; Peltonen et al., 1990). Antibodies to laminin, fibronectin and collagen type IV effectively label these components of basement membranes in both routinely processed and fresh frozen tissues, allowing for the detection of matrix formation by various tumour types in skin (Lee, 1988; Markey et al., 1991; Soini et al., 1989). In particular, linear labelling of the periphery of individual neoplastic cells or groups of cells is typical of tissues exhibiting endothelial, smooth muscle or nerve sheath differentiation (Peltonen et al., 1990). Interruptions of linear matrix deposits underlying neoplastic melanocytes may be evidence of invasion of the papillary dermis by early nodular melanomas, or melanomas arising in lentigo maligna (Havenith et al., 1989). Certain carcinomas may also elaborate matrical elements, including basal cell carcinoma, wherein islands of infiltrating tumour cells are typically surrounded by both collagen type IV and laminin (Markey et al., 1991).

The diagnostic applications of integrins and other cell-adhesion molecules are still undefined in the context of skin pathology, although relationships between various intercellular adhesion molecules (ICAMs), integrins and inflammatory cell populations may provide yet another means of characterizing both benign and malignant lymphoreticular infiltrates, melanocytic lesions, mesenchymal neoplasms, and epidermal tumours in skin (Barker et al., 1990; Garioch et al., 1991; Ralfkiaer et al., 1991).

Oncogenes

The role of oncogene expression in the initiation and modulation of neoplastic growth in cutaneous tissues is the subject of considerable interest, but is a topic that has yet to yield an abundance of practical information. Among the various oncogenes that have been studied in some detail in skin are the epidermal growth factor receptor (EGFR) and the c-*erb*B-*2* (neu) oncogene. The latter is a 185 kD transmembrane glycoprotein with tyrosine kinase activity that is functionally and structurally related to the 175 kD EGFR gene product. Although its role in cell differentiation and proliferation is unknown, it appears to function as a true growth factor receptor when expressed in its native state. In normally differentiated and developing cells, native forms of both EGFR and c-*erb*B-*2* are expressed, but each may be altered or over-expressed in certain epithelial neoplasms.

EGFR expression, not surprisingly, is characteristic of squamous cell carcinomas (Baujnedcht et al., 1985; Nazini et al., 1990; Springer and Robinson, 1991) (Fig.

6.22), but to date there is little evidence that the presence or amount of the native receptor molecule or truncated forms derived from EGFR genic alterations is related to either the grade or clinical behaviour of SCC. EGFR expression has also been detected in BCC, although fewer than half of such lesions are immunoreactive (Nazini et al., 1990; Springer and Robinson, 1991). EGFR may be encountered in benign keratinocytic proliferations, including acrochrodons and seborrheic keratoses. These receptors are increased in the latter lesions in patients who are taking exogenous oestrogenic or progestational hormones, are pregnant, or who have the dysplastic nevus syndrome (Ellis et al., 1990).

Melanocytic lesions also contain EGFR, a finding that may correlate with the expression of HMB-45 antigen through an epidermal growth factor mediated induction (Smoller et al., 1991; Wick, 1991b). There is insufficient evidence to date to correlate the behaviour of malignant melanoma with EGFR-expression, although at least one highly metastatic melanoma cell line (MV3) contains this receptor moiety in abundance (van Muijen et al., 1991).

Over-expression of the c-*erb*B-*2* oncopeptide, although purportedly a marker of higher grade and more clinically aggressive forms of breast carcinoma, does not seem to predict unfavourable behavior in sudoriferous neoplasms (Swanson et al., 1990). In our recent analysis of eccrine carcinoma, five of 23 examples exhibited immunoreactivity, all of which were of low or moderate grade, and none of which metastasized or recurred (Swanson et al., 1990). Extramammary Paget's disease (intraepidermal apocrine carcinomas) may also stain with antibodies to the c-*erb*B-*2* oncopeptide (Wolber et al., 1991), although in our experience, such cases are uncommon compared to similar lesions in mammary skin.

c-*erb*B-*2* expression has been detected in malignant melanomas (Guillen et al., 1991). Although results are preliminary, it has been suggested that intense immunoreactivity for this oncoprotein may correlate with a higher mitotic index among lesions less than 3.0 mm in thickness. Obviously, additional study will be required before any prognostic significance can be atttributed to this phenomenon.

Perhaps the most important lesson that can be learned from our rudimentary understanding of oncogenes and their relationship to cutaneous neoplasms is that we do not yet know how or to what extent a single oncogene

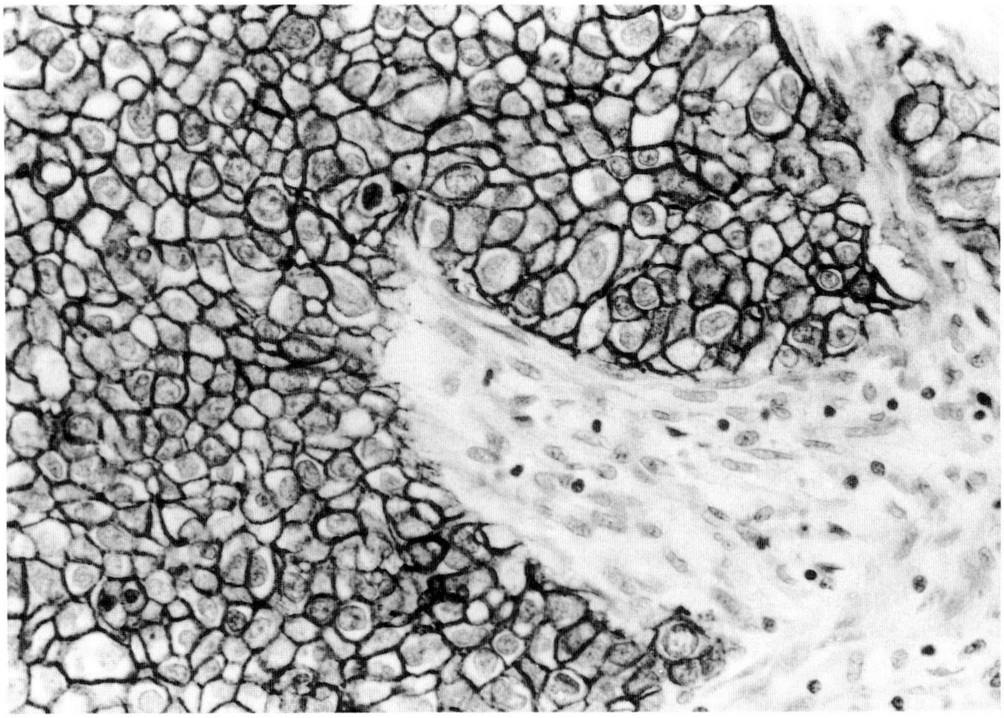

Fig. 6.22. Epidermal growth factor receptor reactivity in squamous cell carcinoma. Crisp membrane staining is encountered in the majority of these tumours.

can initiate or modulate the cascade of events that results in uncontrolled cellular growth. While many of the oncogene products can immortalize cells or maintain the transformed phenotype of cells in culture, the ultimate importance of these effects on the same cell populations in a biological milieu cannot yet be predicted. While there may be validity to claims that expression of the various oncopeptides may relate to the aggressiveness of cutaneous neoplasms, it seems unlikely that any one of them will act alone. Hence, modelling of future immunohistochemical studies designed to correlate oncogene expression with histopathologic or clinical attributes should rely not on analyses of single peptides, but of several oncogene products in concert, in a manner analogous to the immunophenotypic panels that aid the diagnostic pathologist. The interaction of these substances with one another, as well as with various membrane-associated or cytoskeletal determinants, may prove to be as important as their mere presence in a cell.

Conclusion

Based on the foregoing comments, the reader may conclude that we advocate the use of immunostains as a necessary diagnostic adjunct in the majority of cases of cutaneous neoplasia. Surely, immunohistochemistry has contributed considerably to our ability to resolve many diagnostic difficulties in dermatopathology, but such problems arise in only selected or specialized circumstances. In fact, fewer than 5 per cent of cutaneous neoplasms are subjected to immunohistochemical evaluation in our diagnostic practice.

It is important to remember that the immunophenotypic attributes of epithelial, lymphoreticular and mesenchymal neoplasms, when considered alone, may not provide the pathologist with sufficient information to resolve even simple diagnostic problems. A review of the tables presented in this chapter must reinforce in the reader two basic tenets: that different patterns of differentiation may be identified by the presence of selected markers, but that few of these markers are absolutely specific for any one group of neoplasms. Hence, even in settings requiring immunohistochemical analysis, accurate interpretation must still be predicated on a careful consideration of the histopathologic and clinical features in each case. One's skill at interpreting routine histologic material will always yield greater dividends than a cursory knowledge of immunohistochemistry. Indeed, undue emphasis on the content of this chapter or any compendium of immunohistochemistry places the reader at risk for neglecting the fundamental importance of proficiency in diagnostic histopathology.

References

Ahmed, I., Piepkorn, M., Goldgar, D.E. and Cannon-Albright, L.A. (1991). HMB-45 staining of dysplastic melanocytic nevi in melanoma risk groups. *Journal of Cutaneous Pathology* **18**, 257–60.

Aiba, S., Masuko T., Hosokawa, M. and Hashimoto, Y. (1983). Monoclonal antibodies to various morphologic components of human skin. *Journal of Investigative Dermatology* **81**, 498–502.

Alguacil-Garcia, A. (1991). Giant cell fibroblastoma recurring as dermatofibrosarcoma protuberans. *American Journal of Surgical Pathology* **15**, 798–801.

Allen M.H., Barker, J.N.H.N. and MacDonald, D.M. (1991). Keratinocyte expression of CD36 antigen in benign and malignant epidermal cell-derived tumours. *Journal of Cutaneous Pathology* **18**, 198–203.

Alles, J.U. and Bosslet, K. (1986). Immunohistochemical and immunochemical characterization of a new endothelial cell-specific antigen. *Journal of Histochemistry and Cytochemistry* **34**, 209–14.

Amaral, A.L.M.P., Nascimento, A. and Goellner, J.R. (1984). Proliferating pilar (trichilemmal) cyst. Report of two cases, one with carcinomatous transformation, and one with distant metastases. *Archives of Pathology and Laboratory Medicine* **108**, 808–10.

Azumi, N., Ben-Ezra, J. and Battifora, H. (1988). Immunophenotypic diagnosis of leiomyosarcomas and rhabdomyosarcomas with monoclonal antibodies to muscle-specific actin and desmin in formalin-fixed tissue. *Modern Pathology* **1**, 469–74.

Banerjee, S.S., Heald, J. and Harris, M. (1991). Twelve cases of Ki-1 positive anaplastic large cell lymphoma of skin. *Journal of Clinical Pathology* **44**, 119–25.

Banks, P.M. (1985). Lymphoid neoplasms of the skin. In Wick, M.R. (ed.), *Pathology of Unusual Malignant Cutaneous tumours*, Marcel Dekker, New York, pp. 299–356.

Barker, J.N., Allen, M.H. and Macdonald, D.M. (1990). Distribution of intercellular-adhesion molecule-1 (ICAM-1) and lymphocyte-function-asociated antigen-1 (LFA-1) in epidermal tumours. *Clinical and Experimental Dermatology* **15**, 331–4.

Battifora, H. (1984). Recent progress in the immunohistochemistry of solid tumours. *Seminars in Diagnostic Pathology* **1**, 251–71.

Battifora, H. and Silva, E.G. (1986). The use of antikeratin antibodies in the immunohistochemical distinction between neuroendocrine (Merkel cell) carcinoma of the skin, lymphoma, and oat cell carcinoma. *Cancer* **58**, 1040–6.

Baujnedcht, T., Gross, G. and Hagedorn, M. (1985). Epidermal growth factor receptors in different skin tumours. *Dermatologica* **171**, 16–20.

Beckstead,J.H., Wood, G.S. and Fletcher, V. (1985). Evidence for the origin of Kaposi's sarcoma from lymphatic endothelium. *American Journal of Pathology* **119**, 294–300.

Beljaards, R.C., Meijer, C.J. and Scheffer, E. (1989). Prognostic significance of CD30 (Ki-1/Ber-H2) expression in primary cutaneous large-cell lymphoma of T-cell origin. A clinicopathologic and immunohistochemical study in 20 patients. *American Journal of Pathology* **135**, 1169–78.

Berry, C.L. and Amerigo, J. (1983). Blood group antigens in vascular tumours. Evaluation of the immunoperoxidase technique. *Virchows Archives (Pathology and Anatomy)* **388**, 167–74.

Bhawan, J., Bacchetta, C., Joris, I. and Majno, G. (1979). A myofibroblastic tumour. Infantile digital fibroma (recurrent digital fibrous tumour of childhood). *American Journal of Pathology* **94**, 19–28.

Bhawan, J., Wolff, S.M., Ucci, A.A. and Bhan, A.K. (1985). Malignant lymphoma and malignant angioendotheliomatosis: One disease. *Cancer* **55**, 570-6.

Broelaert, D., Goeman, L. and Ramaekers, F.C. (1990). An investigation of cytokeratin expression in skin epithelial cysts and some uncommon types of cystic tumours using chain-specific antibodies. *Archives of Dermatologic Research* **282**, 383–91.

Brooks, J.J. (1986). The significance of double phenotypic patterns and markers in human sarcomas. A new model of mesenchymal differentiation. *American Journal of Pathology* **125**, 113–23.

Burgdorf, W.H.C., Mukai, K. and Rosai, J. (1981). Immunohistochemical identification of factor VIII-related antigen in endothelial cells of cutaneous lesions of alleged vascular nature. *American Journal of Clinical Pathology* **75**, 167–71.

Carroll, T.J., Schelper, R.L., Goeken, J.A. and Kemp, J.D. (1986). Neoplastic angioendotheliomatosis: Immunopathologic and morphologic evidence for intravascular malignant lymphoma. *American Journal of Clinical Pathology* **85**, 169–75.

Caselitz, J., Janner, M., Breitbach, E., Weber, K. and Osborn, M. (1983). Malignant melanomas contain only the vimentin type of intermediate filaments. *Virchows Archives (Pathology and Anatomy)* **400**, 43–51.

Cerio, R., Spaull, J., Oliver, G.F. and Jones, E.W. (1990). A study of factor XIIIa and MAC 387 immunolabelling in normal and pathological skin. *American Journal of Dermatopathology* **12**, 221–33.

Chang, Y., Dehner, L.P. and Egbert, B. (1990). Primary cutaneous rhabdomyosarcoma. *American Journal of Surgical Pathology* **14**, 977–82.

Chase, D.R., Enzinger, F.M., Weiss, S.W. and Langloss, J.M. (1984). Keratin in epithelioid sarcoma. An immunohistochemical study. *American Journal of Surgical Pathology* **8**, 435–41.

Clark, H.B., Minesky, J.J., Agrawal, D. and Agrawal, H.C. (1985). Myelin basic protein and P2 protein are not immunohistochemical markers for Schwann cell neoplasms: A comparative study using antisera to S100, P2, and myelin basic proteins. *American Journal of Pathology* **121**, 96–101.

Cohen, C., DeRose, P.B., Campbell, W.G., Schlosnagle, D.C., and Sgoutas, D. (1990). Estrogen receptor status in malignant melanoma. *American Journal of Dermatopathology* **12**, 562–4.

Cohen, P.R., Rapini, R.P. and Farhood, A. (1991). The expression of the human haematopoietic progenitor cell antigen CD-34 in vascular and spindle cell tumours (abstract). *Journal of Cutaneous Pathology* **18**, 363.

Cramer, S.F. (1990). Epithelial membrane antigen staining of melanocytic nevi. *Human Pathology* **21**, 121–2.

Crocker, J., Burnett, D. and Jones, E.L. (1984). Immunohistochemical demonstration of cathepsin B in the macrophages of benign and malignant lymphoid tissues. *Journal of Pathology* **142**, 87–94.

Dale, B.A., Gown, A.M., Fleckman, P., Kimball, J.R. and Resing, K.A. (1987). Characterization of two monoclonal antibodies to human epidermal keratohyalin: Reactivity with filaggrin and related proteins. *Journal of Investigative Dermatology* **88**, 306–13.

Davaris, D.X.G., Ling, F.C.K. and Prentice, R.S.A. (1991). Congenital self-healing histiocytosis. Report of two cases with histochemical and ultrastructural studies. *American Journal of Dermatopathology* **13**, 481–7.

Delarve, J., Avril, M., Charpentier, P. and Prade, M. (1987). Estrogen receptors in malignant melanoma. *Archives of Dermatology* **123**, 159–60.

Dorfman, R.F. (1986). Kaposi's sarcoma: With special reference to its manifestations in infants and children and to the concepts of Arthur Purdy Stout. *American Journal of Surgical Pathology* **10** (Suppl. 1), 68–77.

Drier, J.K., Swanson, P.E., Cherwitz, D.L. and Wick, M.R. (1987). S100 protein in poorly-differentiated carcinomas: An immunohistochemical comparison with malignant melanomas. *Archives of Pathology and Laboratory Medicine* **111**, 447–52.

DuBoulay, C.E.H. (1982). Demonstration of alpha-1–antitrypsin and alpha-1-antichymotrypsin in the fibrous histiocytomas using the immunoperoxidase technique. *American Journal of Surgical Pathology* **6**, 559–64.

Dymock, R.B., Allen, P.W., Stirling, J.W., Gilbert, E.F. and Thornberry, J.M. (1987). Giant cell fibroblastoma: A distinctive recurrent tumour of childhood. American Journal of Surgical Pathology **11**, 263–8.

Egan, M.J,. Crocker, J., Newman, J. and Collard, M. (1986). Immunohistochemical localization of S100 protein in skin tumours. *Archives of Pathology and Laboratory Medicine* **110**, 765–7.

Ellis, D.L., Nanney, L.B. and King, L.E. Jr. (1990). Increased epidermal growth factor receptors in seborrheic keratoses and acrochordons of patients with the dysplastic nevus syndrome. *Journal of the Academy of Dermatology* **23**, 1070–7.

Enzinger, F.M and Weiss, S.W. (1989). *Soft Tissue Tumours*, 2nd edn. C.V. Mosby, St. Louis.

Enzinger, F.M. and Zhang, R. (1988). Plexiform fibrohistiocytic tumour presenting in children and young adults. An analysis of 65 cases. *American Journal of Surgical Pathology* **12**, 818–26.

Epstein, A.L., Marder, R.J., Winter, J. and Fox, R.I. (1984). Two new monoclonal antibodies (LN-1, LN-2) reactive in B5–fixed, paraffin-embedded tissues with follicular centre cell and mantle zone human B lymphocytes and derived tumours. *Journal of Immunology* **133**, 1028–36.

Eusebi, V., Carcangiu, M.L., Dina, R. and Rosai, J. (1990). Keratin-positive epithelioid angiosarcoma of thyroid. A report of four cases. American Journal of Surgical Pathology **14**, 737–47.

Facchetti, F., Bertalot, G. and Grigolato, P.G. (1991). KP1 (CD 68) staining in malignant melanomas. *Histopathology* **19**, 141–5.

Faure, P., Chittal, S., Gorguet, B. and Caveriviere, P. (1990). Immunohistochemical profile of cutaneous B-cell lymphoma on cryostat and paraffin sections. *American Journal of Dermatopathology* **12**, 122–33.

Feigl, W., Denk, H., Davidovits, A. and Holzner, J.H. (1976). Blood group isoantigens in human benign and malignant vascular tumours. *Virchows Archives (Pathology and Anatomy)* **370**, 323–2.

Fithian, E., Kung, P., Goldstein, G.and Rubenfeld, M. (1981). Reactivity of Langerhans' cells with hybridoma antibody. *Proceedings of the National Academy of Science (USA)* **78**, 2541–4.

Fletcher, C.D.M. (1988). Giant cell fibroblastoma of soft tissue: A clinicopathological and immunohistochemical study. *Histopathology* **13**, 499–503.

Fletcher, C.D.M. (1990). Benign fibrous histiocytoma of subcutaneous and deep soft tissue: A clinicopathologic analysis of 21 cases. *American Journal of Surgical Pathology* **14**, 801–9.

Fletcher, C.D.M., Behan, A., Bekir, S., Clarke, A.M.T. and Marley, N.J.E. (1991a). Epithelioid angiosarcoma of deep soft tissue. A distinctive tumour readily mistaken for an epithelial neoplasm. *American Journal of Surgical Pathology* **15**, 915–24.

Fletcher, C.D.M., Beham, A,. Schmid, C. (1991b). Spindle cell haemangioendothelioma: A clinicopathological and immunohistochemical study indicative of a non-neoplastic lesion. *Histopathology* **18**, 291–301.

Flotte, T.J., Hatcher, V.A. and Friedman-Kien, A.E. (1984). Factor VIII-related antigen in Kaposi's sarcoma in young homosexual men. *Archives of Dermatology* **120**, 180-2.

Flowers, J.L., Seigler, H.F., McCarthy and K.S. Sr. (1987). Absence of estrogen receptor in human melanoma as evaluated by a monoclonal anti-estrogen receptor antibody. *Archives of Dermatology* **123**, 764–5.

Flynn, K.J., Dehner, L.P., Gajl-Peczalska, K.J. and Dahl, M.V. (1982). Regressing atypical histiocytosis: A cutaneous proliferation of atypical neoplastic histiocytes with unexpectedly indolent biological behavior. *Cancer* **49**, 959–70.

Foon, K., Todd, R. (1986). Immunologic classification of leukaemia and lymphoma. *Blood* **68**, 1–31.

From, L., Hanna, W., Kahn, H.J. and Gruss, J. (1983). Origin of the desmoplasia in desmoplastic malignant melanoma. *Human Pathology* **14**, 1072–80.

Fulling, K. and Gersell, D. (1983). Neoplastic angioendotheliomatosis: histologic, immunohistochemical, and ultrastructural findings in two cases. *Cancer* **51**, 1107–18.

Gallagher, R.L. and Helwig, E.B. (1980). Neurothekeoma: A benign cutaneous tumour of nerve sheath origin. *American Journal of Clinical Pathology* **74**, 759–64.

Garioch, J.J., Mackie, R.M., Campbell, I. and Forsyth, A. (1991). Keratinocyte expression of intercellular adhesion molecule 1 (ICAM-1) correlated with infiltration of lymphocyte function associated antigen 1 (LFA-1) positive cells in evolving allergic contact dermatitis reactions. *Histopathology* **19**, 151–4.

George, E., Swanson, P.E. and Wick, M.R. (1989a). Neuroendocrine differentiation in basal cell carcioma. An immunohistochemical study. *American Journal of Dermatopathology* **11**, 131–5.

George, E., Swanson, P.E., Wick, M.R. (1989b). Malignant peripheral nerve sheath tumours of the skin. *American Journal of Dermatopathology* **11**, 213–21.

Gianotti, F., Caputo, R., Ermacora, E. and Gianni, E. (1986). Benign cephalic histiocytosis. *Archives of Dermatology* **122**, 1038–43.

Gonzalez-Crussi, F. and Reyes-Mugica, M. (1991). Cellular haemangiomas ('haemagioendotheliomas') in infants. Light microscopic, immunohistochemical and ultrastructural observations. *American Journal of Surgical Pathology* **15**, 769–8.

Gown, A.M., Vogel, A.M., Hoak, D. and McNutt, M.A. (1986). Monoclonal antibodies specific for melanocytic tumours distinguish subpopulations of melanocytes. *American Journal of Pathology* **123**, 195–203.

Gown, A.M., Boyd, H.C. and Chang, Y. (1988). Smooth muscle cells can express cytokeratins to 'simple' epithelium. Immunohistochemical and biochemical studies in vitro and in vivo. *American Journal of Pathology* **132**, 223–32.

Gray, M.H., Rosenberg, A.E., Dickersin, G.R. and Bhan, A.K. (1989). Glial fibrillary acidic protein and keratin expression by benign and malignant nerve sheath tumours. *Human Pathology* **20**, 1089–96.

Gray, M.H., Rosenberg, A.E., Dickersin, G.R. and Bhan, A.K. (1990a). Cytokeratin expression in epithelioid vascular neoplasms. *Human Pathology* **21**, 212–17.

Gray, M.H., Smoller, B.R., McNutt, N.S. and Hsu, A. (1990b). Neurofibromas and neurotized nevi are immunohistochemicaly distinct neoplasms. *American Journal of Dermatopathology* **12**, 234–41.

Gray, M.H., Smoller, B.R., McNutt, N.S. and Hsu, A. (1990c). Immunohistochemical demonstration of factor XIIIa expression in neurofibromas. A practical means of differentiating these tumours from neurotized melanocytic nevi and schwannomas. *Archives of Dermatology* **126**, 472–6.

Griesser, H., Feller, A.C. and Sterry, W. (1990). T-cell receptor and immunoglobulin gene rearrangements in cutaneous T-cell-rich pseudolymphomas. *Journal of Investigative Dermatology* **95**, 292–5.

Grossniklaus, H.E., Swerlick, R.A. and Solomon, A.R. (1990). IgA and complement immunofluorescent patterns in sebaceous gland carcinoma of the eyelid. *American Journal of Ophthalmology* **109**, 353–5.

Gu, J., Polak, J.M., Van Noorden, S. and Pearse, A.G.E. (1983). Immunostaining of neuron-specific enolase as a diagnostic tool for Merkel cell tumours. *Cancer* **52**, 1039–43.

Guarda, L.G., Silva, E.G., Ordonez, N.G. and Smith, J.L. (1981). Factor VIII in Kaposi's sarcoma. *American Journal of Clinical Pathology* **76**, 197–200.

Guillen, C., Oliver, V., Millan, F. and Marotel, M. (1991). P185 neu expression in malignant melanoma (abstract). *Journal of Cutaneous Pathology* **18**, 372.

Hanson, C.A., Jaszcz, W. and Kersey, J.H. (1989). True histiocytic lymphoma: histopathology, immunophenotypic and genotypic analysis. *British Journal of Haematology* **73**, 187–98.

Hashimoto, K., Eto, H., Matsumoto, M. and Hori, K. (1983). Antikeratin antibodies: Production, specificity, and applications. *Journal of Cutaneous Pathology* **10**, 529–39.

Hashimoto, T., Inamato, N., Nakamura, K. and Harada, R. (1987). Involucrin expression in skin appendage tumours. *British Journal of Dermatology* **117**, 325–32.

Hassab-El-Naby, H.M., Tam, S., White, W.L. and Ackerman, A.B. (1989). Mixed tumours of the skin. A histological and imuonhistochemical study. *American Journal of Dermatopathology* **11**, 413–28.

Havenith, M.G., van Zandvoort, E.H., Cleutjens, J.P. and Bosman, F.T. (1989). Basement membrane deposition in benign and malignant nevo-melanocytic lesions: an immunohistochemical study with antibodies to type IV collagen and laminin. *Journal of Histopathology* **15**, 137–42.

Headington, J.T. (1976). Tumours of the hair follicle: A review. *American Journal of Pathology* **85**, 480-505.

Heenan, P.J., Cole, J.M. and Spagnolo, D.V. (1990). Primary cutaneous neuroendocrine carcinoma (Merkel cell tumour). An adnexal epithelial neoplasm. *American Journal of Dermatopathology* **12**, 7–16.

Heyderman, E., Graham, R.M., Chapman, D.V., Richardson, T.C. and McKee, P.H. (1984). Epithelial markers in primary skin cancer: An immunoperoxidase study of the distribution of epithelial membrane antigen (EMA) and carcinoembryonic antigen (CEA) in 65 primary skin carcinomas. *Histopathology* **8**, 423–34.

Hirose, T., Kudo, E., Hasegawa, T., Abe, J-I. and Hizawa, K. (1989). Expression of intermediate filaments in malignant fibrous histiocytomas. *Human Pathology* **20**, 871–7.

Holden, C.A. (1989). Histogenesis of Kaposi's sarcoma and angiosarcoma of the face and the scalp. *Journal of Investigative Dermatology* **93** (Suppl. 2), 119S–24S.

Holden, C.A., Spaull, J., Williams, R. and Spry, C.J.F. (1986). The distribution of endothelial cell antigens in cutaneous tissue using methacarn and periodate lysine paraformaldehyde fixation. *Journal of Immunologic Methods* **91**, 45–52.

Hui, P.K., Feller, A.C. and Kaiserling, E. (1987). Skin tumour of T accessory cells (interdigitating reticulum cells) with high content of T lymphocytes. *American Journal of Dermatopathology* **9**, 129–37.

Hyder, D.M. and Schnitzer, B. (1986). Utility of Leu M1 monoclonal antibody in the differential diagnosis of Hodgkin's disease. *Archives of Pathology and Laboratory Medicine* **110**, 416–19.

Imam, A., Mitchell, M.S. and Modlin, R.L. (1986). Human monoclonal antibodies that distinguish malignant melanoma from benign nevi in fixed tissue sections. *Journal of Investigative Dermatology* **86**, 145–8.

Imayama, S., Murakamai, Y., Hashimoto, H. and Hori, Y. (1992). Spindle cell haemangioendothelioma exhibits the ultrastructural features of reactive vascular proliferation rather than of angiosarcoma. *American Journal of Clinical Pathology* **97**, 279–87.

Ito, M., Tazawa, T., Ito, K., Shimuzu, N., Katsuumi, K. and Sato, Y. (1986a). Immunological characteristics and histological distribution of human hair fibrous proteins studied with anti-hair monoclonal antibodies HKN-2, HKN-4, and HKN-6. *Journal of Histochemistry and Cytochemistry* **34**, 269–74.

Ito, M., Tazawaa, T. and Shimuzu, N. (1986b). Cell differentiation in human anagen hair and hair follicles studied with anti-hair keratin monoclonal antibodies. *Journal of Investigative Dermatology* **86**, 563–9.

Ito, M., Tazawa, T. and Shimuzu, N. (1988). Intraepidermal pilar epithelioma: a new dermatopathologic interpretation of a skin tumour. *Journal of the American Academy of Dermatology* **18**, 123–32.

Jacinto, C.M., Grant-Kels, J.M., Knibbs, D.R., Daman, L.A. and Piorkowski, R.J. (1991). Malignant primitive neuroectodermal tumour presenting as a scalp nodule. *American Journal of Dermatopathology* **13**, 63–70.

Jimenez-Acosta, F., Planas, L. and Penneys, N.S. (1990). Lipase expression in human skin. *Journal of Dermatological Science* **1**, 195–200.

Kahn, H.J., Marks, A., Thom, H. and Baumal, R. (1983). Role of antibody to S100 protein in diagnostic pathology. *American Journal of Clinical Pathology* **79**, 341–7.

Kanitakis, J., Schmitt, D., Bernard, A., Boumsell, L. and Thivolet, J. (1983). D47: A new monoclonal antibody reacting with the secretory cells of human eccrine sweat glands (abstract). *Journal of Investigative Dermatology* **80**, 338.

Kanitakis, J., Zambruno, G., Viac, J. and Thivolet, J. (1986). Involucrin expression in adnexal skin tumours: An immunohisotchemical study. *Virchows Archiv (Patholoy and Anatomy)* **408**, 527–40.

Kanitakis, J., Zambruno, G., Viac, J., Tommaselli, L. and Thivolet, J. (1989). Expression of an estrogen receptor-associated protein (p29) in epithelial tumours of the skin. *Journal of Cutaneous Pathology* **16**, 272–6.

Kapila, P.K., Grant-Kels, J.M., Allred, C,. Forouhar, F. and Caprigliome, A.M. (1985). Congenital, spontaneously regressing histiocytosis: Case report and review of the literature. *Paediatric Dermatology* **2**, 312–17.

Kaplan, K.I., Weber, D. and Cook, P. (1983). Monoclonal antibodies to E92, an endothelial cell surface antigen. *Arteriosclerosis* **3**, 403–12.

Kaposi, M.: Idiopathisches multiples Pigmentsarkom der Haut (1872). *Archives of Dermatology and Syphiligraphy (Berlin)* **4**, 265–73.

Kariniemi, A.L., Vesterinen, E. and Wahlstrom, T. (1984). Carcinoembryonic antigen in mammary and extramammary Paget's disease. In MacDonald, D.M. (ed.), *Immunodermatology*, Butterworths, London, pp. 61–4.

Kaudewitz, P. and Burg, G. (1991). Lymphomatoid papulosis and Ki-1 (CD30)-positive cutaneous large cell lymphomas. *Seminars in Diagnostic Pathology* **8**, 117–24.

Kaye, V.N. and Dehner, L.P. (1991). Cutaneous glomus tumour. A comparative immunohistochemical study with pseudoangiomatous intradermal melanocytic nevi. *American Journal of Dermatopathology* **13**, 2–6.

Kaye, V.N. and Swanson, P.E. (1991). Evaluation of spindle cell tumours. *Clinics in Dermatology* **9**, 217–26.

Kerl, H. and Smolle, J. (1990). Classification of cutaneous pseudolymphomas. *Current Problems in Dermatology* **19**, 167–75.

Kermarec, J., Canioni, D., Michiels, J.F. and Kullman, B. (1984). L'angioendotheliomatose (maligne) systemique. A propos d'une observation avec etude ultrastructurale et histo-immunologique. *Annales Pathologie (Paris)* **4**, 61–7.

Kindblom, L.F., Jacobsen, G.K. and Jacobsen, M. (1982). Immunohistochemical investigations of tumours of supposed fibroblastic-histiocytic origin. *Human Pathology* **13**, 834–40.

Klein-Szanto, A.J.P., Barr, R.J., Reiners, J.J. and Mamrack, M.D. (1984). Filaggrin distribution in keratoacanthomas and squamous cell carcinomas. *Archives of Pathology and Laboratory Medicine* **108**, 888–90.

Klingel, R., Boukamp, P. and Moll, R. (1990). Expression of epithelial antigens Exo-1 and EPM-1 in human epidermal keratinocyte maturation and benign and malignant neoplasia. *Cancer Research* **50**, 7668–76.

Knowles, D.M. II. (1985). Lymphoid cell markers: Their distribution and usefulness in the immunophenotypic analysis of lymphoid neoplasms. *American Journal of Surgical Pathology* **9** (Suppl.), 85–108.

Kraffert, C., Planus, L. and Pennys, N.S. (1991). Kaposi's sarcoma: Further immunohistologic evidence of a vascular endothelial origin. *Archives of Dermatology* **127**, 1734–5.

Kurtin, P.J. and Pinkus, G.S. (1985). Leukocyte common antigen – a diagnostic discriminant between haematopoietic and nonhaematopoietic neoplasms in paraffin sections using monoclonal antibodies. Correlation with immunologic studies and ultrastructural localization. *Human Pathology* **16**, 353–65.

Kuwano, H., Hashimoto, H. and Enjoji, M. (1985). Atypical fibroxanthoma distinguishable from spindle cell carcinoma in sarcoma-like skin lesions. *Cancer* **55**, 172–80.

Kvedar, J.C., Fewkes, J. and Baden, H.P. (1986). Immunologic detection of markers of keratinocyte differentiation in neoplastic and preneoplastic lesions of skin. *Archives of Pathology and Laboratory Medicine* **110**, 183–8.

Latham, J.A., Redfern, C.P., Thody, A.J. and DeKretzer, J.A. (1989). Immunohistochemical markers of human sebaceous gland differentiation. *Journal of Histochemistry and Cytochemistry* **37**, 729–34.

Lautier, R., Wolff, H.H. and Jones, R.E. (1990). An immunohistochemical study of dermatofibrosarcoma protuberans supports its fibroblastic character and contradicts neuroectodermal or histiocytic components. *American Journal of Dermatopathology* **21**, 25–30.

Layton, G.T., Devine, P.L. and Warren, J.A. (1990). Monoclonal antibodies reactive with the breast carcinoma-associated mucin core protein repeat sequence also recognize the ovarian carcinoma-associated sebaceous gland antigen. *Tumour Biology* **11**, 274–86.

LeBoit, P.E., Barr, R.J. and Burall, S. (1991). Primitive polypoid granular cell tumour and other cutaneous granular cell neoplasms of apparent non-neural origin. *American Journal of Surgical Pathology* **15**, 48–58.

Leader, M., Patel, J., Collins, M. and Henry, K. (1987). Anti-alpha-1–antichymotrypsin staining in 194 sarcomas, 38 carcinomas and 17 malignant melanomas. Its lack of specificity as a tumour marker. *American Journal of Surgical Pathology* **11**, 133–9.

Lee, A.K. (1988). Basement membrane and endothelial antigens: Their role in the evaluation of tumour invasion and metastasis. In DeLellis, R.A. (ed.), *Advances in Immunohistochemistry*, Raven Press, New York, pp. 363–93.

Lever, W.F. and Schaumberg-Lever, G. (1989). *Histopathology of the Skin*, 7th edn, J.B. Lippincott, Philadelphia.

Lisby, S., Ralfkaier, E., Hansen, E.R. and Vejlsgaard, G.L. (1990). Keratinocyte and epidermal leucocyte expression of CD36 (OKM5) in benign and malignant skin diseases. *Acta Dermatologica Venereoligica* **70**, 18–22.

Little, D., Said, J.W. and Siegel, R.J. (1986). Endothelial cell markers in vascular neoplasms: An immunohistochemical study comparing factor VIII-related antigen, blood group specific antigens, 6–keto-PGF1 alpha, and Ulex europaeus I lectin. *Journal of Pathology* **149**, 89–95.

Lloveras, B., Googe, P.B., Goldberg, D.E. and Bhan, A.K. (1991). Estrogen receptors in skin appendage tumours and extrammamary Paget's disease. *Modern Pathology* **4**, 487–90.

Lloyd, R.V. and Wilson, B.S. (1983). Specific endocrine tissue marker defined by a monoclonal antibody. *Science* **222**, 628–30.

Loftus, B., Loh, L.C., Curran, B., Henry, K. and Leader, M. (1991). MAC 387: its non-specificity as a tumour marker or marker of histiocytes. *Histopathology* **17**, 251–5.

Lynch, M.H., O'Guin, M., Hardy, C., Mak, L. and Sun, T-T. (1986). Acidic and basic hair/nail ('hard') keratins: Their colocalization in upper cortical and cuticle cells of the human hair follicle and their relationship to 'soft' keratins. *Journal of Cell Biology* **103**, 2593–606.

Mackie, R.M., Campbell, I. and Turbitt, M. (1984). Use of NKI/C3 monoclonal antibody in the assessment of benign and malignant melanocytic lesions. *Journal of Clinical Pathology* **37**, 367–72.

Maeda, K., Maeda, K. and Jimbow, K. (1989). Positive reactivity of dysplastic melanocytes with a monoclonal antibody against melanoma melanosomes, MoAb HMSA-2. *Journal of Investigative Dermatology* **91**, 247–50.

Manivel, C., Dehner, L.P. and Wick, M.R. (1985). Nonvascular sarcomas of the skin. In Wick, M.R. (ed.), *Pathology of Unusual Malignant Cutaneous Tumours*, Marcel Dekker, New York, pp. 211–79.

Manivel, C., Wick, M.R., Dehner, L.P. and Sibley, R.K. (1987). Epithelioid sarcoma: An immunohistochemical study. *American Journal of Clinical Pathology* **87**, 319–26.

Manivel, C., Wick, M.R. and Mukai, K. (1986). Pilomatrix carcinoma: An immunohistochemical comparison with benign pilomatrixoma and other benign cutaneous lesions of pilar origin. *Journal of Cutaneous Pathology* **13**, 22–9.

Markey, A.C., Tidman, M.J. and Churchill, L.J. (1991). The epidermal basement membrane in basal cell carcinoma: An immunohistochemical study. *British Journal of Dermatology* **125**, 21–6.

Martorelli, M., Calabuig, C., Peydro-Olaya, A. and Llombart-Bosch, A. (1989). Fibroblast and myofibroblast participation in malignant fibrous histiocytoma (MFH) of bone. Ultrastructural study of eight cases with immunohistochemical support. *Pathology Research and Practice* **184**, 582–90.

Maruyama, I., Bell, E. and Majerus, P.W. (1985). Thrombomodulin is found on endothelium of arteries, veins, capillaries and lymphatics, and on syncytiotrophoblast of human placenta. *Journal of Cell Biology* **101**, 363–71.

Mazoujian, G. (1988). Gross cystic disease fluid protein-15 (GCDFP-15). In Wick, M.R. and Siegal, G.P. (eds), *Monoclonal Antibodies in Diagnostic Immunohistochemistry*, Marcel Dekker, New York.

Mazoujian, G. (1990). Immunohistochemistry of GCDFP-24 and zinc alpha-2–glycoprotein in benign sweat gland tumours. *American Journal of Dermatopathology* **12**, 452–7.

Mazoujian, G. and Margolis, R. (1988). Immunohistochemistry of gross cystic disease fluid protein (GCDFP-15) in 65 benign sweat gland tumours of the skin. *American Journal of Dermatopathology* **10**, 28–35.

Mazoujian, G., Pinkus, G.S. and Haagensen, D.E. Jr. (1984). Extramammary Paget's disease – evdence for an apocrine origin. An immunoperoxidase study of gross cystic disease fluid protein-15, carcinoembryonic antigen, and keratin proteins. *American Journal of Surgical Pathology* **8**, 43–50.

Mechterscheimer, G. (1991). Towards the phenotyping of soft tissue tumours by cell surface markers. *Virchows Archives (Pathology and Anatomy)* **419**, 7–28.

Mechterscheimer, G., Staudter, M. and Majdie, O. (1990). Expression of HLA-A,B,C, beta-2–microglobulin, HLA-DR, -DP, -DQ and of HLA-D-associated invariant chain (Ii) in soft tissue tumours. *International Journal of Cancer* **46**, 813–23.

Metze, D., Jurecka, W. and Gebhardt, W. (1989). Immunohistochemical demonstration of immunoglobulin A in human sebaceous and sweat ducts. *Journal of Investigative Dermatology* **92**, 13–17.

Miettinen, M. (1988). Immunoreactivity for cytokeratin and epithelial membrane antigen in leiomyosarcoma. *Archives of Pathology and Laboratory Medicine* **112**, 637–40.

Miettinen, M. (1990). Immunohistochemistry of peripheral nerve sheath sarcomas (abstract). *Laboratory Investigation* **62**, 67A.

Miettinen, M., Holthofer, H., Lehto, V-P., Miettinen, A. and Virtanen, I. (1983). Ulex europaeus I lectin as a marker for tumours derived from endothelial cells. *American Journal of Clinical Pathology* **79**, 32–6.

Miettinen, M., Lehto, V-P., Badley, R.A. and Virtanen, I. (1982). Expression of intermediate filaments in soft tissue sarcomas. *International Journal of Cancer* **30**, 541–6.

Miettinen, M., Lehto, V-P. and Virtanen, I. (1983a). Neuroendocrine carcinoma of the skin (Merkel cell carcinoma): Ultrastructural and immunohistochemical demonstration of neurofilaments. *Ultrastructural Pathology* **4**, 219–25.

Miettinen, M., Lehto, V-P. and Virtanen, I. (1983b). Postmastectomy angiosarcoma (Stewart-Treves syndrome): Light microscopic, immunohistological, and ultrastructural findings of two cases. *American Journal of Surgical Pathology* **7**, 329–39.

Miettinen, M., Lehto, V-P. and Virtanen, I. (1983c). Presence of fibroblastic-type intermediate filaments (vimentin) and absence of neurofilaments in pigmented nevi and malignant melanomas. *Journal of Cutaneous Pathology* **10**, 188–92.

Miettinen, M. and Franssila, K. (1989). Immunohistochemical spectrum of malignant melanoma. The common presence of keratins. *Laboratory Investigation* **61**, 623–8.

Miettinen, M. and Soini, Y. (1989). Malignant fibrous histiocytoma. Heterogeneous patterns of intermediate filament proteins by imunohistochemistry. *Archives of Pathology and Laboratory Medicine* **113**, 1363–6.

Modlin, R.L., Hofman, F.M., Kempf, R.A. and Taylor, C.R. (1983). Kaposi's sarcoma in homosexual men: An immunohistochemical study. *Journal of the American Academy of Dermatology* **8**, 620-7.

Mogollon, R., Penneys, N.S., Albores-Saavedra, J. and Nadji, M. (1984). Malignant schwannoma presenting as a skin mass: Confirmation by the demonstration of myelin basic protein within tumour cells. *Cancer* **53**, 1190-3.

Moll, R., Lowe, A., Laufer, J. and Franke, W.W. (1992). Cytokeratin 20 in human carcinomas. A new histodiagnostic marker detected by monoclonal antibodies. *American Journal of Pathology* **140**, 427–47.

Mori, S,. Itoyama, S., Mohri, N. and Shibuya, A. (1985). Cellular characteristics of neoplastic angioendotheliosis: An immunohistological marker study of 6 cases. *Virchows Archives (Pathology and Anatomy)* **407**, 167–75.

Mukai, K. and Rosai, J. (1984). Factor VIII-related antigen: An endothelial marker. In DeLellis, R.A. (ed.), *Diagnostic Immunohistochemistry*, Masson, New York, pp. 253–61.

Mukai, K., Rosai, J. and Burgdorf, W.H.C. (1980). Localization of factor VIII-related antigen in vascular endothelial cells using an immunoperoxidase method. *American Journal of Surgical Pathology* **4**, 273–6.

Murphy, G.F., Bhan, A.K., Sato, S., Mihm, M.C. Jr. and Harrist , T.J. (1981). A new immunologic marker for human Langerhans' cells. *New England Journal of Medicine* **304**, 791–2.

Murphy, G.F., Flynn, R.C., Rice, R.H. and Pinkus, G.S. (1984). Involucrin expression in normal and neoplastic human skin: A marker for keratinocyte differentiation. *Journal of Investigative Dermatology* **82**, 453–7.

Nadji, M., Morales, A.R., Ziegels-Weissman, J. and Penneys, N.S. (1981). Kaposi's sarcoma: Immunohistologic evidence for an endothelial origin. *Archives of Pathology and Laboratory Medicine* **105**, 274–7.

Nakhleh, R.E., Wick, M.R., Rocamora, A., Swanson, P.E. and Dehner, L.P. (1990a). Morphologic diversity in malignant melanomas. *American Journal of Clinical Pathology* **93**, 731–40.

Nakhleh, R.E., Swanson, P.E. and Wick, M.R. (1990b). Cutaneous adnexal carcinoma with divergent differentiation. *American Journal of Dermatopathology* **12**, 325–34.

Nappi, O., Pettinato, G. and Wick, M.R. (1989). Adenoid (acantholytic) squamous cell carcioma of the skin. *Journal of Cutaneous Pathology* **16**, 114–21.

Nazini, M.N., Dykes, R.I. and Marks, R. (1990). Epidermal growth factor receptors in human epidermal tumours. *British Journal of Dermatology* **123**, 153–61.

Nemes, Z. and Thomazy, V. (1988). Factor XIIIa and the classic histiocytic markers in malignant fibrous histiocytoma. A comparative immunohistochemical study. *Human Pathology* **19**, 822–9.

Nemeth, A.J. and Penneys, N.S. (1989). Factor XIIIa is expressed by fibroblasts in fibrovascular tumours. *Journal of Cutaneous Pathology* **16**, 266–71.

Nickoloff, B.J., Fleischmann, H.E., Carmel, J., Wood, C.C. and Roth, R.J. (1986). Microcystic adnexal carcinoma. Immunohistologic observations suggesting dual (pilar and eccrine) differentiation. *Archives of Dermatology* **122**, 290-4.

Norton, A.J. and Isaacson, P.G. (1989a). Lymphoma phenotyping in formalin-fixed and paraffin wax-embedded tissues. I. Range of antibodies and staining patterns. *Histopathology* **14**, 437–46.

Norton, A.J. and Isaacson, P.G. (1989b). Lymphoma phenotyping in formalin-fixed and paraffin wax-embedded tissues. II. Profiles of reactivity in the various tumour types. *Histopathology* **14**, 557–79.

Norton, A.J,. Ramsay, A.D., Smith, S.H., Beverley, P.C.L. and Isaacson, P.G. (1986). Monoclonal antibody (UCHL-1) that recognizes normal and neoplastic T cells in routinely fixed tissues. *Journal of Clinical Pathology* **39**, 399–405.

Om, A., Ghose, T. and Rowden, G. (1991). Keratin and carcinoembryonic antigen (CEA) in human melanoma cells.

Virchows Archives (Cellular Pathology) **61**, 81–7.

Ordonez, N.G. and Batsakis, J.G. (1984). Comparison of Ulex europaeus I lectin and factor VIII-related antigen in vascular lesions. *Archives of Pathology and Laboratory Medicine* **108**, 129–32.

Ordonez, N.G., Ji, X.L. and Hickey, R.C. (1988). Comparison of HMB45 monoclonal antibody and S100 protein in the immunohistochemical diagnosis of melanoma. *American Journal of Clinical Pathology* **90**, 385–90.

Palazzo, J. and Duray, P.H. (1989). Typical, dysplastic, congenital and Spitz nevi. A comparative immunohistochemical study. *Human Pathology* **20**, 341–6.

Patterson, J.W. and Maygardern, S.J. (1986). Extraskeletal Ewing's sarcoma with cutaneous involvement. *Journal of Cutaneous Pathology* **13**, 46–58.

Peltonen, J., Jaakola, S. and Hsiao, L.L. (1990). Type IV collagen. In situ hybridization and immunohistochemistry reveal abundant mRNA and protein levels in human neurofibromas, schwannoma and mormal peripheral nerve tissues. *Laboratory Investigation* **62**, 487–92.

Penneys, N.S. (1984). Immunohistochemistry of adnexal neoplasms. *Journal of Cutaneous Pathology* **11**, 357–64.

Penneys, N.S., Nadji, M. and Morales, A.R. (1982a). Carcinoembryonic antigen in benign sweat gland tumours. *Archives of Dermatology* **118**, 225–7.

Penneys, N.S., Nadji, M., Ziegels-Weissman, J., Ketabchi, M. and Morales, A.R. (1982b). Carcinoembryonic antigen in sweat gland carcinomas. *Cancer* **50**, 1608–11.

Penneys, N.S., Nadji, M,. Ziegels-Weissman, J. and Morales, A.R. (1983). Prekeratin in spindle cell tumours of the skin. *Archives of Dermatology* **119**, 476–9.

Penneys, N.S., Mogollon, R., Kowalczyk, A,. Nadji, M. and Adachi, K. (1984). A survey of cutaneous neural lesions for the presence of myelin basic protein: an immunohistochemical study. *Archives of Dermatology* **120**, 210-13.

Penneys, N.S. and Zlatkiss, I. (1990). Immunohistochemical demonstration of ferritin in sweat gland and sweat gland neoplasms. *Journal of Cutaneous Pathology* **17**, 32–6.

Perentes, E. and Rubinstein, L. (1985). Immunohistochemical recognition of human nerve sheath tumours by anti-Leu 7 (HNK-1) monoclonal antibody. *Acta Neuropathologica (Berlin)* **68**, 319–24.

Perez, A.R., Achenbach, H. and Lack, E.E. (1986). High-grade epithelioid angiosarcoma of the scalp: An immunohistochemical and ultrastructural study. *American Journal of Dermatopathology* **8**, 411–18.

Pettinato, G., Manivel, J.C., De Rosa, G., Petrella, G. and Jaszcz, W. (1990). Angiomatoid malignant fibrous histiocytoma: Cytologic, immunohistochemical, ultrastructural, and flow cytometric study of 20 cases. *Modern Pathology* **3**, 479–87.

Pinkus, G.S. and Kurtin, P.J. (1985). Epithelial membrane antigen – a diagnostic discriminant in surgical pathology: Immunohistochemical profile in epithelial, mesenchymal, and haematopoietic neoplasms using paraffin sections and monoclonal antibodies. *Human Pathology* **16**, 929–40.

Posnett, D.N., Marboe, C.C. and Knowles, D.M. II. (1984). A membrane antigen (HC1) selectively present on hairy cell leukaemia cells, endothelial cells, and epidermal basal cels. *Journal of Immunology* **132**, 2700–2.

Puches, R., Smolle, J., Rieger, E., Soyer, H.P. and Kerl, H. (1991). Expression of cytoskeletal components in melanocytic skin lesions. An immunohistochemical study. *American Journal of Dermatopathology* **13**, 137–44.

Ralfkiaer, E. (1991). Immunohistological markers for the diagnosis of cutaneous lymphomas. *Seminars in Diagnostic Pathology* **8**, 62–72.

Ralfkiaer, E., Thomsen, K., Agdal, N., Hou-Jensen, K. and Wantzin, G.L. (1989). The development of a Ki-1 positive large cell non-Hodgkin's lymphoma in pagetoid reticulosis. *Acta Dermato-Venereologica* **69**, 206–11.

Ralfkiaer, E., Thonsen, K. and Vejlsgaard, G.L. (1991). Expression of a cell adhesion protein (VLA beta) in normal and diseased skin. *British Journal of Dermatology* **124**, 527–32.

Reed, W., Oppendal, B.R. and Eeg Larson, T. (1990). Immunohistology is valuable in distinguishing between Paget's disease, Bowen's disease and superficial spreading malignant melanoma. *Histopathology* **16**, 583–8.

Rest, E.B. and Horn, T.D. (1991). Immunophenotypic analysis of benign aand malignant cutaneous lymphoid infiltrates. *Clinics in Dermatology* **9**, 261–72.

Ricci, A. Jr., Cartun, R.W. and Zakowski, M.F. (1988). Atypical fibroxanthoma. A study of 14 cases emphasizing the presence of Langerhan's histiocytes with implications for differential diagnosis by antibody panels. *American Journal of Surgical Pathology* **12**, 591–8.

Rijlaarsdam, U. and Willemze, R. (1991). Cutaneous pseudo-T-cell lymphomas. *Seminars in Diagnostic Pathology* **8**, 102–8.

Roholl, P.J.M., Kleyne, J. and Van Unnik, J.A.M. (1985). Characterization of tumour cells in malignant fibrous histiocytoma and other soft tissue tumours in comparison with malignant histiocytes. II. Immunoperoxidase study on cryostat sections. *American Journal of Pathology* **121**, 269–74.

Roholl, P.J.M., Rutgers, D.H., Rademakers, L.H.P.M. and DeWeger, R.A. (1988). Characterization of human soft tissue sarcomas in nude mice. Evidence for histogenic properties of malignant fibrous histiocytomas. *American Journal of Pathology* **131**, 559–68.

Rowden, G., Connelly, E.M. and Winkelmann, R.K. (1983). Cutaneous histiocytosis X: The presence of S100 protein and its use in diagnosis. *Archives of Dermatology* **119**, 553–9.

Rulon, D.B. and Helwig, E.B. (1974). Cutaneous sebaceous neoplasms. *Cancer* **33**, 82–102.

Russell-Jones, R., Spaull, J., Spry, C.J.F. and Wilson-Jones, E. (1986). The histogenesis of Kaposi's sarcoma in patients with and without AIDS. *Journal of Clinical Pathology* **39**, 742–9.

Rutgers, J.L., Wieczorek, R., Bonetti, F. and Kaplan, K.J. (1986). The expression of endothelial cell surface antigens by AIDS-associated Kaposi's sarcoma: Evidence for a vascular endothelial cell origin. *American Journal of Pathology* **122**, 493–9.

Said, J.W., Sassoon, A.F., Shintaku, I.P. and Banks-Schlegel, S. (1984). Involucrin in squamous and basal cell carcinomas of the skin: An immunohistochemical study. *Journal of Investigative Dermatology* **82**, 449–52.

Sakamoto, F., Ito, M., Sato, S. and Sato, Y. (1985). Basal cell tumour with apocrine differentiation: Apocrine epithelioma. *Journal of the American Academy of Dermatology* **13**, 355–63.

Salisbury, J.R. and Isaacson, P.G. (1985). Synovial sarcoma: An immunohistochemical study. *Journal of Pathology* **147**, 49–57.

Sanchez, N.P. and Winkelmann, R.K. (1982). Basal cell tumour with eccrine differentiation (eccrine epithelioma). *Journal of the American Academy of Dermatology* **6**, 514–18.

Schlingemann, R.O., Dingjan, G.M., Emeis, J.J. and Blok, J. (1985). Monoclonal antibody PAL-E specific for endothelium. *Laboratory Investigation* **52**, 71–6.

Schmookler, B.M., Enzinger, F.M. and Weiss, S.W. (1989). Giant cell fibroblastoma. A juvenile form of dermatofibrosarcoma protuberans. *Cancer* **64**, 2154–61.

Schurch, W., Seemayer, T.A., Lagace, R. and Gabbiani, G. (1984). The intermediate filament cytoskeleton of myofibroblasts: An immunofluorescence and ultrastructural study. *Virchows Archives (Pathology and Anatomy)* **403**, 323–36.

Scott, G.A. and Rosai, J. (1988). Spindle cell haemangioendothelioma. Report of seven additional cases of a recently described vascular neoplasm. *American Journal of Dermatopathology* **10**, 281–8.

Sharma, S., Sarkar, C., Mathur, M., Dinda, A.K. and Roy, S. (1990). Benign nerve sheath tumours: A light microscopic, electron microscopic and immunohistochemical study of 102 cases. *Pathology* **22**, 191–5.

Sheibani, K., Battifora, H., Burke, J.S. and Rappaport, H. (1986a). Leu M1 antigen in human neoplasms: An immunohistologic study of 400 cases. *American Journal of Surgical Pathology* **10**, 227–36.

Sheibani, K., Battifora, H., Winberg, C.D. and Burke, J.S. (1986b). Further evidence that 'malignant angioendotheliomatosis' is an angiotropic large-cell lymphoma. *New England Journal of Medicine* **314**, 943–8.

Shimizu, N., Ito, M., Tazawa, T. and Sato, Y. (1989). Immunohistochemical study of keratin expression in certain cutaneous epithelial neoplasms. Basal cell carcinoma, pilomatricoma, and seborrheic keratosis. *American Journal of Dermatopathology* **11**, 534–40.

Sibley, R.K. and Dahl, D. (1985). Neuroendocrine (Merkel cell?) carcinoma of the skin. II. An immunocytochemical study of 21 cases. *American Journal of Surgical Pathology* **9**, 109–16.

Sibley, R.K., Rosai, J., Foucar, E., Dehner, L.P. and Bosl, G. (1980). Neuroendocrine (Merkel cell) carcinoma of the skin: A histologic and ultrastructural study of two cases. *American Journal of Surgical Pathology* **4**, 211–21.

Sieber, S.C., Lopez, V., Rosai, J. and Buckley, P.J .(1990). Primary tumour of spleen with morphologic features of malignant fibrous histiocytoma. Immunohistochemical evidence for a macrophage origin. *American Journal of Surgical Pathology* **14**, 1061–70.

Silvis, N.G., Swanson, P.E., Manivel, J.C., Kaye, V.N. and Wick, M.R. (1988). Spindle-cell and pleomorphic neoplasms of the skin. A clinicopathologic and immunohistochemical study of 30 cases, with emphasis on 'atypical fibroxanthomas'. *American Journal of Dermatopathology* **10**, 9–19.

Smith, M.E.F., Costa, M.J. and Weiss, S.W. (1991). Evaluation of CD68 and other histiocytic antigens in angiomatoid malignant fibrous histiocytoma. *American Journal of Surgical Pathology* **15**, 757–63.

Smolle, J., Konrad, K. and Kerl, H. (1985). Granular cell tumours contain myelin-associated glycoprotein. *Virchows Archives (Pathology and Anatomy)* **406**, 1–5.

Smolle, J., Soyer, H-P. and Kerl, H. (1990a). Tubulin expression in melanocytic skin tumours. An immunohistochemical study. *American Journal of Dermatopathology* **12**, 17–24.

Smolle, J., Torne, R., Soyer, H.P. and Kerl, H. (1990b). Immunohistochemical classification of cutaneous pseudolymphomas: Delineation of distinct patterns. *Journal of Cutaneous Pathology* **17**, 149–59.

Smoller, B.R. (1991). Immunohistochemistry in the diagnosis of malignant melanomas. *Clinics in Dermatology* **9**, 235–41.

Smoller, B.R., Hsu, A. and Krueger, J.(1991). HMB-45 monoclonal antibody recognizes an inducible and reversible melanocytic cytoplasmic protein. *Journal of Cutaneous Pathology* **18**, 315–22.

Smoller, B.R., Kwan, T.H. and Said, J.W. (1986). Keratoacanthoma and squamous cell carcinoma of the skin. Immunohistochemical localization of involucrin and keratin proteins. *Journal of the American Academy of Dermatology* **14**, 225–36.

Smoller, B.R., McNutt, N.S. and Hsu, A. (1989). HMB-45 recognizes stimulated melanocytes. *Journal of Cutaneous Pathology* **16**, 49–53.

Snover, D.C. and Rosai, J. (1985). Vascular sarcomas of the skin. In Wick, M.R. (ed.), *Pathology of Unusual Malignant Cutaneous Tumours*, Marcel Dekker, New York, pp. 181–210.

Soini, Y. (1990). Cell differentiation in benign cutaneous fibrous histiocytomas. An immunohistochemical study with antibodies to histiomonocytic cells and intermediate filament proteins. *American Journal of Dermatopathology* **12**, 134–40.

Soini, Y., Autio-Harmainen, H. and Miettinen, M. (1989). Immunoreactivity for laminin and type IV collagen in malignant and benign fibrous histiocytoma. *Journal of Pathology* **158**, 223–8.

Springall, D.R., Gu, J., Cocchia, D. and Michetti, F. (1983). The value of S100 immunostaining as a diagnostic tool in human malignant melanomas. *Virchows Archives (Pathology and Anatomy)* **400**, 331–44.

Springer, E.A. and Robinson, J.K. (1991). Patterns of epidermal growth factor receptors in basal cell carcinomas and squamous cell carcinomas. *Journal of Dermatological Surgery and Oncology* **17**, 20–4.

Stanton, C., Perentes, E., Collins, V. and Rubinstein, L. (1987). GFA protein reactivity in nerve sheath tumours: A polyvalent and monoclonal antibody study. *Journal of Neuropathology and Experimental Neurology* **46**, 634–41.

Starink, T.M., Blonjous, C.E., Stoof, T.J. and Van Der Linden, J.C. (1990). Clear cell basal cell carcinoma. *Histopathology* **17**, 401–5.

Stefansson, K. and Wollman, R.L. (1982). S100 protein in granular cell tumours (granular cell myoblastomas). *Cancer* **49**, 1834–8.

Stefansson, K., Wollman, R.L. and Jenkovic, M. (1982). S100 protein in soft tissue tumours derived from Schwann cells and melanocytes. *American Journal of Pathology* **106**, 261–8.

Strauchen, J.A. and Dimitriu-Bona, A. (1986). Malignant fibrous histiocytoma: expression of monocyte/macrophage differentiation antigens detected with monoclonal antibodies. *American Journal of Pathology* **124**, 303–9.

Sun, J., Morton, T.H. and Gown, A.M. (1990). Antibody HMB-45 identifies the cells of blue nevi. An immunohistochemical study on paraffin sections. *American Journal of Surgical Pathology* **14**, 748–51.

Suzuki, Y., Hashimoto, K. and Kato, I. (1989). A monoclonal antibody, SKH1, reacts with 40 kD sweat gland-associated antigen. *Journal of Cutaneous Pathology* **16**, 66–71.

Swanson, P.E. (1990). Cytokeratin(-like) immunoreactivity in soft tissue sarcoma (abstract). *Journal of Histochemistry and Cytochemistry* **38**, 1065.

Swanson, P.E. (1991). Heffalumps, jagulars and cheshire cats. A commentary on cytokeratins and soft tissue sarcomas. *American Journal of Clinical Pathology* **95** (Suppl.), S2–S7.

Swanson, P.E., Cherwitz, D.L., Neumann, M.P. and Wick, M.R. (1987a). Eccrine sweat gland carcinoma: A histologic and immunohistochemical study of 32 cases. *Journal of Cutaneous Pathology* **14**, 65–86.

Swanson, P.E. and Dehner, L.P. (1991). Pathology of soft tissue sarcomas in children and adolescents. In Maurer, H.M., Ruymaqnn, F.B., Pochedly, C.E. (eds.), *Rhabdomyosarcoma and Related Tumours in Children and Adolescents*, CRC Press, New York, pp. 385–420.

Swanson, P.E., Manivel, J.C., Scheithauer, B.W. and Wick, M.R. (1989). Epithelial membrane antigen reactivity in mesenchymal neoplasms. An immunohistochemical study of 306 soft tissue sarcomas. *Surgical Pathology* **2**, 313–22.

Swanson, P.E., Manivel, J.C. and Wick, M.R. (1987b). Leu 7–immunoreactivity in neurofibrosarcomas and other spindle-cell sarcomas of soft tissue. *American Journal of Pathology* **126**, 546–60.

Swanson, P.E., Mazoujian, G., Mills, S.E., Campbell, R.J. and Wick, M.R. (1991). Immunoreactivity for estrogen receptor protein in sweat gland tumours. *American Journal of Surgical Pathology* **15**, 835–41.

Swanson, P.E., Niehans, G.A. and Wick, M.R. (1990). Immunoreactivity for c-erbB-2 (neu) oncopeptide in eccrine carcinoma (abstract). *Journal of Cutaneous Pathology* **17**, 321.

Swanson, P.E. and Sirgi, S.E. (1992). CD34 and tumour associated glycoprotein immunoreactivity in epithelioid soft tissue sarcomas (abstract). *Modern Pathology* **5**, 11A.

Swanson, P.E., Stanley, M.W., Scheithauer, B.W. and Wick, M.R. (1988a). Primary cutaneous leiomyosarcoma. A histologic and immunohistochemical study of nine cases, with ultrastructural correlation. *Journal of Cutaneous Pathology* **15**, 129–41.

Swanson, P.E. and Wick, M.R. (1990). HLA-DR (Ia-like) reactivity in tumours of bone and soft tissue. An immunohistochemical comparison of monoclonal antibodies LN3 and LK8D3 in routinely-processed specimens. *Modern Pathology* **3**, 113–19.

Swanson, P.E. and Wick, M.R. (1991). Immunohistochemical evaluation of vascular neoplasms. *Clinics in Dermatology* **9**, 243–54.

Swanson, P.E., Sun, T-T., Smoller, B.R. and Wick, M.R. (1988b): Immunoreactivity for 'hard keratins' in cutaneous neoplasms (abstract). *Journal of Cutaneous Pathology* **15**, 346.

Szadowska, A., Wozniak, L., Lasota, J. and Giryn, I. (1989). Neuroendocrine (Merkel cell) carcinoma of the skin: A clinico-morphological study of 13 cases. *Histopathology* **15**, 483–93.

Takata, M., Hirone, T. and Matsumura, H. (1989). Beta-2–microglobulin expression in normal melanocytes, nevocellular nevi, and malignant melanomas. *Journal of Investigative Dermatology* **92** (Suppl. 5), 243s–47s.

Tateyama, H., Eimoto, T., Tada, T. and Niwa, T. (1992). Malignant pilomatrixoma. An immunohistochemical study with antihair keratin antibody. *Cancer* **69**, 127–32.

Taylor, C.R., Hofman, F.M., Modlin, R.L. and Rea, T.H. (1983). Immunoperoxidase techniques applied to dermatopathology.

Journal of Cutaneous Pathology **10**, 145–63.

Toker, C. (1972). Trabecular carcinoma of the skin. *Archives of Dermatology* **105**, 107–10.

Tokura, Y., Yoshikuni, K. and Teraki, Y. (1989). Immunohistochemically detectable duct-like structures in benign and malignant eccrine poromas: CEA and involucrin immunostaining. *Journal of Dermatology* **16**, 133–41.

Traweek, S.T., Kandalaft, P.L., Mehta, P. and Battifora, H. (1991). The human haematopoietic progenitor cell antigen (CD34) in vascular neoplasia. *American Journal of Clinical Pathology* **96**, 25–31.

Tsubura, A., Morii, S. and Veda, S. (1987). Immunohistochemical demonstration of MAM-3 and MAM-6 antigen in normal human skin appendages and their tumours. *Archives of Dermatologic Research* **279**, 550–7.

Tsukuda, T., McNutt, M.A., Ross, R. and Gown, A.M. (1987). HHF35, a muscle actin-specific monoclonal antibody. II. Reactivity in normal, reactive, and neoplastic human tissue. *American Journal of Pathology* **127**, 389–402.

Turner, R.R., Wood, G.S., Beckstead, J.H. and Colby, T.V. (1984). Histiocytic malignancies: Morphologic, immunologic, and enzymatic heterogeneity. *American Journal of Surgical Pathology* **8**, 485–500.

Ushigome, S., Tadakuna, T. and Hyuga, M. (1986). Perineurial cell tumour and the significance of the perineurial cells in neurofibroma. *Acta Pathologica Japonica* **36**, 973–81.

van Muijen, G.N.P., Ruiter, D.J., Ponec, M., Huiskens-Van der Mey, C. and Varnaar, S.O. (1984). Monoclonal antibodies with different specificities against cytokeratins: An immunohistochemical study of normal tissues and tumours. *American Journal of Pathology* **114**, 9–17.

van Muijen, G.N., Jansen, K.F. and Cornelissen, I.M.(1991). Establishment and characterization of a human melanoma cell line (MV3) which is highly metastatic in nude mice. *International Journal of Cancer* **48**, 85–91.

van Vreeswijk, H., Ruiter, D.J., Broeker, E-B., Welvaart, K. and Ferrone, S. (1988). Differential expression of HLA-DR, DQ and DP antigens in primary and metastatic melanoma. *Journal of Investigative Dermatology* **90**, 755–61.

Visona, A., Ronconi, G., Montaguti, A., Stracca-Pansa, V. and Azzopardi, J.G. (1987). Juvenile hyaline fibromatosis. Case report and review of the literature. *Pathologica* **79**, 357–66.

von Kuster, L.C., Liwnicz, B.H. and Ward, D.E. (1986). Concanavalin A- and Lens culinaris agglutinin binding patterns in normal and neoplastic sebaceous epithelium. *Journal of Cutaneous Pathology* **13**, 274–84.

Voytek, T.M., Ricci, A. Jr. and Cartun, R.W. (1991). Estrogen and progesterone receptors in primary eccrine carcinoma. *Modern Pathology* **4**, 582–5.

Warner, T.F.C.S., Uno, H., Hafez, R. and Burgess, J. (1983). Merkel cells and Merkel cell tumours. Ultrastructure, immunocytochemistry, and review of the literature. *Cancer* **52**, 238–45.

Weiss, L.M., Trela, M.J., Cleary, M.L. and Turner, R.R. (1985). Frequent immunoglobulin and T-cell receptor gene rearrangements in 'histiocytic' neoplasms. *American Journal of Pathology* **121**, 369–73.

Weiss, S.W. and Enzinger, F.M. (1982). Epithelioid haemangioendothelioma: A vascular tumour often mistaken for a carcinoma. *Cancer* **50**, 970-81.

Weiss, S.W. and Enzinger, F.M. (1986). Spindle-cell haemangioendothelioma. A low grade angiosarcoma resembling a cavernous haemangioma and Kaposi's sarcoma. *American Journal of Surgical Pathology* **10**, 521–30.

White, W.L., Tam, S.T., Mitchell, M.S., Yu, M.C. and Kan-Mitchell, J. (1991). Evaluation of human monoclonal antibody (2–139–1) in cutaneous melanocytic neoplasms in fixed tissue sections. *Journal of Histochemistry and Cytochemistry* **39**, 777–85.

Wick, M.R. (1988). Monoclonal antibodies to carcinoembryonic antigen in diagnostic immunohistochemistry. In Wick, M.R. and Siegal, G.P. (eds), *Monoclonal Antibodies in Diagnostic Immunohistochemistry*. Marcel Dekker, New York.

Wick, M.R. (1991a). Kaposi's sarcoma unrelated to the acquired immunodeficiency syndrome. *Current Opinions in Oncology* **3**, 377–83.

Wick, M.R. (1991b). HMB-45: A clue to the biology of malignant melanoma? *Journal of Cutaneous Pathology* **18**, 315–22.

Wick, M.R. and Coffin, C.M. (1985). Sweat gland and pilar carcinomas. In Wick, M.R. (ed.), *Pathology of Unusual Malignant Cutaneous Tumours*. Marcel Dekker, New York, pp. 1–76.

Wick, M.R., Cooper, P.H., Swanson, P.E., Kaye, V.N. and Sun, T.T. (1990). Microcystic adnexal carcinoma. An immunohistochemical comparison with other cutaneous appendage tumours. *Archives of Dermatology* **126**, 189–94.

Wick, M.R., Hagen, K.A. and Frizzera, G. (1987a). Three immunostaining techniques for the localization of leukocyte common antigen in formalin-fixed, paraffin-embedded dermatological biopsy specimens. *American Journal of Dermatopathology* **9**, 250–5.

Wick, M.R., Kaye, V.N., Sibley, R.K., Tyler, R. and Frizzera, G. (1986a). Primary neuroendocrine carcinoma and small-cell malignant lymphoma of the skin: A discriminant immunohistochemical comparison. *Journal of Cutaneous Pathology* **13**, 347–58.

Wick, M.R. and Kaye, V.N. (1986). The role of diagnostic immunohistochemistry in dermatology. *Seminars in Dermatology* **5**, 346–58.

Wick, M.R. and Manivel, J.C. (1986). Epithelioid sarcoma and isolated necrobiotic granuloma: A comparative immunohistochemical study. *Journal of Cutaneous Pathology* **13**,

253–60.

Wick, M.R. and Manivel, J.C. (1987). Epithelioid sarcoma and epithelioid haemangioendothelioma: An immunohistochemical and lectin-histochemical comparison. *Virchows Archives (Pathology and Anatomy)* **410**, 309–16.

Wick, M.R., Millns, J.L., Sibley, R.K., Pittelkow, M.R. and Winkelmann, R.K. (1985). Secondary neuroendocrine carcinomas of the skin: An immunohistochemical comparison with primary neuroendocrine carcinomas of the skin ('Merkel cell' carcinomas). *Journal of the American Academy of Dermatology* **13**, 134–42.

Wick, M.R. and Mills, S.E. (1991). Intravascular lymphomatosis: clinicopathologic features and differential diagnosis. *Seminars in Diagnostic Pathology* **8**, 91–101.

Wick, M.R., Mills, S.E., Scheithauer, B.W. and Cooper, P.H. (1986b). Reassessment of 'malignant angioendotheliomatosis': Evidence for its reclassification as 'intravascular lymphomatosis.' *American Journal of Surgical Pathology* **10**, 112–23.

Wick, M.R. and Scheithauer, B.W. (1985). Primary neuroendocrine carcinoma of the skin. In Wick, M.R. (ed.), *Pathology of Unusual Malignant Cutaneous Tumours*, Marcel Dekker, New York, pp. 107–80.

Wick, M.R., Scheithauer, B.W. and Kovacs, K. (1983). Neuron-specific enolase in neuroendocrine tumours of the thymus, bronchus, and skin. *American Journal of Clinical Pathology* **79**, 703–07.

Wick, M.R. and Swanson, P.E. (1986). Primary adenoid cystic carcinoma of the skin: A clinical, histologic, and immunohistochemical comparison with adenoid cystic carcinoma of salivary glands, and adenoid basal cell carcinoma. *American Journal of Dermatopathology* **8**, 2–13.

Wick, M.R. and Swanson, P.E. (1991). Cutaneous Adnexal Tumours. *A Guide to Pathologic Diagnosis*, ASCP Press, Chicago.

Wick, M.R., Swanson, P.E., Leboit, P.E., Strickler, J.G. and Cooper, P.H. (1991). Lymphoepithelioma-like carcinoma of the skin with adnexal differentiation. *Journal of Cutaneous Pathology* **18**, 93–102.

Wick, M.R., Swanson, P.E., Scheithauer, B.W. and Manivel, J.C. (1987b). Malignant peripheral nerve sheath tumour: An immunohistochemical study of 62 cases. *American Journal of Clinical Pathology* **87**, 425–33.

Wick, M.R., Swanson, P.E. and Rocamora, A. (1988). Recognition of malignant melanoma by the monoclonal antibody HMB-45. *Journal of Cutaneous Pathology* **15**, 201–8.

Wilson, B.S., Herzig, M.A. and Lloyd, R.V. (1984). Immunoperoxidase staining for Ia-like antigens in paraffin-embedded tissues from human melanoma and lung carcinoma. *American Journal of Pathology* **115**, 102–16.

Wilson, B.S. and Lloyd, R.V. (1984). Detection of chromogranin in neuroendocrine cells with monoclonal antibody. *American Journal of Pathology* **115**, 458–68.

Wolber, R.A., Dupuis, B.A. and Wick, M.R. (1991). Expression of c-erbB-2 oncoprotein in mammary and extramamary Paget's disease. *American Journal of Clinical Pathology* **96**, 243–7.

Wood, G.S., Beckstead, J.H., Turner, R.R. and Hendrickson, M.R. (1986). Malignant fibrous histiocytoma tumour cells resemble fibroblasts. *American Journal of Surgical Pathology* **10**, 323–35.

Wood, W.S. and Tron, V.A. (1991). Analysis of HMB-45 immunoreactivity in common and cellular blue nevi. *Journal of Cutaneous Pathology* **18**, 261–3.

Wrotnowski, U., Mills, S.E. and Cooper, P.H. (1985). Malignant angioendotheliomatosis: An angiotropic lymphoma? *American Journal of Clinical Pathology* **83**, 244–8.

Yonezawa, S., Maruyama, I. and Sakae, K. (1987). Thrombomodulin as a marker for vascular tumours: Comparative study with factor VIII and Ulex europaeus I lectin. *American Journal of Clinical Pathology* **88**, 405–11.

Zarbo, R.J., Crissman, J.D., Venkat, H. and Weiss, M.A. (1986). Spindle-cell carcinoma of the upper aerodigestive tract mucosa. An immunohistologic and ultrastructural study of 18 biphasic tumours and comparison with seven monophasic spindle-cell tumours. *American Journal of Surgical Pathology* **10**, 741–53.

Zarbo, R.J., Gown, A.M., Nagle, R.B., Visscher, D.W. and Crissman, J.C. (1990). Anomolous cytokeratin expression in malignant melanoma: One and two dimensional western blot analysis and immunohistochemical survey of 100 melanomas. *Modern Pathology* **3**, 494–501.

Zhao, Y., Chen, H. and He, C. (1991). Reactivity of monoclonal antibody OKM5 with sebaceous carcinoma. *Journal of Cutaneous Pathology* **18**, 323–7.

7 ◆ *Central nervous system diseases and tumours*

Michael F. Gonzales

Introduction

As in other systems, immunohistochemistry has uniquely contributed to the present sophistication of knowledge about disease processes affecting the nervous system. In both diagnostic neuropathology and neuroscience research, the techniques of direct and indirect immunofluorescence, peroxidase-antiperoxidase, avidin-biotin and immunogold-silver histochemistry have established their niche alongside the very powerful techniques of modern molecular biology. The rapid expansion in the neurosciences in the past decade has greatly extended the coterie of nervous system antigens that have been isolated and characterized. Neuropathologists now have an extremely powerful array of monoclonal and polyclonal antibodies to employ in both diagnostic and research settings.

This chapter emphasizes the role of immunohistochemistry in facilitating the diagnosis of infectious, degenerative and neoplastic diseases of the central nervous system. Where appropriate, research applications are also discussed. Unless otherwise indicated, the patterns of immunoreactivity that are discussed and illustrated apply to formalin-fixed, paraffin-embedded tissue.

Infectious and inflammatory/reactive disorders

Herpes simplex encephalitis

Herpes simplex Type I (HSV-I) is a DNA virus which causes a necrotizing meningoencephalitis, predominantly affecting the white matter of the frontal and temporal lobes. Because the appearances on computerized tomographic (CT) scanning and magnetic resonance imaging (MRI) are diagnostic in the majority of patients, open brain biopsy has become uncommon. However, occasional patients have an atypical clinical presentation or CT and MRI findings and in these circumstances, open biopsy is required for definitive diagnosis. Direct immunofluorescence, performed on frozen sections of fresh tissue provides the most rapid and accurate method of identifying viral antigen in neurones and glial cells (Fig. 7.1). Rapid peroxidase-antiperoxidase (PAP) immunohistochemistry can also be used. Because HSV-II and Herpes Varicella Zoster virus (VZV) may occasionally cause a similar encephalitis and encephalomyelitis (Devinsky et al., 1991), antibodies against each of these viruses should be included in the immunohistochemistry protocol.

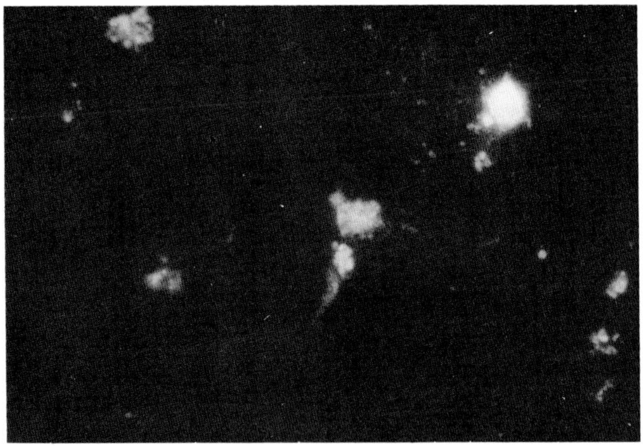

Fig. 7.1. Herpes simplex encephalitis: HSV antigen identified in glial cells and neurons by direct immunofluorescence with a fluorescein labelled anti-HSV 1 antibody (×400 frozen section).

Human immunodeficiency virus (HIV) subacute encephalitis

A subacute encephalitis, characterized pathologically by microglial nodules containing multinucleated giant cells, vacuolation of white matter (vacuolar myelopathy) and diffuse gliosis is the commonest central nervous system complication of human immunodeficiency virus (HIV) infection (Gonzales and Davis, 1988). It is the pathology that underlies the dementia associated with the acquired immunodeficiency syndrome (AIDS-dementia complex; ADC). Antibodies against a variety of HIV epitopes, in particular the p17 and p24 nucleocapsid proteins and the gp120 and gp41 envelope glycoproteins are now available for diagnostic use. HIV antigen has been most frequently identified in multinucleated giant cells and endothelial cells in brains with established subacute encephalitis (Fig. 7.2; Wiley et al., 1986) and in perivascular microglial cells in brains without the pathological features of subacute encephalitis. Multinucleated giant cells, either as a component of or separate from microglial nodules are pathognomonic of HIV infection of the central nervous system (Budka, 1986). These and mononuclear cells of monocyte/macrophage lineage appear to be productively infected by HIV, resulting in

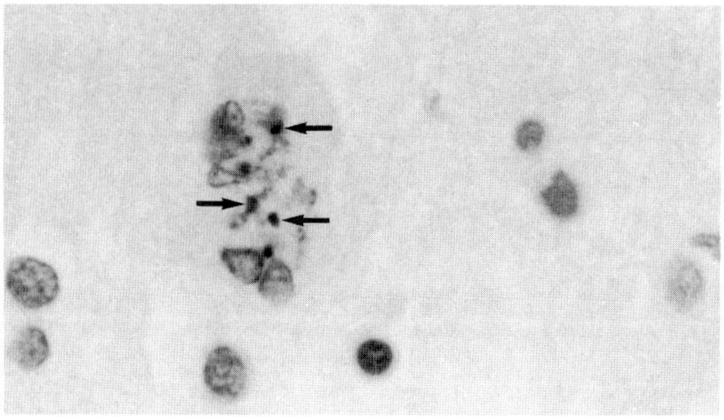

Fig. 7.2. HIV sub-acute encephalitis: HIV gp120 antigen (arrows) in cytoplasm of multinucleated giant cell in cerebral white matter (HIV gp120/PAP/ Haematoxylin; x1000).

the secretion of soluble factors that induce neuronal and oligodendroglial dysfunction (Giulian et al., 1990).

Cytomegalovirus infection

Cytomegalovirus (CMV) has rarely been proven to cause an acute encephalitis without concomitant immune-suppression (Phillips et al., 1977). Intrauterine infection is a recognized cause of several congenital malformations. Since the mid-1980s, opportunistic CMV infection of the central nervous system in patients with HIV-induced immune-suppression has been increasingly reported. Evidence of coinfection with cytomegalovirus (CMV) is found in approximately 25 per cent of brains with HIV subacute encephalitis. Five distinct types of pathology may result from opportunistic CMV infection of the brain and spinal cord (Morgello et al., 1987) and in each of these, CMV antigen can be readily detected by immunohistochemistry (Fig. 7.3). The most frequent manifestation is an encephalitis in which microglial nodules often containing CMV inclusions but without multinucleated giant cells are present in grey matter. Necrotizing ependymitis, isolated cells containing CMV inclusions, necrotizing myelitis and radiculomyelitis may also occur.

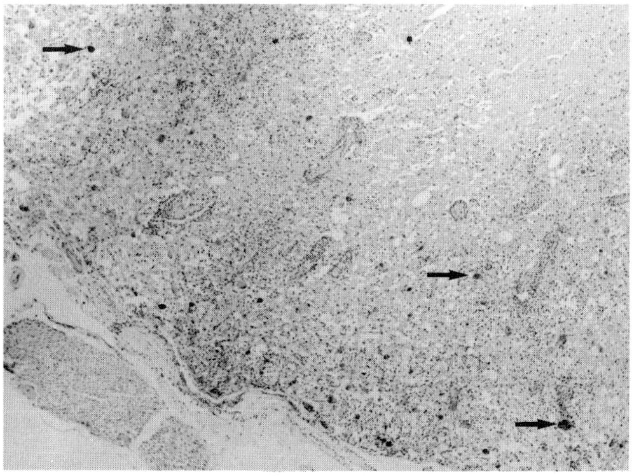

Fig. 7.3. Cytomegalovirus (CMV) necrotizing radiculomyelitis involving anterior nerve root exit zone of thoracic spinal cord in a patient with acquired immunodeficiency syndrome (AIDS). CMV antigen (arrows) identified by PAP immunohistochemistry (×40).

Progressive multifocal leucoencephalopathy (PML)

Infection of the central nervous system by the JC serotype of human papovavirus results in multiple small foci of demyelination (Astrom et al., 1958). These are particularly obvious in white matter immediately subjacent to the cerebral cortex but may also be seen in the white matter of the brain stem, cerebellum and spinal cord. Progressive multifocal leucoencephalopathy usually occurs as an opportunistic infection in patients with disseminated malignancy (in particular lymphoma), AIDS, neurosarcoidosis and iatrogenic immune suppression such as is associated with organ transplantation. Viral antigen can be identified immunohistochemically in the nuclei of atypical oligodendrocytes and astrocytes particularly at the margins of the lesions (Fig. 7.4A). The typical filamentous and icosahedral arrangement of JC virions can be identified by electron microscopy (Fig. 7.4B) and the virus is also detectable by DNA:DNA hybridization (Hulette et al., 1991).

Sub-acute sclerosing panencephalitis (SSPE)

Subacute sclerosing panencephalitis is an uncommon, slowly developing encephalitis that results from infection by a defective measles virus (Greenfield, 1950). It is clinically and pathologically distinct from the acute post-infectious form of measles encephalitis. Patients with SSPE do not produce antibody against viral M protein which is necessary for the release and subsequent neutralization of the virus (Hall et al., 1978). The pathology in the brain varies according to the length of survival.

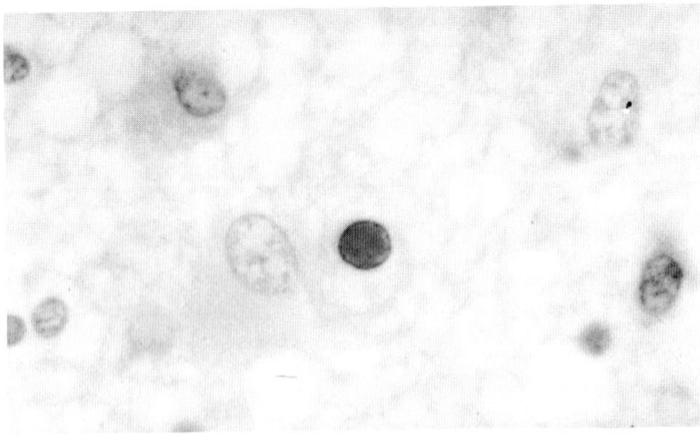

A

Fig. 7.4. Progressive multifocal leucoencephalopathy (PML): JC virus inclusion in the nucleus of an oligodendrocyte identified (A) by PAP immunohistochemistry (×1000) and (B) by electron microscopy (Uranyl acetate/Lead citrate; Bar = 200 nanometres).

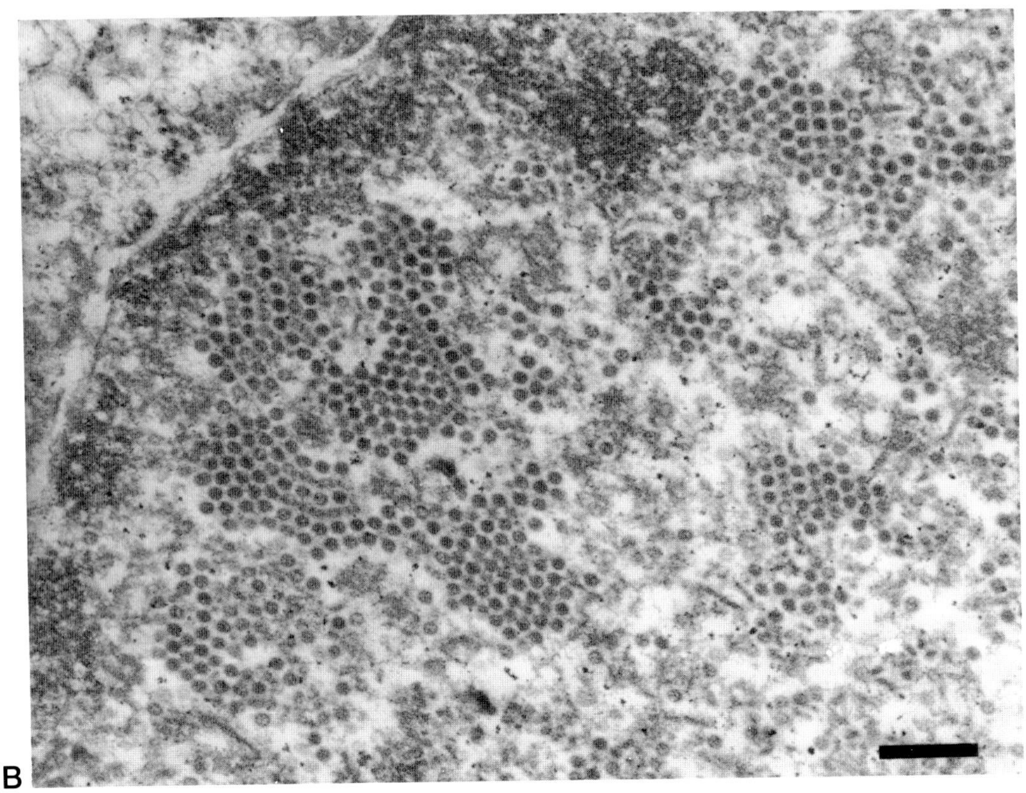

B

The mean age at presentation is 7 years but most patients have had documented measles infection before the age of 2 years (Modlin et al., 1977). The brains of patients with relatively short survival show the classical triad of pathological changes associated with viral encephalitis: perivascular mononuclear cell infiltration, neuronophagia and intranuclear inclusion bodies, predominantly in oligodendrocytes but also in neurones and astrocytes. These can be confirmed as measles virus inclusions by immunohistochemistry. Inclusion bodies are extremely difficult to find in the brains of patients surviving for long periods after presentation, but measles virus antigen may still be identified immunohistochemically. In long survivors, diffuse and often intense astrocytic gliosis and demyelination are prominent features.

Numerous inclusion bodies are seen in the nuclei of cortical neurones and oligodendrocytes in measles encephalitis occurring in immunosuppressed individuals.

Miscellaneous infections of the central nervous system

Other central nervous system infections in which immunohistochemical identification of antigen establishes the diagnosis include rabies, toxoplasmosis and amoebiasis (Acanthamoebae). In addition a variety of viral antigens and genomic sequences has been identified in and adjacent to the plaques of multiple sclerosis (for review see Rodriguez, 1989). These include HSV-I, CMV, mumps virus, measles virus and human T-cell leukaemia virus Type I (HTLV-1). Although the presence of these antigens supports a viral aetiopathogenesis of multiple sclerosis, conclusive proof of a cause–effect relationship remains to be established.

Reactive astrocytic and microglial proliferation

Non-neoplastic reactive proliferation of fibrous astrocytes is a fundamental reparative process in the central nervous system. In the past, this proliferation was often referred to as glial scarring analogous to replacement of parenchymal cells in other organs by collagen. The most florid examples of this process in the brain are the established plaque of multiple sclerosis and the firm rim of white matter adjacent to a remote infarct. Reactive astrocytic gliosis is also seen adjacent to mass lesions such as neoplasms, abscesses and haematomata, in the margins of penetrating wounds and in the cortical and sub-cortical grey matter following the neuronal drop-out that characterizes some neurodegenerative diseases. In these reactive states the increase in the number of astrocytes and prominence of their fibrillary processes can only be fully appreciated by the demonstration of immuno-reactivity for glial fibrillary acidic protein (Fig. 7.5), a component of astrocyte intermediate filaments.

More recently, the possible role of activated astrocytes and microglial cells in central nervous system immunity has come under increasing scrutiny. Immunohistochemistry has been central in clarifying these phenomena. Microglial cells were first described in 1919 by del Rio-Hortega who grouped them with the neuroglia because he found they had the same affinity for heavy metals as astrocytes, oligodendrocytes, ependymal cells and neurones. However, they are now recognized as the resident macrophages of the brain, equivalent to the Kupffer cells of the liver and alveolar macrophages of the lung. Their true identity was proven by the immunohistochemical demonstration that activated microglia express the same surface markers as peripheral blood and peritoneal macrophages, in particular Fc, CD4 and complement receptor 3 (CR3) and secrete the

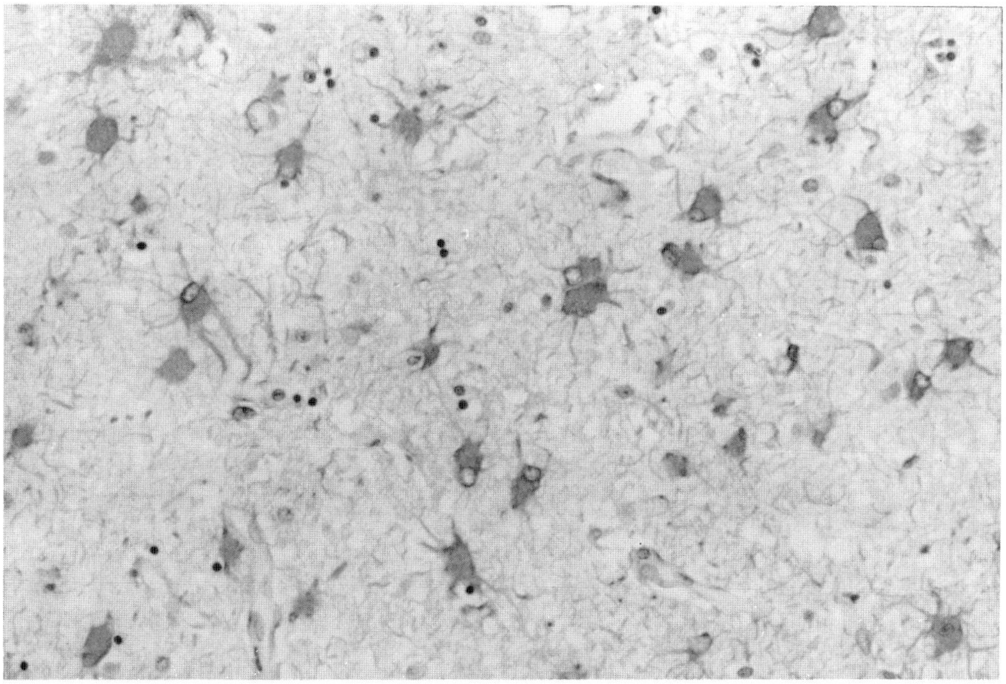

Fig. 7.5. Reactive astrocytic proliferation (gliosis) in cerebral white matter adjacent to a long-standing infarct. The processes of astrocytes are highlighted by their reactivity with an antibody against glial fibrillary acidic protein (GFAP). (GFAP/PAP; x200).

same soluble factors, interleukin-1 (IL-1) and tumour necrosis factor (TNF) They also react with antibodies raised against ferritin (Kaneko et al., 1989). Using these markers, traffic of cells from peripheral blood across the blood-brain barrier into perivascular spaces and eventually into the cerebrospinal fluid has been mapped (Hickey and Kimura, 1989; Perry and Gordon, 1988). Surface expression of major histocompatibility class II (MHC II) molecules by microglia under a variety of *in vivo* and *in vitro* conditions has been demonstrated, thereby identifying them as putative antigen presenting cells.

Expression of MHC molecules on the cell surfaces of reactive astrocytes can also be recognized immunohistochemically. This phenomenon, as well as the ability to release cytokines, carry out phagocytosis and the complement of lysosomal enzymes suggest that reactive astrocytes act as accessory immune cells, in particular as processors and presenters of antigen in association with microglia. It is unclear whether neoplastic astrocytes express MHC molecules and secrete cytokines such as IL-1 and other factors such as apolipoprotein-E. Demonstration of restricted expression of these factors to reactive astrocytes would provide a solution to the frequent dilemma of distinguishing them from neoplastic astrocytes.

Degenerative diseases of the central nervous system

Table 7.1 sets out a simple classification of the common degenerative diseases that affect the central nervous system. These disorders have a number of pathological features in common: loss of specific groups of neurones, retrograde or 'dying-back' axonal degeneration and alterations in the neuronal cytoskeleton. The cytoskeletal pathology results in such features as neurofibrillary tangles, Lewy bodies and other neuronal inclusions such as those seen in Pick's lobar atrophy and amyotrophic lateral sclerosis. Immunohistochemical techniques have played a pivotal role in clarifying the pathogenesis of these cytoskeletal changes, in particular the accumulation of altered cytoskeletal proteins. The identity and function of neurones that are lost in some neurodegenerative diseases such as Huntington's disease have also been determined by immunohistochemical techniques, utilizing antibodies against specific neurotransmitters and neuropeptides.

Alzheimer's disease

First described in 1898, Alzheimer's disease is now the commonest cause of dementia worldwide. The brain

Table 7.1. Classification of neurodegenerative diseases

Site of pathology	Dominant clinical features	Disease
Cerebral cortex	Dementia	Alzheimer's disease Pick's disease Diffuse Lewy body disease* Prion Diseases (see text)
Basal ganglia	Movement disorders +/−dementia	Parkinson's disease Parkinson's/dementia/ALS complex of Guam (see text) Progressive supranuclear palsy Huntington's disease
Spinal cord	Muscle weakness	Motor neuron disease/ALS
Multisystem atrophy	Ataxia	Olivopontocerebellar atrophy cerebellar cortical Degeneration Friedreich's ataxia Striato-nigral degeneration Pallido-luysian degeneration

* Lewy bodies present in cortical and sub-cortical neurons.

macroscopically appears atrophic and weighs 1000 grams or less in the unfixed state. However, in an unselected population, correlation between the degree of atrophy and presence of the microscopic changes of Alzheimer's disease is poor. The dominant microscopic abnormalities are the presence of numerous neuritic plaques in the cerebral cortex and accumulation of amyloid in the walls of small cortical arteries and meningeal vessels.

Neuritic plaques appear as focal disturbances of the neuropil. These pass through a developmental sequence which has been determined with the aid of immunohistochemical techniques (Probst et al., 1991). In the fully developed state, they comprise a corona of club-like swellings of neurites, particularly dendrites, a central core of amyloid and are infiltrated peripherally by reactive astrocytes and microglial cells. Functionally they result in de-afferentation of neurons. Neuritic plaques are particularly numerous in the temporal cortex and hippocampus and in associative cortical areas. Other histopathological abnormalities include neurofibrillary tangles, granulo-vacuolar degeneration and intraneuronal Hirano bodies (Probst et al., 1991). Similar microscopic abnormalities can be present in the brains of non-demented elderly individuals and the histopathological diagnosis of Alzheimer's disease is based on a set of quantitative criteria that have been established from clinico-pathological correlative studies (Khachaturian, 1985).

A significant body of data has now accumulated indicating that the pathogenesis of Alzheimer's disease involves the abnormal cleavage of a protein that spans the synaptic membrane resulting in the deposition of amyloid in the extracellular space and walls of cerebral vessels. This membrane-spanning protein has been designated the amyloid precursor protein (APP). To date, three different APP isoforms with 695, 751 and 770 amino-acid residues respectively have been identified (Kitaguchi et al., 1988; Ponte et al., 1988, Tanzi et al., 1988). The 751 amino-acid polypeptide (APP 751) differs from APP 695 by a 56 amino-acid domain which has 50 per cent homology with the Kunitz family of serine protease inhibitors. The APP 770 polypeptide contains an additional 19 amino-acid sequence immediately adjacent to the protease inhibitor domain of APP 751. Abnormal proteolytic cleavage of APP 695, which is thought to result from the absence of a protease inhibitor in this isoform, releases a 42–43 amino-acid polypeptide with a relative mass of 4 kD. This has been designated the beta-A4 (βA4) protein and it

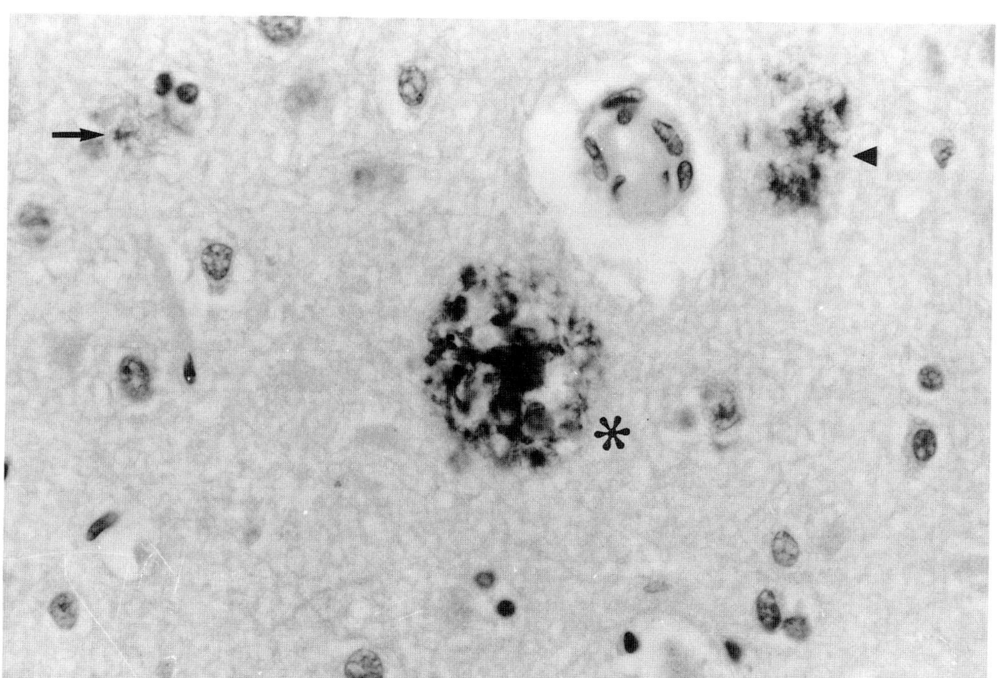

Fig. 7.6. Alzheimer's disease: section of cerebral cortex reacted with an antibody against the beta-A4 protein. An early or diffuse plaque, appearing only as a focal disturbance of the neuropil (arrow), a plaque with A4-reactive dystrophic neurites (arrowhead) and a mature plaque (asterisk) with a central amyloid, A4-reactive core as well as a corona of A4-reactive dystrophic neurites are highlighted (beta A-4/PAP; x200).

constitutes the major component of the amyloid fibril in the cores of the neuritic plaques and walls of cortical and meningeal blood vessels in both Alzheimer's disease and Down's syndrome (Masters et al., 1985; Vinters et al., 1988).

A number of antibodies raised against the βA4 protein are presently available. These have become invaluable in accurately applying the quantitative criteria for the pathological diagnosis of Alzheimer's disease (Davies et al., 1988) because they have facilitated the detection of diffuse plaques i.e. plaques that are in an early stage of development and lack amyloid cores (Fig. 7.6). In helping to confirm the βA4 component of definitive plaque cores (Fig. 7.6) and cerebral vascular amyloid (Fig. 7.7) they are useful adjuncts to the more conventional techniques of Bielchowsky silver impregnation and Congo red staining.

Whereas neuritic plaques are primarily due to amyloid deposition, the other histopathological manifestations of Alzheimer's disease, neurofibrillary tangles, granulo-vacuolar degeneration and Hirano bodies result from degeneration of the neuronal cytoskeleton. The major components of the neuronal cytoskeleton are alpha and beta tubulin, the microtubule-associated proteins (MAP), the neurofilament or neuronal intermediate filament proteins and actin which forms the microfilaments (for review see Henderson and Finch, 1989). Alpha and beta tubulin are 54 and 56 kD monomers respectively that polymerize into 24 nm microtubules. Two subgroups of MAP proteins have been identified: the high relative mass, phosphorylated MAP-1 and MAP-2 (300 kD and 270 kD respectively) and the low molecular weight, non-phosphorylated tau protein with a relative mass of 55 kD. The tubulins and MAP proteins are involved in fast axonal transport. Antibodies against these proteins have shown that tau is normally present only in axons, MAP-1 in axons and dendrites and MAP-2 in both cell bodies and dendrites. Neurofilaments, which are responsible for the slow component of axonal transport, have been shown to consist of three subunits with relative masses of 200 kD, 160 kD and 70 kD respectively (Hoffman and Lasek, 1975). These have been designated NFH, NFM and NFL. All three exist in both phosphorylated and non-phosphorylated states. Non-phosphorylated forms are found only in cell bodies and become phosphorylated on entering the axon (Sternberger and Sternberger, 1983). Neuronal microfilaments are composed of actin subunits.

Ultrastructural studies have shown that neurofibrillary tangles are composed of a helical arrangement of paired filaments, hence the designation 'paired helical filaments' (PHF). The individual filaments have a thickness of 10 nm and the half-periodicity of the helix is 80–100 nm. Immunoblot and immunohistochemical studies have shown that the major component of paired helical filaments is an abnormally phosphorylated form of the tau protein (Iqbal et al., 1984; Ihara et al., 1986). A variety of antibodies against phosphorylated neurofilament proteins have been shown to cross-react with phosphorylated epitopes on tau (Perry et al., 1985; Cork et al., 1986). Antibodies against ubiquitin, one of the family of stress or acute phase reactive proteins have also been shown to be immunoreactive with PHF's (Mori et al., 1987; Perry et al., 1987). In the diagnostic setting, neurofibrillary tangles can be demonstrated by Bielchowsky or Bodian silver impregnation (Fig. 7.8A) and immunohistochemically with antibodies against phosphorylated tau epitopes (Fig. 7.8B) and ubiquitin (Fig. 7.8C). Reactivity of neurofibrillary tangles with antibodies against a 68 kD antigen termed 'Alz-50' has been reported (Wolozin and Davies, 1986). Alz-50 immunoreactivity is also seen in dystrophic neurites forming the corona of neuritic plaques and in subsets of neurones that do not contain neurofibrillary tangles. There is a marked increase in the Alz-50 content of Alzheimer's brains compared with age-matched controls. However, the frequently observed cross-reactivity of antigens with both anti-tau and anti-Alz-50 antibodies has heightened speculation that Alz-50 is an isoform of tau.

Hirano bodies and the granules that are characteristic of granulo-vacuolar degeneration are immunoreactive with antibodies against actin, alpha-actinin, tau and tropomysin but their identification by immunohistochemical means is academic since their presence is not essential for the pathological diagnosis of Alzheimer's disease.

Pick's lobar atrophy

Pick's disease is a rare cause of dementia in which frontal signs accompany the more usual cognitive deficits. In some patients, the features of frontal lobe dysfunction may be dominant. The characteristic macroscopic abnormality is the presence of very sharply circumscribed areas of atrophy of one or more lobes with the border between normal and atrophic brain sometimes being in the long

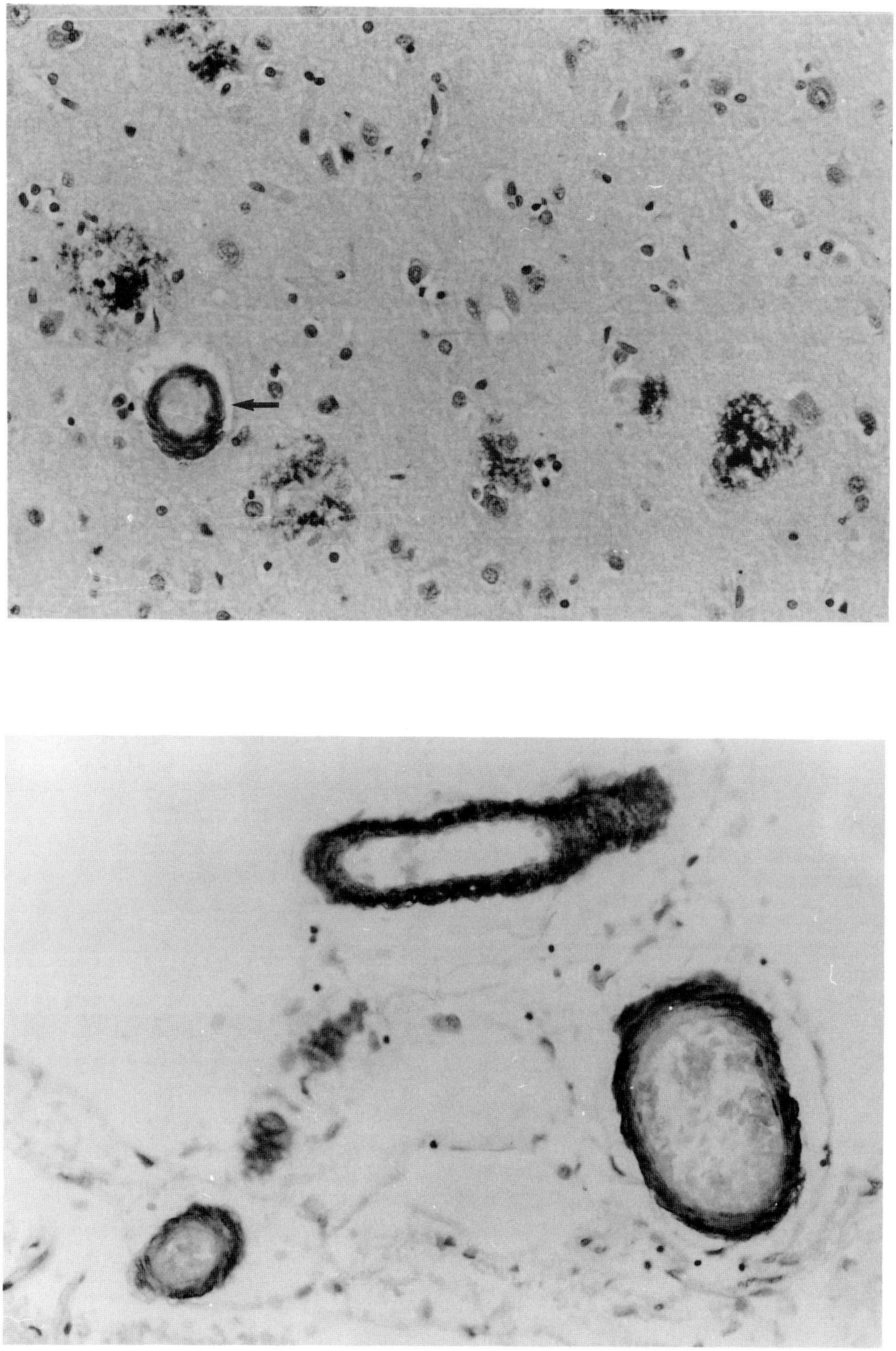

A

B

Fig. 7.7. Alzheimer's disease: Vascular beta-A4 immunoreactivity (A) in wall of a small cortical arteriole (arrow) (×200), and (B) in the walls of leptomeningeal arteries and arterioles (×400).

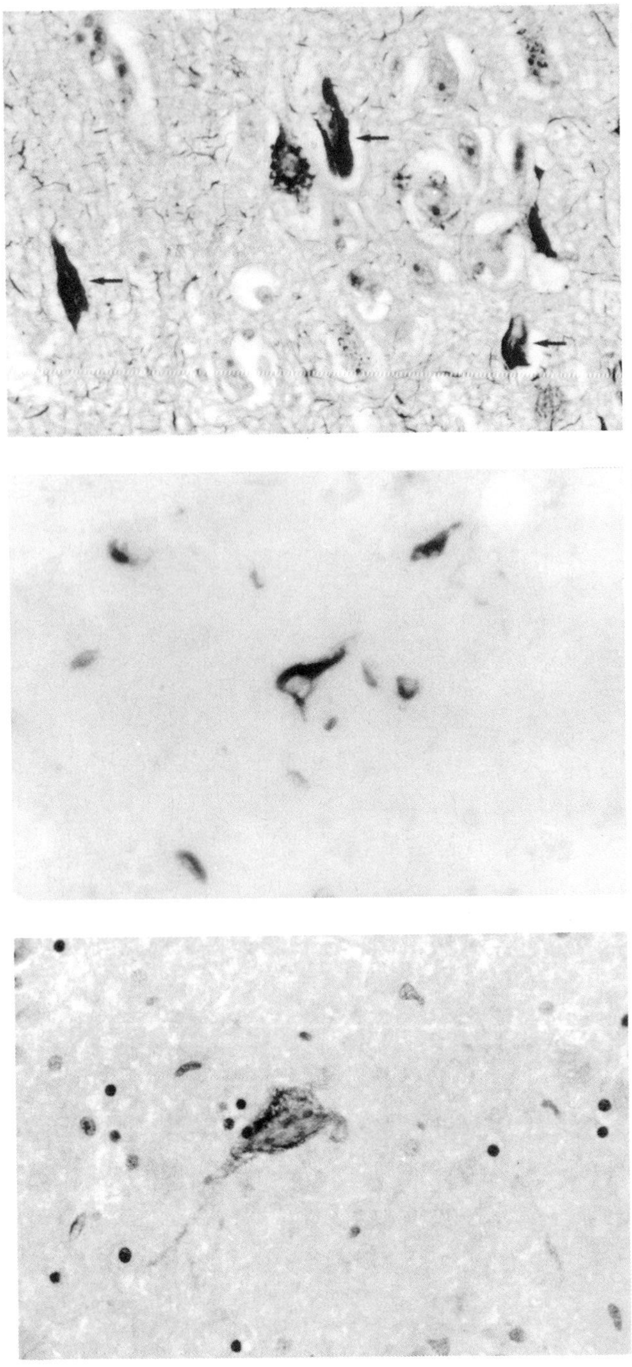

Fig. 7.8. Alzheimer's disease: neurofibrillary tangles (arrows) in cortical neurones. (A) Bielchowsky silver impregnation (×400), (B) Tau immunoreactivity (×400). (C). Ubiquitin immunoreactivity (×400).

axis of one gyrus. Involvement of one or both frontal lobes and atrophy of the superior temporal gyrus are almost universal. Microscopic examination reveals silver-positive inclusions in cortical neurons. These are usually immunoreactive with antibodies against ubiquitin (Fig. 7.9; Lowe et al., 1988) and phosphorylated neurofilament protein, in particular NFH.

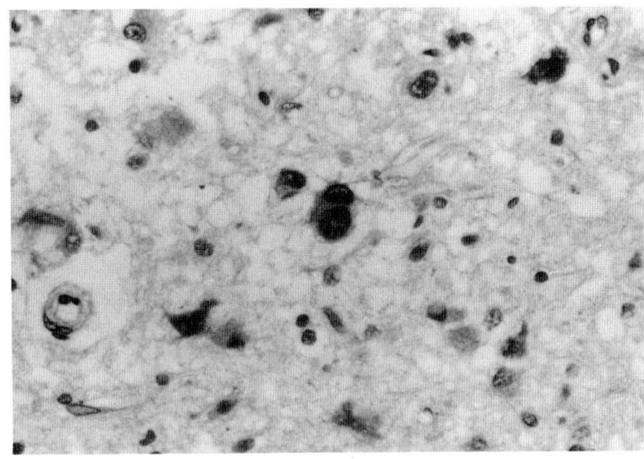

Fig. 7.9. Pick's disease: ubiquitin-reactive inclusion body (Pick body) in cortical neurones (ubiquitin/PAP; x400).

Diffuse Lewy body disease

A rare form of dementia, sometimes with a much earlier onset than the commoner dementias has recently been recognized. This disorder, in which classical Lewy bodies and Lewy-like bodies are present diffusely in cortical and subcortical neurons has been called cortical or diffuse Lewy body disease (Gibbs et al., 1989). Clinically, affected patients exhibit Parkinsonism in addition to their cognitive disorder and on neuropathological examination, classical Lewy bodies are usually present in pigmented neurones of the substantia nigra. These and the Lewy-like bodies in cortical and other neurones represent abnormal accumulations of neuronal cytoskeletal proteins. They can be demonstrated by conventional silver impregnation techniques and are immunoreactive with antibodies against ubiquitin and neurofilament protein (NFH and NFM) (Fig. 7.10).

The prion diseases

The isolation of a sialoglycoprotein from the brains of animals with scrapie and humans with Creutzfeld–Jakob disease (CJD) and the subsequent demonstration in animal experiments that it could transmit these diseases has provided a novel insight into the

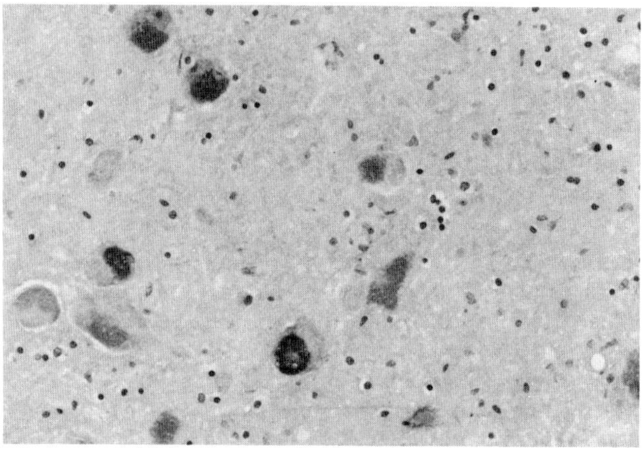

Fig. 7.10. Diffuse Lewy body disease: ubiquitin-reactive inclusion bodies in cortical neurones (ubiquitin/PAP; x200).

pathogenesis of some neurodegenerative diseases (for reviews see Prusiner, 1987; Prusiner and DeArmond, 1987). This sialoglycoprotein has been termed the 'prion' protein (proteinaceous infectious particle – PrP). Besides scrapie in sheep and CJD in humans, the prion protein also causes the Gerstmann–Straussler–Sheinker Syndrome and Kuru in humans and bovine spongiform encephalopathy (BSE), transmissible mink encephalopathy and chronic wasting disease of mule, deer and elk.

Three PrP isoforms have been identified. The brains of normal individuals contain a 33–35 kD isoform (PrP^{C}) that can be completely digested by proteinase K. The function of PrP^{C} is not known but amino-acid sequencing has revealed a cell surface receptor-like structure. A second isoform, also with a relative mass of 33–35 kD and termed PrP^{Sc}, has been isolated from the brains of hamsters infected with a scrapie isolate and from CJD brains. This isoform is incompletely digested by proteinase K to a smaller, third isoform with a relative mass of 27–30 kD, designated PrP^{27-30}. In animal experiments designed to investigate transmissibility, both PrP^{Sc} and PrP^{27-30} have been found to be inseparable from infectivity. Only brain homogenates containing these isoforms transmit the disease while homogenates from which they have been removed are incapable of transmission. Antibodies raised against PrP^{27-30} have also demonstrated that this isoform assimilates into amyloid rods in the extracellular space and vessel walls (DeArmond et al., 1985). These extracellular accumulations appear as plaques in the Gerstmann-Straussler-Scheinker Syndrome (Fig. 7.11) and to a lesser degree in CJD in humans and experimental scrapie in hamsters. Plaques with PrP immuno-reactivity are seen in up to 20 per cent of cases of CJD but immuno--reactivity in vessel walls (Fig. 7.12) is more common. Both sporadic and familial forms of CJD are recognized and in the majority of these, single point mutations in the PrP gene have been identified (for review see Brown et al., 1991). Alterations in the secondary and tertiary structure of PrP brought about by these mutations contribute to the adoption of a β-pleated configuration and subsequent amyloid deposition.

Open or stereotactic brain biopsies are occasionally performed on patients with rapidly progressive dementia

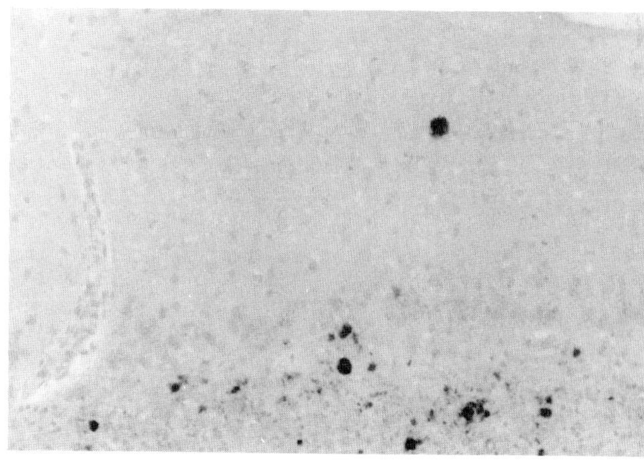

Fig. 7.11. Gerstmann-Straussler-Sheinker Syndrome: plaques in cerebellar cortex showing reactivity with an antibody against the 27–30 kDa isoform of the prion protein (PrP/PAP; ×200).

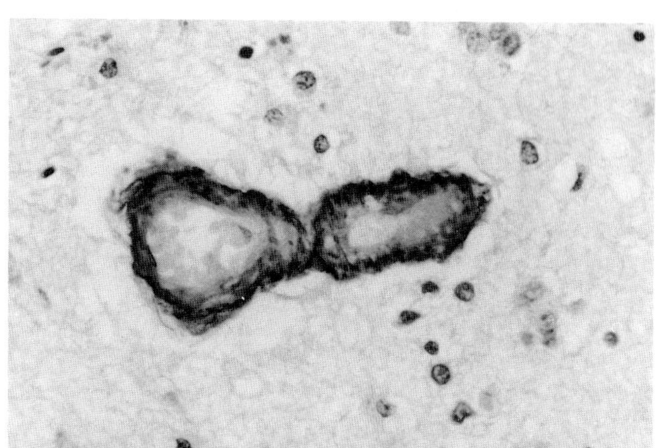

Fig. 7.12. Creutzfeld–Jakob disease: PrP reactivity in the walls of cerebral cortical arterioles (PrP/PAP; x400).

and myoclonus in the hope of confirming CJD. The classical histopathological features are diffuse spongiform degeneration with loss of cortical neurons and exuberant astrocytic gliosis. Immunoreactivity for PrP may be demonstrated in the walls of vessels.

Idiopathic Parkinson's disease and Parkinsonian syndromes

As in Alzheimer's disease, degeneration of the neuronal cytoskeleton is fundamental to the pathogenesis of idiopathic Parkinson's disease and a variety of Parkinsonian syndromes. These latter syndromes include diffuse Lewy body disease, progressive supranuclear palsy (Steele–Richardson–Olzewski syndrome), post-infectious Parkinsonism (encephalitis lethargica), Shy–Drager syndrome, striato-nigral degeneration and the Parkinson's/dementia/amyotrophic lateral sclerosis (ALS) complex described in Guam, the Philippines and parts of Japan. The classical Lewy bodies of idiopathic Parkinson's disease, seen particularly in pigmented neurons of the substantia nigra and locus caeruleus have been identified as accumulations of ubiquinated neurofilament proteins (Pappolla, 1986; Lowe et al., 1988; Bancher et al., 1989). Although easily seen in sections stained with haematoxylin and eosin, they are strikingly immunoreactive with ubiquitin and neurofilament protein antibodies (Fig. 7.13). Similarly, ubiquitin antibodies highlight the neurofibrillary tangles in neurones of the substantia nigra and brainstem nuclei in progressive supranuclear palsy, Shy–Drager syndrome, post-infectious Parkinsonism and the Parkinson's/dementia/ALS complex. The neurofibrillary tangles in these conditions are composed of straight filaments, not paired helical filaments as in Alzheimer's disease. They are, nevertheless, immunoreactive with Alz-50 antibodies (Tabaton et al., 1988) as are tangles composed of paired helical filaments.

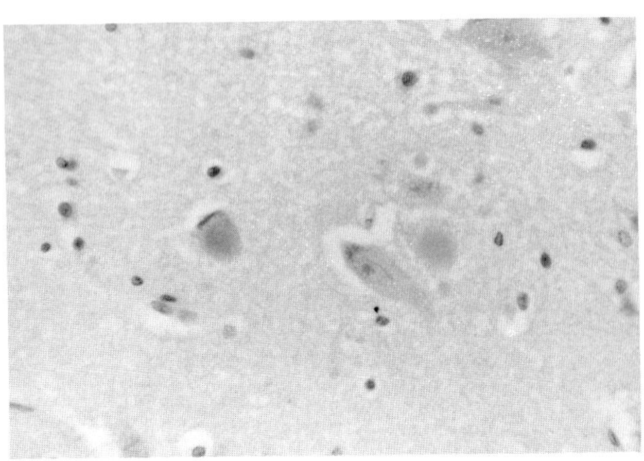

Fig. 7.13. Idiopathic Parkinson's disease: ubiquitin-reactive Lewy bodies in neurones of the substantia nigra (ubiquitin/PAP; x400).

Approximately 15 per cent of brains with the classical pathology of idiopathic Parkinson's disease also have sufficient neuritic plaques, demonstrated by Bielchowsky silver impregnation and β-A4 immunostaining for a pathological diagnosis of Alzheimer's disease.

Huntington's disease

The major role of immunohistochemistry in the neuropathological assessment of Huntington's disease is to assist in grading severity and identifying subsets of neurones that are depleted. Five pathological grades of severity (O-IV) are presently recognized (Vonsattel et al., 1985); the assessment includes both macroscopic and microscopic features. Particular subpopulations of neurones appear to be lost from the corpus striatum at different stages in the evolution of the disease. In the early choreic phase, neurones containing gamma-amino-butyric acid (GABA) and met-enkephalin are depleted from the globus pallidus externa, while GABA-ergic/substance-P neurones of the globus pallidus interna are preserved. Later, in the phase of the illness characterized clinically by rigidity and braddykinesia, GABA-ergic/ substance P neurones of the globus pallidus interna are also depleted. Alterations in the relative density these different subsets of neurones can be demonstrated immunohistochemically with antibodies against a variety of neuropeptides, in particular, substance P, met-enkephalin, neuropeptide Y, somatastatin, calcineurin and NADPH-diaphorase (Grafe et al., 1985; Kowall et al., 1987; Goto et al., 1989). Neuronal loss is accompanied by reactive proliferation of astrocytes which can be highlighted with antibodies against glial fibrillary acidic protein (GFAP).

Motor neurone disease/amyotrophic lateral sclerosis (ALS)

This disorder, which is manifest clinically by progressive weakness and spasticity of limb muscles is another neurodegenerative disease resulting from alterations in neuronal cytoskeleton. Pathological examination of the brain and spinal cord reveals loss of neurones from the lower cranial nerve nuclei, particularly the XIIth. nucleus and from anterior horn grey matter of the cervical and lumbosacral segments. Surviving neurones frequently contain irregular inclusions in the perikaryon and axonal swellings, termed spheroids, are present in white matter tracts, often concentrated in the anterolateral funiculi of the spinal cord. The perikaryonal inclusions have variable morphology but have been shown by immunohistochemistry to be composed of ubiquinited neurofilament proteins (Fig. 7.14; Martin et al., 1990). Both phosphorylated and non-phosphorylated forms of neurofilament proteins have been identified (Manetto et al., 1988; Leigh et al., 1989).

Axonal spheroids appear to be aggregations of predominantly non-phosphorylated neurofilament proteins (Toyoshima et al., 1989). In the Guamanian form of motor neurone disease, granulo-vacuolar degeneration of motor neurons may also be a prominent feature (Hirano et al., 1968).

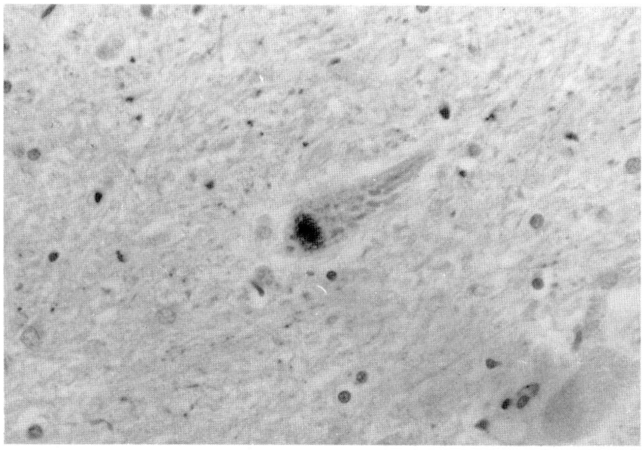

Fig. 7.14. Motor neurone disease: inclusion in cell body of a cervical anterior horn neurone showing reactivity with an antibody against ubiquitin (ubiquitin/PAP; x400).

Multisystem atrophy

A number of neurodegenerative disorders, known collectively as multisystem atrophy result from retrograde or dying-back axonal degeneration and dropout of specific groups of neurones. The predominant clinical feature is ataxia and both sporadic and familial forms occur. Neuronal loss from areas such as the cerebellar cortex and tract degeneration can usually be demonstrated by silver impregnation and myelin staining. Immunohistochemical techniques are rarely called upon in the diagnostic setting. However, as in Huntington's disease, immunohistochemistry has helped identify subsets of neurons that undergo degeneration, for example, loss of substance P-containing neurones from the dorsal horns in Friedreich's ataxia.

Table 7.2 summarizes the morphological features of the neurodegenerative diseases that can be detected and enhanced by immunohistochemistry.

Tumours of the central nervous system

Immunohistochemistry is indispensable in the diagnosis of central nervous system neoplasms. It is now possible to determine the cell lineage of most tumours by immunohistochemical techniques and the range of lineage-specific antibodies is continually expanding. These techniques can also detect over-expression of oncogenes and assist in the measurement of proliferative indices, phenomena which appear to be predictive of biological behaviour.

Neuroepithelial tumours

Gliomas

Gliomas are tumours of the non-neuronal supporting cells of the brain and spinal cord. They may be of astrocytic, oligodendroglial or ependymal lineage and mixed forms are also encountered. The most common is the astrocytoma, of which three histological grades are recognized: well-differentiated, anaplastic and glioblastoma multiforme (Ringertz, 1950). In well-differentiated tumours, the astrocytic lineage is usually apparent from cell morphology, particularly in smears prepared from fresh biopsy tissue. In these, the characteristic fibrillary processes of tumour cells and their tendency to aggregate around the walls of blood vessels can be more easily appreciated than in histological sections. Immunohistochemistry can also be applied to smear preparations (Fig. 7.15). Determination of astrocytic lineage in anaplastic astrocytomas and glioblastomas multiforme can present considerable difficulty and in this situation, immunohistochemistry is invaluable.

Table 7.2: Immunohistochemical reactions in neurodegenerative disease

Disorder	Antibody	Feature highlighted
Alzheimer's disease	beta-A4	Early/diffuse plaques
		Amyloid plaque cores
		Vascular amyloid
	tau	NFTs
	Ubiquitin	NFTs
	Alz-50	NFTs; dystrophic neurites
Pick's disease	Ubiquitin	Intra-neuronal inclusions
Prion diseases	PrP	Occasional plaque in CJD
		Plaques in GSS
		Vascular amyloid
	GFAP	Cortical gliosis
Parkinson's disease	Ubiquitin	Classical Lewy bodies
Cortical/diffuse Lewy body disease	Ubiquitin	Classical Lewy bodies Intra-neuronal inclusions
Huntington's disease	Substance P Met-enkephalin Neuropeptide Y Somatastatin Calcineurin	Loss of subsets of neurons from corpus striatum
Amyotrophic lateral sclerosis	Ubiquitin	Intra-neuronal inclusions anterior horn neurons

Notes: NFT = neurofibrillary tangle
CJD = Creutzfeldt–Jakob Disease
GS = Gerstmann–Straussler–Sheinker Syndrome

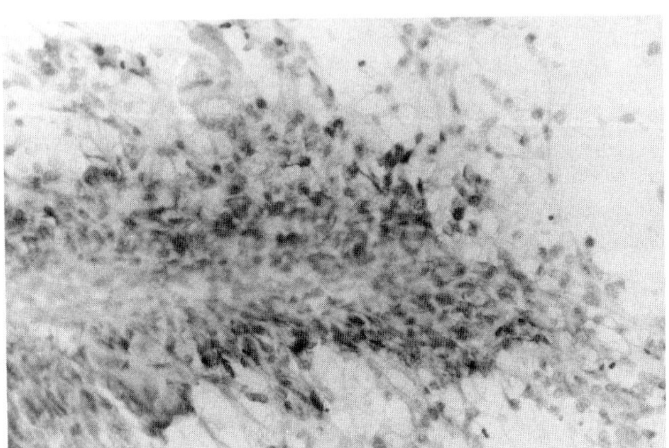

Fig. 7.15. Smear of an anaplastic astrocytoma prepared from fresh biopsy material and reacted with an anti-GFAP antibody by PAP immunohistochemistry. Aggregation of tumour cells around blood vessels (gliovascular structuring) is characteristic in these preparations. Fibrillary cytoplasmic processes of tumour cells are highlighted by GFAP immunoreactivity (×200).

Antibodies against components of astrocytic intermediate filaments are commonly applied to this task. The first of these components to be isolated and characterized was glial fibrillary acidic protein (GFAP; Bignami and Dahl, 1975). Vimentin was later identified as another intermediate filament protein in astrocytes, developing neurons and cells of mesenchymal lineage (Gabbianni et al., 1981; Osborn et al., Bignami et al., 1982). The profile of GFAP and vimentin immuno-reactivity in astrocytomas varies with the degree of differentiation. Well-differentiated astrocytomas are usually strongly immunoreactive for GFAP (Fig. 7.16) and weakly immmunoreactive for vimentin. In glioblastoma multiforme, this pattern is frequently reversed (Fig. 7.17) and the pattern is intermediate in anaplastic astrocytomas. The lack of GFAP expression in high grade astrocytomas is explained by the frequent loss of all or part of chromosome 17 (Fults et al., 1990), the locus of the human GFAP gene (Bongcam-Rudloff et al., 1991). Stem cells of the developing nervous system have recently been shown to express a novel intermediate filament protein which has been called nestin (Lendahl et al., 1990). Immunoreactivity for nestin has been described in a variety of gliomas (Toyohama et

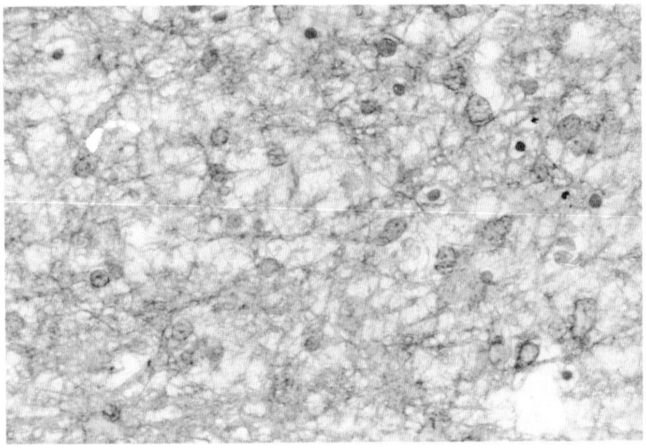

Fig. 7.16. Well-differentiated astrocytoma: section of formalin-fixed, paraffin-embedded tissue showing fibrillary cytoplasmic processes reactive with an anti-GFAP antibody (GFAP/PAP; x400).

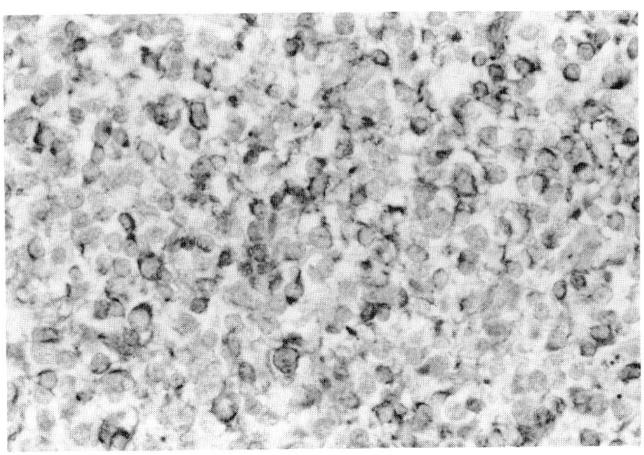

Fig. 7.17. Glioblastoma multiforme showing reactivity of tumour cells with an anti-vimentin antibody (vimentin/PAP; ×400)

al., 1991) and its usefulness appears to be in detecting glial lineage rather than in separating glioma subtypes.

High grade astrocytomas may contain a spindle-cell component derived either from the adventitia of tumour vessels or from the leptomeninges where these are invaded. This component may become sarcomatous (gliosarcoma). The spindle cells are GFAP negative but often show immunoreactivity for vimentin and fibronectin and, occasionally for desmin. Astrocytomas show variable, non-specific immunoreactivity for high molecular weight cytokeratins (AE1/AE3), the protease inhibitors alpha-1-anti-trypsin and alpha-1-anti-chymotrypsin (Zuccarello et al., 1987), S100 protein (Haglid et al., 1973), gamma-enolase or neurone-specific enolase (Haglid et al., 1973; Schmechel et al., 1978) and Leu7 and Leu19, both markers of natural killer T-lymphocytes (Motoi et al., 1985; Nawrotzki et al., 1990).

Similar patterns of immunoreactivity for the majority of antibodies are also seen in reactive astrocytes and, despite intensive research, a tumour-specific antigen has yet to be isolated. Although GFAP is a useful marker of glial tumours, immunoreactivity has also been demonstrated in a variety of non-glial CNS tumours. These include pineocytomas (Herrick and Rubinstein, 1979), choroid plexus papillomas (Rubinstein and Brucher, 1981), some pituitary adenomas and cerebellar haemangioblastomas (Kepes et al., 1979). The GFAP-positive cells in pineocytomas and pituitary adenomas are regarded as stromal cells of astrocytic lineage that are incorporated in the tumour and not neoplastic.

Because of their particular histological appearances, some astrocytomas are categorized separately from their well-differentiated, anaplastic and glioblastoma multiforme counterparts. These include juvenile pilocytic astrocytoma, pleomorphic xanthoastrocytoma and subependymal giant cell astrocytoma which occurs almost exclusively in association with tuberous sclerosis. Immunoreactivity for GFAP is intense in juvenile pilocytic astrocytoma but highly variable in subependymal giant cell astrocytoma and pleomorphic xanthoastrocytoma (Rubinstein, 1982). Subependymal giant cell astrocytoma may also show focal neurofilament immuno-reactivity. By convention, none of these subtypes is graded histologically and all have a favourable prognosis.

Oligodendrogliomas have proven difficult to characterize by immunohistochemical techniques. The likely explanation is that oligodendroglial markers, such as carbonic anhydrase isoenzyme II, β-galactocerebrosidase and myelin-associated glycoprotein are expressed during myelin assembly and in definitive myelin sheath formation. This process does not occur in oligodendrogliomas and so these markers are rarely detected by immunohistochemistry (Nakagawa et al., 1986). There have been several studies showing immuno-reactivity of oligodendrogliomas for Leu7 and Leu19 (Motoi et al., 1985; Nakagawa et al., 1986 and Nawrotzki et al., 1990). The majority of oligodendrogliomas are Leu7 and Leu19 immunoreactive but reactivity is also seen in astrocytomas medulloblastomas and some meningiomas. Most oligodendrogliomas are low grade at first presentation (Ludwig et al., 1986). In higher grade oligodendrogliomas an astrocytic component is often present, accounting for the GFAP immunoreactivity (Fig. 7.18) that has been reported in oligodendrogliomas. These are correctly designated as mixed tumours and further progression of the astrocytic component to anaplastic astrocytoma and glioblastoma multiforme is a common occurrence.

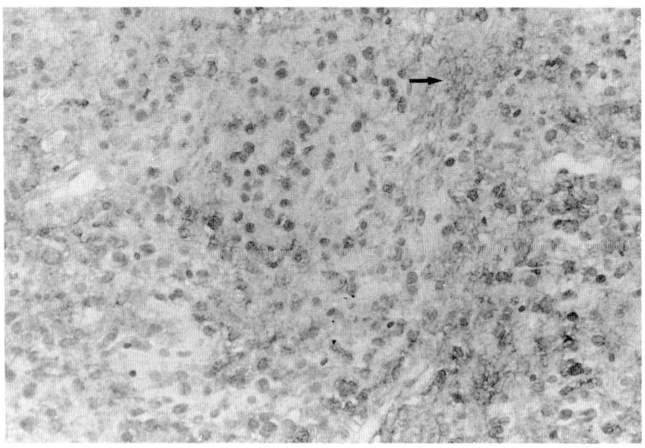

Fig. 7.18. Mixed oligodendroglioma/astrocytoma: focal GFAP immunoreactivity of astrocytic cell processes is seen (arrow). The majority of cells, which are of oligodendroglial lineage are non-reactive GFAP/PAP; x200).

Ependymomas are similar to astrocytomas in their expression of intermediate filament components (Rubinstein, 1982). Cells comprising the perivascular pseudo-rosettes and occasional ependymal canals and rosettes of well-differentiated ependymomas show variable but usually detectable GFAP immunoreactivity. In the less well-differentiated cellular ependymoma, GFAP immunoreactivity is unusual, but reactivity for vimentin is often present. Like astrocytomas and oligodendrogliomas, ependymomas may also cross react with Leu7 antibodies (Motoi et al., 1985). Two variants of ependymoma are recognized: subependymoma, a pedunculated intraventricular tumour which may be an incidental CT, MRI, operative or autopsy finding and myxo-papillary ependymoma of the filum terminal. Both are immunoreactive for GFAP (Rubinstein, 1982).

The immuno-reactivity patterns of glial tumours are summarized in Table 7.3.

Table 7.3: Immunohistochemical reactions of gliomas

	GFAP	Vimentin	CK	CAII	AAT/AACT	S100	NSE	Leu7	Leu19	Nestin
Astrocytoma										
WD	+++	+/−	++	+	+/++	++	+	+	+++	+
Anaplastic	++	++	+	+	+/−	++	+	+	+++	+
GM	+	+++	+	+/−	+/−	++	+	+	+++	+
JPA	+++	+/−	+	+/−	+/−	++	+	+	+++	+
PXA	+/−	+/−	+/−	−	−	+	+	+/−	++	+
SEGCA	+/−	+/−	+/−	−	−	+	+	+/−	+/−	+
Oligo-dendroglioma	−	−	−	−	−	+	−	+	+	+
Mixed O/A	+	+	+	+	+	+	+	+	+	+
Ependymoma	++	++	+	−	+	+	+/−	−	−	+
Subependymoma	+/−	+/−	+/−	−	+/−	+	+/−	−	−	+
Myxo-papillary ependymoma	+	+	+	−	+/−	+	+/−	−	−	+

Notes:
WD = well-differentiated
GM = glioblastoma multiforme
JPA = juvenile pilocytic astrocytoma
PXA = pleomorphic xanthoastrocytoma
SEGCA = subependymal giant cell astrocytoma
O/A = oligo-astrocytoma
GFAP = glial fibrillary acidic protein
CK = cytokeratin
CA II = carbonic anhydrase isoenzyme II
AAT/AACT = alpha-1-antitrypsin/anti-chymotrypsin
NSE = neurone-specific enolase

Tumours of neurones and neurone precursor cells

This category includes neurocytoma, cerebral neuroblastoma, medulloblastoma, medulloepithelioma and ganglioglioma.

Neurocytoma

Central neurocytoma usually presents as an intraventricular tumour whose histopathological appearance can be confused with oligodendroglioma (Nishio et al., 1988). Immunohistochemistry has demonstrated a range of neuronal markers, in particular, synaptophysin which reacts with a component of synaptic membranes (Fig. 7.19; Gould et al., 1987; von Deimling et al., 1990). Electron microscopy has confirmed the neuronal lineage of this neoplasm by demonstrating synaptic vesicles and membrane-bound granules (Nishio et al., 1988). Occasional incorporated, reactive astrocytes are detected with GFAP antibodies and most neurocytomas show non-specific immunoreactivity for neurone-specific enolase and Leu7 (Kubota et al., 1991). The distinction from oligodendroglioma is important because of the benign nature of neurocytoma.

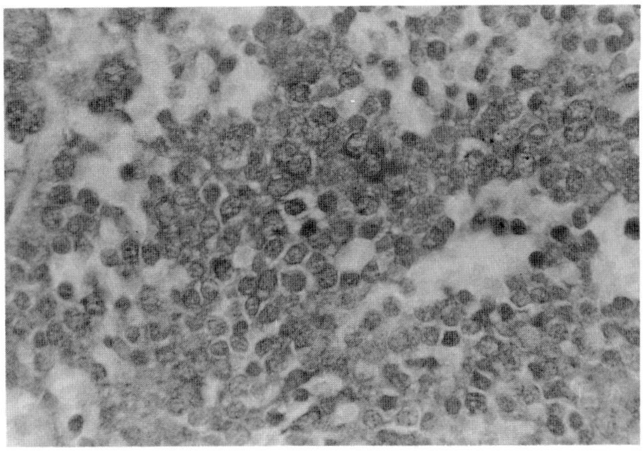

Fig. 7.19. Central neurocytoma: reactivity of tumour cells with an antibody against synaptophysin (synaptophysin/PAP; x400).

Cerebral neuroblastoma

Although exceedingly rare, cerebral neuroblastoma has to be considered in the differential diagnosis of cerebral tumours composed of small round lymphocyte-like cells (Horten and Rubinstein, 1976). The histopathological diagnosis has traditionally relied on demonstrating neuritic processes by silver impregnation and neurosecretory granules, neurotubules and synapse-like structures by electron microscopy. Some neuroblastomas have a desmoplastic stroma while others display ganglionic differentiation. Variable synaptophysin immunoreactivity is often present in some but not all cells and neuritic processes, if present, can be highlighted by antibodies against phosphorylated neurofilament protein epitopes. Antibodies against non-phosphorylated neurofilaments will identify ganglion cells. Immunoreactivity for the gamma subunit of neurone-specific enolase and S100 protein is usual but non-specific. Expression of the N-myc oncogene can be assessed by immunogold-silver histochemistry and semi-quantified by grain counting. The degree of N-myc amplification has been shown to be predictive of behaviour in peripheral neuroblastomas (Seeger et al., 1985). However, no data relating N-myc amplification to biological behaviour are available for cerebral neuroblastoma.

Medulloblastoma and medulloepithelioma

The histopathological recognition of medulloblastoma usually presents little difficulty and the role of immunohistochemistry in the neuropathological assessment of this tumour has been to detect evidence of neuronal or glial lineage in subsets of tumour cells. The presence of cells of astrocytic lineage showing GFAP immunoreactivity has been associated with a more favourable prognosis in one study (Goldberg-Stern et al., 1991). Approximately 30 per cent of medulloblastomas show regional GFAP immunoreactivity in tumour cells, and between 80 and 90 per cent show immunoreactivity for neuronal markers (Cruz-Sanchez et al., 1989). Evidence of photoreceptor cell lineage has been reported in a small number of medulloblastomas (Kramm et al., 1991). Immunoreactivity for vimentin and S100 protein is present in a minority of medulloblastomas (Cruz-Sanchez et al., 1989). The desmoplastic type of medulloblastoma is less-frequently immunoreactive for GFAP, vimentin and neuronal markers (Cruz-Sanchez et al., 1989).

Medulloepithelioma is an exceedingly rare tumour arising from primitive cells of the medullary plate and neural tube (Rubinstein, 1972). One immunohistochemical study of this tumour has reported immunoreactivity for GFAP, vimentin, class II β-tubulin, MAP-2 and neurone-specific enolase (Caccamo et al., 1989).

Ganglioglioma

There has been much controversy regarding the histopathological features that constitute a ganglioglioma and whether true gangliogliomas should be classified as a neoplasm or a hamartoma (Rorke et al., 1985). The major difficulty is determining if ganglion cells or neurones are an integral component of the tumour. The ganglion cells may sometimes be confused with gemistocytic astrocytes in haematoxylin and eosin-stained sections. However, they usually react strongly with antibodies against non-phosphorylated neurofilament proteins (Fig. 7.20) and are GFAP negative. The glial component is usually astrocytic and GFAP reactive. There is increasing evidence that where the astrocytic component can be graded as anaplastic, the subsequent biological behaviour is according to that component. At the opposite end of the spectrum where a well-differentiated ganglion cell component is dominant, the behaviour of the tumour, almost without exception, will be benign.

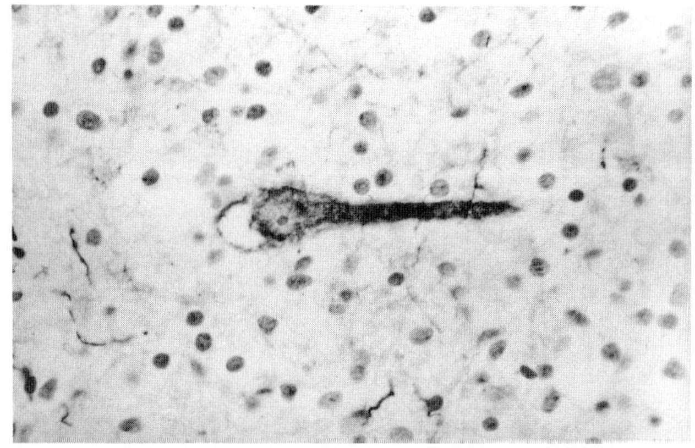

Fig. 7.20. Ganglioglioma: cell of neuronal lineage shows reactivity with an antibody against the 200 kDa neurofilament protein (NFP/PAP; x400).

Primitive neuroectodermal tumour (PNET)

The true status of primitive neuroectodermal tumour (PNET) and what tumours should be designated as such has been another long-standing controversy in neuro-oncology (Rubinstein, 1985). The term PNET is applied to tumours composed of cells with morphology resembling that of germinal matrix (Rorke et al., 1985). The majority of these occur before the end of the first decade and display aggressive biological behaviour. Much of the controversy has centred on whether tumours such as medulloblastoma, ependymoblastoma, pineoblastoma, retinoblastoma and the small cell variant of glioblastoma multiforme should be designated as PNETs and if the term PNET can still be applied if neuronal or glial differentiation is demonstrated immunohistochemically. Demonstration of such differentiation has been the major application of immunohistochemistry in the neuropathological work-up of PNETs. The majority of PNETs are immunoreactive for synaptophysin, neurofilament protein, vimentin, GFAP and a variety of neuropeptides: bombesin, somatostatin, substance P and vasoactive intestinal polypeptide (Gould et al., 1990). This antigenic heterogeneity probably reflects a propensity for differentiation along several lines and illustrates the difficulty of classifying these tumours.

Dysembryoplastic neuroepithelial tumour (DENET)

The designation 'dysembryoplastic neuroepithelial tumour' (DENET), has recently been proposed for a complex tumour composed of astrocytes, oligodendrocytes, neurones and cells of uncertain lineage. The mean age at presentation in the series of 39 patients reported by Daumas-Duport et al. in 1988 was 9 years. The majority of patients had a history of intractable complex partial seizures. All DENET's thus far reported have been confined to the cerebral cortex, some with an exophytic component projecting from the brain surface. The temporal lobe has been the most common anatomical location. Unlike PNET, the astrocytic, oligodendroglial and neuronal components of DENET are readily apparent in haematoxylin and eosin (H & E)-stained sections. Immunoreactivity for GFAP and neurofilament protein is present in the cells of astrocytic and neuronal lineage respectively. Some atypical and bi-nucleate neurones are often present. Immunostaining for neurofilament protein also highlights the dysplasia that is characteristically seen in the adjacent cerebral cortex. The biological behaviour of DENET has been uniformly benign.

Tumours of mesenchymal origin

Meningioma

Meningiomas exhibit such a wide range of histological appearances that confusion with a variety of non-meningeal tumours in H & E-stained sections is likely (Scheithauer, 1990). In addition to this range of histological appearances, they have a spectrum of biological behaviour that is difficult to predict on the basis of histopathological features (Scheithauer, 1990). Irrespective of histological subtype, meningiomas express a combination of epithelial and mesenchymal markers (Table 7.4). Difficulty is often encountered in clearly differentiating a meningioma without classical histopathological features that is vimentin-positive but epithelial membrane antigen epithelial membrane antigen (EMA) -negative from a high grade astrocytoma, infiltrating leptomeninges that is also vimentin-positive but GFAP-negative. Both tumours may be immunoreactive for S100 protein and cytokeratin. Similar difficulties can arise in determining the lineage of a cerebello-pontine angle tumour in which the features of meningioma and neurilemmoma ('Schwannoma') may be inseparable in an H & E-stained section. Both will be immunoreactive for vimentin and S100 protein and may be negative for other markers such as EMA and cytokeratin. In both situations, electron microscopy offers a means of determining cell lineage. Complex interdigitating cytoplasmic processes and desmosomes are characteristic of meningiomas. A thin but often incomplete layer of basal lamina-like material may also be seen separating adjacent cell membranes. Neurilemmomas show less complex interdigitation of cytoplasmic processes than meningiomas, a well-formed basal lamina and prominent long-space collagen; desmosomes are not seen.

Mesenchymal, non-meningothelial tumours

A variety of non-meningothelial tumours of mesenchymal lineage involve the leptomeninges (Jellinger and Paulus, 1991). The most frequently encountered is the meningeal haemangiopericytoma, formerly classified as a subtype of angioblastic meningioma. Usually, the histopathological features of slit-like and 'stag-horn' vascular spaces, the dense cellularity and a characteristic reticulin pattern suggest the diagnosis. Meningeal haemangiopericytomas are usually diffusely immunoreactive for vimentin but show only focal reactivity for EMA and S100 protein. In contrast, conventional meningiomas usually show diffuse immunoreactivity for both vimentin and EMA. Immunoreactivity for desmin, muscle actin, alpha-actinin, laminin and type IV collagen may occasionally be seen in meningeal haemangiopericytoma. Other non-meningothelial mesenchymal tumours include, malignant fibrous histiocytoma, fibrosarcoma, liposarcoma, leiomyosarcoma, rhabdomyosarcoma and chondrosarcoma. All are extremely rare. Each of these tumours usually shows immunoreactivity for vimentin and occasionally for S100 protein, desmin and EMA (Jellinger and Paulus, 1991).

Haemangioblastoma

The cell lineage of capillary haemangioblastoma of the cerebellum has still to be determined. This tumour has two components. Capillary spaces lined by endothelial cells which are immunoreactive for Factor VIII make up one component. The second consists of the stromal cells which separate individual capillaries. The immunohistochemical profile of stromal cells, in particular, reactivity for neurone-specific enolase, synaptophysin, substance P and neuropeptide YY (Becker et al., 1989), suggests a neuroendocrine lineage. Focal reactivity for GFAP, vimentin, neurofilament protein, cytokeratin and erythropoietin has also been reported (Kepes et al., 1979; Böhlig et al., 1987). Capillary haemangioblastomas may rarely involve the supratentorial leptomeninges (Ishwar et al., 1971). In this anatomical location they were formerly classified as

Table 7.4: Immunohistochemical reactions of meningioma and tumours included in the differential diagnosis

Antibody	Meningioma	Arachnoid cells	Glioma	Chordoma	Carcinoma	Neurilemmoma
EMA	++	++	–	+	+	–
Cytokeratin	+ (5–15%)	–	+	+	+	–
S100 protein	++	++	+	+	±	++
Vimentin	++	++	+	+	±	+
GFAP	–	–	+	–	±	±

a variety of angioblastic meningioma (Zülch, 1979). Supra-tentorial haemangioblastomas exhibit the same range of immunohistochemical reactions as the more common cerebellar variety.

Nerve sheath tumours

Neurilemmoma (Schwannoma) of the acoustic nerve is the commonest nerve sheath tumour of the central nervous system. The majority occur as single neoplasms but multiple intracranial neurilemmomas, involving the optic and trigeminal nerves in addition to the acoustic nerve are seen in patients with central neurofibromatosis. The tumour is composed almost entirely of Schwann cells which are strongly immunoreactive for S100 protein. Focal GFAP immunoreactivity may also be present. As already discussed, distinguishing between meningioma and neurilemmoma can sometimes prove difficult, even by immunohistochemistry and requires electron microscopy. Malignant neurilemmoma occasionally occurs in the central nervous system (McLean et al., 1990) and shows reduced S100 immunoreactivity probably reflecting lack of differentiation.

The cells of an occasional neurilemmoma may contain melanin pigment. These have been designated melanotic Schwannomas and their distinction from metastatic melanoma can sometimes be problematic. Both are immunoreactive for S100 protein and, similar to melanoma, the melanotic Schwannoma may be reactive for vimentin. The two tumours may sometimes be distinguished by the lack of immunoreactivity for melanoma-specific markers such as HMB-45 that is usual in melanotic Schwannoma. However, this can only be exploited when the metastatic melanoma is HMB-45 immunoreactive. Electron microscopy is required to identify the basal lamina that indicates the Schwann cell lineage of melanotic Schwannoma.

Neurofibromas and myxoid tumours of nerve sheath are rarely seen in the central nervous system, but can involve the trigeminal ganglion and spinal nerves. Both are S100 immunoreactive. Silver impregnation identifies the delicate neurites that are characteristic of neurofibroma.

Tumours of the choroid plexus

Although composed primarily of cells derived from primitive medullary epithelium, tumours of the choroid plexus have traditionally been classified as vascular tumours (Zülch, 1979). Papillomas and the very occasional carcinoma form the bulk of these tumours. Immunohistochemical studies have been limited but have shown immunoreactivity of normal choroid epithelial cells and choroid plexus papilloma for cytokeratin, S100 protein, neurone-specific enolase and GFAP (Rubinstein and Brucher, 1981; Coffin et al., 1986; Miettinen et al., 1986). The focal immunoreactivity for GFAP has been interpreted as ependymal differentiation (Rubinstein and Brucher, 1981). Immunoreactivity for transthyretin (TTR), a carrier protein that facilitates entry of thyroid hormone into the central nervous system has been demonstrated in normal choroid epithelium and choroid plexus papillomas and carcinomas. It is synthesized in choroid epithelial cells and reaches its highest concentration in cerebrospinal fluid (Aleshire et al., 1983). Immunoreactivity for transthyretin in choroid plexus epithelium allows choroid plexus papilloma to be distinguished from papillary ependymoma and choroid plexus carcinoma from metastatic adenocarcinoma.

The stroma of the choroid may be expanded as a result of extramedullary haemopoiesis and is also one of the central nervous system sites of leukaemic infiltration.

Angiosarcoma and Kaposi's sarcoma may occur very rarely in the central nervous system. In published reports, angiosarcoma has involved the parenchyma in preference to the leptomeninges (Charman et al., 1988) while Kaposi's sarcoma has usually presented as a meningeal tumour in patients with acquired immunodeficiency syndrome (Levy, Bredeson and Rosenblum, 1985). The endothelial cell component in each of these tumours is immunoreactive for Factor VIII.

Pituitary tumours

Adenoma

Pituitary adenomas are subdivided into the two categories of endocrine-active and endocrine-inactive or 'null cell'. Determination and characterization of the type of hormone secreted by an adenoma is dependant on immunohistochemistry and antibodies against all anterior pituitary hormones are readily available. The present classification of pituitary adenomas is based on both immunohistochemical and ultrastructural features (Scheithauer, 1984a and b). The majority of endocrine-active adenomas secrete prolactin. However, in contrast to growth hormone (GH) and adrenocorticotrophin

(ACTH)-secreting adenomas, which are strongly immunoreactive with GH and ACTH antibodies prolactinomas are often weakly immunoreactive. This is postulated to be due to lack of storage of prolactin within cells once it is synthesized. All pituitary adenomas, except those that secrete ACTH are also immunoreactive for chromogranin which is expressed on the surface of membrane-bound secretory granules (Lloyd, 1987). Immunoreactivity for cytokeratin and GFAP is commonly seen in the Crooke's hyaline that is present in many of the cells of ACTH-secreting adenomas. Focal immunoreactivity for GFAP is also common in all adenomas.

Craniopharyngioma

The morphological features of craniopharyngioma are usually instantaneously recognizable and immunohistochemistry is only occasionally required to confirm the diagnosis. The epithelial component is immunoreactive for cytokeratin and where adjacent brain parenchyma is included, GFAP immunoreactivity highlights the often florid reactive astrocytic gliosis.

Pineal tumours

Tumours of the pineal are usually divided into the two broad categories of germ cell and pineal parenchymal. The former group includes, germinoma, embryonal carcinoma, endodermal sinus tumour (yolk sac tumour), teratoma and choriocarcinoma while pineocytoma, pineoblastoma, astrocytoma and meningioma comprise the latter. Non-pineal germ cell tumours can also occur in the pituitary fossa, region of the third ventricle and in the lateral ventricle. Immunohistochemistry is essential in the work-up of pineal tumours, in particular of germ cell tumours. A panel of antibodies comprising β-human chorionic gonadotrophin (β-HCG), alpha fetoprotein (AFP), carcinoembryonic antigen (CEA), alpha-1-antitrypsin/anti-chymotrypsin (AAT/AACT), ferritin and placental alkaline phosphatase (PLAP) should be employed. The profile of immunoreactivity of intracranial germ cell tumours is almost identical to that of gonadal germ cell tumours (Table 7.5.; Bjornsson et al., 1985; Taylor, 1986). Choriocarcinoma is usually intensely immunoreactive for β-HCG but rarely reacts with other antibodies. However, any of the other germ cell tumours can have a syncytio-trophoblast component which will be immunoreactive for β-HCG. Immunoreactivity for AFP is seen in endodermal sinus tumour, embryonal carcinoma and immature teratoma. Embryonal carcinoma may also show reactivity for CEA and AAT/AACT, while germinomas usually react with antibodies against ferritin and placental alkaline phosphatase. The components of a teratoma may be more accurately identified using antibodies against cytokeratin, EMA, neurofilament protein and GFAP in

Table 7.5: Immunohistochemical reactions of intracranial germ cell tumours

	β-HCG	AFP	CEA	AAT/AACT	Ferritin	PLAP
Choriocarcinoma	+++	–	–	–	–	–
Germinoma	(+)*	–	–	–	++	++
Embryonal carcinoma	(+)*	++	+	+	–	–
Endodermal sinus Tumour	(+)*	++	–	–	–	–
Teratoma#						
Mature	–	–	±	–	–	–
Immature	(+)*	++	±	–	–	–

Notes: * Reactivity depends on the presence of syncytiotrophoblast # Teratomas may show immunoreactivity for a variety of epithelial, mesenchymal and glial markers depending on maturity

β–HCG: = beta subunit of human chorionic gonadotrophin
AFP: = alpha-fetoprotein
CEA: = carcinoembryonic antigen
AAT/AACT: = alpha-1-antitrypsin/antichymotrypsin
PLAP: = placental alkaline phosphatase

addition to those in the germ cell tumour panel. Accurate identification of epithelial and mesenchymal elements is essential to assessing the maturity of a teratoma.

Pineocytomas and pineoblastomas can both show concomitant neuronal and astrocytic differentiation, determined by immunoreactivity for GFAP and synaptophysin. Some pineal parenchymal tumours have been shown to be immunoreactive for S-antigen and rhodopsin suggesting retinal differentiation (Perentes et al., 1986). This supports a previous contention of an association between retinoblastoma and pineoblastoma.

Primary central nervous system lymphoma

Although its incidence rate is increasing, lymphoma remains an uncommon central nervous system tumour (Adams and Howatson, 1990). It presently comprises approximately 1 per cent of primary central nervous system neoplasms. There is still considerable debate whether primary CNS lymphoma develops from resident microglial cells or from cells which leave the circulation and become established as a neoplasm in the brain parenchyma. In tissue fixed in B-5 solution (Fig. 7.21A), tumour cells are immunoreactive for common leucocyte antigen (LCA). Further immunohistochemical phenotyping has shown that the majority of primary central nervous system lymphomas are of B-cell lineage (Table 7.6; Figure 7.21B) and that a population of small T-lymphocytes is frequently present (Fig. 7.21C). The presence of bizarre, reactive astrocytes intermingled with lymphoma cells is a common feature. These can be highlighted with GFAP antibodies; they may also show cross-reactivity with some T-lymphocyte and monocyte/macrophage markers.

An unusual form of lymphoma in which tumour cells remain within the lumina of vessels may present initially with central nervous system dysfunction. This has been termed intravascular lymphoma or malignant angioendotheliomatosis. The central nervous system manifestations have usually been dementia or stroke due

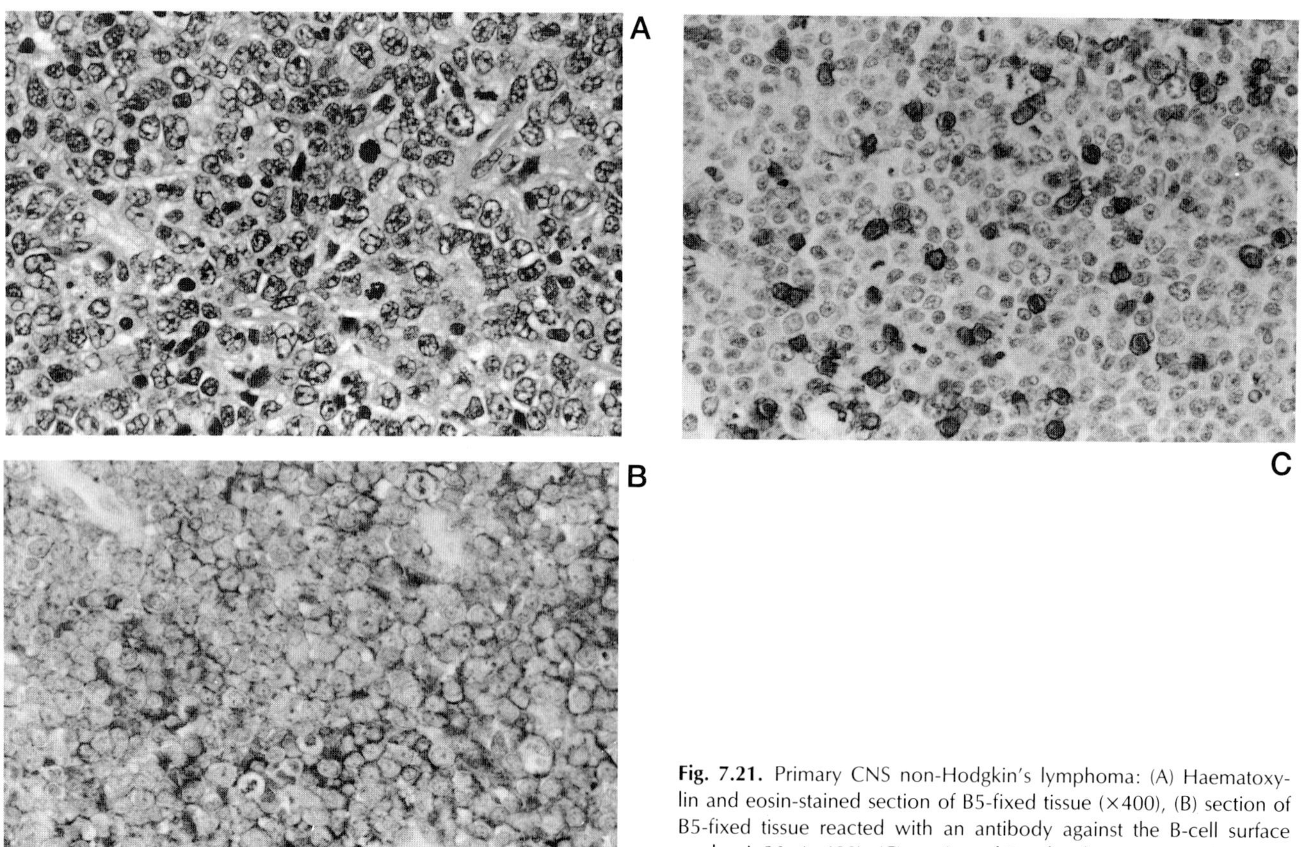

Fig. 7.21. Primary CNS non-Hodgkin's lymphoma: (A) Haematoxylin and eosin-stained section of B5-fixed tissue (×400), (B) section of B5-fixed tissue reacted with an antibody against the B-cell surface marker L-26. (×400), (C) section of B5- fixed tissue reacted with an antibody against the T-cell surface marker UCHL-1 (×400).

Table 7.6: Immunoreactivity of 10 primary CNS lymphomas – The Royal Melbourne Hospital 1987–91

Antibody	Number of tumours showing immunoreactivity	
Leucocyte common antigen	10	
B-cell markers:		
L26	10	
4KB5	9	
T-cell markers:		
UCHL-1	8	minor population of small lymphocytes
Leu22	8	
Monocyte/macrophage markers:		
KP1	7	some cross-reactivity with microglial cells and reactive astrocytes
LeuM1	5	

to vascular luminal occlusion by tumour cells (Wick et al., 1982; Ojeda et al., 1984). Immunophenotyping has shown that tumour cells are of B-lymphocyte lineage (Bhawan et al., 1985).

Chordoma

A linear streak of notochordal tissue in the dorsal midline of the 18-day embryo is the first indication of central nervous system development. Remnants of this tissue are present definitively in the nucleus pulposus of intervertebral discs, in the region of the spheno-occipital syndesmosis, vertebral bodies and portions of the sacrum and ilium adjacent to the sacroiliac joint. This pattern explains the anatomical distribution of chordomas which arise from these notochordal remnants. Chordomas express markers which reflect the origin of notochord from embryonic ectoderm. There is usually strong immunoreactivity for low molecular weight cytokeratin, e.g. CAM 5.2 (Fig. 7.22A) and epithelial membrane antigen with less intense reactivity for vimentin and S100 protein (Scheithauer, 1990). Immunoreactivity for cytokeratin is useful in distinguishing chordoma from chondrosarcoma which is usually non-reactive with cytokeratin antibodies. Reactivity for GFAP is occasionally seen in chordoma, probably resulting from cross-reactivity with keratin epitopes. The presence of desmosomes on electron microscopic examination (Fig. 7.22B) also reflects the epithelial lineage of chordomas.

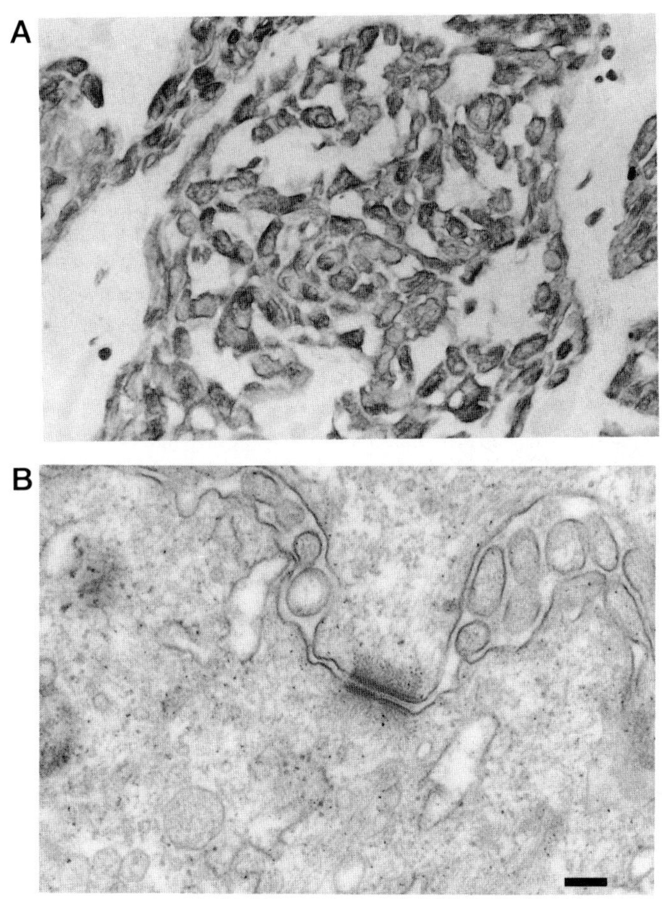

Fig. 7.22. Chordoma: (A) reactivity of tumour cells with an antibody against low relative mass cytokeratin (CAM 5.2) (×400), (B) electron micrograph of a chordoma showing formation of a desmosome between adjacent cells reflecting the ectodermal lineage of this tumour (Uranyl acetate/Lead citrate; Bar=100 nanometres).

Cysts

A number of both simple and complex acquired cysts occur in the central nervous system and the challenge for the neuropathologist is to accurately determine their lineage. Dermoid, epidermoid and Rathke's pouch cysts are of ectodermal origin (Leech and Olafson, 1977). Third ventricular colloid cysts, however, remain controversial and an origin from such tissues as paraphysis, primitive neuroepithelium, ependyma and choroid plexus epithelium has been proposed.

Colloid cysts are lined by simple cuboidal or columnar epithelium anchored to a prominent layer of collagen. Some cells may be ciliated and goblet cells may also be present. The lining cells are consistently immunoreactive for cytokeratin and epithelial membrane antigen and non-reactive for GFAP and vimentin (Mackenzie and Gilbert, 1991). Reactivity for carcinoembryonic antigen is also frequently observed. This immunohistochemical profile and some ultrastructural features favour an origin from endoderm of the primitive foregut, similar to the enterogenous or neuroenteric cysts of the spinal canal (Mackenzie and Gilbert, 1991, Yagashita et al., 1984). Immunoreactivity of lining cells for transthyretin in some colloid cysts suggests an origin from choroid epithelium.

Arachnoid cysts, which are thought to develop as pulsion diverticulae that invaginate the underlying cerebral tissue are composed of a thin layer of arachnoid cells which are focally hyperplastic. These are immunoreactive for epithelial membrane antigen (EMA) and vimentin. Cysts lined by ependymal cells are the least common. These are usually supra-tentorial and subarachnoid in location but may also present within the substance of the spinal cord (Robertson et al., 1991). They are lined by a layer of ciliated cuboidal cells that show focal immunoreactivity for GFAP.

Metastatic tumours

Metastatic tumours of the central nervous system occur in the United States at a rate of approximately 8.3/100,000/year compared with 8.2/100,000/year for primary tumours (Walker et al., 1985). The majority of these arise from carcinoma of the bronchus, but a considerable number are metastases of breast carcinoma and malignant melanoma. Compression of the spinal cord is frequently due to osseous metastases of prostatic and breast carcinoma and spread of systemic lymphoma to the extradural space. In addition, carcinoma of the paranasal sinuses may directly invade the floor of the anterior and middle cranial fossae and involve leptomeninges and brain parenchyma.

Two distinct patterns of involvement of the central nervous system by metastatic tumours have been recognized. The majority become established as well-circumscribed parenchymal lesions, centred on the junction between cerebral cortex and white matter in the distribution of the middle cerebral artery. Alternatively, seeding of the leptomeninges resulting in diffuse thickening and step-wise cranial nerve paralysis may occur. This pattern, known as meningitis carcinomatosa or leptomeningeal carcinomatosis can also involve the spinal leptomeninges either separate from or in addition to involvement of the cranial leptomeninges.

With the exception of central nervous system involvement by systemic lymphoma, metastatic tumours are almost without exception of epithelial lineage and are immunoreactive with antibodies raised against epithelial antigens. Standard among these are the cytokeratins, epithelial membrane antigen, anti-human tumour-associated glycoprotein-72 (MAb B72.3) and carcino-embryonic antigen (Pinkus and Kurtin, 1985; Thomas and Battifora, 1987; Prey et al., 1991). Reactivity for intestinal mucins assists in the identification of the gastrointestinal origin of some metastatic adenocarcinomas. Immunoreactivity for prostate-specific antigen (PSA) and prostatic acid phosphatase (PSAP) should be determined in osseous metastases, particularly those involving vertebrae. Metastases from small cell carcinoma of lung may be immunoreactive for neurone-specific enolase and synaptophysin. Immunoreactivity of extradural tumours for lymphoid markers should also be sought to exclude lymphoma.

Central nervous system metastases of malignant melanoma are frequently either amelanotic or poorly melanized. Diagnosis is facilitated by the demonstration of immunoreactivity for S100 protein and vimentin. Immunoreactivity for GFAP is not seen in tumour cells but will highlight reactive astrocytes in adjacent brain. A number of putative melanoma-specific markers have been described (Gown et al., 1986). Of these, HMB-45 appears to be the most specific (Wick et al., 1988). However, although primary malignant melanomas usually show strong immunoreactivity for HMB-45, reactivity in metastases is frequently absent.

Some tumours of epithelial lineage are immunoreactive for GFAP (Gustaffson et al., 1989). However, their metastases usually show a degree of differentiation that is sufficient for their distinction from primary gliomas. Metastasis of systemic carcinoma to a primary central nervous system tumour has occasionally been reported (Osterberg, 1957; Poskinoff and Stratford, 1960; Farnsworth, 1972). In this situation, recognition of the metastasis is aided by cytokeratin, epithelial membrane antigen and carcinoembryonic antigen immunoreactivity and non-reactivity for glial fibrillary acidic protein. Some difficulty may arise where metastasis to a meningioma has occurred. Both the metastasis and meningioma will be reactive for epithelial membrane antigen and the metastasis may react with antibodies against vimentin. Non-reactivity of the meningioma with antibodies against carcinoembryonic antigen may allow separation provided the metastasis is reactive.

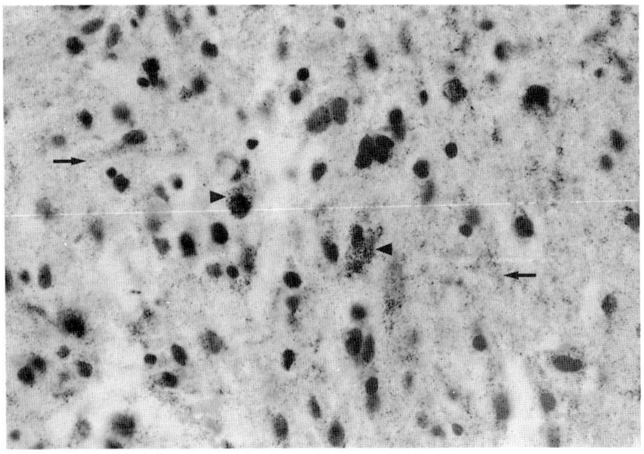

Fig. 7.23. Over-expression of the c-Ha-ras oncogene in an anaplastic astrocytoma. ·Expression of the ras oncoprotein is detected by silver granules over peri-nuclear cytoplasm (arrowheads) and cell processes (arrows) (immunogold-silver/Nuclear Fast Red B counterstain; ×200; for method see Orian et al., 1992).

Proliferative potential of central nervous system tumours

Several markers of the proliferative potential of central nervous system and other tumours have been identified. Detection and quantitation of expression of these markers has been found to be useful in more accurately determining the likely biological behaviour of a particular tumour. A variety of techniques have been utilized including immunohistochemistry, immunoblotting, *in situ* hybridization, Southern and Northern blotting and the polymerase chain reaction. Of these, immunohistochemistry is the most appropriate technique for tissue sections.

Indices of the number of cells in the DNA synthetic phase of the cell cycle have been found to be the most accurate predictors of biological behaviour. Several indices, namely bromodeoxyuridine (BuDR) uptake, Ki-67 nuclear antigen, proliferating cell nuclear antigen (PCNA) and DNA polymerase all detectable and quantifiable by immunohistochemistry, have been found to correlate with the histological grade of astrocytic tumours (Labrousse et al., 1991; Raghavan et al., 1990). The BuDR labelling index has also been found to be predictive of recurrence of meningiomas (Cho et al., 1987).

Expression of the protein products of oncogenes by tumour cells can be detected by immunohistochemistry, in particular immunogold-silver histochemistry which also permits semi-quantitation of expression (Fig. 7.23). The profile and degree of over-expression of a number of oncogenes correlates with histological grade in astrocytomas (Bigner et al., 1988; Orian et al., 1992). Glioblastomas multiforme over-express up to four oncogenes, in particular, *c-erbB*-1, *c-myc*, c-Ha/N-ras and *c-fos*, while low grade astrocytomas, in particular juvenile pilocytic astrocytoma frequently over-express the combination of *c-erbB-1/c-fos* (Orian et al., 1992). The detection of over-expression of three or more oncogenes in a glioma that appears well-differentiated on histological criteria would suggest a high propensity for progression to higher grades of malignancy.

In addition to over-expression of specific oncogenes, loss or mutational inactivation of other genes, termed tumour suppressor genes, can now be detected by immunohistochemistry. Mutations of the p53 tumour suppressor gene located on chromosome 17 are the most common genetic alteration in a wide variety of human cancers including astrocytic tumours (Levine et al., 1991). Such mutations result in a prolonged half-life of the mutant gene product which can then be detected in tissue sections with specific antibodies. Because the wild-type p53 gene product has an extremely short half-life, cross reactivity with wild-type product does not occur and immunohistochemistry can reliably detect mutations. Mutations of p53 have been linked to progression of anaplastic astrocytomas to glioblastoma multiforme (Fults et al., 1992). Detection of overexpression of oncogenes such as ras and *c-myc*, together with mutations of p53 and chromosome 10 alterations will, in future, become an integral part of the surgical pathology work-up of glial tumours and provide a more accurate assessment of likely biological behaviour than is possible by histological criteria alone.

The pattern of ganglioside expression by glioma cells has also been suggested to correlate with histological grade and may provide another means of predicting biological behaviour. Gangliosides are acidic glycosphingolipids composed of sialic acid, oligosaccharide, sphingosine and fatty acid domains which project from the surface of most mammalian cells. They reach their highest concentration in grey matter and are particularly abundant in synaptic membranes. They are also a component of the membranes of cytoplasmic organelles such as Golgi, endoplasmic reticulum and lysosomes. Thin layer chromatographic analyses of gangliosides from different grades of astrocytomas have shown simplification of their molecular structure in higher grade tumours (Jenneman et al., 1990). Specific monoclonal antibodies, capable of detecting these alterations have been developed and may, in the future, be of use in grading astrocytomas.

References

Adams, H.J. and Howatson, A.G. (1990). Cerebral lymphomas: A review of 70 cases. *Journal of Clinical Pathology* **43**, 544–7.

Aleshire, S.L., Bradley, C.A., Richardson, L.D. and Parl, F.F. (1983). Localization of human pre-albumin in choroid plexus epithelium. *Journal of Histochemistry* **31**, 608–12.

Astrom, K-E., Mancall, E.L. and Richardson, E.P. (1958) Progressive multifocal leukoencephalopathy: A hitherto unrecognized complication of chronic lymphatic leukemia and Hodgkin's disease. *Brain* **81**, 93–111.

Bancher, C., Lassman, H., Budka, H., Jellinger, K., Grundke-Iqbal, I., Iqbal, K., Wiche, G., Seitelberger, F. and Wisniewski, H.K. (1989). An antigenic profile of Lewy bodies: Immunocytochemical indication for protein phosphorylation and ubiquitination. *Journal of Neuropathology and Experimental Neurology* **48**, 81–93.

Becker, N., Paulus, W. and Roggendorf, W. (1989). Histogenesis of stromal cells in cerebellar hemangioblastomas. An immunohistochemical study. *American Journal of Pathology* **134**, 271–5.

Bhawan, J., Wolff, S.M., Ucci, A.A. and Bhan, A.K. (1985). Malignant lymphoma and malignant angioendotheliomatosis: One disease. *Cancer* **55**, 570–6.

Bignami, A. and Dahl, D. (1975). Degradation of glial fibrillary acidic protein in multiple sclerosis plaques. *Laboratory Investigation* **32**, 442–7.

Bignami, A., Raju, T. and Dahl, D. (1982). Localization of vimentin, the non-specific intermediate filament protein, in embryonal glia and in early differentiating neurons. *In vivo* and *in vitro* immunofluorescence study of the rat embryo with vimentin and neurofilament antisera. *Developmental Biology* **91**, 286–92.

Bigner, S.H., Burger, P.C., Wong, A,J., Werner, M.H., Hamilton, S.R., Muhlbaier, L.H., Vogelstein, B. and Bigner, D.B. (1988). Gene amplification in malignant human gliomas: Clinical and histopathologic aspects. *Journal of Neuropathology and Experimental Neurology* **47**, 191–205.

Bjornsson, J., Scheithauer, B.W., Okazaki, H. and Leech, R.W. (1985). Intracranial germ cell tumours: Pathobiological and immunohistochemical aspects of 70 cases. *Journal of Neuropathology and Experimental Neurology* **44**, 32–46.

Böhlig, T., Haltia, M., Rosenlöff, F. and Fyhrquist, F. (1987). Erythropoietin in capillary hemangioblastomas. *Acta Neuropathologica (Berlin)* **74**, 324–8.

Bongcam-Rudloff, E., Nister, M., Betsholtz, C., Wang, J-L., Stenman, G., Huebner, K., Croce, C.M. and Westermark, B. (1991). Human glial fibrillary acidic protein: Complementary DNA cloning, chromosomal localization, and messenger RNA expression in human glioma cell lines of various phenotypes. *Cancer Research* **51**, 1553–60.

Brown, P., Goldfarb, L.G. and Gajdusek, D.C. (1991). The new biology of spongiform encephalopathy: Infectious amyloidoses with a genetic twist. *Lancet* **337**, 1019–22.

Budka, H. (1986). Multinucleated giant cells in brain: A hallmark of acquired immunodeficiency syndrome. *Acta Neuropathologica* **69**, 253–8.

Caccamo, D.V., Herman, M.M. and Rubinstein, L.J. (1989). An immunohistochemical study of the primitive and maturing elements of human cerebral medulloepitheliomas. *Acta Neuropathologica (Berlin)* **79**, 248–54.

Charman, H.P., Lowenstein, D.H., Cho, K.G., DeArmond, S.J. and Wilson, C.B. (1988). Primary cerebral angiosarcoma. *Journal of Neurosurgery* **68**, 806–10.

Cho, K.G., Hoshino, T., Nagashima, T. and Davis, R.L. (1987). Proliferative potential of malignant and non-malignant meningiomas. In Chate, M., Darcel, F. and Pecker, J. (eds), *Brain Oncology*, Martinus Nijhoff, Dordrecht, pp. 79–81.

Coffin, C.M., Wick, M.R., Braun, J.T. and Dehner, L.P.

(1986). Choroid plexus neoplasms. Clinicopathological and immunohistochemical studies. *American Journal of Surgical Pathology* **10**, 394–404.

Cork, L.C., Sternberger, N.H., Sternberger, L.A., Casanova, M.F., Strubel, R.G. and Price, D.L. (1986). Phosphorylated neurofilament antigens in neurofibrillary tangles in Alzheimer's disease. *Journal of Neuropathology and Experimental Neurology* **45**, 56–64.

Cruz-Sanchez, F.F., Rossi, M.L., Hughes, J.T., Esiri, M.M. and Coakham, H.B. (1989). Medulloblastoma: An immunohistochemical study of 50 cases. *Acta Neuropathologica* **79**, 205–10.

Daumas-Duport, C., Scheithauer, B.W., Chodkiewicz, J-P, Laws, E.R., Jnr. and Vedrenne, C. (1988). Dysembryoplastic neuroepithelial tumour: A surgically curable tumour of young patients with intractable partial seizures. Report of thirty-nine cases. *Neurosurgery* **23**, 545–56.

Davies, L., Wolska, B., Hilbich, C., Multhaup, G., Martins, R., Simms, G., Beyreuther, K. and Masters, C.L. (1988). A4 amyloid protein deposition and the diagnosis of Alzheimer's disease. Prevalence in brains determined by immuno cytochemistry compared with conventional neuropathologic techniques. *Neurology* **38**, 1688–93.

DeArmond, S.J., McKinley, M.P., Barry, R.A., Braunfield, M.B., McColloch, J.R. and Prusiner, S.B. (1985). Identification of prion amyloid filaments in scrapie-infected brain. *Cell* **41**, 221–35.

Devinsky, O., Cho, E-S., Petito, C.K. and Price, R.W. (1991). Herpes zoster myelitis. *Brain* **114**, 1181–96.

Farnsworth, J. (1972). Regressing melanoma metastazing to an oligodendroglioma. *Pathology* **4**, 253–7.

Fults, D., Pedone, C.A., Thomas, G.A. and White, R. (1990). Allelotype of hurnan malignant astrocytoma. *Cancer Research* **50**, 5784–9.

Fults, D., Brockmeyer, D., Tullous, M.W., Pedone, C.A. and Cawthorn. R.W. (1992). p53 mutation and loss of heterozygosity on chromosomes 17 and 10 during human astrocytoma progression. *Cancer Research* **52**, 674–9.

Gabbianni, G., Kapanci, Y., Barazzone, P. and Franke, W.W. (1981). Immmunochemical identification of intermediate-sized filaments in human neoplastic cells: A diagnostic aid for the surgical pathologist. *American Journal of Pathology* **104**, 206–16.

Gibbs, W.R.G., Luthert, P.J., Janota, I. and Lantos, P.L. (1989). Cortical Lewy body dementia: Clinical features and classification. *Journal of Neurology, Neurosurgery, and Psychiatry* **52**, 185–92.

Giulian, D., Vaca, K. and Noonan, C.A. (1990). Secretion of neurotoxins by mononuclear phagocytes infected with HIV-1. *Science* **250**, 1593–6.

Goldberg-Stern, H., Gadoth, N., Stern, S., Cohen, I.J., Zaizov, R. and Sandbank, U. (1991). The prognostic significance of glial fibrillary acidic protein staining in medulloblastoma. *Cancer* **68**, 568–73.

Gonzales, M.F. and Davis, R.L. (1988). Neuropathology of Acquired Immunodeficiency Syndrome. *Neuropathology and Applied Neurobiology* **14**, 345–63.

Goto, S., Hirano, A. and Rojas-Corona, R.R. (1989). An immunohistochemical investigation of the human neostriatum in Huntington's disease. *Annals of Neurology* **25**, 298–304.

Gould V.E., Jansson, D.S., Molenaar, .M., Rorke, L.B., Trojanowski, J.Q., Lee, V.M., Packer, R.J. and Franke, W.W. (1990). Primitive neuroectodermal tumors of the central nervous system. Patterns of expression of neuroendocrine markers, and all classes of intermediate filament proteins. *Laboratory Investigation* **62**, 498–508.

Gould, V.E., Wiedenmmann, B., Lee, I., Scchwechheimer, K., Dockhorn, J.A., Moll, R. and Franke, W. (1987). Synaptophysin expression in neuroendocrine neoplasms as determined by immunocytochemistry. *American Journal of Pathology* **126**, 243–57.

Gown, A.M., Vogel, A.M., Hoak, D., Gough, F. and McNutt, M.A. (1986). Monoclonal antibodies specific for melanocytic tumours distinguish subpopulations of melanocytes. *American Journal of Pathology* **123**, 195–203.

Grafe, M.R., Forno, L.S. and Eng, L.F. (1985). Immunocytochemical studies of substance P and met-enkephalin in the basal ganglia and substantia nigra in Huntington's, Parkinson's and Alzheimer's diseases. *Journal of Neuropathology and Experimental Neurology* **44**, 47–59.

Greenfield, J.G. (1950). Encephalitis and encephalomyelitis in England and Wales during the last decade. *Brain* **73**, 141–66.

Gustaffson, H., Virtanen, I. and Thornell, L-E. (1989). Glial fibrillary acidic protein and desmin in salivary neoplasms. Expression of four different types of intermediate filament proteins within the same cell type. *Virchows Archives B Cellular Pathology* **57**, 303–13.

Haglid, K., Carlsson, C.A. and Stavrou, D. (1973). An immunological study of human brain tumours concerning the brain specific proteins S-100 and 14.3.2. *Acta Neuropathologica (Berlin)* **24**, 187–93.

Hall, W.W., Lamb, R.A. and Choppin, P.W. (1979). Measles and SSPE virus proteins: Lack of antibodies to the M protein in patients with subacute sclerosing panencephalitis. *Proceedings of the National Academy of Sciences USA* **76**, 2047–51.

Henderson, V.E. and Finch, C.E. (1989). The neurobiology of Alzheimer's disease. *Journal of Neurosurgery* **70**, 335–53.

Herrick, M.K. and Rubinstein, L.J. (1979). The cytological differentiating potential of pineal parenchymal neoplasms (true pinealomas). A clinicopathological study of 28 tumours. *Brain* **102**, 289–20.

Hickey, W.F. and Kimura, H. (1989). Perivascular microglial cells of the CNS are bone marrow-derived and present antigen in vivo. *Science* **239**, 290–92.

Hirano, A., Decubitzer, H.M., Kurland, L.T. and Zimmerman, H.M. (1968). The fine structure of some intraganglionic alterations. *Journal of Neuropathology and Experimental Neurology* **27**, 167–87.

Hoffman, P.N. and Lasek R.J. (1975). The slow component of transport: Identification of major structural polypeptides of the axon and their generality among mammalian neurons. *Journal of Cell Biology* **66**, 351–66.

Horten, B.C. and Rubinstein, L.J. (1976). Primary cerebral neuroblastoma. A clinicopathological study of 35 cases. *Brain* **99**, 735–56.

Hulette, C.M., Downey, B.T. and Burger, P.C. (1991). Progressive multifocal leukoencephalopathy. Diagnosis by in situ hybridization with a biotinylated JC virus DNA probe using an automated histomatic code-on slide stainer. *American Journal of Surgical Pathology* **15**, 791–7.

Hume-Adams, H. and Howatson, A.G. (1990). Cerebral lymphomas: A review of 70 cases. *Journal of Clinical Pathology* **43**, 544–7.

Ihara, Y., Nukina, N. and Miura, R. (1986). Phosphorylated tau protein is integrated into paired helical filaments in Alzheimer's disease. *Journal of Biochemistry* **99**, 1807–10.

Iqbal, K., Zaidi, T. and Thompson, C.H. (1984). Alzheimer's paired helical filaments: Bulk isolation, solubility, and protein composition. *Acta Neuropathologica* **62**, 167–77.

Ishwar, S., Taniguichi, R.M. and Vogel, F.S. (1971). Multiple supratentorial haemangioblastomas. Case study and ultrastructural characteristics. *Journal of Neurosurgery* **35**, 396–405.

Jellinger, K. and Paulus, W. (1991). Mesenchymal non-meningothelial tumours of the central nervous system. *Brain Pathology* **1**, 79–87.

Jenneman, R., Roden, A., Bauer, B., Mennel, H-D. and Weigandt, H. (1990). *Glycosphingolipids of human gliomas Cancer Research* **50**, 7444–9.

Kaneko, Y., Kitamoto, T., Tateishi, J. and Yamaguchi, K. (1989). Ferritin immunohistochemistry as a marker for microglia. *Acta Neuropathologica* **79**, 129–36.

Kepes, J.J., Rengachary, S.S. and Lee, S.H. (1979). Astrocytes in hemangioblastomas of the central nervous system and their relationship to stromal cells. *Acta Neuropathologica (Berlin)* **47**, 99–104.

Khachaturian, Z.S. (1985). Diagnosis of Alzheimer's disease. *Archives of Neurology* **42**, 1097–105.

Kitaguchi, N., Takahashi, Y., Tokushima, Y., Shiojiri, S. and Ito, H. 1988). Novel precursor of Alzheimer's disease amyloid protein shows protease inhibitory activity. *Nature* **331**, 530–2.

Kowall, N.W., Ferrante. R.J. and Martin J.B. (1987). Patterns of cell loss in Huntington's disease. *Trends in Neuroscience* **10**, 24–9.

Kramm, C.M., Korf, H-W., Czerwionka, M., Schachenmayr, W. and de Grip, W.J. (1991). Photoreceptor differentiation in cerebellar medulloblastoma: Evidence for a functional photopigment and authentic S-antigen (arrestin). *Acta Neuropathologica (Berlin)* **81**, 296–302.

Kubota, T., Hayashi, M., Kawano, H., Kabuto, M., Sato, K., Ishise, J., Kawamoto, K., Shirataki, K., Iizuka, H., Tsunoda, S. and Katsuyama, J. (1991). Central neurocytoma: Immunohistochemical and ultrastructural study. *Acta Neuropathologica (Berlin)* **81**, 418–27.

Labrousse, F., Daumas-Duport, C., Batorski, L. and Hoshino, T. (1991). Histological grading and bromodeoxyuridine labelling index of astrocytomas. Comparative study in a series of 60 cases. *Journal of Neurosurgery* **75**, 202–5.

Leech, R.W. and Olafson, R.A. (1977). Epithelial cysts of the neuraxis. *Archives of Pathology and Laboratory Medicine* **101**, 196–202.

Leigh, P.N., Probst, A., Dale, G.E., Power, D.P., Brion, J-P., Dodson, A. and Anderton, B.H. (1989). New aspects of the pathology of neurodegenerative disorders as revealed by ubiquitin antibodies. *Acta Neuropathologica* **79**, 61–72.

Lendahl, U., Zimmerman, L.B. and McKay, D.G. (1990). CNS stem cells express a new class of intermediate filament protein. *Cell* **60**, 585–95.

Levine, A.J., Momand, J. and Finlay, C.A. (1991). The p53 tumour suppressor gene. *Nature* **351**, 453–56.

Levy, R.M., Bredeson, D.E. and Rosenblum, M.L. (1985). Neurological manifestations of the acquired immunodeficiency syndrome (AIDS): Experience at UCSF and review of the literature. *Journal of Neurosurgery* **62**, 475–95.

Lloyd, R.V. (1987). Immunohistochemical localization of chromogranin in normal and neoplastic endocrine tissues. In Rosen, P.P. and Fechner, R.E. (eds), *Pathology Annual*, Part 2. Appleton-Century-Crofts. Norwalk, Connecticut, pp. 69–90.

Lowe, J., Blanchard, A., Morrell, K., Lennox, G., Reynolds, L., Billet, M., Landon, M. and Mayer R.J. (1988). Ubiquitin is a common factor in intermediate filament inclusion bodies of diverse type in man, including those of Parkinson's disease, Pick's disease, and Alzheimer's disease, as well as Rosenthal fibres in cerebellar astrocytomas, cytoplasmic bodies in muscle, and Mallory bodies in alcoholic liver disease. *Journal of Pathology* **155**, 9–15.

Ludwig, C.L., Smith, M.T., Godfrey, A.D. and Armbrustmacher, V.W. (1986). A clinicopathological study of 323 patients with oligodendrogliomas. *Annals of Neurology* **19**, 15–21.

McLean, C.A., Laidlaw, J.D., Brownbill, D.S.B. and Gonzales, M.F. (1990). Recurrence of acoustic neurilemmoma as a malignant spindle-cell neoplasm. Case report. *Journal of Neurosurgery* **73**, 946–50.

Mackenzie, I.R.A. and Gilbert, J.J. (1991). Cysts of the neuraxis of endodermal origin. *Journal of Neurology, Neurosurgery and Psychiatry* **54**, 572–5.

Manetto, V., Perry, G., Tabaton, M., Mullvihill, P., Fried, V.A., Smith, H.T., Gambetti, P. and Autilio-Gambetti, L. (1988). Ubiquitin is associated with abnormal cytoplasmic filaments characteristic of neurodegenerative diseases. *Proceedings of the National Academy of Science (USA)* **85**, 4501–5.

Martin, J.E., Swash, M. and Schwartz, M.S. (1990). Annotation. New insights in motor neuron disease. *Neuropathology and Applied Neurobiology* **16**, 97–110.

Masters, C.L., Simms, G. and Weinman, N.A. (1985). Amyloid plaque core protein in Alzheimer's disease and Down's syndrome. *Proceedings of the National Academy of Sciences* **82**, 4245–9.

Miettinen, M., Clark, R. and Virtanen, J. (1986). Intermediate filament proteins in choroid plexus and ependyma and their tumours. *American Journal of Pathology* **123**, 231–40.

Modlin, J.F., Jabbour, J.T., Witte, J.J. and Halsey, N.A. (1977) Epidemiological studies of measles, measles vaccine and subacute sclerosing panencephalitis. *Pediatrics* **59**, 505–12.

Morgello, S., Cho, E-S., Nielsen, S., Devinsky, O. and Petito, C.K. (1987). Cytomegalovirus encephalitis in patients with acquired immunodeficiency syndrome: An autopsy study of 30 cases and a review of the literature. *Human Pathology* **18**, 289–97.

Mori, H., Kondo, J. and Ihara, Y. (1987). Ubiquitin component of paired helical filaments in Alzheimer's disease. *Science* **235**, 1641–4.

Motoi, M., Yoshino, T., Hayashi, K., Nose, S., Horie, Y. and Ogawa, K. (1985). Immunohistochemical studies on human brain tumours using anti-Leu 7 monoclonal antibody in paraffin-embedded specimens. *Acta Neuropathologica (Berlin)* **66**, 75–7.

Nakagawa, Y., Perentes, E. and Rubinstein, L.J. (1986). Immunohistochemical characterization of oligodendrogliomas: An analysis of multiple markers. *Acta Neuropathologica (Berlin)* **72**, 15–22.

Nawrotzki, R., Starzinski-Powitz, A., Weber, F. and Schröder, R. (1990). Cross reactivity of monoclonal antibody Leu-19 with some neuroectodermal and other non-immune tissues. *Acta Neuropathologica (Berlin)* **79**, 520–7.

Nishio, S., Tashima, T., Takeshita, I. and Fukui, M. (1988). Intraventricular neurocytoma: Clinicopathological features of six cases. *Journal of Neurosurgery* **68**, 665–70.

Ojeda, V.J., Soopa, J., Cala, L.A. and Kakulas, B.A. (1984). Multifocal progressive neurological disorder caused by neoplastic angioendotheliosis. *Medical Journal of Australia* **141**, 246–9.

Orian, J.M., Vasilopoulos. K., Yoshida. S., Kaye. A.H., Chow. C.W. and Gonzales. M.F. (1992). Overexpression of multiple oncogenes related to histological grade of astrocytic glioma. *British Journal of Cancer* **66**, 106–12.

Osborn, M., Ludwig-Festl, M. and Weber, K. (1981). Expression of glial and vimentin type intermediate filaments in cultures derived from human glial material. *Differentiation* **19**, 161–7.

Osterberg, D.H. (1957). Metastasis of carcinoma to meningioma. *Journal of Neurosurgery* **13**, 337.

Pappolla, M.A. (1986). Lewy bodies of Parkinson's disease. Immune electron microscopic demonstration of neurofilament antigens in constituent filaments. *Archives of Pathology and Laboratory Medicine* **100**, 1160–3.

Perentes, E., Rubinstein, L.J., Herman, M.M. and Donoso, L.A. (1986). S-antigen immuno-reactivity in human pineal glands and pineal parenchymal tumours. A monoclonal antibody study. *Acta Neuropathologica (Berlin)* **71**, 224–7.

Perry, G., Rizzuto, N., Autilio-Gambetti, L. and Gambetti, P. (1985). Paired helical filaments from Alzheimer's disease patients contain cytoskeletal components. *Proceedings of the National Academy of Sciences* **82**, 3916–20.

Perry, G., Friedmen, R., Shaw, G and Chau, V. (1987). Ubiquitin is detected in neurofibrillary tangles and senile plaque neurites of Alzheimer's disease brains. *Proceedings of the National Academy of Sciences (USA)* **84**, 3033–6.

Perry, V.H. and Gordon, S. (1988). Macrophages and microglia in the nervous system. *Trends in Neuroscience* **11**, 273–7.

Phillips, C.A., Fanning, W.L., Gump, D.W. and Phillips, C.F. (1977). Cytomegalovirus encephalitis in immunologically normal adults. Successful treatment with vidarabine. *Journal of the American Medical Association* **238**, 299–300.

Pinkus, G.S. and Kurtin, P.J. (1985). Epithelial membrane antigen – a diagnostic discriminant in surgical pathology: Immunohistochemical profile of epithelial, mesenchymal and haematopoietic neoplasms using paraffin sections and monoclonal antibodies. *Human Pathology* **16**, 929–40.

Ponte,P., Gonzalez-DeWhitt, J., Schilling, J., Miller, J., Hsu, D., Greenberg, B., Davis, K., Wallace, A., Lieburg, I., Fuller, F. and Cordell, B. (1988). A new A4 amyloid mRNA contains a domain homologous to serine protease inhibitors. *Nature* **331**, 525–7.

Poskinoff, J. and Stratford, J. (1960). Carcinoma metastasis to malignant glioma. *Archives of Neurology* **5**, 93/559–97/563.

Prey, M.U., Bedrossian, C.W.M. and Masood, S. (1991). The value of monoclonal antibody B72.3 for the diagnosis of breast carcinoma: Experience with the first commercially available source. *Human Pathology* **22**, 598–602.

Probst, A., Langui, D. and Ulrich, J. (1991). Alzheimer's disease: A description of structural lesions. *Brain Pathology* **1**, 229–39.

Prusiner, S.B. (1987). Prions and neurodegenerative diseases. *The New England Journal of Medicine* **317**, 1571–81.

Prusiner, S.B. and DeArmond, S.J. (1987). Biology of Disease. Prions causing nervous system degeneration. *Laboratory*

Investigation **56**, 349–63.

Raghavan, R., Steart, P.V. and Weller. R.O. (1990). Cell proliferation patterns in the diagnosis of astrocytomas, anaplastic astrocytomas and glioblastoma multiforme: A Ki-67 study. *Neuropathology and Applied Neurobiology* **16**, 123–33.

Ringertz, N. (1950). Grading of gliomas. *Acta Pathologica Microbiologica Scandinavica* **27**, 51–65.

del Rio-Hortega, P. (1919). El tercer elemento de los centros nerviosos. I. La microglia. II. Intervencion de la microglia en los procesos patologicas. III. Naturaleza probable de la microglia. *Boletin de la Sociedad espanola de biologica* **9**, 69–120.

Robertson, D.P., Kirkpatrick, J.B., Harper, R.I. and Mawad, M.E. (1991). Spinal intramedullary ependymal cyst. Report of three cases. *Journal of Neurosurgery* **75**, 312–16.

Rodriguez, M. (1989). Multiple sclerosis: Basic concepts and hypothesis. *Mayo Clinic Proceedings* **64**, 570–6.

Rorke, L.B., Gilles, F.H., Davis, R.L. and Becker, L.E. (1985). Revision of the World Health Organization classification of brain tumours for childhood brain tumours. *Cancer* **56**, 1869–86.

Rubinstein, L.J. (1972). In *Tumours of the Central Nervous System*, Fascicle 6. Armed Forces Institute of Pathology, Washington DC, pp. 127–9.

Rubinstein, L.J. (1982). Diagnostic applicability of GFA protein immunoperoxidase staining. In *Tumours of the Central Nervous System*. Suppl. to Fascicle 6. Armed Forces Institute of Pathology. Washington, DC, p. S–25.

Rubinstein, L.J. (1985). Embryonal central neuroepithelial tumours and their differentiating potential. A cytogenetic view of a complex neuro-oncological problem. *Journal of Neurosurgery* **62**, 795–805.

Rubinstein, L.J. and Brucher, J.M. (1981). Focal ependymal differentiation in choroid plexus papilloma. An immunoperoxidase study. *Acta Neuropathologica* **53**, 29–33.

Scheithauer, B.W. (1984a). Surgical pathology of the pituitary: The adenomas, Part I. In Sommers, S.C. and Rosen, P.P. (eds), *Pathology Annual*, Part I. Appleton-Century-Crofts/Norwalk, Connecticut, pp. 317–74.

Scheithauer, B.W. (1984b). Surgical pathology of the pituitary: The adenomas, Part II. In Sommers, S.C. and Rosen, P.P. (eds), *Pathology Annual*, Part 2, Appleton-Century-Crofts/Norwalk, Connecticut, pp. 269–330.

Scheithauer, B.W. (1990). Tumours of the meninges: Proposed modifications of the World Health Organization classification. *Acta Neuropathologica* **80**, 343–54.

Schmechel, D., Marangos, P.J., Zis, A.P., Brightman, M.W. and Goodwin, F.K. (1978). Brain enolase as specific markers of neuronal and glial cells. *Science* **199**, 313–15.

Seeger, R.C., Brodeur, G.M., Sather, H., Dalton, A., Siegel, S.E., Wang, K.Y and Hammond, D. (1985). Association of multiple copies of the N-myc oncogene with rapid progression of neuroblastomas. *New England Journal of Medicine* **313**, 1111–16.

Sternberger, L.A. and Sternberger, N.H. (1983). Monoclonal antibodies distinguish phosphorylated and nonphosphorylated forms of neurofilaments in situ. *Proceedings of the National Academy of Sciences (USA)* **80**, 6126–30.

Tabaton, M., Whitehouse, P.J., Perry, G., Davies, P., Autilio-Gambetti, L. and Gambetti, P. (1988). Alz 50 recognizes abnormal filaments in Alzheimer's disease and progressive supranuclear palsy. *Annals of Neurology* **24**, 407–13.

Tanzi, R.E., McClatchey, A.I., Lamperti, E.D., Villa-Komaroff, L., Gusella, J.F. and Neave R.L. (1988). Protease inhibitor domain encoded by an amyloid protein precursor mRNA associated with Alzheimer's disease. *Nature* **331**, 528–30.

Taylor, C.R. (1986). Tumours of the ovary and testis. In Taylor, C.R. and Benington, J.C. (eds), *Major Problems in Pathology. Immunomicroscopy: A Diagnostic Tool for the Surgical Pathologist.* W.B.Saunders, Philadelphia, pp. 203–21.

Thomas, P. and Battifora, H. (1987). Keratins versus epithelial membrane antigen in tumour diagnosis: An immunocytochemical comparison of five monoclonal antibodies. *Human Pathology* **18**, 728–34.

Toyoshima, I., Yamamoto, A., Masamune, O. and Satake, M. (1989). Phosphorylation of neurofilament proteins and localization of axonal swellings in motor neuron disease. *Journal of Neurological Sciences* **89**, 269–77.

Toyohama, T., Lee, V.M-Y, Rorke, L.B., Marvin, M., McKay, R.D.G. and Trojanowski, J.Q. (1991). Nestin expression in human neuroepithelial development and tumours. *Journal of Neuropathology and Experimental Neurology* **50**, 292 (Abstract).

Vinters, H.V., Partridge, W.M. and Yang, J. (1988). Immunohistochemical study of cerebral amyloid angiopathy: Use of an antiserum to a synthetic 28–amino-acid peptide fragment of the Alzheimer's disease amyloid precursor. *Human Pathology* **19**, 214–22.

von Deimling, A., Janzer, R., Kleihues, P. and Wiestler, O.D. (1990). Patterns of differentiation in central neurocytoma. An immunohistochemical study of eleven biopsies. *Acta Neuropathologica (Berlin)* **79**, 473–9.

Vonsattel, J-D., Myers, R.H., Stevens, T.J., Ferrante, R.J., Bird, E.D. and Richardson, E.P.Jnr. (1985). Neuropathologic classification of Huntington's disease. *Journal of Neuropathology and Experimental Neurology* **44**, 559–77.

Walker, A.E., Robins, M. and Weinfeld, F.D. (1985). Epidemiology of brain tumours: The national survey of intracranial neoplasms. *Neurology* **35**, 219–26.

Wick, M.R., Scheithauer, B.W., Okazaki, H. and Thomas, J.E. (1982). Cerebral angioendotheliomatosis. *Archives of Pathology and Laboratory Medicine* **106**, 342–6.

Wick, M.R., Stanley, S.J. and Swanson, P.E. (1988). Immunohistochemical diagnosis of sinonasal melanoma, carcinoma and neuroblastoma with monoclonal antibodies against HMB-45 and anti-synaptophysin. *Archives of Pathology and Laboratory Medicine* **112**, 616–20.

Wiley, C.A., Schrier, R.D., Nelson, J.A., Lampert, P.W. and Oldstone, M.B.A. (1986). Cellular localization of human immunodeficiency virus infection within the brains of acquired immunodeficiency syndrome patients. *Proceedings of the National Academy of Science (USA)* **83**, 7089–93.

Wolozin, B. and Davies, P. (1986). A neuronal antigen in the brains of Alzheimer's patients. *Science* **232**, 648–50.

Yagashita, S., Itoh, Y., Shiozawa, T. and Tanaka, T. (1984). Ultrastructural observation on a colloid cyst of the third ventricle. *Acta Neuropathologica (Berlin)* **65**, 41–5.

Zuccarello, M., Sawaya, R. and Ray, M.B. (1987). Immunohistochemical demonstration of alpha-1–proteinase inhibitor in brain tumours. *Cancer* **60**, 804–09.

Zülch, K.J. (1979). Histological classification of tumours. *WHO* No. 21. Geneva.

8 ◆ *Immunocytochemistry applied to cytological specimens*

Carlos W.M. Bedrossian and Shahla Masood

Introduction

Oncologic pathology relies ever more frequently on cytologic specimens for early cancer diagnosis. The non-invasive nature of endoscopic procedures and fine needle aspiration biopsies enables sampling of virtually every organ of the body. As a result, cytopathology is called upon for the diagnosis and confirmation of solid tumours as well as haematologic malignancies. Routine stains such as Papanicolaou and May–Grunwald–Giemsa's methods are sufficient for establishing a diagnosis of malignancy. However, classification of tumours is more difficult and benefits from ancillary techniques (Coleman and Omerod, 1983). Both, electron microscopy and immunocytochemistry have been used for tumour classification based on patterns of differentiation (Bedrossian, 1992). This is easily accomplished by the combination of cytomorphology with immunocytochemistry/immunocytopathology (Bedrossian, 1990). For prognostication, some progress has been realized with the study of cytologic specimens by flow cytometry and image analysis (Koss et al., 1989). More recently, the use of hormone receptor assays and proliferative markers has expanded our repertoire in predicting prognosis.

The greatest advantage of cytopathology is in the follow-up of malignancy, by repeat collection of cytologic samples. The usefulness of cytopathology can be further expanded by correlating qualitative with quantitative information derived from flow cytometry and image analysis, both of which utilize immunologic markers. However, this approach may still fall short of answering prognostic and therapeutic questions, hence the upsurge of cell stem assays and hormone receptor assays in clinical practice. That these techniques have been adopted for the study of cytologic samples is a logical progression, a consequence of clinical needs and innovation in technology. In a sense, as cytopathology matures, it is becoming more clinically relevant and more scientifically precise. Rather than a paradox, this evolution should be viewed as a bridge between cell biology and clinical medicine. In this chapter, we will discuss the value of immunocytochemistry, both as an adjunct to cytopathology and hormone receptor assays, and as the basis for quantitative techniques, such as flow cytometry, image analysis.

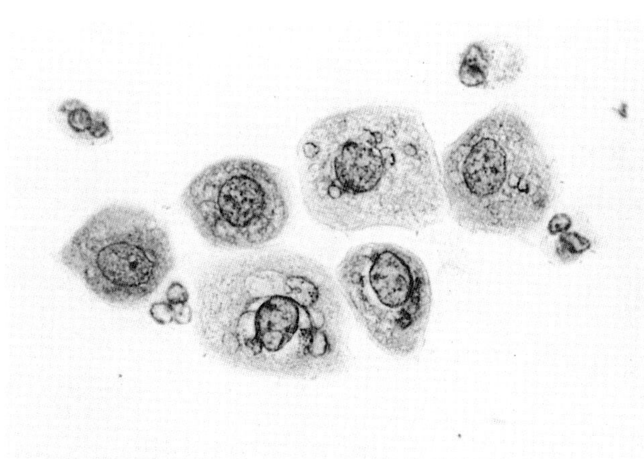

Fig. 8.1. Groups of cells stained for Chlamydia. Note immunopositivity in elementary bodies and vacuoles throughout the cytoplasm. (Courtesy of Prabodh Gupta, MD).

Immunocytopathology

Introduction

The evaluation of cellular activity is at the core of cytologic diagnosis. Reactive, hyperplastic and neoplastic cells display nuclear features that allow their recognition. Much more difficult, however, is the recognition of transformed cells, particularly when the neoplastic process masks or erodes their histogenetic derivation. Immunocytopathology is helpful in this regard by identifying cytoplasmic substances which may have been formed as a result of malignant transformation. Positivity for various markers, however, has to be correlated with morphologic features, particularly the manner by which the tumour cells relate to one another. Not to be forgotten is the wide application of immunocytopathology in the detection and classification of pathogenic organism in cytologic specimens (Fig. 8.1).

Ultrastructural basis of cell groupings

Cells of epithelial origin have a tendency to attach to their neighbours, and exfoliate in a cohesive fashion, either naturally or when retrieved artificially, by scraping, brushing or negative-pressure aspiration. When examined ultrastructurally, the boundaries between epithelial cells can assume certain configurations which are typical of their origin. Squamous cells have spaces between them, except where their prickly processes touch each other and are fastened by well-formed desmosomes. These correspond to the intercellular bridges seen by light microscopy. To fulfill acceptable criteria, desmosomes must be separated by a space no larger than 24 nm and small filaments must be seen, converging upon the lamina densa (hemidesmosomes) of each cell of the pair. Squamous cells invariably connect to other cells around their entire perimeter whereas columnar cells are more likely to show at least one free pole. In undisturbed sheets, squamous cells appear roughly as lozenges which demonstrate wide intercellular gaps but do not form true extracellular acinar spaces. Glandular cells, on the other hand, frequently form intracellular and extracellular lumina, into which microvilli or cilia will abut. Near the apex, these cells are fastened by long, tortuous terminal bars, which should not be confused with the terminal plates noted at the base of ciliated surfaces. At their sides, in a columnar row, glandular cells are always closely apposed to each other and their boundaries may appear either as straight lines or complex interdigitating lines of demarcation. The latter, particularly in cell clusters, resemble masonry work held together without the need of mortar, simply by their tight fit and inconspicuous pegs. Upon closer inspection these 'pegs' correspond to junctional complexes with no more than 5–10 nm between the two adjoining cell membranes. Even in cells relating to each other by straight membranes, small dilatations of the intercellular space may occur, which do not qualify as acini, but may resemble the bile canaliculi of liver cells. The presence of microvilli on the cell surface is not sufficient to substantiate glandular differentiation, unless they project into a space. For all practical purposes, cilia in a cytologic sample should be regarded as indicative of benignancy. However, ovarian and lung neoplasms often demonstrate cilia at the ultrastructural level, and occasionally these can be observed by light microscopy as well.

The cells of mesothelioma form very large clusters, connected to each other by tight junctions or true desmosomes. Their distinct surface characteristic is the presence of florid microvilli, very long and very slender (Fig. 8.2). These microvilli which may be noted even in the so-called 'mesenchymal' type of mesothelioma can also be outlined by epithelial membrane antigen (EMA) (Leong et al., 1990). The cytoplasm of mesothelial cells is rich in keratin proteins with minimal or no expression of carcinoembryonic antigen (CEA) (Warhol, 1984). When correlated to ultrastructural findings, these cytochemical features allow for the most reliable diagnosis of

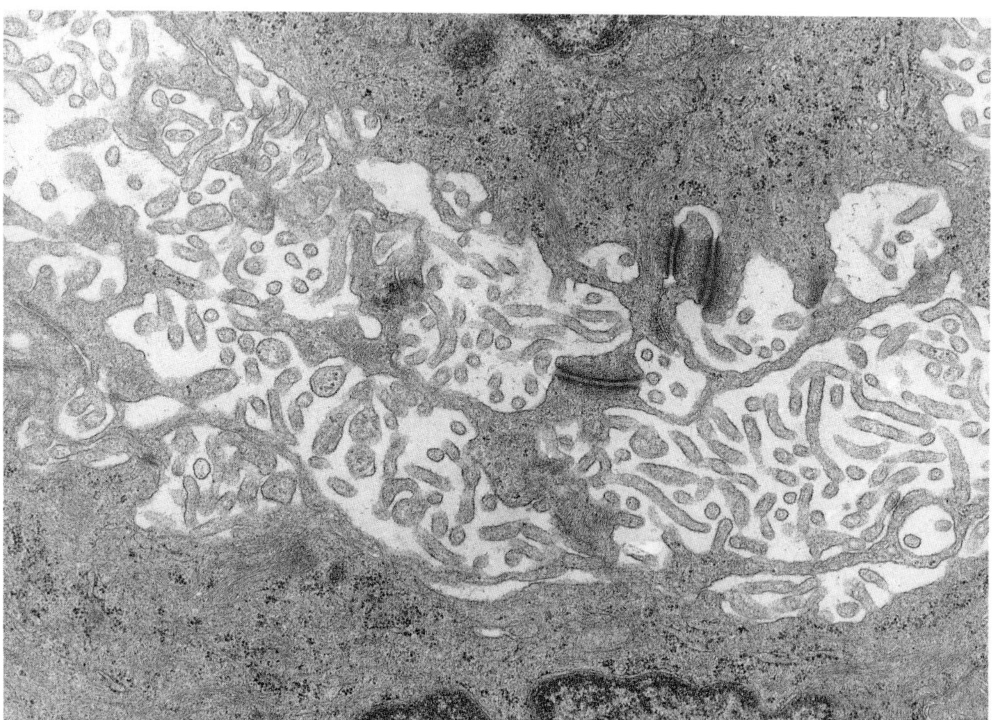

Fig. 8.2. Desmosome-like cell junction between two mesotheliomatous cells. The space traversed by slender microvilli corresponds to the thick membrane pattern of immunostain with EMA.

mesothelioma (Bedrossian et al., 1992). In malignant effusions, immunocytochemical panels aid in the distinction between mesothelioma and adenocarcinoma and in pin-pointing the primary site of metastatic malignancies (Mason et al., 1987).

Cells of non-epithelial origin shed in a non-cohesive fashion and lack cell junctions at the ultrastructural level. Macrophage have cytoplasmic projections of extreme irregular size and shape (pseudopods). Immature histiocytic cells may approximate up to 69 nm. They may display paired subplasmalemmal linear densities, but they never form true desmosomes. The same applies to lymphocytes which usually have relatively smooth surfaces, except in hairy cell leukemia where the cells have prominent filopodia. The greatest level of complexity in the contact between cells is exhibited by tumours of neuronal differentiation. Classical of this is the neuropil of neuroblastoma, but to a certain extent neuroendocrine cells (Kultchitsky cells of the gut and Kultchitsky-like cells of the lung) also have intertwined cytoplasmic process which do not need specialized functional structures to hold them together. Further identification of cell types require close scrutiny of the cell shape and the contents of the cytoplasm. Cytopathology is far superior to histopathology for this purpose. However, one should not regard them as competing disciplines, but rather as a complement to one another. The entire basis of morphologic diagnosis has to do with microscopic and ultrastructural level. There are antibodies directed against desmoplakin, the cement-like substance between two hemidesmosomes which have found some application in diagnostic pathology (Moll et al., 1986). Other antibodies can detect different cell surface markers, a practice highly in vogue among lymphoma specialists, interested in the immunologic classification of such neoplasms. Still another important category of antibodies enabled the elucidation of various cytoskeletal components responsible for the cells ability to acquire different shape, according to its function (Altmannsberger et al., 1984).

Cytoskeletal determinants of cell shape

The cytoskeleton is responsible for the structural integrity of the cell and serves as a supportive matrix for cytoplasmic organelles. A constant for all mammalian cells, the cytoskeleton is composed of structural proteins that vary according to the function of various cell types. With appropriate antibodies cytoskeletal components have been well characterized, ranging from 6 nm in thickness (microfilaments) to 25 nm (microtubules). In between, a wide variety of 10 nm 'intermediate' filaments have been recognized, and classified according to the tissues from which they were isolated: neurofilaments (neurons); glial filaments (astrocytes), vimentin (mesenchymal cells), desmin (muscle cells) and keratin (epithelial cells) (Table 8.1). Epithelial cells contain intermediate filaments in the cytoplasm, known as keratins. This complex family of proteins of various molecular weights can be detected by antibodies raised to a mixture of keratins (polyclonal antibodies) as well as to high or low molecular weight keratins (monoclonal antibodies). Even though theoretically possible, broad-spectrum, monoclonal antibodies directed against all Keratins are not currently available. In our practice we utilize two different polyclonal antibodies raised against epidermis, and two monoclonal antibodies, low molecular weight (35-B-H11) and high molecular weight (34-B-E12) cytokeratins. Battifora, since 1980, has successfully utilized two other monoclonal antibodies, AE1 and AE3, which recognize, respectively, low molecular weight and high molecular weight keratins. A number of antibodies with restricted specificity have also been utilized but their use depends on commercial availability of reagents, which varies in different markets. Useful applications of keratin antibodies includes: 1) detection of micrometastasis in lymph nodes and bone marrow biopsies; 2) diagnosis of thymoma in FNAs with small and large cells; and 3) diagnosis of mesothelioma in tumours with

Table 8.1. Classification of intermediate filaments

Epithelial	Keratin 40,000–68,000 daltons	Keratinizing and non-keratinizing epithelia
Neuronal	Neurofilament 68,000, 160,000 200,000 daltons	Neurons (CNS) Peripheral nerve
Glial	GFAP 55,000 daltons	Glia
Muscular	Desmin 53,000 daltons	Sarcomeric muscle
Mesenchymal	Vimentin 57,000 daltons	Fibroblasts; chondrocytes, macrophages; endothelial cells

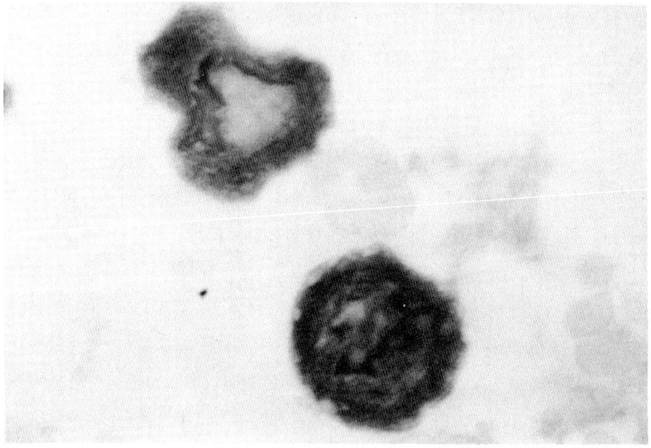

Fig. 8.3. Single cells from squamous carcinoma. Positivity for keratin outlines nuclei with sharp borders.

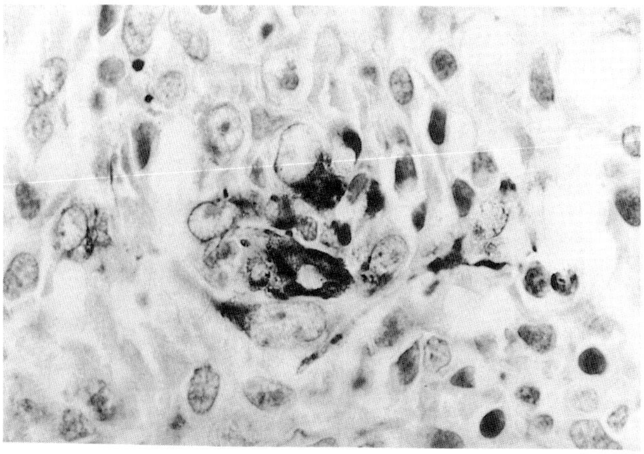

Fig. 8.4. Cell block from an FNA showing angio-sarcoma. Focal positivity for vimentin is noted in cells showing prominent nucleoli.

a predominant spindle-cell pattern and 4) distinction between carcinoma and lymphoma in effusions and aspirates. The latter application is particularly crucial when the cytologic sample shows only a few suspicious cells (Fig. 8.3).

The distribution of vimentin and keratin correlates very closely to the morphologic appearance of various cell types when visualized cytologically and by electron microscopy. Thus, spindle mesenchymal cells may show parallel intermediate filaments which curve to surround the nucleus and fuse at both ends of the cell. These will invariably stain for vimentin, and, depending on the direction of their differentiation for desmin, as well as actin and/or myosin. Keratin, on the other hand, creates a very dense perinuclear ring responsible for the neat endoplasmic ectoplasmic demarcation demonstrated by mesothelial cells. In cytologic samples, however, distribution of vimentin is not uniform within every tumour cell (Fig. 8.4). Vimentin cannot be taken as a marker of non-epithelial differentiation since it is positive in various carcinomas including those of the thyroid gland (Davila, 1988). Occasionally, in small cell carcinoma of the lung, intermediate filaments will form dense tufts next to the nuclei, the significance of which is not clear at present. The presence of neurofilament in small cell carcinomas of the lung and other neuroendocrine tumours is highly disputed. If proven correct, this would lend support to the theory of neural crest derivation for these neoplasms. However, more recent evidence suggests that all lung tumours derive from the same precursor: immature, small-granular mucous cells, the true reserve cells of the bronchial mucosa. These cells are totipotential, capable of evolving into ciliated, goblet, Kultchitsky-like and metaplastic squamous cells.

Differentiation markers

Cytoplasmic organelles are dispersed amongst the cytoskeleton and provide clues as to the origin of the cell, its degree of differentiation, as well as its functional state. The distribution and concentration of these organelles actually define the cell type as for example the parallel stacks of rough endoplasmic reticulum, indicative of immunoglobulin synthesis characteristic of plasma cells. Fibroblasts also display prominently dilated cisternae when synthesizing collagen, a property shared by other mesenchymal cells but not shared by plasma cells. By utilizing the proper histochemical and/or immunocytochemical stains, one can determine the direction of differentiation taken by various cell types and consequently elicit more specific diagnoses. This is particularly important when attempting to establish the primary origin of metastatic neoplasms.

Undifferentiated neoplasms

Malignant cells regress to a very primitive stage rendering their histogenesis impossible to discern by morphologic means. Alongside neoplastic transformation, synthesis of abnormal proteins may occur in the cytoplasm, partially resembling embryonic protein synthesis. Because carcinoembryonic antigen (CEA) was first detected in colonic neoplasms, it was believed to be specific for this type of tumour. Now we know that

CEA occurs in other tumours, particularly adenocarcinomas, regardless of the site of origin (Fig. 8.5). Other oncofetal markers (alpha-fetoprotein (AFP), human chorionic gonadotrophin (hCG), and human placental lactogen (hPL)) are expressed widely in neoplasms of various origins. CEA is a reliable marker to distinguish epithelial cells from lymphocytes and histiocytes in lymph nodes and epithelial cells from mesothelial cells in effusions and tissue sections (Silverman, 1987).

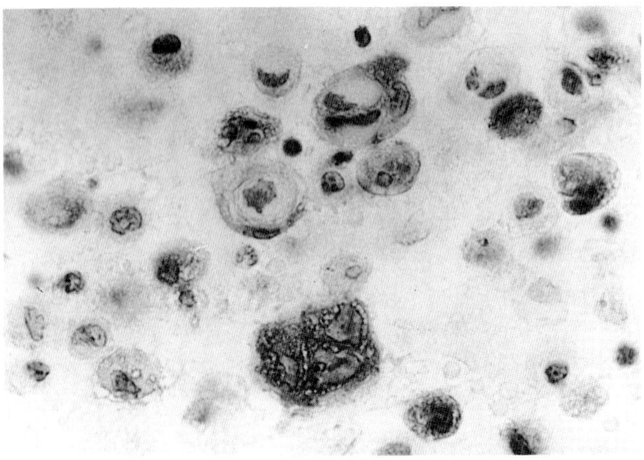

Fig. 8.5. Gastric carcinoma in pleural effusion. Notice CEA positive cells, some of which show the signet-ring appearance (PAP).

Germ cell tumours

A number of oncofetal markers permit the identification of germ cell tumours in gonadal and extragonadal sites, and to a certain extent, their subclassification (Szymendera et al., 1981). Thus, dysgerminoma is not associated with either AFP or hCG. The mononuclear cells which predominate in embryonal carcinoma contain AFP but not hCG; and the syncytiocytotrophoblastic giant cells of choriocarcinoma are positive for hCG but not AFP. Mononuclear cells show no immunostaining for hCG and the positivity for AFP is focal rather than diffuse, in the endodermal sinus tumour. The presence of oncofetal markers in a mediastinal tumour is not proof of extragonadal germ cell derivation. Carcinoma of the lung needs to be ruled out, since this tumour may occasionally be positive for AFP and hCG. Another oncofetal marker present in germ cell tumours is alpha-1-antitrypsin (A1AT) (Permanetter and Wiesinger, 1987). Interpretation of A1AT is problematic in poorly differentiated, large-cell, tumours of the mediastinum and retroperitoneum. In these cases the A1AT positivity is not helpful in distinguishing between carcinoma of the lung, histiocytic malignancy or a germ cell tumour with undifferentiated large cells. In general, CEA and the other oncofetal markers are more useful when utilized as part of a panel. This is exemplified by the differential diagnosis between germ cell tumours from carcinoma, lymphomas and histiocytic processes (Table 8.2).

Malignant lymphomas

Haematopoietic malignancies were the first neoplasms to be classified immunocytochemically by antibodies against surface markers. This approach however, is best applied to frozen sections or cell suspensions of unfixed material (Forbes and Leong, 1987). The latter can either be concentrated onto slides by cytocentrifugation, or dispersed further into a continuous flow of single cells which are paraded through the flow cytometer. Cytocentrifuged preparations may be stained with fluorescent dye and examined under the ultraviolet microscope. In flow cytometry, the individual cells are first tagged

Table 8.2. Differential diagnosis of germ cell neoplasms

	Germ cell tumour	Poor differential carcinoma	Histiocytic neoplasm	B-cell lymphoma
CEA	±	+	−	−
Keratin	−	+	−	−
Vimentin	−	−	±	−
LCA	−	−	+	+
AFP	+	±	−	−
Lysozyme	−	−	+	−
Lectin	−	−	+	−

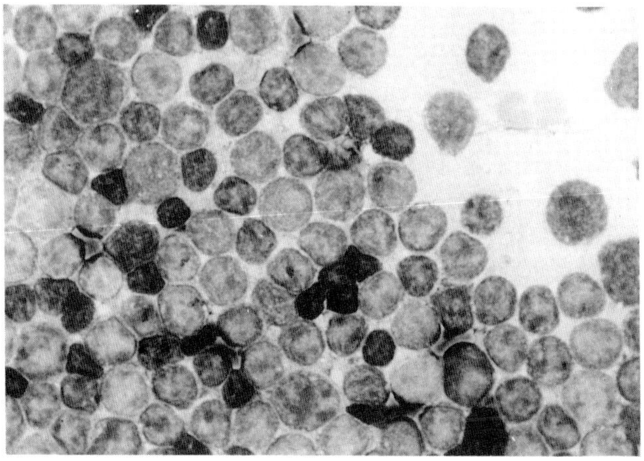

Fig. 8.6. B-cell lymphoma in pleural effusion. Notice large lymphocytes stained by the MGG technique (MGG X400).

with fluorescent probes and excited with argon or laser light source and the fluorescence measured by computer. Cytologically, a sizeable cell population of abnormal lymphocytes is noted in lymphoma (Fig. 8.6). In large cell lymphoma, monoclonality can be established by quantitatively determining the expression of light chains (Fig. 8.7). T-cell lymphomas are more difficult to recognize cytologically (Fig. 8.8). More than one light source can be used with different dyes suitable for multiparameter evaluation and, in this fashion, a large number of surface markers can be measured simultaneously, thus providing the phenotype of the lymphoma (Fig. 8.9). The advantage of flow cytometer is that it can measure many properties other than fluorescence with great sensitivity, objectivity and speed (10^5 cells/min). Disadvantage is that the cell being measured cannot be visually inspected as it is true in image analysis. Despite the powerful tool represented by flow cytometry, care should be taken in not over interpreting results. Positivity for a given mononuclear antibody by itself, is not indicative of malignancy, lymphoma, or even a subtype of lymphoma. Malignancy is best diagnosed by correlating tumour behaviour with architectural abnormalities in impeccable histologic sections of lymph node. The diagnosis of lymphoma is confirmed when non-neoplastic and metastatic processes are excluded by

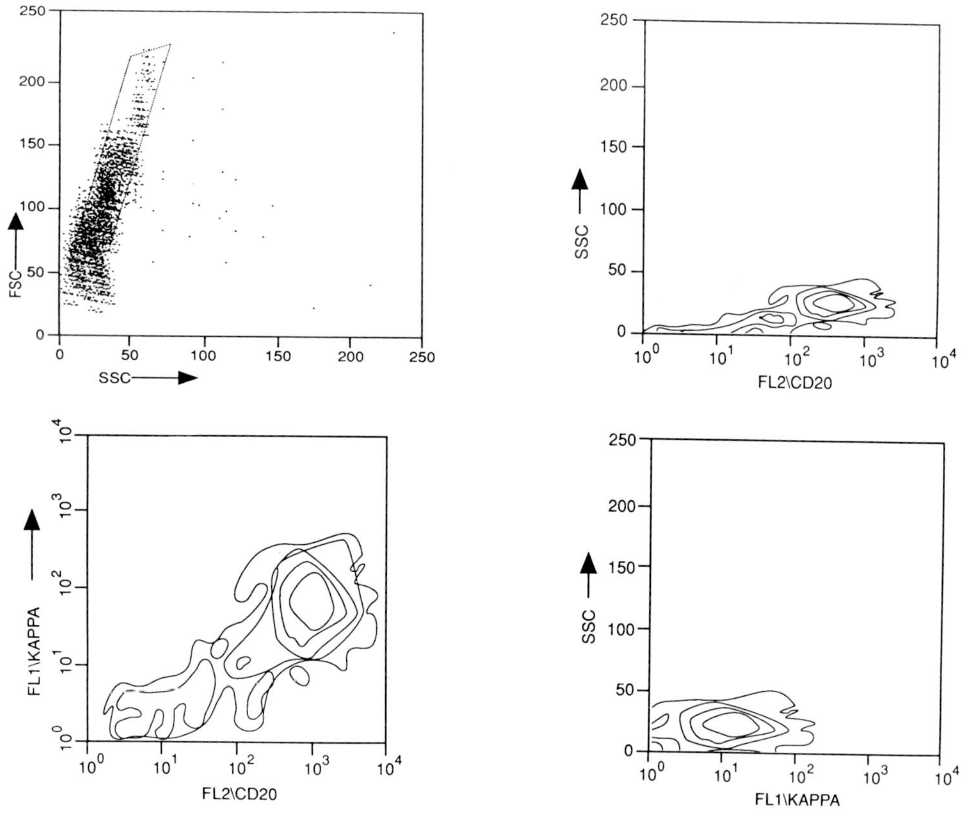

Fig. 8.7. Four-panel dot and contour plots of same large cell lymphoma shown in Fig. 8.6. Note expression of CD20 and Kappa light chain typical of B-cell lineage.

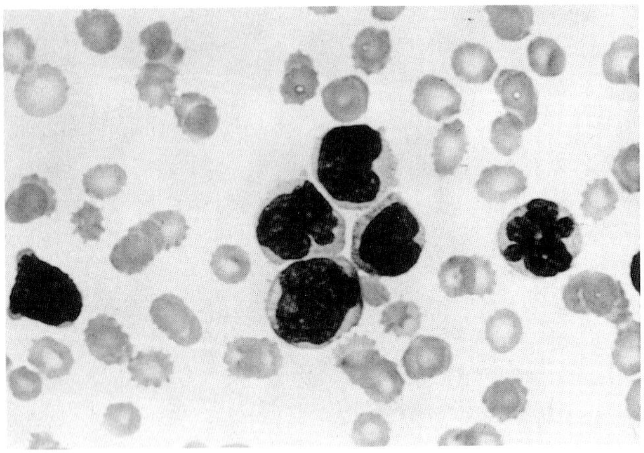

Fig. 8.8. T-cell lymphoma in pericardial fluid. Notice the irregular shape of the nuclei and negligible amount of cytoplasm – (MGG ×400).

cytomorphologic criteria and monoclonality is established by appropriate antibodies. The pattern of positivity in a battery of monoclonal antibodies in frozen sections and cell suspensions but not in formaldehyde fixed paraffin-embedded sections permits the subtyping of lymphomas.

The futility of utilizing monoclonal antibodies in paraffin sections of lymphoma cannot be overemphasized. Surface immunoglobulins are not detected at all, and cytoplasmic immunoglobulins are recognized with difficulty. This limits the use of paraffin sections only to the detection of immunoglobulins and light chains in large cell lymphomas. However, formaldehyde denatures immunoglobulins so that their occurrence in a tumour is totally unpredictable, and therefore meaningless for the purpose of classification. One leukocyte common antigen (T200) gives positive results in B5-fixed paraffin embedded tissues. IL1 and IL2 antibodies also work in paraffin-embedded tissues and recognize B cell lymphomas. The use of trypsinization has been utilized in an attempt to uncover antigenic sites on the surface cells. In our experience, trypsinization, often fails to accomplish this goal and may result in floating of the tissue section and uneven distribution of the immunostain.

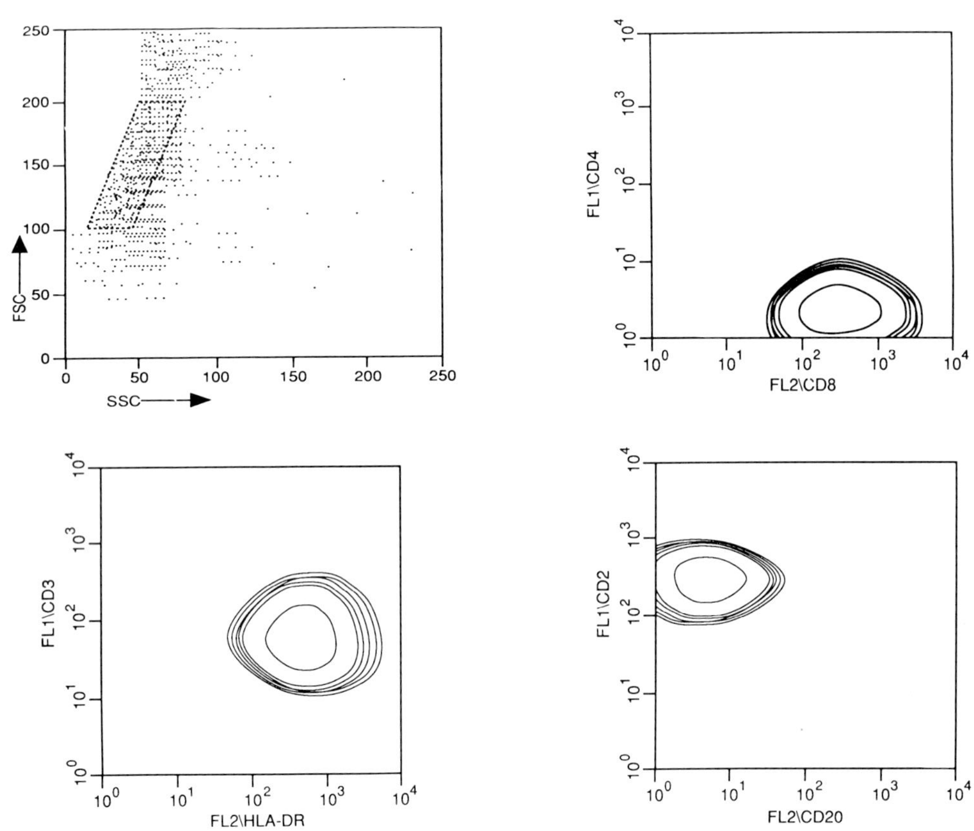

Fig. 8.9. Same T-cell lymphoma shown in Fig. 8.8 submitted for flow cytometry. The contour-plot distribution reveals expression of HLA-DR and CD8.

Table 8.3. Differential diagnosis of small cell carcinoma

	Small cell carcinoma	T-cell lymphoma	Neuro-blastoma	Rhabdomyo-sarcoma
CEA	–	–	–	–
Keratin (LMW)	+	–	–	–
NSE	+		+	–
Vimentin	–	–	–	+
LCA (T200)	–	+	–	–
Neuro-filament	–	–	+	–

There are, however, many polyclonal antibodies which can be utilized in routine paraffin sections and are helpful in the separation between lymphomas and other epithelial and non-epithelial small cell neoplasms (Table 8.3).

Immunocytochemical markers are not replacements for skilful histopathologic interpretation and careful clinicopathologic correlations in cases suspected of being lymphomas. Caution should be increased in interpreting lymphocytic processes occurring at extranodal sites because classification of lymphoma requires observation of the pattern of involvement of the lymph node architecture. In cytologic specimens it is often possible to diagnose lymphoma and classify it into large and small cell types. Further subclassification, however, is best accomplished by immunomarkers and flow cytometry.

Table 8.4. Ultrastructural distinction between mesothelioma and adenocarcinoma

Location	Mesothelioma	Adenocarcinoma
Cell surface	Microvilli evenly distributed around entire cell	Microvilli concentrated at poles
	Slender bushy microvilli	Short stubby microvilli
	No glycocalyceal bodies	Glycocalyceal bodies noted
Cell junctions	Apical tight junctions	Terminal bars near lumen
	Well-developed desmosomes	Poorly developed junctions
Cytoplasm	Tonofilaments surrounding the nucleus	Irregularly distributed intermediate filaments
	Abundant glycogen	Variable amount of glycogen
	No secretory granules	Numerous secretory granules

Adenocarcinomas

Mucin secretion is easily demonstrated by histochemical means and constitutes good evidence of glandular differentiation, a feature typical of adenocarcinomas. There are several ultrastructural features that support the diagnosis of adenocarcinoma (Table 8.4). Likewise, a number of markers exist that allow the recognition of adenocarcinoma in cytologic material. This is an important step in excluding mesothelioma. Ultrastructurally, it is not always possible to subtype adenocarcinomas but bronchioloalveolar carcinomas can be separated into mucinous Clara cell and Type II cell subtypes. Clara cell-derived neoplasms display large electron dense granules limited by a single membrane. Type II cell neoplasma – the rarest of the three variants – contain lamellated inclusion bodies, typical of the surfactant substance they produce. These products can also be demonstrated by histochemical and immunocytochemical methods. CEA is a good indicator of glandular differentiation and is present in virtually all adenocarcinomas, particularly colon and lung. EMA also distinguishes adenocarcinomas including papillary non-secreting tumours, without regard to its site of origin (Fig. 8.10). Secretory piece, initially described in breast carcinoma, is another general

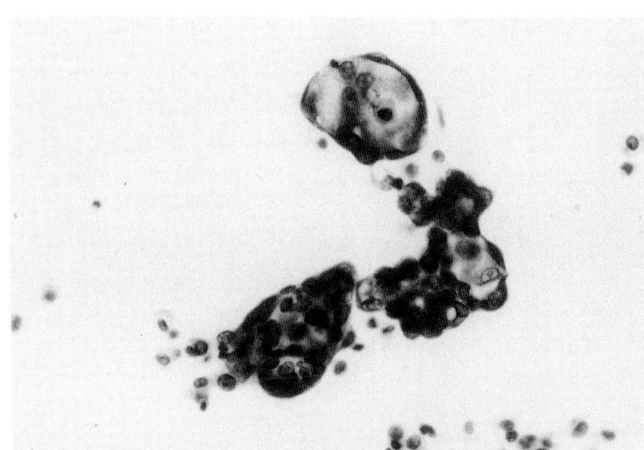

Fig. 8.10. Papillary group of cells form ovarian carcinoma stained for EMA. Note strong cytoplasmic positivity in contrast to the negative cells in the background.

marker for adenocarcinomas, but is not as frequently positive as CEA. In our hands, this marker has been consistently positive in renal cell carcinomas. By electron microscopy these tumours demonstrate abundant glycogen and lipid droplets. Even though mesothelioma also contains glycogen and lipid, these substances occur in small amounts and this tumour displays hyaluronic acid (Table 8.4).

Neuroendocrine tumours

Until relatively recently, the neural crest was believed to be histogenetically related to a number of diverse neoplasms capable of endocrine activity or at least, of elaborating neuroendocrine substances. Current theory, however, favours the existence of totipotential cells in various tissues, capable of neuroendocrine differentiation, without intervention of the neural crest or another neuroendocrine structure per se. This concept is more easily reconciled with the recognition of neuroendocrine tumours outside the endocrine system and in virtually every major organ of the body. The unifying characteristic of these tumours is not embryologic, but morphologically expressed at the ultrastructural and functional level. Neuroendocrine tumours share a common cytomorphology represented by small, blue round cells. By electron microscopy, these cells contain variable amounts of neuroendocrine granules (Akhtar et al., 1992). Immunocytochemically, neuroendocrine activity is expressed in terms of an enzymatic apparatus (neuron-specific enolase); a protein-matrix in granular form (chromogranins); and various substances with neuroendocrine activity (polypeptides, biologically active proteins, hormones, neurotransmitters). All of these have been explored as markers of neuroendocrine differentiation in cytologic material. A useful test is to utilize chromogranin positivity to confirm the diagnosis of islet cell tumour in a fine needle aspirate (Fig. 8.11). Melanomas can be diagnosed immunocytochemically by demonstrating S100 or HMB45 in cells that lack pigment or may otherwise simulate other tumours (Martinez et al., 1990).

Non-epithelial neoplasms

In comparison with epithelial antibodies, mesenchymal markers are less numerous and much more poorly understood. The Factor VIII-related antigen was initially heralded as an endothelial cell marker but it has been detected in other mesenchymal neoplasms. Angiotensin converting enzyme (ACE) is another endothelial cell marker but its utilization in surgical pathology has not been tested as yet. Myogenic differentiation can be detected by the presence of desmin, a broad indicator of cytoplasmic contractile differentiation (Fig. 8.12). The marker is positive in smooth and striated muscle cells as well as myoepithelial cells. Desmin is most consistently positive in smooth muscle, even though striated muscle cells will reveal a faint blush. A common problem in oncologic pathology is the differential between embryonal rhabdomyosarcoma, malignant melanoma or a histiocytic malignancy. Vimentin is of no help since it will stain all three of these neoplasms. The skeletal muscle markers are consistently negative in melanoma and histiocytic

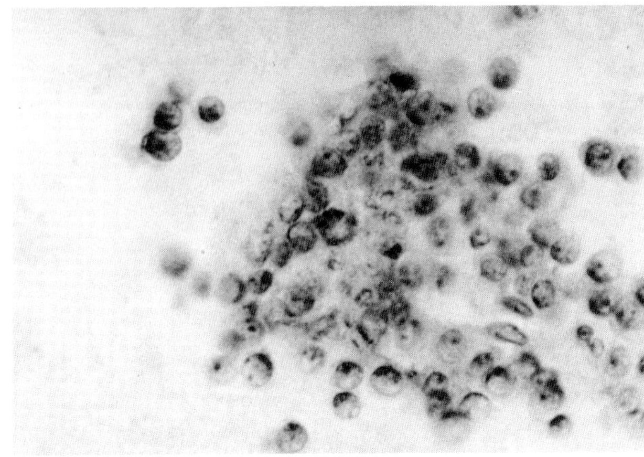

Fig. 8.11. Islet cell tumour stained for chromogranin. Note small cohesive cells with a granular pattern of positivity in the cytoplasm.

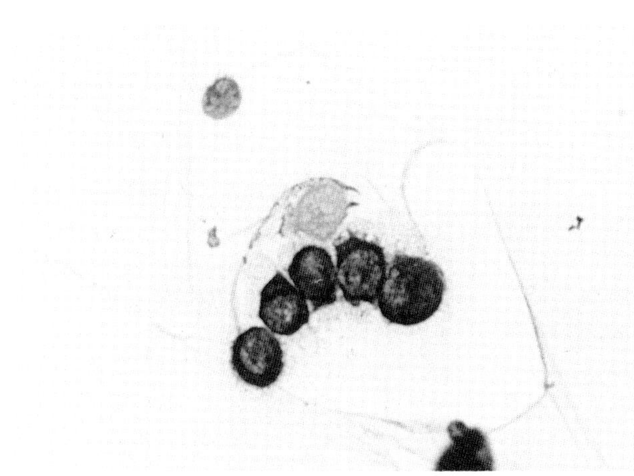

Fig. 8.12. Embryonal rhabdomyosarcoma stained for desmin. Notice high N/C ratio and strong cytoplasmic positivity of the tumour cells.

neoplasms. S100, however, has been of dubious help, since it will occasionally be positive in histiocytes as well as large lymphocytes (Vanstapel et al., 1986). Naevi, melanomas, neurofibromas and Schwannomas have been consistently positive with S100. There is currently a profusion of 'specific' cell markers, described at the rate of one per issue of at least one journal every month. However, until their utility withstands the test of time, one should refrain from stockpiling an arsenal of antibodies, in search of magic markers.

Most sarcomas diagnosed cytologically are derived from fine needle aspirations (FNAs), and more rarely, malignant effusions. These preparations show non-cohesive malignant cells which appear anaplastic. It is helpful to classify these tumours into morphologic categories. According to the predominant cell type: spindle, pleomorphic or epithelioid. Further classification into high grade and low grade may be of assistance in the treatment of the lesion, but is difficult to accomplish. since the neoplasms may be heterogeneous. FNAs from multiple sites may be more preferable than a single incisional biopsy in evaluating the degree of heterogeneity. The latter may not be representative and may ruin the chances for a limb-saving form of therapy by disturbing the vascular supplies. Sarcomas may be classified also, according to their ultrastructural and immunocytochemical feature (Table 8.5).

Table 8.5. Staining characteristics of mesothelioma and adenocarcinoma

Type of stain	Mesothelioma	Adenocarcinoma
Routine stain	Two-tone appearance with Papanicolaou stain	Homogeneously distributed stain
	Peripheral blebs with Romanowski's stain	No peripheral blebs noted
Special stains	Cytoplasm contains PAS (+) digestible material (glycogen)	Glycogen content is variable
	Extracellular space contains Alcian blue (+) material removable by hyaluronidase	No hyaluronic acid present in extracellular space
Immuno-stains	CEA consistently negative	CEA consistently positive
	EMA variably positive with frequently 'thick' membrane pattern	EMA frequently positive in cytoplasm and cell periphery
	Both low and high molecular weights keratin positive	Positive only with low molecular weight keratin

Note: CEA = carcinoembryonic antigen; EMA = epithelial membrane antigen; PAS = periodic acid-Schiff

The metastatic work-up

Cytopathologists can play a very important role in elucidating the primary site of widely metastatic tumours. This can be accomplished by the use of fine needle aspiration (FNA) in conjunction with immunocytochemistry and electron microscopy. The cytopathologist is frequently called to task, in elucidating tumours that spread to lymph nodes, the liver or the retroperitoneum. The same applies to lymph nodes of the supraclavicular and mediastinal areas where the combination of cytomorphology, ultrastructure and immunocytochemistry can pay handsome dividends. The differential diagnosis of tumours found in lymph nodes may be quite extensive (Table 8.6).

Table 8.6. Metastatic work-up

Primary neoplasm	Immuno-diagnostic markers	Ultrastructural features
Prostate	PSA PAP	Short microvilli Abundant organelles
Thyroid	Thyroglobulin Calcitonin	Amorphous material Electron-dense granules
Breast	Lactalbumin Lactoferrin	Intracytoplasmic lumina
Lung	CEA Surfactant	Fluffy granules Lamellar bodies
Kidney	Secretory piece	Glycogen granules Lipid droplets
Liver	AFP, HBSA	Bile canaliculi Bizarre mitochondria
Pancreas	DV Pan 2	Small secretory granules Short microvilli
Ovary	CA 125	Peripheral granules Abundant microvilli
Adrenal	Monoclonals	Mitochondria with tubulovesicular crystal
Thymus	Keratin LCA	Many cell junctions Paucity of organelles
Testicle	AFP PLP Spl, BhCG	Multidirectional differentiation Nucleolonema

Fine needle aspirates

On-site, immediate evaluation of FNAs allow utilization of the material for special studies. Rapid evaluation of the adequacy of the biopsy in accomplished by examination of a drop of the aspirated material by means of Diff-Quik or the fast Papanicolaou method. The remainder of the material should remain in suspension for further study by electron microscopy and immunocytochemistry. Tumours of the head and neck may be classified in FNAs (Bedrossian et al., 1989). Occasionally, immunocytochemical detections of calcitonin allows confirmation of the diagnosis of medullary carcinoma of the thyroid (Fig. 8.13). Retroperitoneal FNAs should be assayed for prostatic markers in the male and markers of ovarian neoplasia in the female. In the liver, the finding of cells with squamous differentiation invariably represent metastatic lung carcinoma in male or female smokers. Second in frequency is cervical carcinoma in the female or oesophageal carcinoma in the male. Metastatic adenocarcinoma must be differentiated from hepatocellular carcinomas, a task made possible by the use of immunocytochemistry (Bedrossian, 1989). This can also be accomplished by electron microscopy, with demonstration of bizarre mitochondria and bile canaliculi in primary liver cell tumours which are often positive for alpha fetoprotein (AFP). Adenocarcinomas from lung and the GI tract are usually CEA positive, whereas lactalbumin positivity favours breast carcinoma. None of these markers can be interpreted in absolute terms. In contrast, thyroglobulin is virtually pathognomonic for origin from follicular cells of the thyroid (Davila, 1988). Other very specific cell markers include: prostate-specific antigen and prostatic acid phosphatase, positive in prostatic carcinoma; GFAP, positive in tumours of glial origin, and surfactant apoprotein, positive in type II cell neoplasms of the lung.

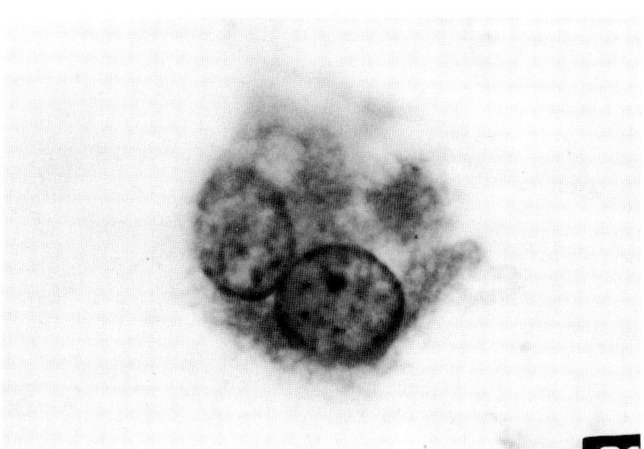

Fig. 8.13. Calcitonin-positive cell in medullary carcinoma of the thyroid. Note binucleation and square shape of abundant cytoplasm.

Malignant effusions

One of the greatest challenges to the cytopathologist is the differentiation between mesothelioma and adenocarcinoma. This difficulty extends to surgical pathology where both papillary and tubulo–acinar neoplasms can be encountered in very minute tissue biopsies. In cytologic samples, the presence of very large individual cells with clear demarcation between endoplasm and ectoplasm favours mesothelioma. However, in cell clusters, adenocarcinoma and mesothelioma may form tridimensional structures which are very difficult to distinguish from one another. The presence of intracytoplasmic lumina is not an absolute criterion for mesothelioma since adenocarcinomas, particularly of breast and lung origin, may also demonstrate this feature. By electron microscopy, however, such lumina as well as the apical pole of mesothelial cells are rich in long, slender and intertwining microvilli, not commonly seen in adenocarcinomas. By immunocytochemistry, mesotheliomas are negative for CEA, show a two-tone positivity for cytokeratin and display a thick rim of positivity for EMA (Leong and Stevens, 1991; Bedrossian et al., 1992) (Fig. 8.14). Adenocarcinomas are strongly positive for CEA and

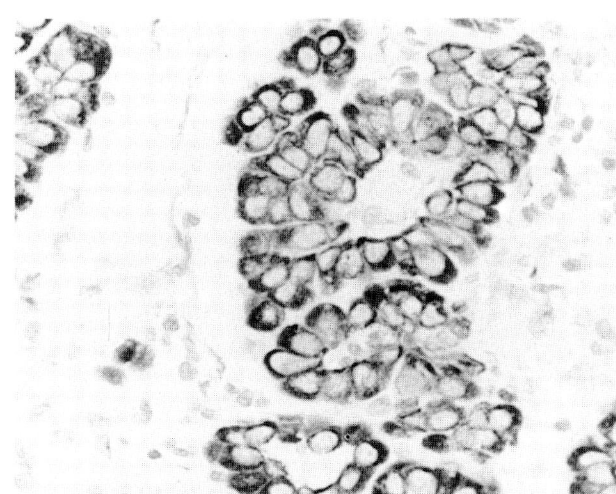

Fig. 8.14. Mesothelioma stained for EMA. The nuclei are spared but the immunostain outlines the cytoplasm in a thick membrane-like pattern.

lack the thick membrane pattern with EMA (Mason et al., 1987). Squamous cell carcinomas exfoliate single cells but are rare in effusions. The CEA is negative in squamous cell tumours whereas high and low molecular weight cytokeratins are positive, but lack the two-tone quality. The EMA is weakly positive in squamous cell carcinoma but without the thick membrane pattern noted in mesothelioma. Because mesothelioma carries such a high risk of medicolegal litigation a combination of cytomorphologic, histochemical immunocytochemical and ultrastructural features ensures the greatest reliability in its diagnosis (Fig. 8.15).

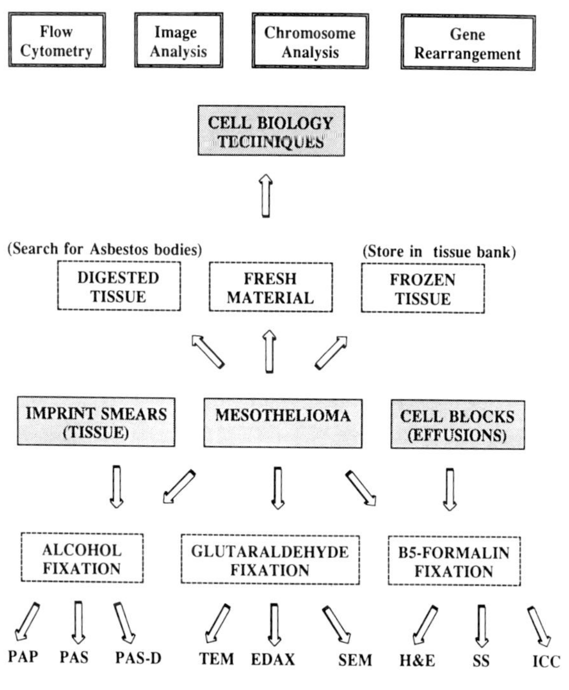

PAP: Pap Stain; PAS: Periodic acid Schiff; PAS-D: Periodic acid Schiff with diastase digestion; TEM: Transmission EM; EDAX: Energy dispersive analysis; SEM: scanning EM; H&E: Hematoxylin and Eosin; SS: Special Stains; ICC: Immunocytochemistry

Fig. 8.15. Multimodal approach to the diagnosis of mesothelioma. The combination of methods shown above can be applied to cytologic as well as to tissue specimens.

Technical considerations

Effusions of the serous cavities and FNAs are the ideal target for the use of immunocytochemistry in cytologic specimens. Cytocentrifuge and cell block preparations are preferred over smears since the cells of interest are concentrated more facilitating the contact of antibodies and their target. We favour cell blocks because multiple section can be obtained. The results are more easily comparable with existing tissue sections and histotechnologist are more familiar with cell blocks than with smears. Alcohol-fixed cytospins and B5-formalin when utilized, provide a nice balance of fixation. Intermediate filament results are lost in the cytospins while differentiation markers give good results in the cell blocks. The counterstain is of greater importance in cytologic preparations than in tissue sections because it enables a definition of malignant features in groups that are positive or negative for immunocytochemistry even in cell blocks when the architecture of cell groups is better preserved. The counterstain is extremely helpful in enhancing the nuclear detail of the positive cells.

Oestrogen and progesterone receptors

It has been known for many years that sex steroid hormones play a role in the development growth and behaviour of certain tumours. Hormonal manipulation has been shown to be effective in the management of a significant number of patients with breast, prostate and gynaecological malignancies.

Hormone receptor analysis is traditionally performed on surgically removed specimens. However, there are situations where surgical specimens are not available or suitable for such analysis. In these circumstances, cytologic material such as FNAs, imprints and exfoliated cells in malignant effusions can be utilized for oestrogen and progesterone receptor analysis. Fine needle aspiration biopsy offers a suitable alternative for hormone receptor analysis in several circumstances. First, in inoperable cases and metastatic or recurrent tumours in which the size and the accessibility to surgical biopsy presents a problems; secondly, in selected cases in which preoperative irradiation or presurgical therapy are the initial treatment options; thirdly, in advanced tumours where serial hormone receptor studies may potentially provide information regarding response to therapy. Fine needle aspiration biopsy is an easy, cost-effective and non-traumatic procedure which permits sampling of several areas of the same tumour and allows better assessment of hormone receptor heterogeneity (Masood, 1989; Katz et al., 1990; Masood, 1991).

Imprint preparations have also been utilized for hormone receptor analysis and are recommended for tumours that are too small or ill-defined to permit conventional sampling for hormone receptor analysis (Masood and Johnson, 1987; Masood, 1988). It has also been possible to show expression of hormone receptors in cytologic preparation obtained from malignant effusions (McCarty et al., 1980; Masood, 1990).

This review summarizes the characteristics of oestrogen and progesterone receptors with emphasis on the application of cytochemical techniques in assessment of sex steroid hormone receptors in cytologic samples.

Definition and characteristics of oestrogen and progesterone receptors

Oestrogen, in common with other steroid hormones, regulate gene expression in target cells through their interaction with specific macromolecular binding proteins called 'receptors.' Receptors are normally found in target tissue such as breast and female reproductive organs. Recent studies suggest that the oestrogen-free receptor is localized predominantly in the nucleus, where it is loosely bound until its association with oestradiol converts the receptor to an active form with the ability to bind tightly in the genome (Welshons et al., 1984). Initially, the oestrogen receptor (ER) associates with low affinity type II receptors within the cytoplasm and then enters the nucleus by virtue of the high affinity receptors in the nucleus. The activated ER-complex is believed to bind with chromatin, resulting in specific changes in gene expression, leading to synthesis of new messenger RNA an proteins characteristic of the hormone's cellular effect. Activation of ER stimulates transcription of progesterone receptor mRNA. Binding of progesterone receptor (PgR) with progesterone then induces synthesis of up to 100 proteins, including growth and mitogenic factors (Martin and Sheridan, 1982).

Pattern of expression and prognostic value

Among many tumours tested for the presence of ER, PgR and other steroid hormone receptors, breast and gynaecological tumours have shown the most consistent pattern of expression. The prognostic, diagnostic and therapeutic implications of hormone receptors in management and follow up of patients with breast and gynaecological malignancies are also well established.

Breast

In American women with breast cancer, expression of ER is seen in 77 per cent of cases, while the frequency of PgR positivity is 55 per cent. Basically, tumours that are both ER+ and PgR+ are regarded as being hormone responsive, while cancers that are hormonally non-responsive are often ER− and PgR−. Tumours that are of a more dubious hormone responsive nature are either ER+, PgR− or ER− and PgR+. Determination of hormone receptor also provides valuable information in predicting the risk of recurrence and metastasis in primary breast tumours (Chevalier et al., 1988); and for choosing both adjuvant regimes and hormone therapy for patients with disseminated disease (Osborne, 1984).

Ovary

In the last few years, it has been recognized that many primary ovarian carcinomas and their metastasis are rich in oestrogen and progesterone receptors (Lautta, 1984). Since then, the prognostic and therapeutic value of sex steroid hormone receptors in ovarian tumours have been under intense investigation. However, the results of these studies have been controversial and no clear guidelines are yet available. Nevertheless, cooperative studies with large numbers of patients are required to definitely evaluate the role of oestrogen and progesterone receptors in management of patients with ovarian cancer (Richman et al., 1988). Meanwhile, assessment of hormone receptors may be of some value in determining the primary site of tumours of unknown origin as well as providing a basis for possible new therapeutic modalities such as the use of radiolabelled ER ligands for imaging and treatment of hormone receptor rich tumours (Lorincz et al., 1985).

Endometrium

Clinical evidence reported in the literature supports the concept that response to hormonal therapy and prognosis in endometrial cancer are related to the steroid hormone receptor status of these tumours. While some investigators have demonstrated a better prognosis for ER positive and PgR positive endometrial cancer, others have (1988) reported significant relationship only between PgR content and survival (Creasman et al., 1985; Ehrlich et al., 1988). The role of progesterone receptor in management of advanced or recurrent endometrial cancer is also supported by the others. In the cumulative world literature, the response to progestin for PgR positive endometrial cancer has been reported to be 72 per cent, while the response rate for PgR negative endometrial cancer is reportedly 12 per cent (Bernradd et al., 1980).

Cervix

Oestrogen and progesterone receptors have been demonstrated in normal, premalignant lesions and neoplastic processes of the cervix. Sporadic reports in the literature regarding prognostic significance of hormone receptors in cervical cancer has shown mixed results. Nevertheless, Potish et al. (1986) suggested that clinical stage hormone receptor level independently predicts survival in patients with cervical cancer. Despite the independent prognostic value of receptors in cervical cancer, their therapeutic utility remains to be proven. Generally, cervical cancer is refractory to endocrine therapy. Thus, the value of oestrogen and progesterone receptor determination in cervical cancer may be limited to select poor prognostic groups of patients for inclusion into a more aggressive chemotherapy regimen.

Hormone receptor analysis

Biochemical assays

Biochemical assays were among the first to be developed and are now the 'standard' by which other methods are compared. These assays utilize a tumour extract in which radioligands combine with receptors to form a steroid-receptor complex. Following separation of bound from unbound radioligands, the bound hormone is measured and the quantity of hormone receptor calculated. Separation may be accomplished either by absorption to dextran-coated charcoal (DCC) or by sucrose density gradient centrifugation. The DCC technique is the most commonly used.

Current biochemical assays suffer form some inherent disadvantages. Interlaboratory variation in biochemical assays may be considerable factors such as dissociation of the non-covalently bound marker, contamination by traces of heavy metal or degradation of the receptor in storage or processing may influence the procedure. Furthermore, anti-oestrogen therapy, high dose oestrogen therapy, non-specific binding and exogenous oestradiol may alter the results.

Additionally, the biochemical methods require ultracentrifugation equipment, scintillation counters and radiolabelled hormones. Thus, they are suitable only for large laboratories. Furthermore, biochemical assays cannot accurately assess tumour heterogeneity and may be completely unsuitable for small lesions or cases where only a small amount of tumour tissue is available. Above all, the predictive value of the biochemical assays is less than sterling, since only 55–60 per cent of patients with biochemical receptor positive tumours respond to endocrine therapy and about 10 per cent of patients with receptor negative tumours respond. Thus, the need for practical tests that are simpler, less expensive and less sensitive to variation than the commonly used biochemical assays has been well recognized.

Cytochemical assays

Fluorescent technique The fluorescent technique introduced by Lee (1978) employs oestradiol linked to bovine serum albumin (BSA), coupled to fluorescein isothiocyanate (FITC). Progesterone is linked to BSA and coupled to tetramethylrhodamine isothiocyanate (TMRITC). This procedure is now patented as Fluoro-Cep (Zeus Technologies, Inc., Raritan, New Jersey). In a number of studies, the fluorescent technique has shown good correlation with the biochemical assay. Indeed, reported sensitivity, specificity as well as positive and negative predictive values for prediction of the clinical response rate are almost comparable to those reported for the biochemical assay (Chen et al., 1989; Lee, 1984).

The fluorescent technique may identify the lower affinity type II cytoplasmic oestrogen binding proteins rather than the high affinity/type I nuclear oestrogen receptor measured biochemically. This latter issue has been raised as a strong point against the fluorescent technique. However, the good results of this assay as reported in the literature may be explained by the frequent coexistence of cytoplasmic and nuclear ER receptors, as demonstrated by Lee (1984). He clearly showed that, for comparative purposes, both the cytoplasmic and nuclear ER assay appear to be useful for identification for ER positive tumours, demonstrating 94–97 per cent concordance (Fig. 8.16).

Immunoperoxidase technique

This technique, utilizing monoclonal antibody to nuclear ER or PgR receptors and peroxidase-

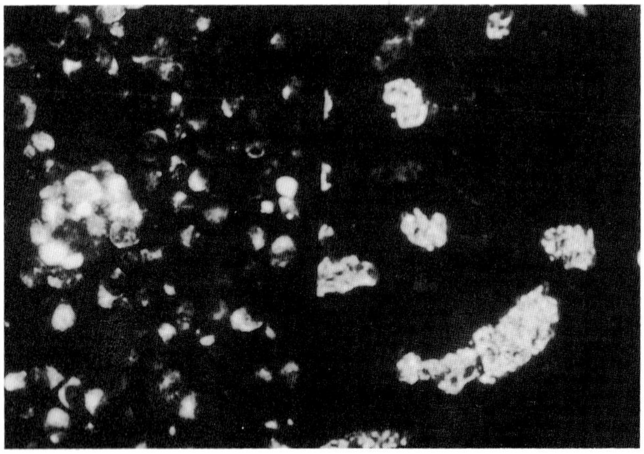

Fig. 8.16. Breast carcinoma. (A) (right) malignant effusion with positive cells for ER, by immunofluorescence. (B) (left) corresponding tissue section showing immunofluorescent nests of ER-positive cells.

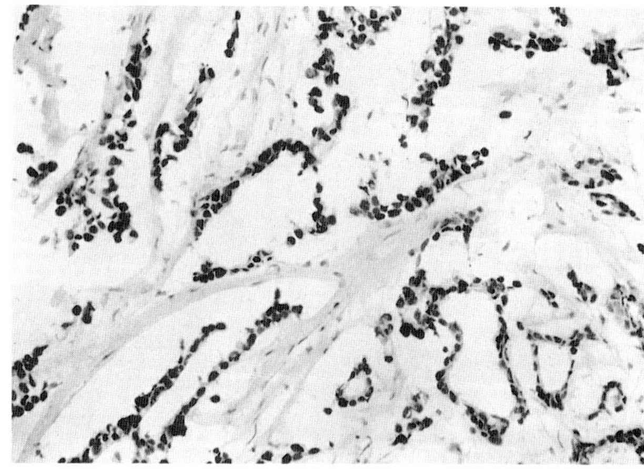

Fig. 8.17. Same neoplasm shown in Fig. 8.16B. Note ER-positivity by the immunoperoxidase technique in neoplastic ductal cells.

antiperoxidase for visualization, is applicable to paraffin or frozen tissue sections and to cytologic preparations. ER monoclonal antibodies are produced by hybridomas utilizing rats immunized with purified receptor from MCG-7 type human breast cancer cell (Green et al., 1980). Typically, a rat monoclonal antibody binds to human oestrophilin in tissue or cells on a microscope slide. A goat antibody forms a bridge between the anti-oestrophilin monoclonal antibody and a rat antibody bound to horseradish peroxidase. After washing, the bound enzyme bearing complex reacts with a chromogenic substance to form a coloured substance at the receptor site, yielding brown nuclear staining. This procedure is available through a commercial kit (ER-ICA) Abbott Laboratories, Chicago, Illinois. More recently, a similar kit has been made available for progesterone receptor (PgR-ICA). Data concerning concordance of hormone receptor immunocytochemical assay with the biochemical procedure are numerous and the results are excellent (Masood, 1991a).

The immunoperoxidase technique is attractive not only for its binding to the nuclear ER or PgR receptors but also for the ability to utilize fresh, frozen or formalin-fixed paraffin embedded specimens. This technique is also easily adaptable to cytologic material including FNAs (Fig. 8.17).

The use of paraffin block material is well suited for retrospective studies. For example, utilizing protease and paraffin-embedded material, Barnes and Masood (1991) demonstrated a strong correlation between ER patterns in *in situ* and invasive breast carcinoma within the same breast. This method also offers a reliable alternative when tissue is unavailable or not suitable for biochemical assay or conventional immunocytochemical assay on frozen tissue.

Cytologic preparations for hormone receptor assays

Imprint preparations

Imprint cytology, introduced by Dudgeon and Patrick in 1927, has been applied to a wide variety of organs and tissues. The value of this technique in now firmly established and it is utilized in some institutions as an adjunct to frozen sections. Steroid hormone receptors can be analysed in imprint preparations with either the fluorescent or immunoperoxidase technique. It is already demonstrated that assessment of ER and PgR using imprint preparation is comparable to that obtained from conventional cytochemical techniques on frozen sections as well as with DCC (Table 8.7). The first report by Masood and Johnson on the value of imprint cytology in cytochemical detection of steroid hormone receptors in breast cancer appeared in 1987. They utilized the fluorescent cytochemical method to study ER and PgR receptors in frozen sections and imprint preparations. The imprint method yielded a 90 per cent concordance with the DCC biochemical method in this respect was superior to the frozen sections. Another study demonstrated good concordance with the DCC biochemical method using

Table 8.7. Summary of concordance between cytochemical hormone receptor assay on imprint preparations and biochemical assay of excised surgical specimen

Authors	No. of cases	Site	Concordance ER(%)	PgR(%)	Technique
Masood and Johnson (1987)	42	Breast	90	90	Fluoro-Cep
Masood (1992)	45	Ovary	91	93	Fluoro-Cep
DeRosa et al. (1989)	47	Breast	92.3	92.3	ER-ICA PgR-ICA
Masood (1992)	214	Breast	95	94	ER-ICA PgR-ICA
Total	348		92	92	

Notes
ER = Oestrogen receptor
PgR = Progesterone receptor
Fluoro-Cep = Fluorescent cytochemical technique
ER-ICA = Oestrogen receptor immunocytochemical assay
PgR-ICA = Progesterone receptor immunocytochemical assay

Source: From Masood, S. (1992). Sex hormone receptors in cytologic material, *Cytopathology annual* **4**, 77-102.

imprint preparation in ovarian cancer (Masood, 1988). These studies demonstrated that cytologic material is adequate to depict the presence of hormone receptors using the fluorescent technique.

More recently, good results have been demonstrated with the immunoperoxidase technique for ER and Pgr assays in touch preparations (DeRosa et al., 1989). It is also shown that storage at −80°C for up to 56 weeks is possible without loss of reactivity, potentially making assays more flexible and economical.

Thus, imprint preparations are suitable for sex steroid hormone receptor analysis. Imprint preparations may be particularly useful for small specimens such as clinically early or occult breast carcinomas and for small metastatic lesions. In such cases it may not be possible to submit a portion of the biopsy specimen for hormone receptor analysis without jeopardizing the histologic diagnosis.

With increasing emphasis on the diagnosis of clinically occult breast carcinomas as the result of refinements in mammography, the value of cytochemical hormone receptor assays in imprint preparations will become more recognized.

Fine needle aspiration biopsy

Over the past several years, FNA biopsy (FNAB) has been increasingly recognized as a valuable tool for the diagnosis of cancer. Although FNAB does not eliminate the need for surgical biopsy, therapy in some cases may be based on FNA results without either open biopsy or frozen section. In addition to the application of established cytologic criteria, the ability to identify specific markers has enhanced the diagnostic and therapeutic utility of FNAB.

Because of the small quantity of material obtained, biochemical DCC analysis cannot be performed on FNAB material. Recently, cytochemical hormone receptor assays have been employed in FNAB material. Good correlation with the biochemical method performed on tissue adjacent to or near the FNAB site has been demonstrated for both the fluorescent and the immunoperoxidase techniques (Curtin et al., 1982; Keshgegian et al., 1988) (Table 8.8).

Table 8.8. Summary of concordance between cytochemical hormone receptor analysis on fine needle aspirates and biochemical assays of the excised surgical specimen

Authors	No. of cases	Concordance ER(%)	PgR(%)	Technique
Azevedo et al. (1986)	31	90		ER-ICA
Curtin et al. (1982)	41	83	87	Fluoro-Cep
Flowers et al. (1986)	33	85		ER-ICA
Keshgegian et al. (1988)	58	76		ER-ICA
Lozowski et al. (1987)	25	92		ER-ICA
Lundy et al. (1990)	96	87.5	91.6	ER-ICA
Masood (1989)	62	92		ER-ICA
Masood (1990)	71		89	PgR-ICA
Masood (1991)	56	89	86	Fluoro-Cep
Katz (1990)	27	94		ER-ICA
Total	500	87.6	88.4	

Notes:
ER = Oestrogen receptor
PgR = Progesterone receptor
Fluoro-Cep = Fluorescent cytochemical technique
ER-ICA = Oestrogen receptor immunocytochemical assay
PgR-ICA = Progesterone receptor immunocytochemical assay

Source: From Masood, S. (1992). Sex hormone receptors in cytologic material. *Cytopathology Annual*, **4**, 77–102.

With the fluorescent method, heterogeneity of cytoplasmic staining is frequently prominent and tumours interpreted as positive should demonstrate bright green and red fluorescence for ER and PgR in 30 per cent of cells examined. With the immunoperoxidase technique, nuclear staining in 20 per cent of tumour cells is regarded as positive (Fig. 8.18).

Although the fluorescent method may be more economical, the immunoperoxidase technique offers great flexibility in that it may be successfully applied to direct smears, cytospin preparations and to paraffin-embedded cell block material.

Using a simple score based on heterogeneity and staining intensity it is also possible to show statistically significant correlation between receptor levels assayed biochemically and those estimated by cytochemical hormone receptor assay. Thus, semiquantitation of hormone receptor values may be possible (Masood and Johnson, 1987). For breast cancer patients in whom surgery might not be performed, such as in advanced localized and recurrent or metastatic disease, sex steroid receptor analysis of FNAB material can eliminate the need for open biopsy. These techniques may also be applied to mammographically guided fine needle aspirates (Masood et al., 1991b). Provided that adequate and representative material is obtained, FNA may be utilized to identify breast cancer patients most likely to respond to hormone therapy.

Malignant effusions

The value of ER and PgR as important predictors of response to hormone therapy has been established for both breast and gynaecologic malignancies. In advanced disease, however, receptor analysis may be more difficult due to inaccessibility of metastatic tumour. Patients with advanced disease, however, may have pleural or peritoneal effusions in which cytologic material is readily obtainable. Quantitative biochemical hormone receptor assays have been employed in detection of hormone receptors in tumour cells exfoliated in malignant effusion (McCarty et al., 1980). However, these studies are sparse and report only a small number of cases. Quantitative biochemical assay on malignant effusion is also limited by a need for highly cellular material. Immunocytochemical assays require less cellular material and are well suited for assessment of hormone receptors in the cells derived from malignant effusion (Fig. 8.18). Hormone receptor analysis has been performed on tumour cells obtained from patients with malignant effusion using both the fluorescent and immunoperoxidase techniques (Masood, 1990). In studies where biochemical values of primary tumours are available, a satisfactory correlation was obtained between the two results (Table 8.9).

Direct smears, cytospin preparations or cell block material may be utilized for hormone receptor analysis. In our experience, CytospinR (Shandon, Inc., Pittsburgh, Pennsylvania 15275) preparation technique allowed use of effusions with small volume or limited number of tumour cells. In none of the cases studied, was there a problem obtaining adequate cellular material for hormone receptor analysis.

Assessment of ER and PgR in malignant effusions is clinically significant, especially when the hormone receptor status of the primary tumour is unknown. In ovarian

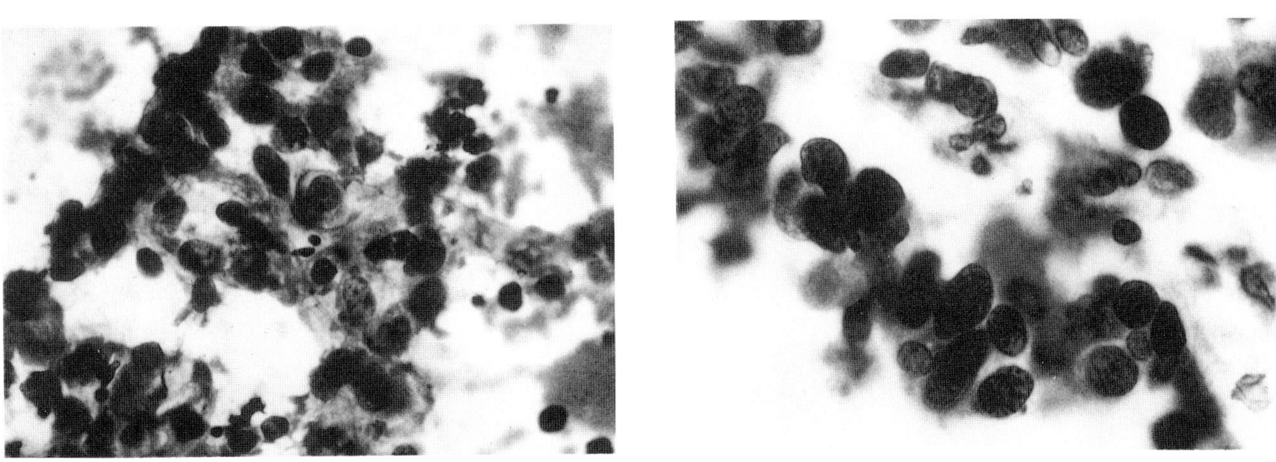

Fig. 8.18. ER-positive breast carcinoma: (A) (left) cells from FNA show nuclear features of malignancy. (B) (right) immunoperoxidase stained preparation shows strong, opaque positivity of some but not all nuclei.

Table 8.9. Summary of concordance between cytochemical hormone receptor analysis on malignant effusions and the biochemical assay of the primary tumours

Authors	No. of cases	Concordance ER(%)	PgR(%)	Technique
Masood (1990)	41	88	83	ER-ICA PgR-ICA
Masood (1990)	28	82	90	PgR-ICA
Total	69	85	86.5	

Notes: ER = ER Oestrogen receptor
PgR = Progesterone receptor
Fluoro-Cep = Fluorescent cytochemical technique
ER-ICA = Oestrogen receptor immunocytochemical assay
PgR-ICA = Progesterone receptor immunocytochemical assay

Source: From Masood, S. (1992). Sex hormone receptors in cytologic material. *Cytopathology Annual*, **4**, 77–102.

tumours, oestrogen receptor expression continues in patients with advanced disease and even after chemotherapy, whereas PgR is lower if the patient has received chemotherapy. Thus, assessment of ER status in patients with ovarian tumours that have been treated medically, may provide the basis for possible new therapeutic modalities. Overall, with a defined hormone receptor status, in advanced breast and gynaecological malignancies, appropriate therapy can be initiated with enhanced confidence of response to hormone therapy (Schwartz et al., 1982; Cannelos et al., 1976).

In addition to prognostic or therapeutic significance, assessment of hormone receptors may be of diagnostic assistance in patients presenting with unknown primary cancers or with metastatic undifferentiated tumour (Golomb and Thomsen, 1975; Kiang and Kennedy, 1977).

Specimen preparation

Imprints

Soon after the fresh tumour tissue is received, a portion of tissue is selected for imprint preparation. The cut surface of the portion of the lesion selected is touched with a clear glass slide to make multiple imprints. Sparsely cellular lesions are scraped gently with a scalpel blade and direct smears are made. Some of the imprints should be stained with Diff-Quik or H & E to determine adequacy.

Fluorescent technique The imprints are placed at 4°C for 1 h in a frost-free refrigerator to dry. They are either processed immediately or stored at −70°C for later processing. The exact test procedure is as suggested by the supplier.

Immunoperoxidase technique Polylysine-treated slides are used for smears or imprint preparations and are fixed immediately in 3.7 per cent formaldehyde-phosphate buffered saline for 15 min. After a minimum 5 min wash in 0.01M, pH7.4 PBS, slides are placed in −10°C methanol and acetone for 3 minutes and then rinsed in cold PBS for 5 minutes. Slides may then be stored at −20°C in PBS-glycerol prior to immunostaining. The rest of the procedure is as outlined by the supplier.

Fine needle aspiration biopsy

Fine needle aspiration (FNA) is performed, utilizing standard procedure. A Diff-Quick stain is employed for immediate evaluation. If malignant cells are present on the Diff-Quik smears, a portion of the aspirate is used for hormone receptor assay, prepared in one of two ways.

Direct smear preparation Polylysine treated slides are utilized for the immunoperoxidase technique and regular glass slides for the fluorescent technique. Fixation and storage procedures are the same as for imprint preparation.

Cytospin preparation For the immunoperoxidase technique, FNAs are rinsed into conical 50 ml centrifuge tube containing about 20 ml of fresh 3.7 formaldehyde-PBA at room temperature. Within 15 min the fixed material is centrifuged at 2400 rpm for 10 min. Supernatant is removed leaving 1–2 ml liquid in which the pellet is resuspended. Two to four cytospin slides are prepared, using about 5–7 drops suspension per slide. The slides require tissue adhesive as specified in the ER or PgR-ICA kit.

Body fluids

The fluids should be processed as soon as possible following thoracentesis or paracentesis. Following centrifugation, direct smears are processed and interpreted following staining with Diff-Quik. If adequate malignant cell present, part of the sediment is rinsed into a 50 ml conical centrifuge tube and processed as described under cytospin preparation technique.

Advantages and limitations of cytochemical hormone receptor assays

The cytochemical assays greatly expand the potential for hormone receptor analysis on cytologic material, since they frequently can be performed on the limited sources obtained by cytologic techniques. The cytochemical assays correlate very well with the biochemical assays and are generally less expensive and easier to perform in the smaller laboratories. The immunoperoxidase technique has been successfully automated. Masood (1989) applied the automated 'code-on' immunology system (Instrumentation Laboratory, Lexington, Massachusetts) for assessment of hormone receptors and demonstrated the potential of this system to conserve monoclonal antibodies and reduce the cost of the test substantially. Adaptability of the immunoperoxidase technique in detection of hormone receptor in formalin-fixed, paraffin-embedded tumours is another attractive advantage. Furthermore, cytochemical assays provide information about tumour hormone receptor heterogeneity in contrast to biochemical assay. This information remains a worthwhile goal, not only with respect to understanding the biology of tumours, but also with regard to explaining difference in response to endocrine therapy that is commonly observed in clinical practice.

Overall, special attention should be given to the results of hormone receptors by biochemical assays. These assays cannot distinguish between tumour tissue, stromal and benign epithelial components, whereas immunocytochemical assays tend to correct this deficiency. This is particularly important in gynaecological situations with positive DCC and negative immunocytochemical assay, we have demonstrated the presence of hormone receptor expression in non-malignant components of the lesion only. This, associated with other factors may explain the reported discrepancies between the DCC and the cytochemical assays.

On the other hand, lack of adequate standardization and quantitation remain limiting factors in the use of cytochemical hormone receptor assays. As the result, many national cancer therapy protocol studies still require biochemical assays for determination of hormone receptor proteins. Only recently, immunocytochemical hormone receptor assay for ER and PgR has been started in the NSABP (National Surgical Adjuvant Breast Project).

Biochemical assays provide quantitative value which is not yet available with cytochemical assay. Continuous efforts have been made to quantitate hormone receptor proteins in cytochemical assays, however, the interpretations are subjective and the measurements are at best semi-quantitative (Perschurk et al., 1987). Sporadic reports in the literature give promise to the use of computerized image analysis system in quantitation of hormone receptors Bacus et al., 1988; Sklarew et al., 1987). Sklarew et al. (1987) produced a pattern oriented approach called 'receptogram analysis' to evaluate ER status or a potential response predictor to hormone therapy. Despite these efforts, difficulties with quantitation in cytochemical hormone receptor assays remain. Overall, it has not been shown that quantitative values beyond a defined level are helpful in selecting treatment options. However, many investigators feel that quantitation may be of prognostic value (DeSombre and Jensen, 1980; Paridaens et al., 1980).

Nevertheless, currently, the cytochemical hormone receptor assays are most adaptable to cytologic material. Also, it seems reasonable to assume that with inherent advantages in the cytochemical hormone receptor assays, these procedures will continue to evolve and may eventually displace the biochemical assays.

Quantitative immunocytochemistry

Proliferative markers

Introduction

In contrast to immunocytopathology which provides diagnostic information, determination of oestrogen and progesterone receptors conveys prognostic data, useful in the treatment of breast cancer. However, other neoplasms that lack these receptors must be evaluated by other means. For instance, one of the most useful indicators of prognosis is the proliferative rate of tumours, as determined by quantitative methods. It has been known for many years that mitotic activity or thymidine labelling index are important predictors of tumour behaviour.

More recently, with the use flow cytometry, a technique is available to determine the proliferative rate as the percentage of cells in the DNA synthetic cells (S-phase) of the cell cycle and the status of the DNA content of tumour cells. Tumour cells with normal DNA content are called 'diploid'. Aneuploidy refers to the presence of tumour cells with abnormal DNA content. Aneuploidy can also be determined by static cytophotometry (image analysis).

Proliferative rate and DNA ploidy

Data from several groups suggests that both ploidy status and S-phase fraction are important prognostic variables in breast cancer (Bedrossian et al., 1981; Raber et al., 1982). Most investigators agree that abnormal DNA content in a tumour is associated with shorter disease-free survival or shortened overall survival. Clark et al. (1988) measured both ploidy and S-phase values in 395 node-negative breast cancer patients with medium follow-up or 95 months. In their study, they showed that the probability of tumour recurrence within five years was 12 per cent in patients with diploid tumours and 26 per cent in patients with aneuploid tumours ($P = 0.02$). Statistically significant difference in probability of tumour recurrence and overall survival was also found between patients with diploid tumours and high S-phase versus those patients with diploid tumours and low S-phase values. It has also been shown that S-phase can discriminate between a high and low probability of relapse within node-negative population with aneuploid tumours.

The importance of S-phase values as a reliable prognostic factor has been further confirmed by other studies on a large series of breast cancer patients. This information has already influenced the selection of different therapeutic modalities in node-negative breast cancer patients (Silverman, 1991; Kline, 1988). Recent production of antibodies against proliferating cells such as Ki-67 and proliferating cell nuclear antigen (PCNA) has also provided another means for evaluation of proliferative activity of tumour cells (Kuenen-Boumester et al., 1989; Garcia et al., 1989).

HER-2/neu oncogene

The neu oncogene, originally isolated from rat neuroblastomas, encodes a 185 kD surface glycoprotein which exhibits tyrosine kinase activity and is structurally similar to the epidermal growth factor receptor. The human homologue of C-neu, which is termed *c-erbB-2* is reported to be amplified in human breast cancer (Slamon et al., 1987) including samples obtained by FNA (Fig. 8.19). This amplification has been correlated with decreased disease-free survival and lower overall survival (Schechter et al., 1984). The oncogene has also been called HER-2/neu. The value of HER-2/neu oncogene expression in ANN patients is still under intense investigation. Confusion remains in the interpretation of the results of the studies on HER-2 protein expression measured by the Western blot technique, or by immunocytochemistry. Immunocytochemistry is being utilized to detect the protein's presence in frozen and paraffin-embedded sections (Fig. 8.20).

Epidermal growth factor receptors

Epidermal growth factor receptor (EGFR) is another oestrogen dependent protein which is regulated by oestro-

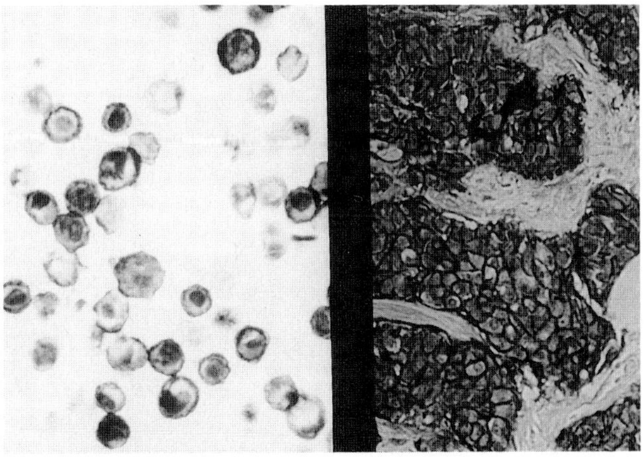

Fig. 8.19. FNA of breast. (A) (Left) single malignant cells showing positivity for antibody against c-erbB-2. (B) (right): corresponding tissue section of breast carcinoma strongly positive for *c-erbB-2*.

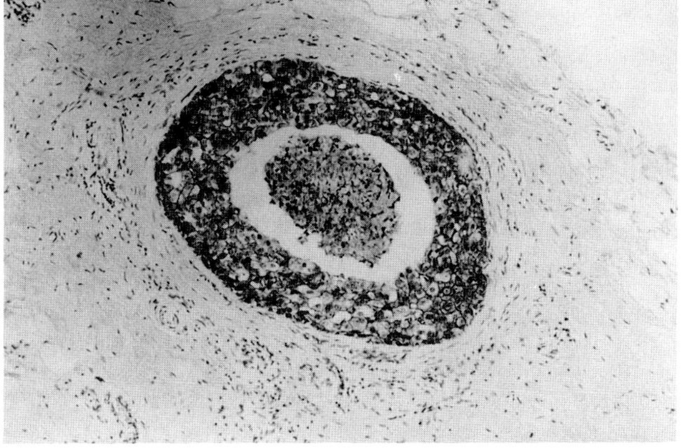

Fig. 8.20. Paraffin section of breast carcinoma stained for *c-erbB-2*. Notice strong positivity of intraductal carcinoma extending also into the comedo component in the center. (Courtesy of Daniel Visscher MD)

gen in breast tumours. EGFR is a single polypeptide chain with Mr = 6000 that is highly stable and is known to occur in a number of organs in the body, including the reproductive tissue. EGFR has been reported in human breast cancer and it is suggested that there is an inverse relationship between EGFR and oestrogen receptor concentration. Elevated levels of EGFR have been associated with a shorter disease-free interval and diminished overall survival for breast cancer patients (Fitzpatrick et al., 1984). EGFR can be detected by biochemical methods as well as by immunocytochemical assays. The immunoperoxidase technique is easily adaptable to breast fine needle aspirates (Fig. 8.21).

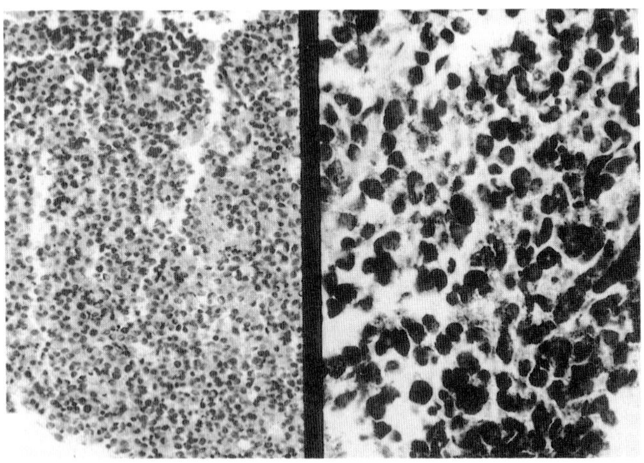

Fig. 8.21. Breast carcinoma in pleural effusion. (A) (left) monotonous population of single malignant cells. (B) (right) malignant cells showing strong positivity for ·epidermal growth factor receptor.

Ki-67 antibody and proliferating cell nuclear antigen (PCNA)

Ki-67 is a human nuclear antigen expressed on all proliferating cells and appears to stain G_1, S G_2, and M-phase cells. Resting (G_0) phase cells are negative. Ki-67 can be detected by immunocytochemical assay on FNAs and on fresh tissue and shows predominantly nuclear staining. There is a high correlation between the reaction of Ki-67 positive cells in breast tumours and the nuclear histologic grade and the mitotic rate. It is also suggested that the degree of Ki-67 staining may have some prognostic significance (Kuenen-Boumester et al., 1989). PCNA is an intranuclear polypeptide, whose synthesis reaches its maximum during the S-phase of the cell cycle. It may be used both on cytological preparation and on formalin-fixed paraffin-embedded section (Garcia et al., 1989). Results are rather promising in FNA of the breast (Fig. 8.22).

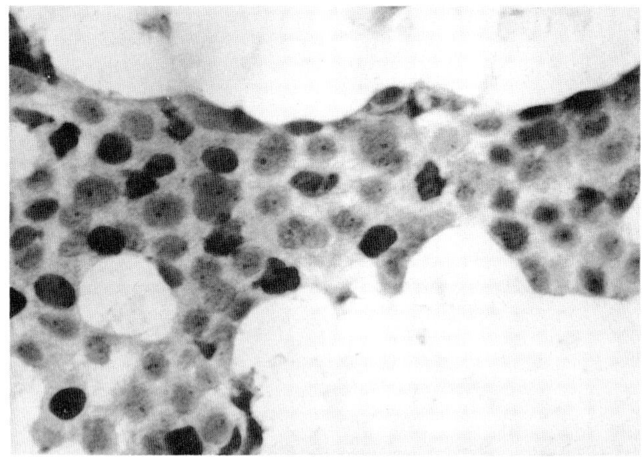

Fig. 8.22. Breast FNA stained with Ki-67 antibody. Numerous positive nuclei attest to the high proliferative activity of the neoplasm (courtesy of Michael Stanley, MD).

Cathepsin-D

Cathepsin-D, a protease 52 kD is an oestrogen-regulated protein which has been originally identified in breast cancer cells. It is proposed that Cathepsin-D might facilitate cancer cell migration and invasion by digesting the basement membrane, extracellular matrix and connective tissue. Patients with high concentrations of Cathepsin-D have shorter disease-free survival and tend for shorter overall survival (Thorpe et al., 1989). Recent studies suggest that Cathepsin-D status is a good predictor of metastatic disease especially in node-negative breast cancer patients. Results in FNAs are comparable to those obtained in tissues (Fig. 8.23).

p53

The p53, a tumour suppressor gene product is found predominantly in the nuclei of different tumours. Due to an increased half-life and an altered confrontational structure, the mutant form of p53 protein accumulates within malignant cells and thus, can be detected.

Recent studies suggest that there is an association between p53 expression and oestrogen receptor negativity, poor histologic grade, and a reduced metastasis-free and overall survival in breast cancer patients (Thor, 1991).

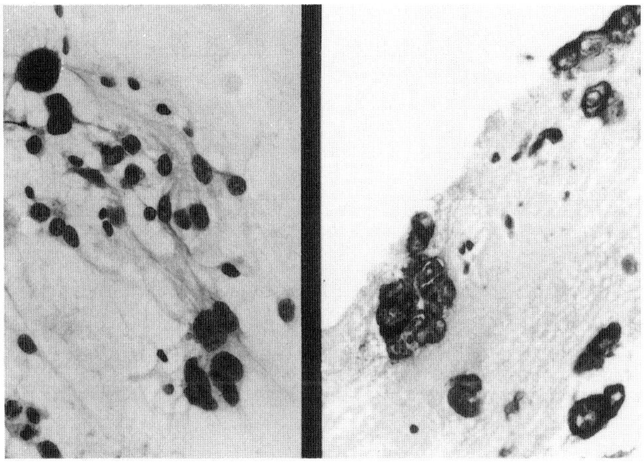

Fig. 8.23. Breast FNA. (A) (left) malignant cells, singly and in small groups. (B) (right) corresponding preparation stained for Cathepsin-D. Notice strong cytoplasmic positivity of tumour cells.

pS2

pS2 is a 6.5 kD oestrogen-inducible, cytoplasmic polypeptide of unknown function. It is suggested that pS2 protein might serve as an additional marker of a functional oestrogen regulatory system and defines another subset of ER/PgR positive patients that may display a better response to endocrine therapy (Molina, 1990). Using an immunoperoxidase technique, Abbondanzo et al. (1992) demonstrated that the expression of pS2 is associated with longer disease-free survival in node-negative breast cancer patients.

NM23

NM23, a suppressor gene was identified on the basis of its reduced steady-state RNA levels in five highly metastatic K-1735 melanoma cell lines, as compared with two related, low metastatic potential K-1735 melanoma cell lines in lines in human breast carcinomas. Low NM23 RNKA levels are correlated with the presence of lymph node metastasis (Steeg et al., 1988; Leone et al., 1991). We have also studied the pattern of NM23 expression in breast cancer vai immunocytochemistry and have shown that low NM23 protein expression correlated with reduced patient survival (Barnes, et al., 1991).

Others

Metastasis-associated laminin receptor, collagenase IV, and the status of angiogenesis have also been suggested as prognostic factors in breast cancer. Assessment of multidrug resistance (P-glycoprotein) in breast cancer may provide information regarding response to chemotherapy. A non-immunocytochemical method of assessing prognostic behaviours is represented by AgNOR counts. The method is similar to antinucleolar antibodies in which the nucleolar organizing region is impregnated by silver (Fig. 8.24). The number and intensity of AgNOR positive markings is proportional to the degree of invasiveness or to a poorer prognosis (Fig. 8.25).

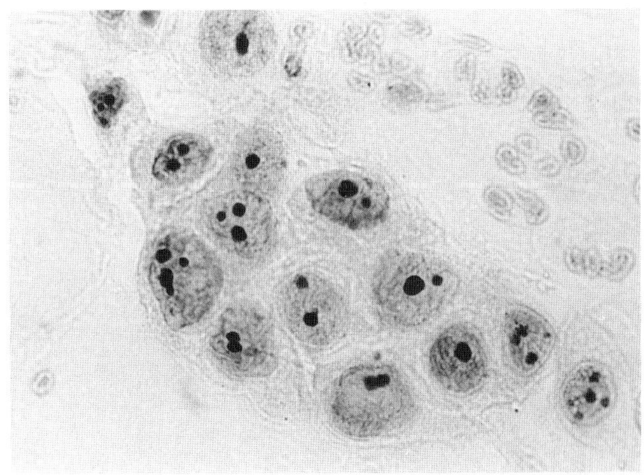

Fig. 8.24. Cervical smear in moderate dysplasia. Numerous AgNORs are highlighted by silver impregnation of dyskaryortic nuclei. (Courtesy Maria R. Cardillo, MD.)

Flow cytometry

Introduction

Flow cytometry is a relatively new method of cell analysis made possible by advances in a number of fields. The method has found important and practical applications in cancer diagnosis (O'Hara et al., 1983). Genetic and immunologic properties as well as cytokinetic parameters can be measured by flow cytometry. Multiple physical characteristics of single cells are measured simultaneously. These measurements are made on a per cell basis at rates of 5,004,000 or more cells per second. The cells are individually dispersed in a moving, flowing stream. As each cell passes through a sensing area, a series of signals are generated. These may represent fluorescence, light scatter, light absorbance or electrical resistance of cells and are accurately measured. The information is then stored and analysed.

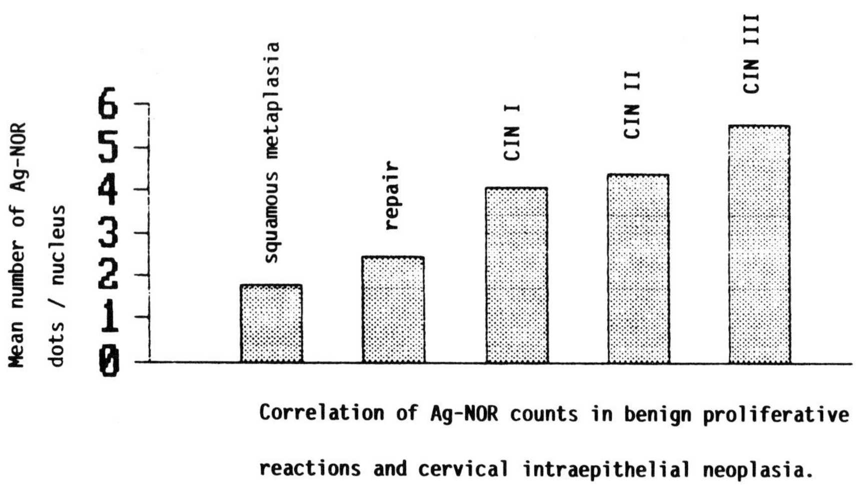

Fig. 8.25. Correlation between AgNORs and squamous intraepithelial lesions. Note increased counts in progressively more severe degrees of nuclear abnormalities. (Courtesy Maria R. Cardillo, MD.)

Many different biochemical and physical properties can be determined, including cell size, nucleic acid content, and presence of antigens or enzymes. Fluorochromes coupled to monoclonal antibodies are frequently used to label the cellular component of interest, fluorochromes omit fluorescence when excited by the illuminating laser beam or mercury are light, yielding information on the expression of target molecules within single cells. Some flow cytometres have 'cell sorting capability' and can isolate and collect specific cell populations for special studies.

Single cell suspensions, required for flow cytometry, may be easily prepared from blood, bone marrow, body fluids, bladder washings, cultured cells and cerebrospinal fluid. Specimens containing small tissue fragments, such as gynaecologic or sputum material may be more difficult to prepare. Solid tumours may require chelating agents or enzymatic digestion to obtain a single cell suspension. Fine needle aspiration samples may be analysed by flow cytometry and have been utilized for DNA analysis and cell surface marker studies in a variety of conditions. Numerous cellular constituents can be analysed by flow cytometry. Cell surface antigens and nucleic acids are currently the most useful for diagnostic pathology. Detailed protocols for the preparation of such specimens for flow cytometry analyses are provided in the Appendix.

Cell surface marker studies

Flow cytometry provides a powerful investigative tool for exploring structural and functional properties of immunoresponsive cells. Specific cell subpopulations may be classified according to phenotype by identification of specific cell surface antigen or receptors with monoclonal antibodies conjugated to fluorescent dye. T- and B- lymphocyte subclasses as well as lymphocyte precursors may be identified. Many antibodies are commercially available, including ones which recognize differentiation antigens on T- and B-lymphocytes, monocytes, granulocytes and platelets. These antibodies are widely used for immunophenotyping of leukaemias and lymphomas, for determination of immune status and for monitoring organ allograft recipients (Reinherz et al., 1979).

DNA measurement and cell cycle analysis

The DNA content of tumours can be rapidly precisely analysed by flow cytometry, providing information potentially of clinical importance. First, measurement of the percentage of cells in the S-phase of DNA replication reflect the rate of tumour growth. Secondly, quantitative measure of abnormal DNA content, if any, provides a determination of ploidy. Meticulous attention to sample preparation is necessary. Major considerations include isolation of nuclei, DNA specific staining of DNA in fresh, frozen and formalin fixed tissues, as well as adequate sampling and use of standardized technique (details provided in the Appendix).

Initially, DNA analysis by flow cytometry relied upon either fresh or frozen-stored tissue and thus was limited in its usefulness. Hedley et al. (1983) described a method utilizing formalin-fixed, paraffin-embedded tissue for DNA flow cytometry study. This latter method is particularly useful for retrospective studies of tumours in patients whose clinical outcome is already known. In addition, obtaining a separate, fresh specimen for DNA at the time of surgery is often inconvenient and may be impossible when the surgical specimen is too small. The need for DNA analysis may not be apparent until after the tissue has been embedded and diagnosis is made. DNA analysis of formalin-fixed, paraffin-embedded tissue also allows selection of the best area of the specimen for analysis. Several investigators have demonstrated a close correlation between DNA index in deparaffinized and fresh specimens from the same tumour (Fossa et al., 1986; Hedley et al., 1983).

DNA content has been studied in a variety of human tumours, allowing classification as diploid or aneuploid. By definition, diploid tumours have normal DNA content, while aneuploid tumours have an 'abnormal' (hypodiploid, hyperdiploid) amount of DNA. DNA content abnormality or aneuploidy is usually expressed as the DNA index, the ratio of the DNA content of the G_0/G_1 cells in the abnormal population to the G_0/G_1 cells of a normal diploid population.

After a cell has completed mitosis, it enters the presynthetic, or G_1 phase of cell growth, in which the nucleus has a diploid or 2N amount of DNA (i.e.: 23 chromosomes pairs) (Fig. 8.26). These cells are cycling. Cells in G_0 are in 'resting' state and have normal amount of DNA. At some point, the cells begin to duplicate their DNA, (S-phase, synthetic phase) where the cells have an intermediate amount of DNA, between 2N and 4N. After DNA replication is complete, the cells enter the post-synthetic or G_2 growth phase in which they have a 4N amount of DNA. In flow cytometry, there is no distinction between G_2 nuclei from M nuclei, as they both have a 4N amount of DNA, and the term 'G_2+M' phase is used.

Flow cytometry is an approach to the measurement of DNA within a nucleus by using fluorescent dyes that bind with the DNA. The fluorescence intensity given off by each cell is proportional to its DNA content. By compiling the DNA content in several thousand nuclei, a histogram can be generated by the DNA content of the cell population being analysed.

Figure 8.27 demonstrates a histogram of a diploid tumour. To the left is a small peak created by chicken erythrocyte nucleus (CEN) which are added to the sample as the fluorescence standard. The majority of cells contain only a diploid amount of DNA and are in G_0/G_1 phase (91.2 per cent). A small percentage (3.2 per cent) of tumour cells contain exactly twice the diploid DNA content and represent cells in G_2 phase as undergoing mitosis. Cells with intermediate DNA

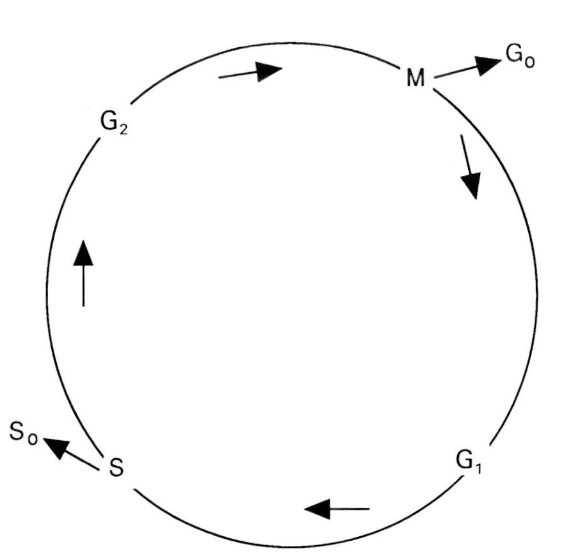

Fig. 8.26. Schematic representation of a cell cycle. G_0/G_1 represents presynthetic stage. S is the synthetic stage and G_2/M identifies postsynthetic stage.

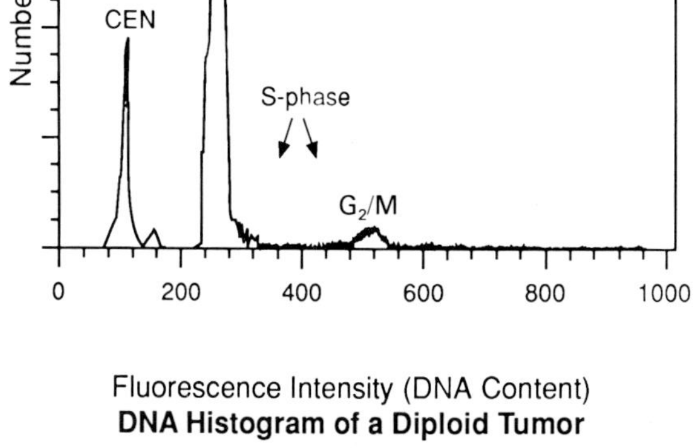

Fig. 8.27. Histogram of diploid tumour. Note similarity of peaks between the tumour and the control (CEN).

content are in S-phase (5.7 per cent). DNA index is 1.0 (ranging from 0.9–1.10) representing normal DNA content. Hyperdiploid tumours have a DNA index > 1.10 and hypodiploid tumours have a DNA index < 1.9. Tetraploid tumours have a DNA index of 2.00.

Figure 8.28 is an example of a histogram of an aneuploid tumour. On the left a normal diploid G_0/G_1 peak is seen. The aneuploid G_0/G_1 population of these tumour cells is displaced to the right of the diploid G_0/G_1 population, reflecting a higher amount of DNA per nucleus.

$$\text{DNA index} = \frac{G_0/G_1 \text{ fluorescence (channel no.) of aneuploid cells (410)}}{G_0/G_1 \text{ fluorescence (channel no.) of diploid cells (275)}} = 1.5$$

Aneuploid tumour cell population constitutes 64.8 per cent of cells examined. S-phase is 18.4 per cent and 16.8 per cent are in G_2M phase. Cell cycle distribution within clonal populations is calculated by variety of computer programs available and models have been suggested for estimation of the distribution of cells within different cell cycle compartments from flow cytometry-generated DNA histograms.

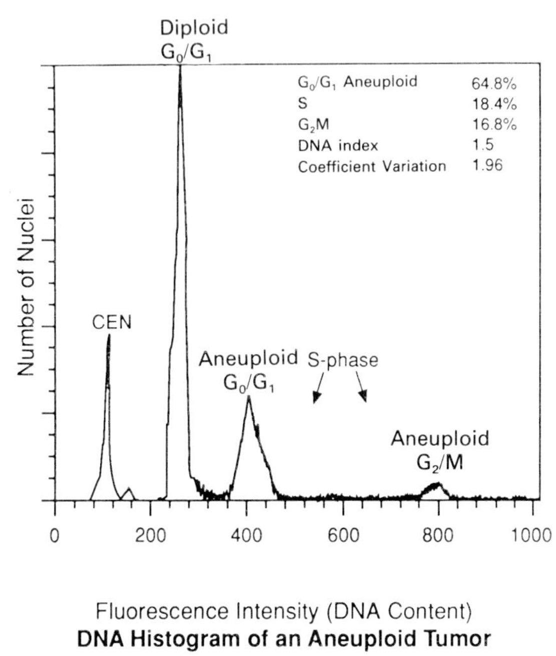

Fig. 8.28. Histogram of aneuploid tumour, markedly dissimilar to the control ·peaks. The DNA index (1.5) unequal to 1.0 is typical of aneuploidy.

Prognostic value of DNA analysis

Patients with diploid tumours have a more favourable prognosis than those with an aneuploid pattern (Fig. 8.29). Diploid tumours are more frequently well differentiated. However, the prognostic significance of ploidy pattern is not constant and may vary with the site of origin and the histologic type of the tumour (Koss et al., 1989).

DNA analysis may provide prognostic information for a variety of malignancies that present with aneuploidy (Fig. 8.30, Table 8.10). Aneuploid DNA content is associated with less favourable prognosis in early breast cancer (McGuire et al., 1985) non-small cell lung cancer (Volm and Mattern, 1985) colorectal carcinoma (Kokal et al., 1986), superficial carcinoma and carcinoma *in situ* in the bladder (Gustafson et al., 1982a, 1982b),

Table 8.10. The relationship between aneupoloidy and prognosis in adult and childhood malignancies

Tumour	DNA pattern	Prognosis
Adult malignancies		
Breast cancer	Aneuploid	Decreases overall survival
Breast cancer, stage I or II node-negative	Aneuploid or diploid with high S-phase	Decreases survival
Non-small cell lung carcinoma	Aneuploid	Worsens survival
Colonic carcinoma	Aneuploid	Decreases survival
Bladder carcinoma, superficial early stage	Aneuploid	Increases risk of progression to invasive carcinoma
Prostate cancer	Aneuploid	Worsens survival
Ovarian epithelial	Aneuploid	Worsens survival
Endometrial carcinoma	Aneuploid	Worsens survival
Cervical cancer	Aneuploid	Increases risk of recurrence after radiation therapy
Melanoma stage I	Aneuploid	Higher risk of relapse
Paediatric malignancies		
Acute lymphoblastic leukaemia	Aneuploid	Improves survival
Neuroblastoma	Aneuploid	Improves survival
Medulloblastoma	Aneuploid	Improves survival
Wilm's tumour	Aneuploid	Worsens survival

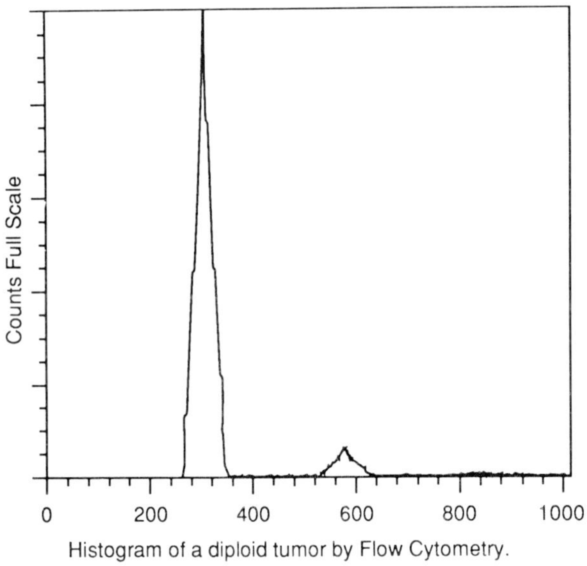

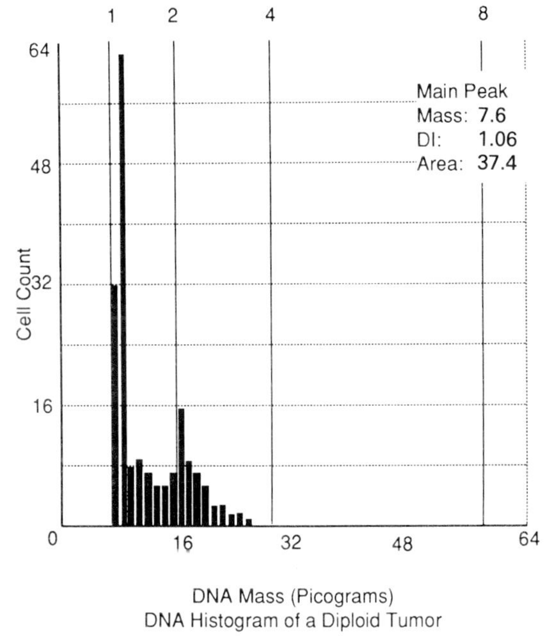

Fig. 8.29. Comparison between flow cytometry and image analysis in a diploid tumour. Note close correspondence of peaks between two techniques. (A) (left) (flow cytometry). (B) (right) (image analysis).

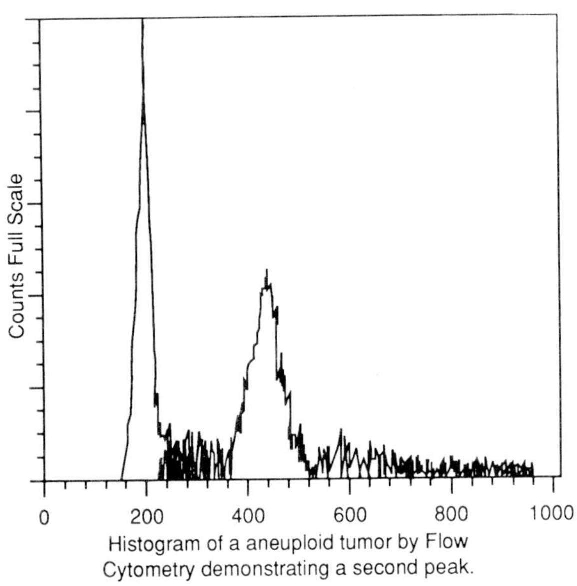

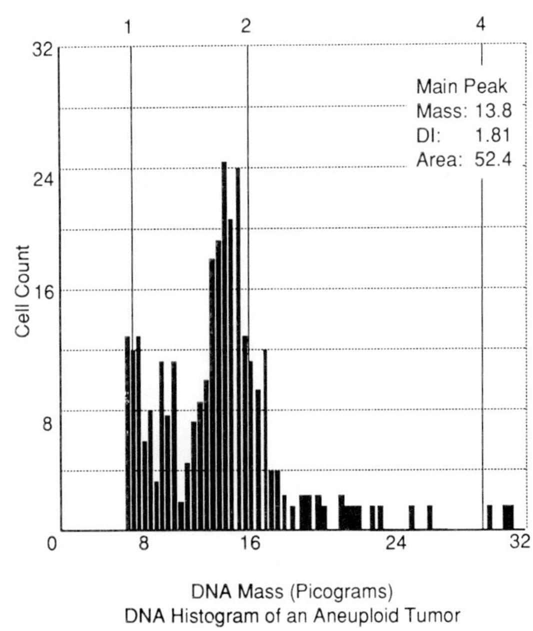

Fig. 8.30. Same neoplasm analysed by flow cytometry and image analysis. (A) (left): flow cytometry showing two peaks. (B) (right): image analysis closely parallels the two peaks.

ovarian cancer (Friedlander et al, 1984) and cervical carcinomas (Jacobsen, 1984). Aneuploidy may also be a marker for prognosis in malignant melanoma (von Roenn et al., 1986), prostate cancer (Fordham, 1986) endometrial and renal cell carcinoma (Koss et al, 1989). Aneuploidy is associated with a good prognosis in paediatric malignancies such as acute lymphoblastic leukaemia neuroblastoma and medulloblastoma but with an unfavourable prognosis in Wilm's tumour (Douglass et al., 1986; Look et al., 1984, 1985; Tomila et al., 1988).

Flow cytometry in cytology

Cytologic material such as bronchoalveolar lavage fluid effusions, bladder washings and fine needle aspirates have also been extensively utilized in flow cytometry study. Yoss (1989) studied the usefulness of flow cytometric analysis of bronchial washings and lavage in 59 patients with a variety of pulmonary disorders. They suggested that flow cytometry analysis not only has the potential to increase the diagnostic yield of bronchoscopy in the diagnosis of lung cancer, but has practical benefit, particularly in patients in whom more invasive procedures such as transbronchial biopsies cannot be performed. In this study, they concluded that the presence of aneuploidy in bronchoalveolar lavage fluid is highly specific for the presence of malignancy but lacked sensitivity. When combined with cytologic studies, the sensitivity improved (to 85 per cent) with only a slight decrease in specificity (91 per cent). Cytologic Studies alone had 100 per cent specificity and 38 per cent sensitivity. The specificity of flow cytometry studies was 91 per cent and sensitivity was 58 per cent. Combining the two studies, the positive predictive value for malignancy was 88 per cent and the negative predictive was also 88 per cent. The effect is important as the addition of flow cytometric analysis does not increase the risk of bronchoscopy, yet may significantly improve the yield.

Reports on flow cytometric analysis of effusions has been rather controversial. Evans et al. (1983) observed aneuploid DNA patterns in all 27 malignant effusions studied. However, all other investigators report that some of the cytologically malignant effusions had a diploid pattern by flow cytometry (Hedley et al., 1984; Katz et al., 1985; Stonesifer et al., 1984; Unger et al., 1983). It is suggested that in a medium such as effusions containing a mixture of broad variety of benign cells and neoplastic cells, the evidence of aneuploidy may be masked in a sample of 10,000 cells studied. Therefore, a much larger sample, careful analysis of predominantly diploid histograms, perhaps in conjunction with sorting of the small proportion of cells with abnormal signals are essential before flow cytometry can be effectively utilized as a diagnostic tool in the assessment of effusions. The use of image cytophotometry on cells stained by the Feulgen method may also be helpful in elucidating DNA distribution patterns in samples of effusions considered diploid or difficult to classify by flow cytometry (Schneller et al., 1987).

Flow cytometry can provide an objective quantitative measure of the exfoliated epithelial cells in bladder washing specimens and may potentially be as sensitive as conventional cytologic studies for the detection of neoplastic cells. It may also be of value in monitoring the course of bladder cancer during treatment and in anticipating recurrence following conservative therapy (Klein et al., 1982). Murphy et al. (1986) compared the roles of urinary cytology and flow cytometry in the evaluation of patients with bladder cancer. When carcinoma was present, it was detected by positive cytology in 75 per cent and by DNA aneuploidy in 78 per cent of the cases. Combination of flow cytometric DNA analysis and urinary cytology increased the diagnosis accuracy to 95 per cent. Flow cytometry was a less method than cytology for detection of abnormalities in treatment of invasive cancers and slightly more sensitive in non-invasive conditions associated with high urothelial cell turnover rates but the concomitant urinary cytology was negative for malignancy. In this study, Murphy et al. (1986) concluded that when used in conjunction with urinary cytology, flow cytometry is a valuable procedure in management of patients with bladder cancer. They also suggest that combination of cytology and flow cytometry may potentially reduce the frequency of cystoscopy and biopsy in selected patients.

Fine needle aspirates are also suitable specimens for both cell surface marker studies and cellular DNA analysis and represent an exciting and potentially expansive integration of a relatively non-invasive diagnostic technique with a more specific modality of interpretation. Preliminary studies in the use of FNAs in assessment of DNA ploidy status of various tumours indicates that; first, sufficient cellular material may be obtained by needle aspiration biopsy to produce good flow cytometric DNA profile and; secondly, DNA analysis by flow cytometry provides objective data that complement the subjective cytologic interpretation of FNAs, allowing a physician to proceed directly to therapy for a malignant tumour and obviating the need for a biopsy (Corkill et al., 1989; Masood and Hart, 1989; Palmer et al., 1988).

In conclusion, flow cytometric analysis of neoplastic and non-neoplastic cells has offered new dimensions of examination and interpretation of disease processes affecting humans. DNA findings of aneuploidy in node negative breast cancer patients has already influenced the selection of different therapeutic modalities (Clark et al., 1988). While the literature recording advances in the is area is relatively young and without total consensus, there is great promise of significant advance in both establishing diagnosis and monitoring therapy of several disorders. Indeed, in a number of tumours, notably lymphomas and leukaemias, flow cytometry has been a standard of interpretation in many medical centres. There is every indication that this trend will continue, probably at an accelerated rate. New innovation such as the integration of image cytophometric analysis with standard flow cytometric methodology will only serve to further improve sensitivity and specificity of this field of diagnostic technology. Flow cytometry represents an exciting advance in the overall fields of both applied medicine and clinical research.

Image analysis

Introduction

Image analysis is obtained by a computerized microscope that is designed to measure a number of cell features on a routine glass slide. It is an effective means of complementing the ability of the pathologists to precisely measure different parameters of an individual cell such as nuclear area and to quantitate stain intensity of different cellular constituents such as DNA by the use of the computer-enhanced, high-resolution digital video camera. The overall goal of cell image analysis is to bring measurement and objectivity to the discipline of pathology (Bacus and Grace, 1987).

In contrast to flow cytometry, image analysis is capable of analysing small numbers of tumour cells and is specifically adaptable to imprint preparation, cytocentrifuge preparations and FNAs. The procedure involves little additional preparatory work over usual cytologic and histologic procedures followed by data collection and analysis. Tumour cells can be identified morphologically and the specimen can be preserved for further analysis (Table 8.11).

Critical aspects for successful cell image analysis include sample preparation, staining consistency, proper controls and standards, precision of microscopic light intensity and pathologists' involvement. Details of preparation and DNA staining provided in the Appendix.

Applications of this methodology include cytophotometry, quantitative DNA analysis, quantitative immunocytochemistry, such as oestrogen and progesterone receptor analysis, analysis of oncogene products (e.g. HER-2/neu), and measurement of cell proliferation rate (Ki-67 antibody).

Table 8.11. Comparison of flow cytometry and cell image analysis

Feature	Flow cytometry	Cell image analysis
Basis of analysis	Fluorescence and/ or light scanner	Morphology and/or cell markers through transmitted light (absorbance)
Specimen preparation	Single cell suspension	Cytocentrifuge preparation imprints, fine needle aspirates, tissue sections (frozen paraffin-embedded)
Morphologic	Absent correlation	Present and will facilitate the identification of specific cells of interest
Morphotometry	Limited to light scatter measurement (size, granularity	Large numbers of direct and derived morphotometric parameters
Rate of analysis	Rapid analysis of large number of cells (10–20,000)	Slow analysis of small number of cells) (100–200)

Cytophotometry

Image analysis allows one to quantitate and analyse morphological differences between individual cells, quickly and easily. It distinguishes texture, size and shape of cell nuclei and alterations in the nuclear-to-cytoplasmic ratio of cells. Cytophotometry has already been applied in distinction between benign and malignant breast lesions (Detweiker et al., 1988), in the differential cytologic diagnosis of lung carcinoma (Burns et al., 1989), and in distinction between benign and malignant cells in effusions (van Molengraft et al., 1982). Attempts have also been made to differentiate between follicular adenomas and carcinomas of thyroid gland (Masuda et al., 1988). Morphometric analysis of cytologic preparations can be employed for the diagnosis of non-Hodgkin's lymphoma (Stevens et al., 1988), gastric tumours (Danno et al, 1976), breast lesions (King et al., 1988) and grading of urinary bladder tumours (Boon et al., 1981).

King et al. (1988) utilized cytophotometry for the classification of premalignant breast disease in FNAs. They were able to correctly diagnose seven proliferative lesions using image analysis, while none of these cases were recognized using conventional cytologic methodology.

Quantitative DNA analysis

Similar to flow cytometry, image analysis can be utilized for ploidy study. The diagnostic and prognostic implications of ploidy study by image analysis is similar to what has already been mentioned for flow cytometry. Overall, DNA ploidy measurement by cell image analysis gives results which are comparable to those obtained by flow cytometry. Diploid tumours will show DNA mass histograms closely parallelling those obtained by flow cytometry of the same neoplasm (Fig. 8.29). The same is true of aneuploid tumours (Fig. 8.30).

In image analysis, DNA quantitation is most often performed on cytologic preparation stained by the Feulgen reaction (Bibbo et al., 1991). This dye binds stoichiometrically to DNA and absorption of light at 560nm is linearly related to total DNA content. This method has the advantage of retrospective study of destained FNA and the other archived material. In addition, smaller samples are utilized and tumour cells can be directly visualized and selected. This is of particular importance in DNA ploidy study of FNAs and imprint preparations of small breast carcinomas often detected by mammography. Furthermore, cell image analysis may have greater sensitivity in detecting small aneuploid and tetraploid populations.

Measurement of cell proliferation rate

Recent studies suggest that in addition to DNA ploidy status, the proliferative activity of malignant tumours has some prognostic significance. This has already been shown to be true in malignant lymphomas (Grogan et al., 1988), breast cancer (Sigurdson et al., 1990) and colon cancer (Sasaki et al., 1988). Since many of the chemotherapeutic agents are cell-cycle specific, assessment of tumour cell proliferation may be of some value in selection of therapy. In addition, study of proliferation rate of a tumour may help in understanding of the tumour biology.

Traditionally, methods such as tritiated thymidine labelling and bromodeoxyuridine incorporation has been used to assess tumour cull proliferation. However, these tests are cumbersome and are not commonly used. In flow cytometry, fluorescent dyes bind stoichiometrically to DNA and labels suspended nuclei, and the DNA histogram is assessed to determine cell cycle phases.

First, it is often difficult to make cell suspension from a solid tumour and there is often loss of tumour cells during preparation. Secondly, dilution of tumour cells by benign epithelial and stromal components, and inflammatory cells are another problem. In addition, lack of morphologic correlation leads to some uncertainty in identifying tumour cells. Furthermore, precise S-phase determination is often difficult. Alternative methods of analysing tumour cell proliferation include using antibodies to nuclear antigens which are cell cycle-specific and quantitating such immunostaining reaction by cell image analysis. Ki-67 antibody is raised against Hodgkin's disease cell line and stains nuclei of proliferating human cells regardless of lineage. Ki-67 antibody stained G1, S G2 and M-phase cells with no reaction to resting (G0) phase cells. Thus, Ki-67 antibody is a direct measurement of proliferative status of tumours which is related to tumour grade and the level of its aggression (Gerdes et al., 1983). The cells in proliferative status by Ki-67 immunostaining show nuclear staining which can be quantitated by image analysis. Not only FNAs (Henry et al., 1991), but imprints and frozen tissue are suitable specimen for this analysis (Clevenger et al., 1987).

Other proliferative associated markers include PCNA/ Cyclin, which is relatively S-phase specific (Garcia, 1989), DNA Polymerase alpha and P-105 antigen, which is mitosis-associated, require further study.

Oestrogen and progesterone receptor analysis

Cell image analysis has been used to quantitate the ER-ICA and PgR-ICA assays be incorporating the percent positivity and intensity value with a quantitative immunocytochemistry (QIC) score. A statistically significant correlation between the QIC score and biochemically determined ER value has been reported with sensitivity of 98 per cent and specificity of 100 per cent. It has also been suggested ·that the presence of greater than 10 per cent ER-positive nuclei correlates with biochemical levels greater than 10 mol/mg protein (Fig. 8.31). Thus, cell image analysis has the potentiality of quantitating ER and PgR and assessment of the heterogeneity of hormone receptor expression (Bacus et al., 1988). This is particularly important in the assessment of ER-negative tumours that may have only a small but fluctuating amount of

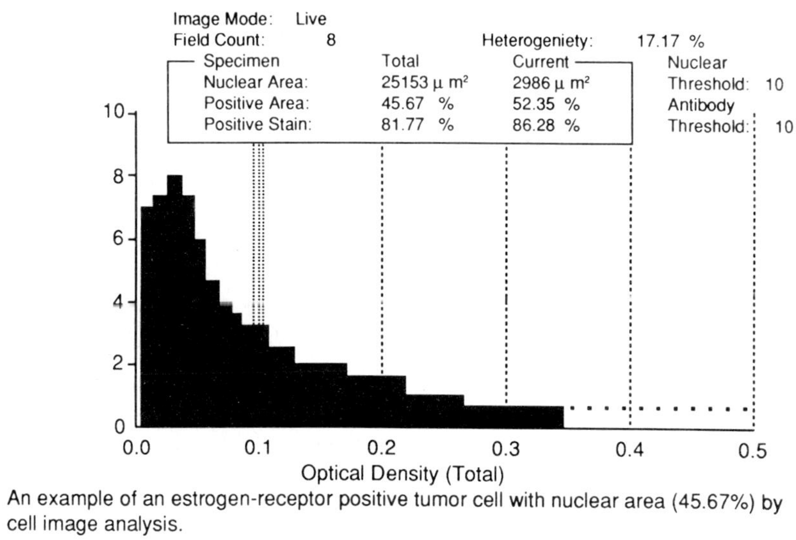

Fig. 8.31. Oestrogen receptor positive tumour submitted for image analysis. Almost half of the nuclear area shows positivity.

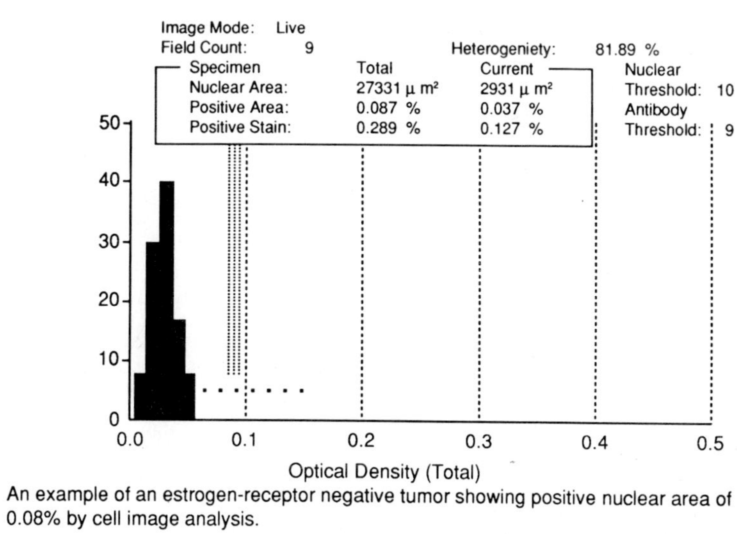

Fig. 8.32. This tumour was negative for oestrogen receptor by image analysis, a small peak corresponds to less than 1 per cent of cells, positive for ER.

ER positive nuclei, demonstrable by image analysis (Fig. 8.32).

Other prognostic markers

Aside from ploidy study, proliferation rate and hormone receptors, recently developed factors that may have prognostic significance include HER-2/neu oncogenes, cathepsin-D, epidermal growth factor receptors p53, pS2, factor VIII, and the others. Provided that we have adequate cellular material, fine needle aspirates and imprints can be easily utilized in prognostic testing, but this is best accomplished by immunocytochemistry as indicated earlier in the chapter.

References

Abbondanzo, S.L. (1992). Prognostic significance of immunocytochemically determined pS2 in axillary node-negative breast carcinoma. *Breast Cancer Research and Treatment* **16**, 182.

Akhtar, M., Bedrossian, C.W.M., Ashraf, M. and Bakry, M. (1992). Fine-needle aspiration biopsy of pediatric neoplasms: correlation between electron microscopy and immunocytochemistry in diagnosis and classification. *Diagnostic Cytopathology* **8**, 258–65.

Altmannsberger, M., Osborn, M. and Droese, M. (1984). Diagnostic value of intermediate filament antibodies in clinical cytology. *Klinische Wochenschrift* **62**, 114–23.

Bacus, S., Flowers, JL and Press, M.F. (1988). The evaluation of estrogen receptor in primary breast carcinoma by computer-assisted image analysis. *American Journal of Pathology* **90**, 233–9.

Bacus, J.W. and Grace, L.J. (1987). Optical microscope system for standardized cell measurement and analysis. *Applied Optics* **26**, 32–80.

Barnes, R. and Masood, S. (1991). Potential value of hormone receptor assay in carcinoma in situ of breast. *American Journal of Clinical Pathology* **94**(5), 533–7.

Barnes, R., Masood, S. and Barker, E. (1990). Low NM23 protein expression in infiltrating ductal breast carcinomas correlates with reduced patient survival. *American Journal of Pathology* **139**, 245–50.

Battifora, H., Sun, T.-T., Bahu, R.M. and Rao, S. (1980). The use of antikeratin antiserum as a diagnostic tool: thymoma versus lymphoma. *Human Pathology* **11**, 635–41.

Bedrossian, C.W.M. (1990) Immunocytochemistry. In Astarita, R. (ed.), *Practical Cytopathology*. Churchill Livingstone, London, pp. 403–57.

Bedrossian, C.W.M. (1992). Electron microscopy: The neglected tool of cytopathology. *Diagnostic Cytopathology* **8**, 179–88.

Bedrossian, C.W.M., Bonsib, S., Moran, C. (1992). Differential diagnosis between mesothelioma and adenocarcinoma: a multimodal approach based on immunocytochemistry and electron microscopy. *Seminars in Diagnostic Pathology* **9**(2), 124–32.

Bedrossian, C.W.M., Davila, R.M. and Merenda, G. (1989). Immunocytochemical evaluation of liver fine-needle aspirations. *Archives of Pathology and Laboratory Medicine* **113**, 1225–30.

Bedrossian, C.W.M., Martinez F, Silverberg, S. (1988). Fine Needle Aspiration. In Gnepp, D (ed.), *Pathology of the Head and Neck*. Churchill Livingstone, London, pp. 25–99.

Bedrossian, C.W.M., Raber, M. Barlogie, B. (1981). Flow cytometry and cytomorphology in primary resectable breast cancer. *Analytical Qualitative Quantitative Cytology and Histology* **10**, 10–15.

Bernradd, T.J., Friberg, L.G., Koenders, A.J.M. and Kullander, S. (1980). Do estrogen and progesterone receptors (ER and PgR) in metastasizing endometrial cancers predict the response to gestation therapy? *Acta Obstetrics* **59**, 155.

Bibbo, M., Bartels, P.H., Dytch, H.E. and Wied, G.L. (1991). Cell image analysis. In Bibbo, M. (ed.), *Comprehensive Cytopathology*, W.B. Saunders, Philadelphia, pp 965–83.

Boon, M.E., Kurrer, P.H.J., Baak, J.P.A. and Goms, E.C.M. (1981). Morphometric differences between urethral cells in voided urine of patients with grade I and grade II bladder tumours. *Journal of Clinical Pathology* **34**, 612–15.

Burns, T.R., Underwood, R.D., Greenberg, S.D., Teasdale, T.A. and Cartwright, J., Jr. (1989). Cytomorphometry of large cell carcinoma of the lung. *Analytical Quantitative Cytology and Histology* **11**, 48–52.

Cannelos, G.P., Devita, V.T. and Gold, G.L. (1976). Combination chemotherapy for advanced breast cancer: response and effect on survival. *Annual Internal Medicine* **84**, 389–92.

Chen, P., Mei, Z., Yao, X. and Meng, X. (1989). Selection of hormone responsive advanced breast cancer with a cytoplasmic estrogen receptor assay. *Cancer* **63**, 139–42.

Chevalier, B., Heintzmann, G. and Mosseri, V. (1988). Prognostic value of estrogen and progesterone receptors in operable breast cancer. Results of univariate and multivariate analysis. *Cancer* **62**, 2517–24.

Clark, G.M., Dressler, I.G. and Owens, M.A. (1988). Prediction of relapse on survival in patients with node-negative breast cancer by DNA flow cytometry. *Cancer* **62**, 2387–91.

Clevenger, C.V., Epstein, A.L. and Bauer, K.D. (1987). Quantitative analysis of a nuclear antigen in interphase and mitotic cells. *Cytometry* **8**, 280.

Coleman, D. and Omerod, M. (1983). Tumour markers in clinical cytology. In Koss, L. and Coleman, D. (eds), *Advances in Clinical Cytology*, Masson Publishers, New York, pp. 33–47.

Corkill, M., Katz, R.L., Naggar, E.L. and Sneige, N. (1989). Acridine orange flow cytometry of FNAs of breast carcinoma (Abstract). *Modern Pathology* **20A**, 115.

Creasman, W.T., Soper, J.T., McCarty, Jr. K.S., Hinshaw, W. and Clark-Pearson, D.L. (1985). Influence of cytoplasmic steroid receptor content on prognosis of early stage endometrial carcinoma. *American Journal of Obstetrics and Gynecology* **151**, 922–32.

Curtin, C.T., Pertschuk, L. and Mitchell, V. (1982). Histochemical detection of estrogen and progesterone binding in FNAs of breast cancer. *Acta Cytologica* **26**, 841–6.

Danno, M. (1976). Statistical criteria for the cytology and gastric tumour. A proposal distance index. *Acta Cytologica* **20**, 466–8.

Davila, R.M., Bedrossian, C.W., Silverberg, A.B. (1988). Immunocytochemistry of the thyroid in cytologic and surgical specimens *Archives of Pathology and Laboratory Medicine* **112**, 51–6.

DeRosa, C.M., Ozzello, L., Habif, D.V., Konrath, J.G. and Green, G.L. (1989). Immunohistochemical assessment of estrogen and progesterone receptors in stored imprints and cryostat sections of breast carcinoma. *Annual Surgical* **212**, 224–8.

DeSombre, E.R. and Jensen, E.V. (1980). Estrophilin assays in breast cancer: quantitative features and application to the mastectomy specimen. *Cancer* **46**, 2783–8.

Detweiker, R., Zahniser, D.J., Garcia, G.L. and Hutchinson, M. (1988). Contextual analysis complements single-cell analysis in the diagnosis of breast cancer in FNAs. *Analytical Qualitative Quantitative Cytology and Histology* **10**, 10–15.

Douglass, E.C., Look, A.T. and Webber, B. (1986). Hyperdiploidy and chromosomal rearrangements define the anaplastic variant of wilm's tumour. *Journal of Clinical Oncology* **4**, 975–81.

Dudgeon, L.S. and Patrick, C.V. (1927). A new method for rapid microscopical diagnosis of tumours with an account of 200 cases so examined. *British Journal of Surgery* **15**, 250–61.

Ehrlich, C.E., Young, P.C.M., Stehman, F.B., Sutton, G.P. and Alford, M.W. (1988). Steroid receptors and clinical outcome in patients with adenocarcinoma of the endometrium. *American Journal of Obstetrics and Gynecology* **158**, 796–807.

Evans, D.A., Thornthwaite, J.T, Ng, A.B.P. and Sugarbaker, E.V. (1983). DNA flow cytometry of pleural effusions. *Analytical Quantitative Cytology* **5**, 19–27.

Fitzpatrick, S.L., Brightwell, J.J., Wittliff, J.L., Barrows, G.H. and Schultz, G.S. (1984), Epidermal growth factor binding by human breast tumour biopsies and relationship to estrogen receptor and progesterone receptor levels. *Cancer Research* **44**, 3448–53.

Forbes, I.J. and Leong, A.S-Y (1987). *Essential Oncology of the Lymphocyte.* Springer-Verlag, London, pp. 171–1207.

Fordham, M.V.P., Burde, A.H. and Mathews J. (1986). Prostatic carcinoma cell DNA content measured by flow cytometry and its relation to clinical outcome. *British Journal of Surgery* **73**, 400–3.

Fossa, S.D., Thorud, E, Shoaib, M.E. and Patterson E.O. (1986). DNA flow cytometry of cells obtained from old paraffin embedded specimens. *Pathologic Research in Procedures* **181**, 200.

Friedlander, M.L., Hedley, D.W. and Taylor, W. (1984). Influence of cellular DNA content on survival in advanced ovarian cancer. *Cancer Research* **44**, 397–400.

Garcia, R.L., Coltrera, M.D. and Gown A.M. (1989). Analysis of proliferative grade using anti-PCNA/cyclin monoclonal antibodies in fixed, embedded tissues. Comparison with flow cytometric analysis. *American Journal of Pathology* **134**, 733.

Gerdes, J., Schwab, O. and Lemki, H. (1983). Production of a mouse monoclonal antibody with reactive cell with a human nuclear antigen associated with cell proliferation. *International Journal of Cancer* **31**, 113.

Golomb, H.M. and Thomsen, S. (1975). Estrogen receptor: Therapeutic guide in undifferentiated metastatic carcinoma in women. *Archives of Internal Medicine* **135**, 942–5.

Green, G.L., Nolan, C., Engler, J.P. and Jensen, E.V. (1980). Monoclonal antibodies to human estrogen receptor. *Proceedings of National Academy of Science USA* **77**, 5115–19.

Grogan, T.M., Limpomas, S.M. and Spier, C.M. (1988). Independent prognostic significance of nuclear proliferation antigen in diffuse large cell lymphomas as determined by the monoclonal antibody Ki-67. *Blood* **71**, 1157.

Gustafson, H., Tribukait, B. and Esposti, P.L. (1982a). DNA profile and the progression in patients with superficial bladder tumours. *Urology Research* **10**, 13–18.

Gustafson, H., Tribukait, B., and Esposti, P.L. (1982b). The prognostic value of dna analysis in primary carcinoma in situ of the urinary bladder. *Scandinavian Journal of Urology and Nephrology* **16**, 141–6.

Hedley, D.W., Friedlander, M.L. and Taylor, I.W. (1983). Application of DNA flow cytometry to paraffin embedded archival material for the study of aneuploidy and its clinical significance. *Journal of Histochemistry and Cytochemistry* **31**, 1333–5.

Hedley, D.W., Philips, J. and Rugg, C.A. (1984). Measure of cellular DNA content as an adjunct to diagnostic cytology in malignant effusions. *European Journal of Cancer and Clinical Oncology* **20**, 749–52.

Henry, J.M., Stanley, M.W., Swenson, B, Connolly, J.E. and

Bates, H. (1991). Cytologic assessment of tumour cell kinetics: Applications of monoclonal antibody Ki-67 to fine needle aspiration smears. *Diagnostic Cytopathology* **7**, 591–6.

Jacobsen, A. (1984). Prognostic impact of ploidy level in carcinoma of the cervix. *American Journal of Clinical Oncology* **7**, 475–80.

Keshgegian, A.A., Inverso, K. and Kline, T.S. (1988). Determination of oestrogen receptor by monoclonal antireceptor antibody in aspiration biopsy cytology from breast carcinoma. *American Journal of Clinical Pathology* **89**, 24–9.

Katz, R.L., Johnson, T.S. and Williamson, K.D. (1985). Comparison of cytologic and acridine orange flow cytometric detection of malignant cells in human body cavity fluids. *Analytical Quantitative Cytology* **7**, 227–35.

Katz, R.L., Patel, S., Sneige, N., Fritsche, Jr. H.A., Hortobagyi, G.N., Ames, F.C., Brooks, T. and Ordonez, N.G. (1990). Comparison of immunocytochemical and biochemical assays for estrogen receptor in fine needle aspirates and histologic sections from breast carcinomas. *Breast Cancer Research and Treatment* **15**, 191–203.

Kiang, D.T. and Kennedy, B.J. (1977). Estrogen receptor assay in the differential diagnosis of adenocarcinomas. *Journal of the American Medical Association* **238**, 23–4.

King, E.B., Chen, K.L. and Duarte L. (1988). Image cytometric classification of premalignant breast disease in FNAs. *Cancer* **62**, 114–24.

Klein, F.A., Herr, H.W., Sogani, R.C., Whitmore, W.F. and Melamed, M.R. (1982). Detection and follow-up of carcinoma of the urinary bladder of flow cytometry. *Cancer* **50**, 389–95.

Kline, T.S. (1988). *Handbook of Fine Needle Aspiration Biopsy Cytology*. Mosby C.V., St Louis.

Kokal, W., Sheibani, K. and Terz, J. (1986). Tumour DNA content in the prognosis of colorectal carcinoma. *Journal of the American Medical Association* **255**, 3123–7.

Koss, L.G., Czerniak, B., Herz, F. and Wersto, R.P. (1989). Flow cytometric measurements of DNA and other cell components in human tumours: A critical appraisal. *Human Pathology* **6**, 528–48.

Kuenen-Boumester, V., Van der Kwast, T.H., Van Laarhoven, H.A. and Henzen-Logmans, S.C. (1989). Ki-67 staining in histological subtypes of breast carcinoma and fine needle aspiration smears. *Journal of Clinical Pathology* **134**, 733.

Lautta, M. (1984). Oestradiol and progesterone receptors in normal ovary and ovarian tumours. *Acta Obstetric Gynaecological Scandinavia* **63**, 497–503.

Lee, S.H. (1978). Cytochemical studies of estrogen receptor in human mammary cancer. *American Journal of Clinical Pathology* **70**, 197–203.

Lee, S.H. (1984). Validity of histochemical estrogen receptor assay. *Journal of Histochemical and Cytochemical* **32**, 305–10.

Leone, A., Faltow, U. and King, C.R. (1991). Reduced tumour incidence, metastatic potential and cytokine responsiveness of NM23 Transfected Melanoma cell. *Cell* **65**, 25–35.

Leong, A.S-Y., Parkinson, R. and Milios, J. (1990). 'Thick' cell membranes revealed by immunocytochemical staining: A clue to the diagnosis of malignant mesothelioma. *Diagnostic Cytopathology* **6**, 9–13.

Leong, A.S-Y. and Stevens, M.W. (1991). Cytologic diagnosis of malignant mesothelioma. *American Society of Clinical Pathologists, check sample exercise. Cytopathology* **II**, CII, 91–6.

Leong, A.S-Y., Stevens, M.W. and Mukherjee, T.M. (1992) Malignant Mesothelioma – Cytologic diagnosis with histologic, immunohistochemical and ultrastructural correlation. *Seminars in Diagnostic Pathology* **9**, 141–50.

Look, A.T., Hayes, F.A. and Nitschke, R. (1984). Cellular DNA content as a predictor of response to chemotherapy in infants with unresectable neuroblastoma. *New England Journal of Medicine* **311**, 231–5.

Look, A.T., Roberson, P.K. and Williams, D.L. (1985). Prognostic importance of blast cell DNA content in childhood acute lymphoblastic leukemia. *Blood* **65**, 1079–86.

Lorincz, M.A., Holt, J.A. and Greene, G.L. (1985). Monoclonal antibody recognition of multiple forms of oestrogen receptor tagged with [125I] methoxy-Iodovinyl oestradiol in ovarian carcinomas. *Journal of Endocrinological Metabolism* **61**, 412–17.

Martin, P.M. and Sheridan, P.J. (1982). Towards a new model for the mechanism of action of steroids. *Journal of Steroid Biochemicals* **16**, 215.

Martinez, F, Merenda, G, Bedrossian, C.W.M. (1990). Fine needle aspiration of a lipid-rich metastatic balloon cell melanoma-diagnosis by a multi-modal approach. *Diagnostic Cytopathology* **6**(6), 427–33.

Mason, M, Bedrossian, C.W.M., Fahey, C (1987). Value of immunocytochemistry in the study of malignant effusions. *Diagnostic Cytopathology* **3**, 215–22.

Masood, S. (1988). The potential value of imprint cytology in cytochemical localization of steroid hormone receptors in ovarian cancer. *Diagnostic Cytopathology* **4**, 42–7.

Masood, S. (1989). Use of monoclonal antibody for assessment of estrogen receptor content in fine needle aspiration biopsy specimen from patients with breast cancer. *Archives of Pathological Laboratory Medicine* **113**, 26–30.

Masood, S. (1990). Assessment of progesterone receptor immunocytochemical assay in breast FNAs. *Acta Cytologica* **34**(5), 735.

Masood, S. (1991). Fluorescent cytochemical detection of estrogen and progesterone receptors in breast FNAs. *American Journal of Clinical Pathology* **95**, 35–40.

Masood, S. and Johnson, H. (1987). The value of imprint cytology in cytochemical detection of steroid hormone receptors in breast cancer. *American Journal of Clinical Pathology* **87**, 30–6.

Masood, S. and Hart, N.M. (1989). Utilization of fine needle aspiration biopsy specimens in DNA flow cytometry study (Abstract). *American Journal of Clinical Pathology* **92**, 535.

Masood, S., Dee, S. and Goldstein, J.D. (1991a). Immunocytochemical analysis of progesterone receptors in breast cancer. *American Journal of Clinical Pathology* **96**, 59–63.

Masood, S., Frykberg, E.R., McLellan, G.L. and Bullard, J.B. (1991b). Application of estrogen receptor immunocytochemical assay to aspirates from mammographically guided fine needle biopsy of nonpalpable breast lesions. *Southern Medical Journal* **84(7)**, 857–61.

Masuda, T., Tezuka, F., Konno, H., Togash, A., Itoh, V. and Sugamara, J. (1988). Intraoperative imprint cytology of the thyroid gland with computer-assisted morphometric analysis of cell clusters. *Analytical Quantitative Cytology and Histology* **10**, 294–8.

McCarty, Jr. K.S., Wortman, J. and Moore J.O. (1980). Malignant effusions in recurrent breast cancer: Steroid hormone receptor analysis by effusion fluid derived cells. *Cancer* **45**, 1609–14.

McGuire, W.L., Meyer, J.S. and Barlogie, B. (1985). Impact of flow cytometry on predicting recurrence and survival in breast cancer patients. *Breast Cancer Research Treatment* **5**, 117–28.

Molina, R. (1990). Estrogen-inducible pS2 protein: tumour characteristics and clinical behaviour in breast cancer. *Proceedings Endocrine Society,* **61**.

Moll, R., Cowin, P., Kapprell, H.-P. and Franke, W.W. (1986). Desmosomal proteins: new markers for identification and classification of tumours. *Laboratory Investigation* **54**, 4–25.

Murphy, W., Emerson, L.D., Chandler, R.W., Moinuddin, S.M. and Soloway, M.S. (1986). Flow cytometry versus urinary cytology in the evaluation of patients with bladder cancer. *Journal of Urology* **136**, 815–19.

O'Hara, M., Bedrossian, C.W.M., Johnson, T., Barlugie, B. (1983). Flow cytometry in cancer diagnosis. In Steformini, M (ed.) *Progress in Clinical Pathology*. Grune and Stratton, New York, pp. 135–53.

Osborne, C.K. and McGuire, W.L. (1984). Correlations between estrogen receptor and progesterone receptor and patients' characteristics in human breast cancer. *Journal of Clinical Oncology* **2**, 1102–9.

Palmer, J.O., McDivitt, R.W. and Stones K.R. (1988). Flow cytometry analysis of breast needle aspirates. *Cancer* **62**, 2387–91.

Paridaens, R., Sylvester, R.J. and Ferrazzi, E. (1980). Clinical significance of the quantitative assessment of estrogen. *Cancer* **46**, 2889–95.

Permanetter, W. and Wiesinger, H. (1987). Immunohistochemical study of lysozyme, alpha-1-anti-chymotrypsin, tissue polypeptide, antigen, keratin and carcinoembryonic antigen in effusion sediments. *Acta Cytologica* **31**, 104–12.

Pertschuk, L.P., Eisenberg, R.N. and Carter, A.C. (1987). Estrogen binding with fluoro-cep estrogen. Correlation with biochemical assay, clinical endocrine response and disease-free interval. *Laboratory Investigation* **56**, 59A.

Potish, R.A., Twiggs, L.B., Twiggs, L.B., Adcock, L.L., Prem, K.A., Savage, J.E. and Leung B.S. (1986). Prognostic importance of progesterone and estrogen receptors in cancer of the uterine cervix. *Cancer* **58**, 1709–13.

Raber, M.N., Barlogie, B., Latreille, J., Bedrossian, C.W.N. (1982). Ploidy, proliferative activity and estrogen receptor content in human breast cancer. *Cytometry* **3**, 36–41.

Reinherz, G.L., Rubinstein, A. and Geha, R.F. (1979). Abnormalities of immunoregulatory T cells in disorders of immune function. *New England Journal of Medicine* **301**, 1018–20.

Richman, C.M., Holt, J.A., Lorincz, M.A. and Herbst, A.L. (1985). Persistence and distribution of estrogen receptor in advanced epithelial ovarian carcinoma after chemotherapy. *Obstetrics and Gynecology* **65**, 257–63.

Sasaki, K., Matsuma, K. and Tatsuo, T. (1988). Relationship between labelling indices by Ki-67 and BrdUrd in human malignant tumours. *Cancer* **62**, 989.

Schechter, A.L., Sten, D.F., Vaidyanathan, L., Decker, S.J., Drebin, J.A., Greene, M.J. and Weinber, R.A. (1984). The *neu* oncogene and *erbB*-related gene encoding a 185,000 m tumour antigen. *Nature* **312**, 513–16.

Schneller, J., Eppich, E., Greenbaum, E., Eleguin, F., Shreman, A., Werslo, R. and Ross, I.G. (1987). Flow cytometry and feulgen cytophotometry in evaluation of effusions. *Cancer* **59**, 1307–13.

Schwartz, P.G., Keating, G. and Maclusky N. (1982). Tamoxifen therapy for advanced ovarian cancer. *Obstetrics and Gynecology* **58**, 583–8.

Sigurdson, H., Baldetorp, B. and Borg, A. (1990). Indicators of prognosis in node-negative breast cancer. *New England Journal of Medicine* **322**, 1045–53.

Silverman, J. (1987). The use of immunoperoxidase panels for the cytologic diagnosis of malignancy in serous effusions. *Diagnostic Pathology* **3**, 134–40.

Silverman, J. (1991). *Breast. In Bibbo, M. (ed.), Comprehensive Cytopathology*, W.B. Saunders, Philadelphia, pp. 703–70.

Sklarew, R.J. and Pertschuk, L.P. (1987). Quantitation of immunocytochemical assay for estrogen receptor protein (ER-ICA) in human breast cancer of television image. *Journal of Histochemistry and Cytochemistry* **25**, 1253–9.

Slamon, D.J., Clark, G.M. and Wang, S.G. (1987). Human breast cancer. Correlation of relapse and survival with amplification of the HER-2/neu oncogens. *Science* **235**, 177–82.

Steeg, P.S., Bevilacqua, G. and Kopper, L. (1988). Evidence for a Rovel gene associated with low tumour metastatic potential. *Journal of the National Cancer Institute* **80**, 200–3.

Stevens, M.W., Crowley, K.S., Fazzalari, N.L. and Woods, A.E. (1988). Use of morphometry in cytological preparations for diagnosing follicular non-Hodgkin's lymphomas. *Journal of Clinical Pathology* **41**, 370–7.

Stonesifer, K.J., Ziany, J., Wilkinson, E.J., Benson, N.A. and Braylin, R.C. (1984). Flow cytometric analysis and cytopathology of body fluids. *Acta Cytologica* **28**, 639–40.

Szymendera, J.J., Zborzil, J. and Sikorowad L. (1981). Value of five tumour markers (AFP, CEA, hCG, hPL and SP1) in diagnosis and staging of testicular germ cell tumours. *Oncology* **38**, 222.

Thor, A.D. (1991). Accumulation of tumour suppressor gene p53 is an independent prognostic marker in breast cancer. *Breast Cancer Research and Treatment* **19**(2), 157 (Abstract 1).

Thorpe, S.M., Rochefort, H. and Garcia, M. (1989). Association between high concentration of Mr 52,000 Cathepsin-D and poor prognosis in primary human breast cancer. *Cancer Research* **49**, 6008–14.

Tomila, T., Yasue, M., Engelhard, H.H., McLone, D.G., Gonzalez-Cruzzi, F. and Bauer, K.D. (1988). Flow cytometric DNA analysis of medulloblastoma. Prognostic implication of aneuploidy. *Cancer* **61**, 744–9.

Unger, K.M., Raber, M., Bedrossian, C.W.M., Stein, D.A. and Barlogie, B. (1983). ·Analysis of pleural effusions using automated flow cytometry. *Cancer* **52**, 873–7.

Van Molengraft, F.J.J.M., Van't Hot, M.A., Herman, C.J. and Vooijts, P.G. (1982). Quantitative light microscopy and atypical mesothelial cells and malignant cells in ascitic fluid. *Analytical Quantitative Cytology* **4**, 220.

Vanstapel, M.-J., Gatter, K.C., deWolf-Petter, C., Mason, D.Y. and Desmet, V.D. (1986). New sites of human S-100 immunoreactivity detected with monoclonal antibodies. *American Journal of Clinical Pathology* **85**, 160–8.

Volm, M. and Mattern, J. (1985). DNA distribution of non-small cell lung carcinomas and its relationship to clinical behaviour. *Cytometry* **6**, 348–56.

Von Roenn, J.M., Kheir, S.M. and Wolter, J.M. (1986). Significance of DNA abnormalities in primary malignant melanoma and nevi, a retrospective flow cytometric study. *Canadian Research* **46**, 7192–5.

Warhol, M.J. (1984). The ultrastructural localization of keratin proteins and carcinoembryonic antigen in malignant mesotheliomas. *American Journal of Pathology* **116**, 385–90.

Welshons, W.V., Liberman, M.D. and Grosk, J. (1984). Nuclear localization of unoccupied oestrogen receptors. *Nature* **307**, 747–79.

Yoss, E.B., Berd, D., Cohn, J.R. and Peters, S. (1989). Flow cytometric evaluation of bronchoscopic washings and lavage fluid for DNA aneuploidy as an adjunct in the diagnosis of lung cancer and tumours metastatic to the lung. *Chest* **96**, 54–9.

9 ◆ *Setting up a diagnostic immunohistochemistry service*

Anthony S-Y. Leong

Introduction

The acceptance of immunohistochemistry as an adjunct to morphological examination is well attested to by a survey in the United Kingdom in 1988 (Angel et al., 1988). It was found that 138 pathology laboratories, which included 35 district general hospital and 29 teaching hospital laboratories, performed immunohistochemical stains and expended a total of £5.4 million on the procedure. While smaller service laboratories may prefer to refer their cases to a larger laboratory for immunostaining, it would appear that many laboratories see immunohistochemistry as an extension of the diagnostic service and would prefer to perform the procedure themselves. There is no question that when employed correctly, immunohistochemistry is a very powerful and practical diagnostic tool. It also provides a high level of professional satisfaction for the surgical pathologist as it complements his or her observational skills and extends the boundaries of morphological examination and diagnosis. Its area of greatest application in surgical pathology is in the typing of tumours and it has been estimated that about 15 to 20 per cent of tumours would benefit from immunohistochemical staining (Leong and Wright, 1988; Leong and Wannakairot, 1992).

This chapter lays out in general terms the setting up of a diagnostic service but the remarks and comments made should be considered in the context of the specific requirements of the individual laboratory.

Laboratory and equipment

The requirements of laboratory space for a diagnostic immunohistochemistry service will depend on the availability of space in the laboratory complex and the workload of the individual laboratory.

We have a separate immunohistochemistry laboratory of 27 square metres with total of 15.7 metres length of bench space. It accommodates one part-time and two full-time technologists and various students, research assistants and visitors from time to time, so that it is often very crowded and far from optimum.

The requirements of an immunohistochemistry laboratory are not different to other histopathology laboratories in that bench space, storage shelves and a wash basin with clean running water are necessary. Unless the more toxic chemicals with heavy metals such as cobalt, lead, and nickel are employed and incubations performed at high temperatures which will vaporize such reagents, a fume-extraction chamber is not generally required.

Provided below (Table 9.1) is a list of the main equipment which would be required for a diagnostic immunohistochemistry laboratory. The brand names are provided only as a suggestion, representing the equipment used in our laboratory. Obviously, the list is not comprehensive and can be expanded or reduced in accordance with the specific requirements of the laboratory. Some equipment can be shared with other laboratories.

Table 9.1. Equipment for immunohistochemistry laboratory

Refrigerator 4°C (any domestic type)
Freezer −70°C (Revco)*
Micropipettors – a range of sizes, eg:
0.5–10 μl
10–50 μl
50–200 μl
200–1000 μl (all Nichiryo, Japan)
Water purification unit (Barnstead Nanopure II)
Vortex mixer (Chilterns)
Digital balance, dual range up to 200 grams, accuracy to five decimal places (Mettler E200)
37°C oven (Laborro)
37°C water incubator (Labmaster)
pH meter (Gallenkamp)
Rotary microtome (Leitz Model 1512)
Flotation bath, paraffin section (Electrothermal)
Slide incubation chambers (can be made from perspex sheets to own specifications)

Note: * −70°C freezer would be ideal but a −20°C freezer will also serve the purpose.

Staffing

Immunohistochemistry is more than just another special stain. While the technical ·procedure is well established and relatively straightforward, it is a multi-step procedure with blocking steps and no means of checking until the procedure is completed. The stain can be capricious, with success being dependent on variables such as antigen preservation, proteolytic digestion, enhancement techniques and the appropriateness of antibody and reagent concentrations. Optimal dilutions of reagents need to be determined each time a new antibody is used, cognisant of the immunoenzyme system used in the laboratory and of the method of tissue fixation and preparation.

The markedly different and sometimes variable levels of sensitivities and specificities of primary antibodies as well as secondary and tertiary reagents, makes immunohistochemistry extremely technique-dependent, and, unlike most other laboratory tests, draws on skills that are normally found in at least two different disciplines, namely, immunology and histology. Clearly, familiarity with the staining procedure and the quality and consistency of the stained product is dependent on the volume of work performed by the laboratory and the individual technologist. For these reasons, it would be optimal that a hospital scientist or senior technologist to be fully dedicated to the immunohistochemistry laboratory. While this may not be possible because of personnel resources, it should at least be the case, for consistency and reproducibility of results, that all immunohistochemical procedures, as well as responsibility for the preparation and dilution of reagents, be performed by the same individual. Furthermore, the supervision or guidance of an interested surgical pathologist will greatly enhance the role and development of the laboratory, particularly in the selection of appropriate reagents for purchase and the assessment of their specificities. The supervising pathologist will also play a consultative role in relation to other pathologists who use the service. It cannot be over-emphasized that the results of immunostaining should not be interpreted in isolation, but in conjunction with the morphological and clinical features of the lesion.

Reagents

The range of stains performed by the laboratory would vary with the workload and nature of the surgical pathology laboratory it services. In general, the widest application in surgical pathology would be in the area of tumour diagnosis and classification and prognostication, however, immunohistochemistry can also be employed to renal diseases, the identification of infectious organisms, leukaemia and lymphoma typing, as well as for research. The extent of involvement in these various areas would determine the range of antibodies and reagents used in the laboratory.

Several inherent problems beset good and consistent immunostaining. These include the marked variability of antibody specificities and sensitivities, the sale of similar or identical antibody clones by different commercial sources and under different names and other problems arising from a lack of standardization of reagents. The use of pre-prepared commercial kits may be seen as a method to circumvent some of these problems; however, kits are not without their own drawbacks. Kits that provide pre-diluted antibodies give the illusion of simplicity and consistency and have fostered a false sense of security among its users who may be unfamiliar with the ramifications of immunological reagents that lack defined specificity. Some kits fail to fulfil even the most reasonable expectations and, in this event, it is often difficult to identify the reagent at fault. Kits are sold 'ready-to-use' and are designed to accommodate all of their users. Their reagent concentrations are not necessarily optimal for the individual laboratory and the opportunities for optimizing reagents to individual requirements are limited, so that their results are often suboptimal. Furthermore, they are expensive.

Table 9.2 provides a list of 20 of the most common antibodies employed in our laboratory, and their commercial sources. This list comprises antibodies to low molecular weight cytokeratin (such as CAM5.2), high molecular weight cytokeratin (such as anti-callus keratin), broad spectrum cytokeratin (such as AE1/3 and anti-bovine keratin), vimentin, desmin, muscle-specific actin, leucocyte common antigen, S100, HMB45, prostate-specific antigen, prostatic alkaline phosphatase, thyroglobulin, gross cystic disease fluid protein-15, placental alkaline phosphatase, chromogranin, CD 57 (Leu7, HNK-1), neurofilament triplet proteins, factor VIII-related protein, carcinoembryonic antigen and epithelial membrane antigen. While some of the general applications of these antibodies are also provided in the table, it is emphasized that they are most effective as diagnostic tools when applied as panels directed to a narrow list of differential diagnoses based on the clinical and morphological features of the individual case. It is also important to appreciate that very few antibodies are tissue- or lineage-specific and are best regarded only as 'tissue-associated'.

Budget

In the foregoing discussion, it is clear that unless the laboratory handles sufficient volumes, it would be very difficult to produce and maintain consistent quality, or

Table 9.2. Twenty commonly used antibodies and their sources

Antibody	Source	Some applications*
CAM 5.2	B & D	Detects low molecular weight cytokeratins present in almost all carcinomas.
Anti-callus keratin	Dako	Polyclonal antisera. Detects high molecular weight cytokeratins present in stratified epithelial, especially squamous cell carcinomas.
AE1/3	BM	A cocktail of antibodies to broad spectrum-keratin. Useful as a screen for cytokeratins.
Anti-vimentin	Dako	Vimentin is the intermediate filament of mesenchymal tumours but is also expressed by a limited number of epithelial tumours.
Anti-desmin	Dako	Identifies tumours with skeletal or smooth muscle differentiation.
Anti-muscle specific actin (MSA)	Enzo	Identifies myogenic differentiation and also myoepithelial cells.
Anti-leucocyte common antigen (LCA, CD45)	Dako	Very specific antibody which identifies lymphoid cells as well as leucocytes.
Anti-S100	Dako	A sensitive but not specific marker of naevus cells and melanomas. Also identifies glial and Schwann cells. Has wide distribution in the body in cells which include myoepithelial, Langerhans', dendritic, reticulum, adrenal medullary sustentaticular cells. Also labels chondrocytes and some breast epithelial cells.
HMB45	Enzo	A melanoma-specific antibody. The antigen may be lost with long exposure to formaldehyde.
Anti-prostate specific antigen (PSA)	Dako	An almost lineage-specific antibody to prostatic cells. Probably more specific than PSAP.
Anti-prostatic acid phosphatase (PSAP)	Dako	Detects prostatic tissue. Rarely expressed by islet cell tumours, breast and renal carcinomas.
Anti-thyroglobulin	Dako	Labels thyroglobulin. As with most other anti-hormone and neuro-peptide antibodies, it is useful for the identification of the specific peptides and hormones in endocrine and neuro-endocrine tumours.
Anti-gross cystic disease fluid protein –15 (GCDFP–15)	Signet	Useful for the identification of breast carcinomas. Also labels salivary gland, sweat gland and prostatic tumours.
Anti-placental alkaline phosphatase (PLAP)	Dako	Labels germ cells and their tumours. Particularly useful for identifying intratubular germ cell neoplasms.
Anti-chromogranin	Dako	Specific to acidic polypeptide contained in the neurosecretory granules of neuro-endocrine cells and their tumours.
Leu7 (HNK-1) (CD 57)	B & D	First developed as an antibody to natural killer cells but subsequently recognized to label a myelin-associated glycoprotein in neuroectodermal tissue. The antigen is expressed by some neuroendocrine tumours, peripheral nerve sheath tumours and prostatic tumours.
Anti-neurofilaments	Dako	A cocktail of antibodies to all three subunits of 70 kD, 170 kD and 195 kD molecular weight. Detects the intermediate filaments in neurons, axons and dendrites and their tumours. Also labels some neuroendocrine tumours.
Anti-factor VIII related protein	Dako	A highly specific marker of endothelial cells and their tumours including angiosarcoma, haemangioendothelioma and Kaposi's sarcoma. Unfortunately its sensitivity is low in poorly differentiated tumours.
Anti-carcinoembryonic antigen (CEA)	Dako	Labels most adenocarcinomas from the gastrointestinal tract. Useful in the distinction of mesotheliomas from metastatic adenocarcinomas, the former being negative for CEA.
Anti-epithelial membrane antigen (EMA)	Dako	Useful for the identification of carcinoma but only in conjunction with anti-cytokeratins. Particularly useful in demonstrating the long microvillous processes characteristic of mesothelial cells.

Notes: *Only some general applications of the antibodies are listed. The reagents are most useful when employed as a panel directed against a short list of differential diagnoses based on clinical and histological features.
B & D = Becton Dickinson, California, USA; Dako = Dakopatts, California, USA; BM = Boehringer Mannheim, Australia; Enzo = Enzo Biochem, New York, USA; Signet = Signet Laboratories, Massachusetts, USA.

to acquire reasonable experience with a wide range of reagents. A bank of these antibodies would cost less than $AUS10,000 in initial outlay, the annual running cost being dependent on usage. With careful use of diluted aliquots and storage of the undiluted antibodies at −70°C, this initial bank of antibodies can be made to last many years so that a large proportion of the yearly budget could be used to purchase new antibodies and to expand the range of tests performed.

Diagnostic immunohistochemistry is not an expensive procedure, particularly if the laboratory handles sufficient volumes. In our laboratory, the average cost of reagents per case is less than $AUS5 inclusive of chromogens and linking reagents, but exclusive of labour cost. This sum is very modest, particularly in the context of the current costs of other laboratory tests. The expenses are contained by bulk purchasing of reagents, and up to a point, labour cost is inversely related to the volume of work, the cost per slide reducing as the volume of work increases. The inclusion of other specialized staining procedures, such as lymphocyte marker studies on cryostat sections and cytospin preparations, oestrogen and progesterone receptor studies, oncogene assays, and the investigation of glomerular disease, as part of the diagnostic service, will significantly add to running costs because of the extensive panels involved and the expensive nature of some of the antibodies. The inclusion of positive and negative controls for each test will add further to the expense and this becomes significant if the antibody is used infrequently as each time a positive control is run, it doubles the cost of the test. The purchase of individual reagents will reduce the cost somewhat in comparison to the use of pre-prepared kits. However, it will incur additional labour for titrating and balancing the reagents. In the costing of prepared kits one has also to take into consideration the frequency of use. A kit costing $AUS500 which can be used for 50 tests would appear to cost $AUS10 per test, but with controls, it doubles to $AUS20 per test. If the kit is used only five times before it expires, the reagent cost is $AUS100 per test.

On the balance, for laboratories which employ immunohistochemistry infrequently, that is, less than 10 cases a week, it may be best to initially purchase a limited number of primary antibodies to use with a staining kit which provides the linking and tertiary reagents in prediluted forms. With increasing requirements and familiarity, the range of primary antibodies can be expanded to include all the common ones as listed in Table 9.2, remembering that the use of an incomplete panel of antibodies, particularly in the hands of the inexperienced, can provide more misleading than helpful information.

Labour is the most expensive item on our laboratory budget. Our total work-up cost per case, inclusive of technician's time, is $AUS76. We have two full-time dedicated technical officers who accession some 11,000 slides (1,500 cases) a year. Itemized cost for each antibody employed in our laboratory is provided in the Appendix. The total expense of a diagnostic immunohistochemistry service, therefore, is very small in comparison to the many new technologies employed in tissue diagnosis such as the polymerase chain reaction, in situ hybridization, protein blotting and other molecular biology techniques, as well as more established technologies such as electron microscopy, chromosome analysis and cell culture. The costs are relatively insignificant in terms of patient care and management and in terms of the high level of professional satisfaction derived from this additional dimension to the process of morphological examination.

Requesting of immunostains

In a large department with several pathologists and trainees, the immunohistochemistry laboratory will function as a service arm of general surgical pathology and autopsy and will receive requests for immunostaining from individuals with a wide range of experience. For efficacious function of the laboratory, such requests should contain, in addition to the usual patient data, information concerning the nature of the specimen, the most appropriate tissue block for immunostaining, the nature of the fixative and duration of fixation if different to the routine method employed in the laboratory, and the provisional diagnosis or differential diagnoses. Individuals with less experience in immunohistochemistry should be encouraged to consult the supervising pathologist in the planning of appropriate diagnostic antibody panels. This will significantly improve the effective use of the service.

Quality control

While the ever-increasing range of antibodies and immunohistochemical reagents continues to expand the diagnostic applications of immunohistochemistry, it is not without its own problems. There are currently over 200 vendors of immunological reagents and antibodies and although this allows the purchaser a wider choice, the reagents available are not of uniform sensitivity and specificity. Different clones are claimed to detect similar antigens and the same clone may be sold as concentrates or in pre-diluted forms, as culture supernatants or as ascitic fluid, and the same antibody may be sold under different names, by different companies. The purchaser has to choose one antibody over so many others with purportedly similar specificities and many immune reagents do not necessarily conform to the claims of sensitivity and specificity made by the manufacturers and distributors. Furthermore, all commercial antibodies carry the disclaimer 'not for diagnostic use' despite the fact that they are sold for this very purpose. While it may be construed that the disclaimer reflects the manufacturers' lack of confidence in their own products, it has been said that the disclaimer is made because of the great variability in antigen preservation as a result of the different processing methods and staining procedures employed in different laboratories. Until recently, many publications reported on home-grown or privately held antibodies and this did not allow inter-laboratory comparison of results. The commercialization of monoclonal antibodies is now a major component of the biotechnology arms of many universities and research institutions, so that many of these home-grown products are now commercially available. Indeed, it is not uncommon to find an antibody on sale while the definitive publication describing its specificity and characteristics is not yet in print. Although inter-laboratory comparisons are made easier by the increasing use of well-characterized commercial monoclonal antibodies, the plethora of antibodies on the market can make it equally confusing for the small laboratory which can be quite easily lost in the quagmire of new antibodies and immunoreagents. Laboratories are faced with the decision of expending valuable time and resources on in-house testing of each of these reagents or purchasing on the recommendation of the distributors or just on 'spec'. A similar situation existed with the surge of leucocyte antibodies and this was partly solved only with the institution of international workshops on leucocyte differentiation markers which have resulted in the cluster designation classification system. Laboratories were invited to submit monoclonal antibodies which were then distributed and tested biochemically, immunologically, and histologically by participants. Antibodies which recognized the same or a very similar antigen were assigned to a common cluster designation group. As a similar programme of testing and standardization for non-lymphoid markers has not yet been instituted, it would be advisable, under the present circumstances, for smaller laboratories to seek the expert advice of larger immunohistochemistry laboratories which perform internal quality control and have greater experience over a wider range of commercial reagents. It would also be clearly advisable for laboratories performing immunohistochemistry to subscribe to some form of quality assurance programme which will allow them to compare and maintain an acceptable quality of work.

Internal laboratory quality control should also be performed. It is necessary to check the sensitivity and the specificity of every new reagent purchased and it is also necessary to check the sensitivity of every new batch of reagent as there may be significant batch-to-batch variation of the same reagent. This is best done by the standard checkerboard titration method against known positive tissue conveniently prepared as a multi-tissue sausage roll (Battifora, 1986; Kraaz et al., 1988; Miller and Groothuis, 1991). For positive control, normal tissues may be used, but it is more appropriate to employ tumour tissue where the levels of antigen expression may not be as high as those of normal tissues but more appropriate to the levels of the test tissue.

With every antibody 'run' there should also be appropriate positive and negative controls. If the volume of work is large, there would be considerable savings in costs and labour if only one positive and one negative control for each antibody was performed, instead of doing the same for each slide that is immunostained. These controls could be labelled with the date of immunostaining as identification.

If immunohistochemical interpretation is not reported by a specific pathologist, it would be appropriate for the pathologist supervising the immunohistochemistry laboratory to systemically examine an appropriate number of slides with each stain run as a method of quality audit.

It is paradoxical that although automation of the immunostaining procedure with one of the several commercial machines currently available (Chapter 1) may provide a means of standardization and consistency of results in smaller laboratories, it is probably not cost effective for low workloads. There is really no substitute for good technical experience and skills, cognisance of reagent sensitivity and specificity, and careful interpretation correlated with morphological and clinical features.

Reporting of immunostaining

If immunohistochemistry is considered to be an integral part of the histopathology report representing no more than an extension of the process of morphological examination, then the results of immunostaining should be a component of the histopathology report. In order that there be no undue delays to the main surgical pathology report, the results of immunohistochemistry can be incorporated as supplementary report. It should be documented the preliminary surgical pathology report that immunohistochemical stains are proceeding as a special study. It cannot be over-emphasized that the results of immunohistochemical stains are to be interpreted in the context of the clinical setting and the gross and microscopic findings. The immunohistochemical report should include the following information: the nature of the specimen, the nature of the fixative employed, duration of fixation and should list the antibodies applied, the results of staining and the diagnosis. It goes without saying that all such immunohistochemistry reports should be signed by a pathologist. A two-to three-day turnaround time with an 80 per cent threshold is acceptable.

Laboratory routine

The laboratory routine is largely determined by the volume and pattern of work. Staining can be batched or performed on demand. The latter method will work only with low volume laboratories and is suited to the use of pre-prepared staining kits. Performing immunostaining on demand will be very disruptive to the smooth running of a high volume laboratory which examines a wide range of tissues and uses a large variety of antibodies. Batching of the specimens would be the most ·efficient and economical method of operation for such laboratories.

In the absence of automation, the batching of stains and having 'runs' on alternate days will allow synchronization of section cutting and staining. For example, on Day 1, requests could be collated, paraffin blocks retrieved and sections cut. Appropriate antibodies and controls could be prepared and the necessary steps be conducted prior to overnight incubation with the primary antibody at room temperature. On Day 2, the staining can be taken to completion with delivery of the immunostained slides to the pathologist by about midday. The rest of the day can be used to perform 'housekeeping chores' such as the diluting of reagents, the preparation of control tissues, record keeping, stock taking, ordering of equipment and reagents, etc.

Day 3 is best retained for the preparation and immunostaining of material other than paraffin sections such as cytospin preparations, imprints and frozen sections. Although these procedures are often more involved as they require more extensive panels of antibodies, the incubation periods are shorter and the staining procedure can be completed within the day. As they involve different staining procedures on materials prepared in different ways, it is best to assign this task to a different medical technologist or to perform the tasks on a day separate to that from routine paraffin section immunostaining.

Days 4 and 5 could revert to the staining of paraffin sections in the manner set out for Days 1 and 2 (Table 9.3).

Table 9.3. Suggested work schedule for diagnostic immunohistochemistry laboratory

Day 1	Collate cases. Select appropriate paraffin blocks and prepare sections. Prepare appropriate antibodies and controls. Overnight incubation of primary antibodies at room temperature.
Day 2	Complete staining. Examine slides and record results in laboratory log book prior to delivery of slides to pathologists (quality control). Routine 'housekeeping chores'.
Day 3	Preparation and immunostaining of material other than paraffin sections, e.g. frozen sections, cytospins. Also special procedures such as double immunolabelling, etc.
Days 4 and 5	Staining of paraffin sections as in Days 1 and 2.

There should also be provision for the laboratory to attend to urgent specimens which may arise from time to time and to perform such stains on demand.

It is important for the laboratory to maintain a log of all specimens examined as well as a record of the results of immunostaining. The latter is separate to the immunohistochemistry report and preferably should be entered by the technologist who performed the stain, after examination of the slide with the senior supervising officer or pathologist. This forms an efficient way of quality control as well as educational tool for the technologist.

References

Angel, C.A., Heyderman, E. and Lauder, I. (1989) Use of immunohistochemistry in Britain: EQA Forum Antibody Usage Questionnaire. *Journal of Clinical Pathology* **42**, 1012–17.

Battifora H. (1986). The multitumour (sausage) tissue block. Novel method for immunohistochemical testing. *Laboratory Investigation* **55**, 244–8.

Kraaz, W., Risberg, B. and Haussein, A. (1988). Multiblock: An aid in diagnostic immunohistochemistry. *Journal Clinical Pathology* **41**, 1337.

Miller, R.T. and Groothuis, C.L. (1991). Multitumor 'sausage' blocks in immunohistochemistry. Simplified method of preparation, practical uses and roles in quality assurance. *American Journal of Clinical Pathology* **96**, 228–32.

Leong, A.S-Y. and Wright, J. (1987). The contributions of immunohistochemical staining in tumour diagnosis. *Histopathology* **11**, 1295–305.

Leong, A.S-Y. and Wannakrairot, P. (1992). A retrospective analysis of immunohistochemical staining in identification of anaplastic round cell and spindle cell tumours – Results, reagents and costs. *Pathology* **24**, 254–60.

Appendix: Staining protocols; antibodies, sources, dilutions and costs

Anthony S-Y. Leong with James Milios
and contributions by Carlos W.M. Bedrossian and Shahla Masood

Introduction

In this Appendix we provide details of various preparation, fixation and staining procedures employed in our laboratory. A list of the antibodies used by us, their sources, working dilutions and staining cost per slide is also provided in 18, page 396. The dilutions of reagents indicated are provided only as a guide as each laboratory will have to determine the optimal dilution for the reagents appropriate to their individual methods of tissue fixation and processing.

Procedures

1. Avidin-biotin peroxidase technique for paraffin sections

1. Deparaffinize sections taking through to absolute alcohol.
2. Block endogenous peroxidase with 0.5 per cent H_2O_2 in methanol for 30 min.
3. Air dry, use 'PAP' pen to encircle the sections (Dako Cat No. S2002), followed by quick dip in the peroxide-methanol blocking reagent, and two washes in PBS pH 7.4 for 5 min each.
4. Block with 3 per cent normal horse serum (NHS) for 20 min.
5. Drain off excess NHS and incubate overnight at room temperature (21°C) with primary antibody appropriately diluted with 3 per cent NHS.
6. Two washes in PBS pH 7.4, 3 min each.
7. Incubate with biotinylated secondary antibody (Dakopatts, USA) 1/500, diluted with 3 per cent NHS, for 30 min at room temperature.
8. Two washes in PBS pH 7.4, 3 min each.
9. Incubate with peroxidase conjugated streptavidin (Pierce, USA) 1/1500, diluted with 3 per cent NHS, for 60 min at room temperature.
10. Two washes in PBS pH 7.4, 3 min each.
11. Apply peroxidase substrate solution: 25 mg diaminobenzidine tetrahydrochloride (Sigma, Cat No. D-5637) in 50 ml Tris HCl buffer pH 7.4, and 50 μl of 30 per cent H_2O_2. Control reaction macroscopically/microscopically, about 10–20 min.
12. Rinse in PBS pH 7.4.
13. Lightly counterstain with Mayer's haematoxylin.
14. Dehydrate, clear and mount.

2. Immunostaining of oestrogen receptors in paraffin sections

1. Immerse sample of fresh tissue (10 × 10 × 3 mm) in 10 per cent buffered formalin for 1 hour.
2. Transfer to 70 per cent ethanol until ready for overnight processing through graded ethylalcohol, chloroform and wax in an automated processor. (Note the absence of formaldehyde in processor.)
3. Cut paraffin sections, mount onto coated slides (amino propyltriethoxysilane), dry at 60°C for 10 min.
4. Deparaffinize sections in xylene for 5–10 min.
5. Three washes in 100 per cent ethyl alcohol, 1 min each.
6. Three washes in distilled water, 1 min each.
7. Wash in PBS pH 7.4 at 37°C for 5 min.
8. Prepare PRONASE (Calbiochem, Cat No. 537088), 0.2 mg/ml in PBS pH 7.4, and heat to 37°C.
9. Digest tissue sections in a humid incubator for 20 min at 37°C.
10. Two washes in PBS pH 7.4, 3 min each.
11. Encircle sections with a 'PAP' pen (Dako Cat No. S2002).
12. Block with 3 per cent normal horse serum (NHS), for 20 min.
13. Drain off excess NHS and apply anti-estrogen receptor antibody (Abbotts, Cat No. 3087–18) 1/5 diluted with 3 per cent NHS, incubate overnight at room temperature (21°C).
14. Two washes in PBS pH 7.4, 3 min each.
15. Incubate with biotinylated rabbit anti-rat IgG (Vector, USA. Cat No. BA-4000) 1/250 diluted with 3 per cent NHS for 30 min at room temperature.
16. Two washes of PBS pH 7.4, 3 min each.
17. Incubate with peroxidase conjugated streptavidin (Pierce, USA) 1/1000 diluted with 3 per cent NHS for 60 min at room temperature.
18. Two washes of PBS pH 7.4, 3 min each.
19. Apply peroxidase substrate solution: 25 mg diaminobenzedine tetrahydrochloride (Sigma, Cat No. D-5637) to 50 ml Tris HCl buffer pH 7.4, 50 μl of 30 per cent H_2O_2 and 500 μl of 1M Imidazole. Control reaction macroscopically/microscopically, about 10–20 min.
20. Wash in PBS pH 7.4, for 1 minute.
21. Counterstain lightly with Mayer's haematoxylin.
22. Dehydrate, clear and mount.

3. Immunostaining of progesterone receptors in paraffin sections

1. Immerse sample of fresh tissue (10 × 10 × 3 mm) in 10 per cent buffered formalin for 1 h.
2. Transfer to 70 per cent ethanol until ready for overnight processing through graded ethylalcohol, chloroform and wax in an automated processor. (Note the absence of formaldehyde in processor.)
3. Cut paraffin sections, mount onto coated slides (amino propyltriethoxysilane), dry at 60°C for 10 min.
4. Deparaffinize sections in xylene for 5–10 min.
5. Three washes in 100 per cent ethyl alcohol, 1 min each.
6. Three washes in distilled water, 1 min each.
7. Wash in PBS pH 7.4 at, for 5 min.
8. Encircle sections with a 'PAP' pen (Dako Cat No. S2002).
9. Block with 3 per cent normal horse serum (NHS), for 20 min.
10. Drain off excess NHS and apply anti-estrogen receptor antibody (Abbotts, Cat No. 2808–18) 1/15 diluted with 3 per cent NHS, incubate overnight at room temperature (21°C).
11. Two washes in PBS pH 7.4, 3 min each.
12. Incubate with biotinylated rabbit anti-rat IgG (Vector, USA. Cat No. BA-4000) 1/250 diluted with 3 per cent NHS for 30 min at room temperature.
13. Two washes of PBS pH 7.4, 3 min each.
14. Incubate with peroxidase conjugated streptavidin (Pierce, USA) 1/1000 diluted with 3 per cent NHS for 60 min at room temperature.
15. Two washes of PBS pH 7.4, 3 min each.
16. Apply peroxidase substrate solution: 25 mg diaminobenzedine tetrahydrochloride (Sigma, Cat No. D-5637) to 50 ml Tris HCl buffer pH 7.4, 50 μl of 30 per cent H_2O_2 and 500 μl of 1M Imidazole. Control reaction macroscopically/microscopically, about 10–20 min.
17. Wash in PBS pH 7.4, for 1 min.
18. Counterstain lightly with Mayer's haematoxylin.
19. Dehydrate, clear and mount.

4. Dual antigen staining technique with peroxidase labelled mouse monoclonal antibody and alkaline phosphatase labelled rabbit polyclonal antibody

1. Deparaffinize sections, taking through to absolute alcohol.
2. Block endogenous peroxidase with 0.5 per cent H_2O_2 in methanol for 30 min.
3. Air dry, use 'PAP' pen to encircle the sections (Dako Cat No. S2002), followed by a quick dip in the peroxide-methanol blocking reagent, and two washes in PBS pH 7.4 for 5 min each.
4. Block with 3 per cent normal horse serum (NHS) for 20 min.
5. Drain off excess NHS and incubate with primary mouse monoclonal antibody appropriately diluted with 3 per cent NHS for 30 min at room temperature (21°C).
6. Two washes in PBS pH 7.4, 3 min each.
7. Incubate with biotinylated horse anti-mouse secondary antibody (Vector, USA) 1/250, diluted with 3 per cent NHS, for 30 min at room temperature.
8. Two washes in PBS pH 7.4, 3 min each.
9. Incubate with peroxidase conjugated streptavidin (Pierce, USA) 1/1500, diluted with 3 per cent NHS, for 30 min.
10. Two washes in PBS pH 7.4, 3 min each.
11. Apply peroxidase substrate solution: 25 mg diaminobenzedine tetrahydrochloride (Sigma, Cat No. D-5637) in 50 ml Tris HCl buffer pH 7.4, and 50 μl of 30 per cent H_2O_2. Control reaction macroscopically/microscopically, about 10–20 min.
12. Rinse in distilled water followed by washing in PBS pH 7.4 for 5 min.
13. Block with 3 per cent swine serum for 20 min.
14. Drain off excess swine serum and apply rabbit polyclonal antibody appropriately diluted with swine serum for 30 min at room temperature.
15. Two washes in PBS pH 7.4, 3 min each.
16. Incubate with secondary swine anti-rabbit immunoglobulins (Dakopatts, USA), 1/50 diluted with swine serum, for 30 min at room temperature.
17. Two washes in PBS pH 7.4, 3 min each.
18. Apply rabbit alkaline phosphatase anti-alkaline phosphatase immune complex (Dakopatts, USA) 1/50 diluted with swine serum, for 30 min at room temperature.

19. Two washes in PBS pH 7.4, 3 min each.
20. Incubate with new fuchsin substrate solution as provided below:

Reagents

Solution A: In fume chamber add 0.2 ml of 5 per cent new fuchsin (Merck 4041) in 2N HCl to 0.5 ml of fresh 4 per cent sodium nitrite. Agitate for 30–60 sec. Add 100 ml of 0.05 M Tris buffer, pH 8.7, and 100 μl of 1M levamisole to block endogenous alkaline phosphatase.

Solution B: Dissolve 50 mg naphthol AS-BI phosphate (Sigma N2250) in 0.6 ml N,N-dimethylformamide.

Add solution B to solution A and mix well. Filter directly onto slides.

Incubate for 10–20 min at room temperature, controlling reaction microscopically until intense red staining is obtained.

21. Rinse with distilled water.
22. Counterstain and coverslip with either organic or aqueous based medium.

5. *Microwave-accelerated immunostaining*

1. Deparaffinize sections, taking through to absolute alcohol.
2. Block endogenous peroxidase by placing sections in a plastic Coplin jar containing 50 ml of 0.5 per cent H_2O_2 in methanol and microwave on 'high' setting for 10 sec (Sharp Model 9570, 700 w).
3. Two washes with PBS pH 7.4, 2 min each.
4. Encircle sections with 'PAP' pen (Dako Cat. No. S2002).
   All subsequent incubations are performed in the microwave oven in a closed humid chamber containing 25 ml of water at the bottom of the chamber. Place the chamber in the centre of the carousel of the oven on a 5 cm high piece of polystyrene.
5. Block with the appropriate non-immune serum by covering the sections with the serum and incubating in the oven on a 'low' setting for 1 min 10 sec.
6. Drain off excess serum.
7. Cover the sections with 100–150 μl of primary antibody appropriately diluted with 3 per cent NHS and incubate as below, at 'low' setting for 1 min 10 sec, leaving the antibody on the sections for a further 3 min 50 sec with the power off.
8. Two washes with PBS pH 7.4, 2 min each.
9. Incubate with biotinylated secondary antibody (Dakopatts, USA) 1/500, diluted with 3 per cent NHS in a manner identical to that for the primary antibody, incubation times as before, at 'low' setting for 1 minute 10 seconds, followed by further 3 min 50 sec with the power off.
10. Two washes with PBS pH 7.4, 2 min each.
11. Incubate with streptavidin-biotin peroxidase complex (Pearce, USA) 1/1500, diluted with 3 per cent NHS in the manner identical to that for the primary and secondary antibody, at 'low' setting for 1 min 10 sec, followed by a further 3 min 50 sec incubation with the power off.
12. Two washes with PBS ph 7.4, 2 min each.
13. Apply peroxidase substrate solution: 25 diaminobenzedine tetrahydrochloride (Sigma, Cat No. D-5637) in 50 ml Tris HCl buffer pH 7.4, and 50 μl of 30 per cent H_2O_2. Control reaction macroscopically/microscopically, 10–20 min.
14. Rinse in PBS pH 7.4.
15. Counterstain very lightly with Mayer's haematoxylin.
16. Dehydrate, clear and mount.

Note: At 'low' setting the Sharp Model 9570, 700 watt microwave oven produced 6 sec periods of irradiation followed by 26 sec intervals of no irradiation. In the 1 min 10 sec period, there were three 6 sec periods of irradiation or a total of 18 sec of irradiation. These figures will vary with the model of microwave oven used and can be obtained from the manufacturers of the oven.

6. *Bone marrow aspirates for immunostaining of metastatic carcinoma*

1. Aspirate 2–3 ml of bone marrow tissue into a heparinized syringe.
2. Layer onto a Ficoll–Hypaque gradient and centrifuge at 400 × g for 20 min.
3. Collect interface layer (containing intact mononuclear

cells and viable epithelial cells) and wash twice in PBS pH 7.4.
4. Decanter fluid.
5. Resuspend the pellet in ten times volume of PBS pH 7.4.
6. Prepare smears from suspensions, 50 μl per slide.
7. Fix immediately in 100 per cent ethanol for up to 2 h.
8. Stain with appropriate dilution of antibody (e.g. CAM5.2, AE1/3) using 30 min incubation at room temperature. Similar 30 min incubations employed for secondary and tertiary stages.

7. Imidazole enhancement of DAB reaction product

Reagents

1. 25 mg diaminobenzidine tetrahydrochloride.
2. 50 μl Tris HCl buffer pH 7.6.
3. 50 μl of 30 per cent H_2O_2.
4. 500 μl of 1M Imidazole.

Working solution

Mix reagent 1 and 2 immediately before use followed by reagent 3, mixing well. Add reagent 4, mix well and apply to slides. Control incubation macroscopically/microscopically about 5–10 min.

Results

Antigen – intense brown.
Background – pale to moderate brown.

Note: Imidazole can cause extensive background staining if incubation is too long, particularly so with polyclonal antibodies.

8. Immunostaining of oestrogen receptors in frozen sections

1. Cut frozen sections including controls on the day of staining and keep cold in cryostat.
2. Fix in freshly prepared periodate lysine paraformaldehyde (PLP), for 10 min.
3. Two washes in PBS pH 7.4, 3 min each.
4. Encircle sections with a 'PAP' pen (Dako Cat No. S2002) and incubate with 3 per cent Normal horse serum (NHS), for 10 min.
5. Drain off excess NHS and incubate with ER (Abbotts Cat No. 3087–18) 1/10 diluted with 3 per cent NHS for 30 min, at room temperature.
6. Two washes in PBS pH 7.4, 3 min each.
7. Biotinylated rabbit anti-rat IgG (Vector, USA) 1/250 diluted with NHS for, 30 min.
8. Two washes in PBS pH 7.4, 3 min each.
9. Peroxidase conjugated streptavidin (Pierce, USA) 1/1000 diluted with NHS, for 30 min.
10. Two washes in PBS pH 7.4, 3 min each.
11. Peroxidase substrate solution: 25 mg diaminobenzedine tetrahydrochloride (Sigma, Cat No. D-5637) to 50 ml Tris HCl buffer pH 7.4, 50 μl of 30 per cent H_2O_2 and 500 μl of 1M Imidazole. Control reaction macroscopically/ microscopically, 10–20 min.
12. Rinse in PBS pH 7.4.
13. Counterstain lightly with Mayer's haematoxylin.
14. Dehydrate, clear and mount.

9. Immunostaining of progesterone receptors in frozen sections

1. Cut frozen sections including controls on the day of staining and keep dry in cryostat.
2. Fix in freshly prepared periodate lysine paraformaldehyde (PLP), for 10 min.
3. Two washes in PBS pH 7.4, 3 min each.
4. Encircle the sections with a 'PAP' pen (Dako Cat No. S2002) and incubate with 3 per cent Normal horse serum (NHS), for 10 min.
5. Drain off excess NHS and incubate with PgR (Transbio, France) 1/200 diluted with 3 per cent NHS for 30 min, at room temperature.
6. Two washes in PBS pH 7.4, 3 min each.
7. Biotinylated rabbit anti-mouse IgG (Dakopatts, USA) 1/500 diluted with NHS, for 30 min.
8. Two washes in PBS pH 7.4, 3 min each.
9. Peroxidase conjugated streptavidin (Pierce, USA) 1/1000 diluted with NHS, for 30 min.
10. Two washes in PBS pH 7.4, 3 min each.
11. Peroxidase substrate solution: 25 mg diaminobenzedine tetrahydrochloride (Sigma, Cat No. D-5637)

to 50 ml Tris HCl buffer pH 7.4, 50 μl of 30 per cent H_2O_2 and 500 μl of 1M Imidazole. Control reaction macroscopically/microscopically, 10–20 min.
12. Rinse in PBS pH 7.4.
13. Counterstain lightly with Mayer's haematoxylin.
14. Dehydrate, clear and mount.

10. Immunostaining of Ki-67 in cryostat sections

1. Cut frozen sections, including controls, briefly immerse for 5 sec in acetone at room temperature and air dry overnight. Results are best when sections are stained as soon as dry.
2. Fix in acetone at room temperature for 10 min prior to staining.
3. Air dry and use 'PAP' pen (Dako Cat No. S2002) to encircle the sections.
4. Block with 3 per cent normal horse serum (NHS) for 10 min.
5. Drain off excess NHS and incubate with primary antibody, diluted as appropriate with 3 per cent NHS, for 30 min at room temperature.
6. Two washes in PBS pH 7.4, 3 min each.
7. Incubate with biotinylated rabbit anti-mouse IgG (Dakopatts, USA) 1/500, diluted with 3 per cent NHS, for 30 min at room temperature.
8. Two washes in PBS pH 7.4, 3 min each.
9. Incubate with peroxidase conjugated streptavidin (Pierce, USA) 1/1000, diluted with 3 per cent NHS, for 30 min at room temperature.
10. Two washes in PBS pH 7.4, 3 min each.
11. Apply peroxidase substrate solution: 25 mg diaminobenzedine tetrahydrochloride (Sigma, Cat No. D-5637) in 50 ml Tris HCl buffer pH 7.4, and 50 μl of 30 per cent H_2O_2. Control reaction macroscopically/microscopically, 10–20 min.
12. Rinse in PBS pH 7.4.
13. Counterstain very lightly with Mayer's haematoxylin.
14. Dehydrate, clear and mount.

11. Lymphocyte surface markers in cryostat sections

1. Cut frozen sections, including controls, briefly immerse for 5 sec in acetone at room temperature and air dry. Results are best when sections are stained as soon as dry.
2. Fix in acetone at room temperature for 10 min prior to staining.
3. Air dry and use 'PAP' pen (Dako Cat No. S2002) to encircle the sections.
4. Block with 3 per cent normal horse serum (NHS) for 10 min.
5. Drain off excess NHS and incubate with primary antibody, diluted as appropriate with 3 per cent NHS, for 30 min at room temperature.
6. Two washes in PBS pH 7.4, 3 min each.
7. Incubate with goat anti-mouse IgG and IgM (Tago, USA) 1/100, diluted with 3 per cent NHS, for 30 min at room temperature.
8. Two washes in PBS pH 7.4, 3 min each.
9. Incubate with peroxidase conjugated streptavidin (Pierce, USA) 1/1000, diluted with 3 per cent NHS, for 30 min at room temperature.
10. Two washes in PBS pH 7.4, 3 min each.
11. Apply peroxidase substrate solution: 25 mg diaminobenzedine tetrahydrochloride (Sigma, Cat No. D-5637) in 50 ml Tris HCl buffer pH 7.4, and 50 μl of 30 per cent H_2O_2. Control reaction macroscopically/microscopically, 10–20 min.
12. Rinse in PBS pH 7.4.
13. Counterstain very lightly with Mayer's haematoxylin.
14. Dehydrate, clear and mount.

12. Cytospin preparations of lymphoid tissue and staining

1. Place representative piece of lymphoid tissue in Hanks buffered salt solution and store at 4°C until ready for use.
2. Place the tissue on a stainless steel mesh (1 mm grids) over a petri dish, add several drops of bovine serum albumin (BSA) over the tissue. Macerate the tissue with a scalpel blade, washing the tissue periodically with Hanks buffered salt solution, total volume of 5 ml.
3. Add 1 part BSA to 3 parts of the tissue suspension and mix well.
4. Prepare cytospins by adding 3–4 drops per slide of the mixture, using the Shandon Cytospin II at 250 rpms for 5 min. Concentration of cells: 150 per μl.
5. Remove slides individually from Cytospin II and fix

cytospins immediately in 100 per cent acetone (at room temperature) for 3–5 sec, air dry and store at −20°C until ready for staining.

6. Staining protocol for lymphocyte antigens. Similar to that for cryostat sections provided in Procedure 11.

13. Periodate-lysine-paraformaldehyde (PLP) fixative

Stock reagents (to be used within 24 h of preparation)

50 ml	3 per cent paraformaldehyde
100 ml	distilled water
0.9 g	lysine
0.146 g	sodium periodate
1.46 g	disodium hydrogen orthophosphate

Preparation

Dissolve paraformaldehyde powder in healed distilled water almost to boiling point. The addition of a minute amount of 5N NaOH will dissolve the remaining powder, immediately clearing the cloudy solution.

Add 50 ml of 3 per cent paraformaldehyde solution to 100 ml distilled water and mix well, then add 0.9 g lysine, 0.146 g sodium periodate and 1.46 g disodium hydrogen orthophosphate, mix until completely dissolved. The solution should be used within 24 h of preparation.

14. Preparation of cytology specimens for cell surface marker analysis

Contributed by Carlos W.M. Bedrossian and Shahla Masood.

Principle

A single cell suspension is exposed to monoclonal antibodies conjugated to fluoresceinisothiocyanate (FITC) and/ or phycoerythrin (PE) to detect cells bearing specific membrane antigens. The stained cells are analysed by flow cytometry to allow classification of cell subpopulations according to their phenotype.

Specimen

A. Requirements
   1. The specimen to be analysed must be in a cell suspension containing at least 500,000 cells per marker to be used. The ideal suspension will contribute 1×10^6 cells per marker.
   2. The cells must be viable.

B. Specimen types
   1. Fine needle aspiration biopsy
   2. Tumour scrapings
   3. Body cavity fluids
   4. Cerebrospinal fluid

Reagents

A. Rejuva Bunny – store at 4°C
B. PBS/0.1 per cent sodium azide – store at 4°C
C. Haemocytometer
D. Cover slips
E. Centrifuge
F. Microscope
G. Petri dish
H. Surgical Scissors
I. 52 mm nylon mesh
J. Wire mesh screen (stainless steel)

Procedure

A. Fine needle aspiration biopsy
   1. FNAs should be dispensed directly into 10 ml of Rejuva Bunny and transported directly to laboratory. If a delay in transport is necessary, the specimen in Rejuva Bunny should be place don ice or in a refrigerator. For maximum viability specimens should be processed within 24 h.
   2. The specimen should be treated according to the Ficoll–Paque procedure and the final cell suspension should be in Rejuva Bunny.
   3. Perform a cell count, make cytospin preparations and check for viability.

B. Tumour scrapings
   1. Tumour scrapings should be placed directly into 10 ml of Rejuva Bunny and transported to laboratory.
   2. Specimens with visible clumps or larger pieces of tissue should be minced over a wire mesh to release cells into suspension. This suspension should be filtered through 52 mm nylon mesh.

3. The cell suspension should be treated according to the Ficoll–Paque procedure. The final cell suspension in Rejuva Bunny should be counted, cytospin preparations made and viability determined.

C. Body cavity fluid
1. Body cavity fluids received in large containers should be mixed and poured off into smaller 50 ml centrifuge tubes. Centrifuge for 10 min at 1500 rpm and pour off supernatant. Collect cell buttons and resuspend in Rejuva Bunny.
2. Treat cell suspension by Ficoll–Paque procedure. The final cell suspension in Rejuva Bunny should be counted, cytospin preparations made and viability determined.

D. Cerebrospinal fluid
1. CSF should be centrifuged immediately and the supernatant removed. Resuspend cells in Rejuva Bunny and perform a cell count to determine if enough cells are present.
2. Ficoll–Paque should be used if enough cells are present. Cell suspension should be counted and checked for viability.

15. Preparation of cytology specimens for DNA analysis by flow cytometry

Contributed by Carlos W.M. Bedrossian and Shahla Masood.

Principle

By suspending a single cell suspension in a hypotonic nuclear staining solution the membrane of the cells is consequently lysed exposing the nuclei to propidium iodide. PI excites at 488 nm with an emission of 625 nm. Both DNA and RNA are stained with PI; however, PI is used predominantly as a DNA stain. RNA is removed by treatment with Ribonuclease A 500 units/ml. The amount of dye that binds is directly proportional to the amount of DNA present in the cell. The stained nuclei are analysed by flow cytometry to demonstrate ploidy and cell phases.

Specimen

A. Requirements
1. The specimen to be analysed must be in a cell suspension containing at least 300,000 cells. The ideal suspension is 1.0×10^6 cells/ml.
2. The cells to be analysed must be viable or fixed while in a viable state. (Refer to procedure for alcohol fixation of cell suspension for DNA analysis.)

B. Specimen types
1. Fine needle aspiration biopsy
2. Tumour scrapings
3. Body cavity fluids
4. Cerebrospinal fluid
5. Bladder washings and urine

Reagents

A. Rejuva Bunny – store at 4°C
B. PBS/0.1 per cent sodium azide – store at 4°C
C. Ficoll–Paque media
D. Trypan blue stain

Equipment

A. 15 ml conical centrifuge tube
B. Disposal pipette
C. Haemocytometer
D. Cover slips
E. Centrifuge
F. Microscope
G. Petri dish
H. Surgical scissors
I. 52 mm nylon mesh
J. Wire mesh screen (stainless steel)

Procedure

A. Fine needle aspiration biopsy
1. FNAs should be dispensed directly into 10 ml of Rejuva Bunny and transported directly to laboratory. If a delay in transport is necessary, the specimen in Rejuva Bunny should be place don ice or in a refrigerator. For maximum viability specimens should be processed within 24 h.
2. Specimens that are free from obvious bloody contamination should be centrifuged 1500 rpm for 5 min, supernatant removed and cell suspension made in Rejuva Bunny for cell counting. If large clumps are seen during counting the suspension should be filtered with 52 mm nylon mesh and recounted.
3. Specimens that are to be used for cell surface

marker study or are grossly bloody should be treated using the Ficoll–Paque procedure. Then an appropriate cell suspension should be made and counted. Cytospin preparations should be made also.

B. Tumour scrapings
   1. Tumour scrapings should be placed directly into 10 ml of Rejuva Bunny and transported to laboratory.
   2. Specimens with visible clumps or larger pieces of tissue should be minced over a stainless steel wire mesh in a petri dish. Dispense Rejuva Bunny solution over the mesh to release cells into suspension. This suspension should be filtered through 52 mm nylon mesh into a centrifuge tube.
   3. Bloody specimens should be lysed using the lysing media procedure and then a cell suspension prepared in Rejuva Bunny.
   4. The resulting cell suspension should be counted, tested for viability with trypan blue stain, and cytospin preparations made.

C. Body cavity fluid
   1. Body fluids received in large containers should be mixed and poured off into smaller 50 ml centrifuge tubes. Centrifuge for 10 min at 1500 rpm and pour off supernatant. Collect cell buttons from all tubes and resuspend in Rejuva Bunny.
   2. Bloody specimens should be lysed using the lysing media procedure.
   3. A cell suspension should be prepared in Rejuva Bunny and counted. Make cytospin preparations. Check for viability.

D. Cerebrospinal fluid
   1. CSF should be centrifuged immediately and the supernatant removed. Resuspend cells in Rejuva Bunny and perform a cell count to determine if enough cells are present.
   2. Bloody specimens should be lysed using lysing media and then a cell suspension prepared.
   3. If enough cells for processing are recovered make cytospin preparations also. (Specimens for cell surface marker studies may be treated with Ficoll–Paque if enough cells are present.) Check for viability.

E. Bladder washings and urine
   1. Bladder washings and urine should be concentrated by centrifugation and then a cell suspension prepared with Rejuva Bunny.
   2. Perform a cell count, viability check and make cytospin preparations.

16. Quantitative ploidy analysis staining procedure – Feulgen technique (DNA)

Contributed by Carlos W.M. Bedrossian and Shahla Masood.

Principle

Histochemical stain for DNA to determine ploidy of cell (quantitative ploidy analysis CAS).

Specimen

Preparation: Cytospin imprints and fine needle aspirates.

Reagents

Quantitative DNA stain kit commercially obtained from CAS, Elmhurst, Illinois, Cat. No. 102400–01.

Prepare as follows:

A. Stain solution
   DNA stain powder (kit), 1 vial 0.1N HCl, 100 ml. Cover, mix solution on stir plate for 1 h – filter.

B. Rinse solution
   Rinse powder (kit), 1 vial 0.05N HCl, 300 ml. Upon mixing, the above solutions are stable for 4–6 h.

C. 0.1N HCl solution
   Distilled H_20, 495.7 ml/999.4 ml, concentrated HCl, 4.3 ml/8.6 ml 500 ml, 1000 ml.

D. 0.05N HCl solution
   Distilled H_2O, 499.14 ml/998.28 ml concentrated HCl, 86 ml/1.72 ml 500 ml or 1000 ml.

E. 5N HCl solution
   Distilled H_2O 28.5 ml/85.5 ml concentrated HCl 21.5 ml/64.5 ml or 150 ml.
   1 per cent acid alcohol solution 70 per cent alcohol 99 ml concentrated HCl 1 ml.

Calibration

Use one CAS calibration slide in stain solution per run of slides.

Quality control

Analysis of CAS control slide confirms quality of stain.

Procedure

1. Prepare stain solution.
2. Place slides in 5N HCl solution for one hour at room temperature – cover coplin jar tightly with parafilm.
3. Filter stain solution into coplin jar. Pour 5N HCl solution off slides and replace with filtered stain solution. Cover tightly and incubate for 1 h at room temperature.
4. Prepare rinse solution. Divide solution into three coplin jars – incubate as follows:
   Pour off stain solution: rinse solution 1–30 sec. Rinse solution 2–5 min. Rinse solution 3–10 min.
5. Place slides in running H_2O_2 for 5 min.
6. Transfer slides to 1 per cent acid alcohol for 5 min.
7. Transfer slides to two changes of alcohol for three min each.
8. Clear slides in two changes of xylene.
9. Mount slides in accumount or permount.
   3DNA quantitation by cell image analysis.

17. *Quantitative ploidy analysis (DNA) by cell image analysis*

Contributed by Carlos W.M. Bedrossian and Shahla Masood.

Specimen

Imprint preparation and fine needle aspirates.

Reagents

Above specimens and controls are stained with Feulgen technique prior to image analysis.

Calibration

Instrument as calibrated by using the DNA calibration slide (CAS) that was stained with the batch of slides to be viewed. Refer to procedure for details.

Quality control

DNA calibration slide is used for parameters in calibration of instrument.

Procedure

1. Turn instrument 'ON'. Refer to start up mode (located top right desk of microscope).
2. Using the mouse, select quantitative ploidy analysis on the main menu. Then, start Standard.
3. Label – enter patient name, accession number, DNA Cal.
4. Set light – place CAS stained calibration slide on stage. Focus on cells with 40× objective. Move to clear area of slide and adjust lighting as monitor instructs. Lighting successful will flash when proper lighting adjustments have occurred.
5. Check light – if lighting has been accomplished, the software will allow you to move on with calibration.
6. 'Bkd light' – refers to background light. Can be off or on. Does not interfere with analysis.
7. Set XY – using CAS calibration slide, locate corner of square. Seek out a dot inside the square of a corner. Enter which corner is used. This is performed so the exact area of cells could be analysed time after time.
8. Image mode – use live as it refers to acquiring data from a slide placed on the microscope stage.
9. Measure – using the CAS stained calibration slide, locate group of cells and enter measure. A new screen will appear for reject, accept, automated, etc. Push 'automated' (instrument will seek out cells with 7.18 picagrams DNA – accept or reject as used for individual 'manual' selection. Measure at least 19 cells to continue with menu options.
10. Upon counting 19–50 cells of the calibration slide – the optical density should be >6000, >8000. The CV should be <4.0. The low reading of CV refers to the darkness of stain intensity. This will allow for more contrast when analysing cells. Do not clear this information. This screen can be used for all patients analysed at a sitting.
11. Print the screen of the DNA calibration.
12. Return to label and next to the accession number, remove DNA cal and enter specimen (breast, liver, etc).
13. Return to menu – remove cal slide from stage.
14. Enter analyse – a new screen will appear. Place patient stained slide on stage.

15. 'Chk light' – focus on cells of patient slide with 40× objective. Move to clear area and enter 'chk light'. If lighting needs re-adjusting, follow instructions given on monitor.
16. Bounds – locate the cells to be analysed. Set boundary with little or no background traces of the actual cell. Enter 'increase' (allows for more blue background – removes cell debris, etc.) or enter 'decrease' (allows for less blue background – adds debris). The crisper, cleaner the nuclei, the easier the analysis will be. Exit when complete.
17. Filter–CAS has installed a filter system designed to seek out cells that fit a set criteria for selection. The filter system will appear on the monitor. To load, enter load – select filter name – move cursor to ALLDNA. Press Enter. ALLDNA will appear under filter name. Press OK. Filter menu will reappear. Press Exit. This step is used for the automated procedure. To perform manual, pass up this selection of the menu and continue with classify.
18. Tissue – when using the filter, enter the tissue thickness of 7 (microns), toggle ON, press exit.
19. Classify – locate the cells for analysis. Focus cells on the monitor - filter measure will appear. As you look at the cell, decide if you need to cut.
    a) *to cut* – using the mouse, move arrow to area to cut. Left button on mouse – freehand draw, middle button is a straight line; right button is exit. An example is to place arrow at area of cut – press middle button of mouse one click – a line will appear. As the line is moved to area of complete cut, press right button one click to end the line that was drawn. Press right button once more to exit cut options.
    b) *point and classify* – under this menu, one is allowed to change classification of cells (1–6), delete a cell (D), or request pertinent information about the cell (?). Press exit.
    c) *measure* – before you press measure, make sure all cells in the field are full intact nuclei that are cut properly and encircled complete as the filter has selected. Press measure – count 200 cells or more per patient slide.
20. Select 2nd – move cursor to directional arrows to obtain a readout of the second peak. The number readout should be 2× the amount of the main peak +0.05. This gives you G2M. Upon locating G2M, press exit. The histogram will show a marker at the site.
21. Area ABCD – this step is user specific. Basically, A should be a population of any diploid cells 1.0 or less, B shows next significant group of cells depending on the peak readout. C can demonstrate G2M population or a third population – D is to delete an area not interested in.
22. Overall analysis review is dependent of user interpretation.
23. 'Disappear' – will allow box of options to disappear. Press print screen so the histogram is printed below the DNA cal histogram on the final printout.
24. Press report – move paper on printer to new sheet. A different view of the histogram will appear. Print two of these on two separate sheets. These histograms are used for the final signout.
25. Upon completion of analysis, the patient data is cleared. Enter new patient information under label and repeat the entire process except the analysis of the DNA calibration slide.

Calculations

This area is totally operator dependent. At the end of printout, the technologist will return to select second and enter the number reading of each peak of the original histogram. This information is used by the pathologist for reference.

Reporting results

Histograms and miscellaneous patient information are given to the attending pathologist for final signout.

Results

0.9–1.10 = diploid
<0.9 and >1.10 = aneuploid

18. *List of antibodies, sources, working dilutions and costs*

Antibody	Source	Working dilution	Antisera Vol.(ml) vial	Antisera cost $	Primary cost/slide
Paraffin					
AAT (P)	DAKO	8000	2.0	117	0.001
AE1/3 (M)	BMA	600	0.5	428	0.285
ACT (P)	DAKO	10000	2.0	117	0.001
ACTIN (M)	AMERSHAM	8000	0.1	350	0.175
AFP (M)	DAKO	40	1.0	293	1.465
Bcl-2 (M)	DAKO	50	1.0	195	0.780
Ber-DRC (M)	DAKO	40	1.0	181	0.905
Ber-EP4 (M)	DAKO	200	1.0	222	0.222
Ber-H2 (M)	DAKO	5	2.0	292	5.840
Bovine keratin (P)	DAKO	10000	1.0	222	0.004
Callus keratin (P)	DAKO	8000	1.0	224	0.006
CAM5.2 (M)	B&D	30	2.0	220	0.733
CATHEPSIN D (M)	NOVACASTRA	100	1.0	540	1.080
CD3 (M)	DAKO	300	1.0	200	0.133
CEA (M)	BIOGENEX	2000	0.2	319	0.160
Chromogranin (P)	INC	1750	0.1	480	0.549
Collagen IV (M)	DAKO	300	1.0	351	0.234
C3bR (M)	DAKO	20	1.0	122	1.220
Cytokeratin 19 (M)	ICN	50	1.0	318	1.272
D33 (M)	DAKO	120	2.0	292	0.243
Desmin (M)	DAKO	50	2.0	292	0.584
DF-T1 (M)	DAKO	50	2.0	351	0.702
EMA (P)	SERA LAB	15000	1.0	100	0.001
ErbB-2 (P)	DAKO	600	1.0	260	0.087
Estrogen receptor (M)	ABBOTTS	5	3.0	960	12.800
FACTOR VIII (P)	DAKO	12000	2.0	150	0.001
FACTOR XIIIa (P)	BEHRING	8000	1.0	73	0.002
GASTRIN (P)	DAKO	4000	1.0	216	0.011
GCDFP-15 (M)	SIGNET	200	0.1	495	4.950
GLUCAGON (P)	DAKO	25	7.0	100	0.114
GFAP (M)	DAKO	300	2.0	292	0.097
HIV (M)	DAKO	10	1.0	174	3.480
Hairy cell leukaemia (M)	DAKO	400	1.0	195	0.098
HAM-56 (M)	DAKO	600	1.0	155	0.052
HCG (M)	BIOGENEX	1200	0.2	388	0.323
HEP-B core (P)	DAKO	4000	1.0	104	0.005
HEP-B surface (P)	BEHRING	1000	5.0	125	0.005
HLA-DR (C3/43) (M)	DAKO	4000	1.0	222	0.011
HLA-DR Alpha (M)	DAKO	10	2.0	205	2.050
HMB45 (M)	DAKO	100	1.0	255	0.510
HUMAN placental lactogen (P)	DAKO	7	7.0	100	0.408
HSV (P)	DAKO	10	14.0	259	0.370
IgG (P)	BEHRING	5000	5.0	126	0.001
IgA (P)	BEHRING	1000	1.0	42	0.008
IgM (P)	BEHRING	1000	1.0	42	0.008
IgD (P)	BEHRING	1000	1.0	42	0.008

Insulin (P)	DAKO	10	7.0	100	0.286
JC7OA (M)	DAKO	25	1.0	174	1.392
Kappa (P)	TAGO	4000	1.0	166	0.008
KP1 (M)	DAKO	400	1.0	222	0.111
Lactalbumin (P)	LIPSHAW	3000	0.2	170	0.057
Lambda (P)	TAGO	3000	1.0	166	0.011
Laminin (P)	EY	1000	1.0	300	0.060
LN1 (M)	BIOTEST	6	5.0	234	1.560
LN2 (M)	BIOTEST	6	5.0	234	1.560
LN3 (M)	BIOTEST	6	5.0	234	1.560
L26 (M)	DAKO	300	2.0	380	0.127
LCA (M)	DAKO	40	2.0	205	0.513
LEU7 (M)	B&D	50	2.0	375	0.750
LEU22 (M)	B&D	200	5.0	220	0.044
LEUM1 (M)	B&D	25	2.0	300	1.200
MAC387 (M)	DAKO	100	2.0	263	0.263
Myelin basic protein (P)	DAKO	2000	1.0	378	0.038
Muramidase (P)	DAKO	4000	2.0	117	0.003
MT1 (M)	BIOTEST	40	5.0	234	0.234
MT2 (M)	BIOTEST	5	5.0	234	1.872
MB1 (M)	BIOTEST	5	5.0	234	1.872
MB2 (M)	BIOTEST	5	5.0	234	1.872
Muscle specific actin (M)	ENZO	15000	0.1	465	0.062
Myoglobin (P)	DAKO	4000	1.0	120	0.006
Neurofilament triplet (M)	DAKO	60	2.0	292	0.487
NSE (M)	DAKO	800	1.0	349	0.087
OPD4 (M)	DAKO	40	1.0	190	0.950
Papilloma virus (human) (P)	DAKO	3000	1.0	224	0.015
Parathormone (P)	BIOGENEX	3000	0.2	300	0.100
p53 (M)	NOVACASTRA	100	1.0	485	0.970
pS2 (M)	BIOGENEX	30	1.0	1170	7.800
PCNA (PC10) (M)	DAKO	6000	1.0	425	0.014
PCNA (19A2) (M)	BIOTECH	40000	1.0	300	0.002
PGP9.5 (M)	ULTRA CLONE	3000	0.2	250	0.083
PHE-5 (M)	ENZO	8000	0.1	550	0.138
PLAP (P)	DAKO	2000	2.0	176	0.009
PNA (lectin)	VECTOR	150	1.0	175	0.233
Pneumocystis (M)	DAKO	20	1.0	222	2.220
Progesterone (frozen) (M)	TRANSBIO	200	0.2	1485	7.425
Progesterone (paraffin) (M)	ABBOTTS	15	3.0	960	4.267
PSA (M)	DAKO	20	1.0	103	1.030
PSAP (M)	DAKO	2000	1.0	222	0.022
QBEnd/10 (M)	OXOID	25	1.0	425	3.400
S100 (P)	DAKO	12000	2.0	292	0.002
Serotonin (P)	SEROTEC	4000	0.1	365	0.183
Smooth muscle actin (M)	SIGMA	2000	0.2	211	0.106
Somatostatin (P)	DAKO	7	7.0	100	0.408
SP1 (P)	DAKO	4000	2.0	148	0.004
Synaptophysin (M)	BMA	10	5.0	301	1.204
Thyroglobulin (M)	DAKO	3500	1.0	222	0.013
TU-9 (M)	BIOTEST	20	1.0	222	2.220
UCHL-1 (M)	DAKO	300	2.0	263	0.088

Ulex (lectin)	VECTOR	150	1.0	210	0.280
Vimentin (M)	DAKO	500	2.0	292	0.058
4KB5 (M)	DAKO	100	2.0	263	0.263
1F8 (M)	DAKO	40	1.0	222	1.110
34BE12 (M)	DAKO	150	1.0	194	0.259
35BH11 (M)	DAKO	200	1.0	194	0.194
Frozen					
B1 (M)	COULTER	10	0.5	125	5.00
B2 (M)	COULTER	10	0.5	125	5.00
BA-1 (M)	BMA	15	0.5	300	8.00
BA-2 (M)	BMA	15	0.5	300	8.00
Calla (M)	DAKO	50	2.0	211	0.42
Desmoplakin (M)	SANBIO	10	1.0	135	2.70
DRC-1 (M)	DAKO	20	2.0	176	0.88
HLA-DR (M)	DAKO	40	0.5	420	4.20
IL2 (M)	B&D	10	2.0	375	3.75
IgA (M)	AMD	40	1.0	135	0.68
IgD (M)	DAKO	20	2.0	176	0.88
IgG (M)	AMD	80	1.0	135	0.34
IgM (M)	DAKO	70	2.0	176	0.25
Kappa (M)	DAKO	150	1.0	184	0.25
Ki-1 (M)	DAKO	10	2.0	292	2.92
Ki-67 (M)	DAKO	100	2.0	292	0.29
Lambda (M)	AMD	80	1.0	184	0.46
LEU1 (M)	B&D	20	4.0	580	1.45
LEU2 (M)	B&D	15	4.0	580	1.93
LEU3 (M)	B&D	3	4.0	300	5.00
LEU4 (M)	B&D	40	2.0	300	0.75
LEU5 (M)	B&D	10	2.0	300	3.00
LEU6 (M)	B&D	15	2.0	300	2.00
LEU7 (M)	B&D	10	2.0	375	3.75
LEU8 (M)	B&D	20	2.0	300	1.50
LEU9 (M)	B&D	40	2.0	350	0.88
LEU12 (M)	B&D	5	2.0	300	6.00
LEU14 (M)	B&D	3	4.0	300	5.00
LEUM3 (M)	B&D	20	0.5	300	6.00
Mucosal lymphocyte antigen	DAKO	10	1.0	187	3.74
OKT 10 (M)	ORTHO	40	1.0	420	2.10
OKT 11 (M)	ORTHO	20	1.0	420	4.20
OKT 3 (M)	ORTHO	10	1.0	420	8.40
OKT 4 (M)	ORTHO	20	1.0	420	4.20
OKT 6 (M)	ORTHO	20	1.0	420	4.20
OKT 8 (M)	ORTHO	20	1.0	420	4.20
OKT 9 (M)	ORTHO	20	1.0	420	4.20
PAN B (M)	DAKO	5	2.0	205	4.10

Notes: (P) = polyclonal (M) = monoclonal
The antibodies are separated into paraffin and frozen section groups, with the corresponding antibody dilutions appropriate for each group. The antibodies for paraffin sections are also immunoreactive in frozen sections.

Key to antibody sources

ABBOTTS	Abbott Laboratories, North Chicago, Illinois, USA
AMD	Australian Monoclonal Development, Artarmon, Australia
AMERSHAM	Amersham, Buckinghamshire, UK
B&D	Becton Dickinson, Mountain View, California, USA
BEHRING	Behringwerke AG, Germany
BIOGENEX	Biogenex Laboratories, San Ramon, California, USA
BIOTECH	American Biotech, Plantation, Florida, USA
BIOTEST	Biotest, Dreieich, Germany
BMA	Boeringer Mannheim, Sydney, NSW, Australia
COULTER	Coulter, Hialeah, Florida, USA
CRB	Cambridge Research Laboratories, Cheshire, UK
DAKO	Dakopatts, Santa Barbara, California, USA
ENZO	Enzo Biochem, New York, USA
EY	EY Laboratories, San Mateo, California, USA
ICN	ICN Biochemicals, Costa Mesa, California, USA
INC	Immunonuclear Corporation, Stillwater, Minnesota, USA
LIPSHAW	Lipshaw, Detroit, Michigan, USA
MILES	Miles Inc, Elkhart, Indiana, USA
MMUNOTECH	Immunotech, France
NOVACASTRA	Novacastra Laboratories, Newcastle Upon Tyne, UK
ORTHO	Ortho Diagnostics, Raritan, New Jersey, USA
OXOID	Oxoid Australia, Victoria, Australia
SANBIO	Sanbio, Uden, Netherlands
SERA LAB	Sera Lab, Sussex, UK
SEROTEC	Serotec, Oxford, UK
SIGMA	Sigma Chemicals, St Louis, Maryland, USA
SIGNET	Signet Laboratories, Dedham, Massachusetts, USA
TAGO	Tago Inc, Burlingame, USA
TRANSBIO	Transbio, Paris, France
ULTRA CLONE	Ultra Clone, Cambridge, UK
VECTOR	Vector Laboratories, Burlingame, California, USA

Index

NOTE:
Antibodies are listed under individual antibody names, with the exception of those starting with a numerical or Greek character, in which case they are listed after the entry 'Antibodies'. Page numbers 396–399 (Appendix, Table A.1) have not been included in the index entries for antibodies. It is suggested that readers consulting antibody references also refer to the Appendix, and the relevant antigens.
Antigens are listed under individual antigens. Only antigens with major textual references are included in the index, and principally those present (as opposed to those absent) in specific diseases. Additional references may, however, be found within the text for specific diseases.
Immunophenotype. All disease-related entries refer to the immunophenotype, unless other noted.
vs denotes differential diagnosis.
The index is in a letter-by-letter alphabetical order.

Abbreviations
Abbreviations used in subentries without further clarification include:-

CEA	–	Carcinoembronic antigen
EMA	–	Epithelial membrane antigen
HMFG	–	Human milk fat globulin
IF	–	Intermediate filaments
PCNA	–	Proliferating cell nuclear antigen

Additional abbreviations are referred to in the index.